Birds of Prey:
Health & Disease

Birds of Prey: HEALTH & DISEASE

THIRD EDITION

John E. Cooper
DTVM, FRCPath, FIBiol, FRCVS

With contributions from:
Margaret E. Cooper, LLB, FLS
Oliver Krone, Dr med vet
Ian Newton, OBE, FRS, FRSE
David B. Peakall, PhD, DSc
Paolo Zucca, DVM, PhD

Blackwell
Science

© 2002 by Blackwell Science Ltd, a Blackwell
Publishing Company
Editorial Offices:
Osney Mead, Oxford OX2 0EL, UK
  Tel: +44 (0)1865 206206
Blackwell Science, Inc., 350 Main Street,
Malden, MA 02148-5018, USA
  Tel: +1 781 388 8250
Iowa State Press, a Blackwell Publishing
Company, 2121 State Avenue, Ames, Iowa
50014-8300, USA
  Tel: +1 515 292 0140
Blackwell Science Asia Pty, 54 University
Street, Carlton, Victoria 3053, Australia
  Tel: +61 (0)3 9347 0300
Blackwell Wissenschafts Verlag, Kurfürstendamm 57,
10707
Berlin, Germany
  Tel: +49 (0)30 32 79 060

First Edition published 1978 by
The Standfast Press as *Veterinary Aspects of
Captive Birds of Prey*
Second Edition (with revisions) published 1985 by
The Standfast Press
Third Edition published 2002 by
Blackwell Science Ltd as *Birds of Prey: Health & Disease*

Library of Congress
Cataloging-in-Publication Data

Cooper, J. E. (John Eric), 1944–
   Birds of prey : health & disease/John E. Cooper; with
   contributions by Margeret E. Cooper . . . [*et al.*].
     p. cm.
     Rev. ed. of: Veterinary aspects of captive birds of prey.
   2nd ed. 1978.
     Includes bibliographical references (p.   ).
     ISBN 0-632-05115-9
     1. Birds of prey – Diseases.   2. Birds of prey – Health.
   I. Cooper, J. E. (John Eric), 1944– Veterinary aspects of captive
   birds of prey.   II. Title.
   SF994.5 .C65 2001
   636.6′86939 – dc21

                                            2001043240

ISBN 0-632-05115-9

A catalogue record for this title is available from
the British Library

Set in Galliards 9¼/12 pt
by SNP Best-set Typesetter Ltd., Hong Kong
Printed and bound in Great Britain by
MPG Books Ltd, Bodmin, Cornwall

For further information on
Blackwell Science, visit our website:
www.blackwell-science.com

To my wife, Margaret,
with thanks for all her support, especially on travels and in testing
times – as well as the happy days – in various parts of the world

Shukrani, Mpenzi Wangu!

And to my parents
Dorothy and Eric Cooper, for over half a century's encouragement

'The sober comfort, all the peace which springs
From the large aggregate of little things;
On these small cares of daughter, wife or friend
The almost sacred joys of home depend.'

Hannah More (1745–1833)

Contents

Foreword

PATRICK T. REDIG

Birds of Prey: Health & Disease is a new title for a seriously re-invented book known to the 'old-guard' of raptor medicine and surgery as *Veterinary Aspects of Captive Birds of Prey* by John E. Cooper, first published in hard-cover form in 1978 with republishing and addition of a supplement in 1985. This was the first modern book on raptor medicine – modern in the sense that it took hawk medicine from the hands of the keepers of the birds (*vis-à-vis*) falconers with their centuries' old medications such as peppercorns and alum and placed it in the context of professional veterinarians schooled in the use of anesthetic agents, effective antibiotics, and an understanding of principles of disease processes and treatment modalities. Ever mindful, however, of the contributions of those that have gone before, John Cooper liberally salted the writing with abundant correlations between the old and the new while adding relevance by blending in his first-hand experiences in clinical and pathological investigations. *Birds of Prey: Health & Disease* retains much of the structure and continues to reflect the cited literature and personal experiences, not only of John Cooper, but also a myriad of present-day clinicians and scientists with whom he has professional contact throughout the world. But there is much new content and previously published but still relevant information is not necessarily repeated. Thus, the astute reader is required to have access to previous editions for thoroughness. Breaking from the previous editions, owing to the vast and diverse increases in knowledge base and in keeping with present practices for contemporary works of inviting contributions from other authors, *Birds of Prey: Health & Disease* has an eclectic content from some well-known scientists as well as talented and emerging individuals who will be continuing the advance of raptor medicine into the future. This diverse content serves not only to expand the topical base, but it also animates John's lifelong theme of bridging the disciplines of veterinary medicine and wildlife biology.

This book is a view of raptor medicine from the 5000 meter vantage point; consistent with its predecessors and different from most other books published recently, it is not a clinical manual *per se*. While it contains relevant information on clinical aspects, the author wisely has developed the theoretical aspects of many topics, then referred the reader to pertinent literature for details. While clinicians will find useful information, this book will serve the uses of those involved in professional education as well. Education in avian medicine is expanding in general, and while there are few places where medicine and surgery of raptors is taught as a discreet discipline, a knowledge base of sufficient magnitude is present such that complementary curricula to those now provided in poultry and companion bird medicine are possible. This book will facilitate the assimilation of material pertinent to the study of raptor medicine by the professional student. At the same time it provides the reference and theoretical base to provide a foundation for graduate students' efforts that will develop the new knowledge needed to maintain the advance of raptor medicine and surgery as an emerging discipline. As one of those students who was encouraged and mentored by John Cooper more than a quarter century ago, at the dawn of modern raptor medicine and surgery, I welcome this work to our body of literature and am confident that, like its progenitors, *Birds of Prey: Health & Disease* will stimulate good science and good clinical practice for a new generation of raptor medicine and surgery specialists.

20 October 2001

Foreword to the First Edition (1978), with Tribute –

LESLIE BROWN

Mystery enshrouds the causes of death in most wild birds – including birds of prey – unless they are shot or electrocuted or run down by cars. In a few cases we know that they die of disease, and often, we assume, of starvation. However, the really well-documented causes of death or illness, other than by unnatural means such as shooting, are few; and will probably remain so.

We may assume, however, that some of the ailments that affect wild birds of prey also affect captives. Here we have a solid, thoroughly researched and abundantly documented treatise on the diseases and accidents that may affect captive birds of prey, both diurnal species and owls, by an expert veterinarian with deep and long practical experience of such matters. I knew John Cooper when he was in East Africa and his house was then full of sick or damaged raptors, apparently is so still, and is, according to him, likely to remain so. It is very doubtful if they could have the fortune to fall into better hands.

Mr Cooper firmly removes the treatment of sick or injured birds of prey from the hocus-pocus and abracadabra of old wives' tales and obscure remedies, right into the twentieth century. But he does not neglect to pay tribute to an older generation of falconers, who from practical necessity found ways to cure or ease some of the ills from which their prized birds suffered. Falconers, apparently, used to be reluctant to consult veterinarians who perhaps knew less about it than they did. Here is a book that shows conclusively that any such attitude is out of date: the treatment of birds of prey, sick or injured, has been modernised, and is thoroughly described herein, with details of how to do it, using many of the modern techniques applied in human medicine.

Arabs used to equate the value of a fine falcon with that of a good horse. A good falcon might now be the more valuable of the two, and is certainly a very valuable bird. Some rare specimens in zoos may be priceless, for restrictions on the capture of threatened species such as the Philippine monkey-eating eagle will ensure that no more can be obtained. For such birds it is necessary to have the service of a skilled veterinarian, who knows what he is talking about; and in this book you can find how to look after an injured or sick bird until such a skilled veterinarian can be found, so that he has a better chance of saving its life.

Falconers use many queer but ancient terms of the condition and ailments of birds of prey. Mr Cooper makes simple sense out of all that. 'Snurt' seems to me an entirely appropriate name for a runny nose, or rhinitis, an affliction I often suffer from myself. When next I am constipated I shall complain that I have something wrong with my 'tewel'. We move here straight from the Middle Ages, and earlier, to the twentieth century.

The twelve chapters explain everything from nomenclature, investigation and treatment to nervous disorders, anaesthesia, and surgery. You need not give up hope if your bird has a simple fracture; there is quite a chance that it may fly again. Mr Cooper sums it all up in a valuable chapter on discussion and conclusions and provides many appendices, line drawings by Thea Lloyd and photographs.

He has gathered his information from several hundred references, old and modern. This is a very thoroughly researched book indeed. It will be indispensable not only to those who keep falcons or birds of prey in zoos, but to students of the wild species in the field.

Leslie Brown
June 1978

Author's note

Leslie Brown, who wrote the Foreword above, gave me much personal encouragement during my time in Kenya 1969–73 and, until his death, for some years after. Leslie was one of the pioneers of raptor biology. Like so many of his generation he was an 'amateur' – in the best sense of that word, viz. one who loved his subject but was not specifically trained or employed in that discipline. Leslie Brown's widow, Barbara, who provided essential support in his work, died in South Africa in 1998. Their only son, Charles, was killed in an accident on the day of his graduation some years before. In retaining the original Foreword to this book, my family and I remember not only Leslie's friendship and contributions to birds of prey but also, with sympathy, the sadness that subsequently over-shadowed the life of his family.

J. E. Cooper
2001

Preface

'We must turn to nature itself, to the observations of the body in health and disease to learn the truth'

Hippocrates

I am writing the closing parts of this book in Uganda, where Margaret and I have been teaching. I look out on Lake Victoria, that immense stretch of water that is bordered by the three East African countries that have been so much part of our lives. Black kites soar overhead, an African goshawk darts through the trees and fish eagles call from the water's edge. These sights and sounds are salutary reminders of the beauty and splendour of birds of prey and of the intricate webs of life that comprise biodiversity.

This book has had a long and rather unusual metamorphosis.

Since childhood I have had a fascination with natural history and wildlife. Birds of prey had always excited me but it was not until 1959, when (as a schoolboy aged 15) I found an injured kestrel in Devon, England and took it home for nursing and eventual release, that I first came into close contact with a live raptor. I was introduced by my mentor, the naturalist and broadcaster, Maxwell Knight, to Paul Jacklin who was a practising falconer. Paul taught me how to handle a hawk and subsequently trained me in falconry techniques. As a young veterinary student and Associate of the British Falconers' Club in the early 1960s, I found myself in demand to examine members' birds that had died and to give first aid treatment to hawks that were unwell. There were then very few veterinary surgeons with an interest in the subject – and, sad to relate, even fewer with any special knowledge of birds of prey.

My interest in birds of prey was very much strengthened in my year as a volunteer (VSO) veterinary surgeon in Tanzania, 1966–67, and subsequently in the period 1969–73 when Margaret and I were living in Kenya – an idyllic period, with many raptor 'casualties' brought to us for treatment and opportunities to work with such great names as Leslie Brown, Joy Adamson and members of the Leakey family. It was at that time that my findings were first put together in book form, originally intended as a thesis but eventually published as a bound volume, a limited edition, by the Hawk Trust (now the Hawk and Owl Trust) in the United Kingdom.

A second, more conventionally produced, edition appeared in 1978 and was published by the Standfast Press, with the help and encouragement of its owner Captain Richard Grant-Rennick. By 1985 it was clear that the subject was developing apace and, in an attempt to keep up with those changes, I compiled a Supplement and this was incorporated into the body of the remaining copies.

Fifteen years later, the situation regarding birds of prey has changed almost beyond recognition. Many more people keep raptors and captive-breeding is widespread and well established; to some it represents big business. Falconry continues to be practised in Britain and certain other countries but as my friend and colleague Neil Forbes has pointed out, attitudes have changed and the 'days of purely gentlemen falconers have . . . passed'. What Neil states is perhaps illustrated in a headline (*Cage & Aviary*

Birds, 27 November 1999) 'Birds In, Dogs Out. Why birds of prey have ousted pit bulls', which goes on to say 'Big birds of prey are taking over from pit bull terriers and Rottweilers as the ultimate cool accessory for the image-conscious pet owner'. This may be exceptional but there is no doubt that a broader selection of people keep raptors than ever before. Consequently, while serving the needs of the increasing body of veterinary surgeons who treat birds of prey, this book is likely to command a much wider readership than that of its forerunners. Falconers will still want to have access to it but their ranks will be swollen by other non-veterinarians who either keep or work with raptors – aviculturists, breeders and zoo staff, for example.

In addition, there are now many rehabilitators of raptors. The care of sick and injured birds has never been more popular or widespread and many centres in Europe and North America now employ full-time staff – a far cry from the days when most people did 'raptor rescue' as an adjunct to full-time employment or as a break from household chores! Falconers, breeders, avian researchers, rehabilitators and staff at zoos increasingly value ready access to information, as do veterinarians who treat these species in captivity.

At the same time that these developments concerning captive birds have taken place, raptor biology has evolved into a very significant, *bona fide*, discipline. Studies on the ecology of free-living birds of prey involve people from many backgrounds but few of them have veterinary or medical training. They, too, therefore require data on health and disease and in some cases may need to consider a veterinary input into their projects and protocols.

The first chapter of this book discusses in more detail trends involving captive and free-living birds of prey. Advances over four decades mean that we now know a substantial amount about the biology of birds of the Orders Falconiformes and Strigiformes. Work on these species, ranging from mate selection in the wild to therapeutics in captivity, is an integral part of modern scientific endeavour.

The production of a new edition of my book was prompted by the publishers, Blackwell, who in 1997 invited me to update and to revise the earlier work. The remit of this new edition is to keep pace with the developments of the past two decades while retaining much of the original book's style and orientation. As stressed above, there is a demand from those who work with raptors, both in the wild and in captivity, for information about the health of these birds. Several books have appeared over the past decade that help to meet this need – and relevant scientific papers appear with great regularity. Nevertheless, *Veterinary Aspects of Captive Birds of Prey*, which was the first modern treatise on the diseases of these birds, was always intended to occupy its own specific niche.

Why is this? In *Veterinary Aspects of Captive Birds of Prey*, I sought to provide, as do other more recent books, up-to-date information on diseases and pathology. I also wanted to promote strongly the concept that those who are new to the field need information on the history of the subject, the origins of terms, the evolution of current thinking and a reliable list of primary references for further reading. I have followed a similar philosophy in its successor. While the result is, perhaps, to make my books rather less technical and 'state of the art' than some of their genre, this approach is intended to ensure that they complement the latter rather than compete with them.

My aim is that *Birds of Prey: Health & Disease*, as this new edition has now been christened, should be of use to all those who work with raptors at all levels of experience and expertise. Further, the inclusion in this edition of data on *free-living* birds, largely as a result of the excellent contributions of two internationally recognised authorities, Professor Ian Newton and Dr David Peakall, reflects both my own increased involvement in this subject and the growing need for a multidisciplinary input into such studies.

The breadth of knowledge now required by those who treat birds of prey has led to my including contributions by others. The sections by Margaret Cooper (on law), Oliver Krone (parasitology) and Paolo Zucca (anatomy) provide specialist information on three important subjects. Line drawings by Jackie Belle, Oliver Krone and Paolo Zucca complement the text as do new photographs, many of them taken by Oliver and Paolo as well as by my wife. The majority of the electronmicrographs were prepared by Steve Gschmeissner.

In revising this book I have, as originally requested by the publisher, sought to retain the essential characteristics of earlier editions. Thus, I have used much of the original framework, chapter headings and titles of Appendices. I have also tried to maintain the personal touch, by writing in the first person, by openly expressing opinions and by referring to my own experiences as well as citing published literature. I hope that this approach (it was described as a 'Victorian style', in one review) will still prove acceptable to readers and encourage discussion and exchange of views.

In embarking upon a revision of my book I faced a dilemma. The subject has developed so much that it would have been possible to select a separate author, an expert in his/her own field, for virtually every chapter. To transform the book to this extent into a very different, multi-author, text would, however, have defeated the object of a 'new edition' of my original text. I have, therefore, revised large parts myself and hope that the continuity and consistency that this brings will prove compatible with the contributions of others, referred to above.

The important changes in this edition are, therefore: first, that it includes specific contributions by colleagues which will enhance the book's scientific value. Secondly, because of the extension of my remit to include free-living, as well as captive, raptors it will provide much information of relevance to field workers. My concern for international issues is reflected by the fact that I have attempted to relate raptor studies to global needs, particularly the environmental problems that face so many parts of the world, especially so-called 'developing' countries.

The book is written in British (European/Commonwealth) English but, conscious of differences elsewhere, I have done my best to reduce misunderstandings and ambiguities. Thus, for example, I have avoided using words that are largely unknown or not understood in the USA or have put in parentheses the corresponding term. This has also been the practice in the Index. I have throughout tried to omit words and expressions that can have special meanings in different countries.

The References and Further Reading are a key part of the volume. Many other books on birds, while providing copious illustrations and ample text, have tended to provide only a few supporting references and often these are not primary sources or they include few in languages other than English. I have referred to a wide variety of published works and the journals and books listed at the end should prove a useful guide to the scientific and lay literature. Every effort has been made to provide a reference when an unusual or poorly documented subject is under discussion or when it is probable that the reader will need further information.

The scientific names of raptors are not included in the text. Appendix I lists these, with English names, based on the checklist of Howard and Moore (1994).

As in previous editions, I should like to pay tribute to the many colleagues and friends who have encouraged and assisted me over the years. In particular, I must acknowledge the help of the following who have provided reprints, references, information or, in some cases, ideas or read parts of the book: Tom Bailey, Leon Bennun, Dick Best, John Chitty, Bill Clark, Norman Comben, Ruth Cromie, John Dickson, Christine Dranzoa, Mary Duncan, Chris Dutton, Kevin Eatwell, Mark Evans, Paul Flecknell, Neil Forbes, Helga Gerlach, Bob Green, Nigel Harcourt-Brown, Mike Hart, Jean-Michel Hatt, Erhard F. Kaleta, Josef Kösters, Martin Lawton, Helen Macdonald, Emma Magnus, John N. Maina, Brian Millard, Ranald Munro, Angels Natividad, Peter Naylor, Ian Newton, David Peakall, Pat Redig, Ron Rees Davies, Victoria Roberts, Jaime Samour, Richard Saunders, Peter Scott, Vic Simpson, Alex Stokes, Clem Tacconi, Dick Treleavan, Tony Turk, Baudouin Van den Abeele, Munir Virani, Jason Waine, Petra Wesche, David Williams, Michael Rodway Williams, Edward Wray, Ian Wyllie and Peer Zwart.

In listing the colleagues above, I am also aware of the important contributions made by numerous people, in different parts of the world, to our knowledge of the health and diseases of birds of prey. Some are named above, others include those who feature as authors of publications that I list in the References. Many are veterinarians or biologists but others are falconers, field naturalists or concerned members of the public. I pay tribute to their input and thank them for their support.

It is stimulating to realise that advances in raptor medicine continue to rely upon a combination of the experience and wisdom of older people and the energy and enthusiasm of those who are younger. This book reflects that important synergy. Ian Newton and David Peakall are experts who have contributed to raptor biology on an international scale for many years; they represent that cadre of scientists who unravelled many of the mysteries relating to the ecology of these birds. The new generation is represented by the input of Oliver Krone and Paolo Zucca, both of whom have had personal experience of the care of birds of prey as well as pursuing the formal study of their health and diseases – traits they share with another young European, Manfred Heidenreich. Dr Heidenreich paid me some kind compliments in his book *Birds of Prey: Medicine and Management*, also published by Blackwell, and I am conscious that in my review of that volume in the *Journal of Wildlife Diseases* I was precluded from drawing attention to his own many achievements in raptor medicine.

The interest and involvement in raptor medicine and pathology of so many colleagues from different backgrounds is exciting and together they are doing much to turn a subject rooted in antiquity into a modern scientific discipline. I have been privileged to span 35 years of exciting progress in our understanding of the diseases of birds of prey and to have seen advances that have greatly enhanced the health, welfare and conservation of these magnificent creatures. Long may such work continue!

I carried out much of the rewriting of this book in the Library at the Centre for Ecology and Hydrology (formerly the ITE) at Monks Wood in Cambridgeshire, UK. There, Neil Simmons, Marilyn Schofield and Pam Moorhouse provided help and a friendly welcome, as did Doreen Wade, formerly Personal Assistant to Ian Newton. I am equally indebted to the staff of the libraries of the Institut für Zoo- und Wildtierforschung (Institute for Zoo Biology and Wildlife Research) in Berlin and the Royal College of Veterinary Surgeons (RCVS) in London who also gave me support on many occasions. The value of such libraries, especially when one is researching a broad-based subject,

cannot be overestimated. Their role is being enhanced by the increasing availability of literature, databases and information on the worldwide web and it is to be hoped that it will not be too long before all raptor researchers, even those in less wealthy countries, have full access to these facilities.

Much of the typing of this edition was carried out by Tricia Tacconi and Lorraine Edwards, to both of whom I extend my thanks for their hard work, very often 'burning the midnight oil'. I am also grateful to Daniel Lee, Elena Wickham and Michael Champion who, at an early stage of preparation, sorted my large collection of reprints. Some other acknowledgements are listed at the end of Paolo Zucca's chapter.

As a postscript (October 2001) to this Preface, I must express my gratitude to Brian Millard for reading Chapter 11, following the sad news of David Peakall's death.

This edition is primarily dedicated to my wife but I include in this tribute my parents, Dorothy and Eric Cooper, in order to thank them for their encouragement since I was a child in my interests in natural history and for suggesting that I train as a veterinary surgeon. My own children, Vanessa and Maxwell, grew up (as Leslie Brown's original Foreword reminds us) with birds of prey in the home and they were both, at an early age, able confidently to hold an injured owl or to raise the vein of a fractious avian patient. I owe much to my family for their forbearance and support. *Ninawashukuru sana, wote!*

Raptors have long enthralled the human race. They are indicators not only of the richness of our planet but also of its fragility. The Earth is threatened by pollution, by fragmentation of ecosystems and by human damage and neglect. Study and understanding of the health of birds of prey can assist us in detecting and reversing some of these trends and in so doing, play a part in ensuring the long-term survival of this enchanting world, its animals, its plants and its peoples.

John E. Cooper
Entebbe, Uganda
September 2000

List of Contributors

John E. Cooper, *DTVM, FRCPath, FIBiol, FRCVS*
Durrell Institute of Conservation and Ecology, University of Kent, UK. Department of Wildlife and Animal Resources Management, Faculty of Veterinary Medicine, Makerere University, Uganda
E-mail: NGAGI@compuserve.com *or* NGAGI@vetaid.net

Margaret E. Cooper, *LLB, FLS*
Durrell Institute of Conservation and Ecology, University of Kent, UK. Department of Wildlife and Animal Resources Management, Faculty of Veterinary Medicine, Makerere University, Uganda
E-mail: NGAGI@compuserve.com *or* NGAGI@vetaid.net

Oliver Krone, *Dr med vet*
Institute for Zoo Biology and Wildlife Research (IZW), Alfred-Kowalke-Strasse 17, 10315 Berlin, Germany
E-mail: Krone@izw-berlin.de

Ian Newton, *OBE, FRS, FRSE*
Centre for Ecology and Hydrology, Monks Wood Research Station, Abbots Ripton, Huntingdon, Cambridgeshire, PE 28 2LS, UK
E-mail: ine@ceh.ac.uk

The late David B. Peakall, *PhD, DSc*
(Formerly Senior Scientist, Canadian Wildlife Service)

Patrick T. Redig
Professor and Director, The Raptor Center,
College of Veterinary Medicine, University of Veterinary Medicine, University of Minnesota, United States of America

Paolo Zucca, *DVM, PhD*
Laboratory of Animal Cognition and Comparative Neuroscience, University of Trieste, Italy
E-mail: zucca@univ.trieste.it

Line drawings by:

Jackie Belle, *VN, BSc, DESMan*

Oliver Krone, *Dr med vet*

Paolo Zucca, *DVM, PhD*

Introduction – the History of Raptor Medicine

'The Wisdom of the Ancients is necessary for the Advancement of Learning.'

Benjamin Farrington

In the Cairo Museum, in Egypt, stands one of the oldest surviving artefacts from the First Dynasty (3100 years before the birth of Christ). It depicts 'The Living Horus', the falcon god. Horus was not only sacred to the Ancient Egyptians but later (following the loss of an eye!) he became a Greek god. This is one of the very earliest records of deification of a falcon and a reminder of the significant role played by birds of prey in human culture and tradition.

Owls have long been symbolic in human society. Lilith, the Mesopotamian goddess of death had wings and talons herself, as well as owls at her side. She was probably the inspiration for Pallas Athene, the Greek goddess of wisdom and warfare and the concept of the 'wise owl' continues in much of Europe to this day. Perhaps in that vein, a carved owl in the wall of the Cathedral of Dijon, France, a building of the thirteenth and fourteenth centuries, continues to this day to be considered a source of good fortune to those who touch it.

When the original, very early version, of this book was privately printed in 1972, I expressed surprise at the paucity of published scientific information on the diseases of birds of prey, bearing in mind that the sport of falconry has been practised for over 3000 years. This was not to suggest, however, that there was no knowledge of the subject. Early writings show that many diseases of trained falcons were recognised by the Arabs 1000 or more years ago and

there is a wealth of information in such literature. In a lecture at the International Conference on Falconry in the United Arab Emirates in 1976 Möller discussed Arabic treatises on falconry and drew attention to the many references to diseases of the birds; amongst works he reviewed were some dating from the ninth century AD. In what was probably the first lecture on the subject by an Emiratee, a paper on 'Diseases of the falcon and their treatment' (1976) Shaikh Zaid Bin Sultan Al Nahayan, President of the Emirates, emphasised the number of traditional cures known to the Bedouin. Mark Allen refers to some of these in his delightful and scholarly work *Falconry in Arabia* (1980), making one wish that more information on the contribution made by the Arabs to the subject was generally available.

The first printed book in English on falconry, *The Boke of St Albans* (Berners, 1486), appeared over 500 years ago and this contained a considerable amount of data on the then known diseases of hawks. It is regularly referred to in this volume because of the clarity of the descriptions and the relevance of some of the text to modern day problems. An earlier work on hunting, by William Twiti, edited by Danielsson (1977) included sections on diseases of birds used in falconry. The classic of the period (1240–1250) *De Arte Venandi cum Avibus* by Frederick II of Hohenstaufen provided relatively little on health but is essential reading for all those with an interest in the history of falconry. Earlier translations of *De Arte Venandi cum Avibus* into English (Wood & Fyfe, 1943) and German have recently been augmented by one in French (Paulus & Van den Abeele, 2000).

A large number of other treatises on falconry and hunting appeared between the thirteenth and sixteenth centuries and a particular study of these has been made by some scholars, amongst them Dr Baudouin Van den Abeele, with whom I have had the pleasure to correspond. Van den Abeele published a synthesis of his findings in 1994, in French – *La Fauconnerie au Moyen Age* – and this includes sections on anatomy, pathology and symptomatology and therapeutics. A work that includes interesting, previously unpublished, information on the training of hawks was edited by Burnett (1998) while Hatt (1995) reviewed in German the history of hunting with the aid of falcons and cheetahs. A useful checklist of primary sources concerning falconry and hawking, covering the period 1575–1975, was compiled by Oelgart (1976) and produced as a limited edition of only 400 copies.

There would appear to be a need for a comprehensive analysis of the history of hawk medicine since, as Comben (1969) and Cooper (1979a) pointed out, several of the conditions of trained hawks diagnosed centuries ago, such as 'frounce' and 'cramp', are still readily recognisable and the origins of others may be traceable to earlier times.

Specific references to falconers and to diseases of birds of prey are regularly located in mediaeval and early modern texts: a rather nice example of the latter, dating back to 1586, occurs in a Puritan survey of Warwickshire clergy and describes the vicar of Temple Grafton, John Frith, as 'an old priest and unsound in religion, he can neither prech nor read well, his chiefest trade is to cure hawkes that are hurt or diseased, for which purpose manie doe usuallie repaire to him' (Schoenbaum, 1975). Mr Frith had clearly not heeded the words of William of Wykeham in the fourteenth century who admonished the Abbess of Romsey to discourage her nuns 'from keeping birds, rabbits, hounds and suchlike frivolous creatures to which they have given more heed than to the offices of the church . . . to the grievous peril of their souls'.

The important names in hawk medicine in Europe in the sixteenth and seventeenth centuries included Turberville (1575), Ferreira (1616), Latham (1615) and Bert (1619), all of whom published books on falconry. Bert appears to have been something of a veterinary consultant for in his book *An Approved Treatise of Hawkes and Hawking* he introduced the section on disease as follows:

'Wherein is contained cures for all known diseases, all of which have been practised by my selfe more upon worthy mens Hawkes that have be sent unto me. . . .'

Although much of the information in these books is, inevitably, anecdotal or based on old Greek concepts, some of the techniques described are worthy of note. Attention will be drawn later to Latham's recommended treatment for bumblefoot; his description differs very little from modern surgical techniques and I think we can assume that Latham and his contemporaries achieved some success with the method.

Richard Blome is worthy of mention even though he openly published other men's work under his own name. From the veterinary point of view, his publications are of interest in that he depicted surgical (cauterising) instruments in his book *The Gentleman's Recreation* (1686) and, in the same volume, he included the following very important maxim:

'Diseases are easier prevented than cured: everyone therefore that intends to keep Hawks should be well advised in the first place how to preserve them from Sickness and Maladies, which is of greater concern than to cure them when distempered.'

For all his shortcomings, Blome can be considered one of the earliest proponents of preventive medicine.

The late Anthony Jack's translation from Portuguese into English of Ferreira's *Arte de Caça de Altaneiria* (1616) appeared only recently (Jack, 1996). It contains several pages on the health of hawks, ranging from 'How to clean a falcon of lice' to 'A catalogue of recipes'.

Although the output of literature on falconry in

Europe declined after the seventeenth century, useful contributions to our knowledge of the biology – and to a certain extent of the pathology – of raptors continued to be made by anatomists and zoologists. For example, Steno (1638–1686) made a detailed study of the anatomy of the eagle while Peyer (1653–1712) described the caeca of the kite and performed experiments on the syrinx. A century later the great comparative pathologist John Hunter (1728–1793) carried out experimental work on hawks in connection with his studies on the air sacs and the Hunterian Museum (housed in the Royal College of Surgeons of England) contains 14 surviving specimens from birds of prey (Cooper, 1982a).

Little then appears to have been published of an original nature for over 150 years. Harting's *Hints on the Management of Hawks and Practical Falconry* appeared in Britain in 1898 and it is of interest to note that Harting had little time for the ancient remedies for treating hawks: he stated that 'No English falconers of the present day believe in them, and there can be no doubt that the less medicine given the better'. In 1891 Harting produced his *Bibliotheca Accipitraria* (1891), which reviewed the literature on hawks and falconry, and it is of interest to note that, by that date, 82 such works had appeared in English and many of these dealt in whole or in part with disease. Nevertheless, with the advent of the gun and the enclosure of land (and perhaps also on account of social change), interest in falconry had waned in Britain and the status of the bird of prey had declined from that of a strictly protected bird (with severe penalties for those who killed or took one) to the stage where every bird with a hooked beak was shot mercilessly by landowners and gamekeepers.

In contrast to most other European countries, falconry never completely died out in Britain and a small band of enthusiasts, first named The Old Hawking Club and later the British Falconers' Club, sustained the sport during the difficult period of the late nineteenth and early twentieth centuries. Books continued to appear in small numbers but these mainly repeated many of the age-old remedies and it is obvious that knowledge of hawk diseases did not advance at the same rate as other spheres of vet-

erinary medicine. For example, in his book *The Art and Practice of Hawking* in 1900, Michell described a number of diseases but his suggested remedies were almost entirely taken from the older texts. For 'snurt' (cold in the head), for instance, he referred his readers to Bert's recipe of 'root of wild primrose dried in an oven and powdered'. Blaine (1936), in his book *Falconry*, showed a rather more enlightened approach, in that he described some of the ailments of hawks in twentieth-century English. He retained faith in many of the old falconers' medicines, however, and stated 'For my own part, I feel that great benefit might accrue from the use of many of their quaint remedies, if we only knew how to concoct and apply them.'

The first real scientific advance in raptor medicine probably occurred in the 1930s, when Dr Tom Hare, a veterinary surgeon who was also medically qualified, began to examine birds for the British Falconers' Club. I was fortunate enough to be given, by the late Mr J G Mavrogordato, some letters which he received from Dr Hare and the latter's enthusiasm for the subject ('Many thanks for the specimens – send lots more') is very apparent. Hare was preoccupied with certain conditions, for example capillariasis and coccidiosis (Hare, 1939), but this in no way detracts from his reputation as the first in Britain – and, possibly, anywhere – to utilise modern laboratory techniques, such as parasitology, for the diagnosis of diseases of trained birds of prey.

World War II delayed further progress but advances were made in the succeeding years. Falconers in particular began to realise that veterinary attention for hawks might prove helpful and there was renewed interest in having *post-mortem* examinations carried out: '. . . we might even get to the point of curing some at least of these sick hawks' stated one contributor to *The Falconer* (Anon, 1953). In 1954 Dr R M Stabler in the United States of America (USA) elucidated the cause of 'frounce' and was able to recommend a modern antiprotozoal drug for its treatment; this and other scientific contributions were quoted in the first edition of Woodford's *A Manual of Falconry* (1960). Woodford's book was one of a number to appear in the 1960s but its approach to disease was a scientific one and, while some caution was urged, the use of modern drugs and techniques was unequivocally recommended. Other authors were less than enthusiastic, however, and ap Evans (1960), went so far as to state that:

'. . . there is no doubt it is far better (except in cases of Frounce) to stick to the natural physics which are the basis of these old recipes. Only if they fail should the falconer subject his hawk to the mercy of laboratory remedies.'

With the passing of The Protection of Birds Act, 1954, and subsequent legislation the survival of falconry in Britain was assured and its popularity began to increase there as well as in certain other countries. Soon after, a drastic decline in numbers of certain birds of prey was observed in Europe and North America (Ratcliffe, 1963, 1965; Hickey, 1969) and investigations indicated that pesticides, particularly the chlorinated hydrocarbons, might be responsible (Jefferies & Prestt, 1966; Ratcliffe, 1970). Further work suggested that one effect of such chemicals was a decrease in eggshell weight and hence reduced hatching success (Ratcliffe, 1967, 1970), although other factors involved probably included failure to lay, desertions and embryonic deaths (Newton & Bogan, 1974).

Later investigations suggest that the polychlorinated biphenyls (PCBs) might also be contributing to the decline of some species (Lincer & Peakall, 1970). At that time David Peakall wrote a useful review of the role of pesticides in his article in the *Canadian Field-Naturalist* (Peakall, 1976) (see Chapter 11) and the interested reader is referred to that together with other papers in the same edition. It is important to remember that many species of raptor also became threatened due to destruction or degradation of habitat and human persecution.

In the 1960s and 1970s progressive restrictions were imposed on the use of DDT and certain other pesticides in European countries, the USA and Canada, and these appeared to reverse the trend. However, the status of many species remained precarious and was not helped in some locations by an increase in thefts of eggs and young.

The risk of extinction that threatened some raptors resulted in considerable interest amongst biologists and other scientists in the behaviour, physiology and ecology of birds of prey. Raptor 'management' became an important subject – not the care of birds of prey in captivity but the management of raptors in the wild, which encompasses attention to habitat and minimising disturbance (by, for example, changes in land use) as well as survey, marking and research. This approach is well illustrated in the publication *Raptor Management Techniques Manual* (Pendleton *et al.*, 1987), which should be read by all those with an interest in raptor biology, including health and disease.

Part of this new approach involved the breeding in captivity of raptors for study purposes. In the USA, for example, a colony of American kestrels was established to study the effects of various pesticides (Porter & Wiemeyer, 1970). Likewise in the UK European kestrels kept by the Hawk Trust yielded valuable information on bacteriology, haematology and energetics (Kirkwood, 1979; Kirkwood *et al.*, 1979).

The new art of captive breeding rapidly developed (Cooper, 1984a). Serious attempts to breed the peregrine had commenced in North America in 1970 and met with great success (Cade, 1975) permitting birds to be used for a variety of purposes. Work in Germany and elsewhere in Europe paralleled those advances. Captive breeding was supported by some, although not all, conservationists – for two main reasons.

The first of these was that, by breeding birds in captivity and making the offspring available to falconers and zoological collections, one might be able to reduce pressures on raptors in the wild. This was the point made in the 1976 Recommendation of the European Section of the International Council for Bird Preservation (now BirdLife International).

'That the avicultural societies of Europe promote and encourage breeding programmes in order to lessen the drain of taking birds from wild populations.'

The second justification for captive breeding was that free-living populations might be supplemented by the release of captive-bred birds to the wild, but this argument proved to be controversial in some quarters. The rationale was that the mortality rate of most first-year birds in the wild is very high (Brown & Amadon, 1968; Snow, 1968) and therefore it should be possible to augment free-living populations by breeding, or rearing, young raptors in captivity for their first year and then to release them. This approach was endorsed in an editorial on raptor research and conservation in the *Canadian Field-Naturalist* mentioned earlier, by Ian Newton (1976) who stated: 'Another welcome development of the last five years has been the successful breeding of peregrines in captivity, not just a few birds, but on a scale sufficient for release projects.'

Newton went on to argue that such work had at least ensured the survival of endangered genotypes, albeit in captive populations, and this alone could be an important argument for captive breeding. In North America, in particular, reintroduction of peregrines to the wild proved to be a great success. The controversy elsewhere about release arose largely because restoration of habitat was considered to be more important and relevant than reintroducing birds: recently, this objection to introduction or reintroduction has been strengthened by concerns about the possible dissemination of pathogens in the course of such programmes (Cooper, 1989a).

The past 20 years have seen great advances in captive-breeding of birds of prey and in studies on their behaviour, physiology and ecology. Useful examples and data are to be found in a number of books, in papers and in proceedings of conferences. The role of captive-breeding in the management of endangered species has been recognised and has become an integral part of many programmes – for example, on the Mauritius kestrel, the California condor and the Philippine eagle.

These concerns about free-living birds of prey and interest in captive-breeding involved people from many disciplines. It was not long before veterinarians joined their ranks (Cooper, 1968a,b; 1969a,b; 1970a).

The veterinary profession can contribute to raptor work in six main areas, these being falconry, zoological collections, aviculture, the care of wild bird casualties, studies on free-living populations and research projects. Nevertheless, it was captive birds, especially those kept for falconry, that were the main preoccupation of veterinarians in the first instance.

With an upsurge of interest in falconry in many countries, practising veterinary surgeons increasingly found themselves consulted about sick or injured raptors and this demand has grown. Large numbers of birds of prey are also maintained in captivity in zoos, safari parks and private collections: in Britain alone, in 1994, there were more than 16 000 captive diurnal raptors and similar numbers of owls (Forbes, 2000). Veterinary advice is an important factor in the management of all such birds.

The increasingly active part being played by the veterinary profession in such work is often reflected in legislation (see Appendix XI). In Britain, for instance, both the Wildlife and Countryside Act 1981 and the Zoo Licensing Act 1981 have provided new roles for veterinarians at premises where raptors are kept. Veterinary participation in work with casualty birds has also, to some extent, been encouraged by the provisions of the Wildlife and Countryside Act (see also Appendix XI).

There has long been great concern amongst the public in Britain and elsewhere about the plight of wild bird casualties and many species, including raptors, are presented for veterinary attention (Cooper, 1975a; 1987a). Such care can certainly be justified on humanitarian grounds and, in a few cases, where populations are very small, may be significant in terms of conservation. From the scientific point of view, work with casualties can yield useful information on causes of disease and death in free-living populations. Involvement in the diagnosis and treatment of disease in such birds offers the veterinary surgeon an opportunity to deal with a wide variety of less familiar species and to gain expertise in avian surgery and medicine.

Veterinary input into work on free-living birds of prey was traditionally limited – a handful of enthusiasts usually assisting biologists at their own expense. In recent years, however, veterinarians have collaborated much more closely with raptor biologists (Cooper, 1993a) and concern about the decline or mass mortality of some species, e.g. vultures in India (Cunningham, 2000) and Eleonora's falcons in Crete (Ristow & Xirouchakis, 2000) has recently prompted an even greater input.

Veterinary input into raptor release and translocation programmes is becoming routine, prompted partly by the need to monitor ('screen') such birds (see Appendix VII). The *post-mortem* examination of raptors that are found dead after translocation can yield valuable information and such necropsies are best carried out by a veterinarian with knowledge of pathology. This has been the case, for example, in Sardinia and Sicily where restocking and reintroduction (respectively) of griffon vultures has taken place over many years and pathologists have been part of the team.

As a result of greater interest in the biology of predatory birds veterinary advice on such subjects as immobilisation, surgery and disease diagnosis is proving of increasing importance to scientists who are engaged in such studies (Cooper, 1993a; Greenwood, 1996). It prompted, for example, the inclusion of chapters or sections on pathology, haematology and blood chemistry in the (North American) *Raptor Management Techniques Manual* (Pendleton *et al.*, 1987) to which reference was made earlier. Such liaison between veterinarians and biologists is not entirely new; Ratcliffe (1970) consulted avian pathologists on possible differential diagnoses for eggshell thinning in British raptors when carrying out his seminal work on pesticide residues.

Under this heading of interdisciplinary collaboration, one can include work on birds of prey that are maintained for experimental purposes. Raptors have been used for bacteriological (Blancou & Rajaonarison, 1972) and toxicological studies (Fimreite & Karstad, 1971; Porter & Wiemeyer, 1972; Yamamoto & Santolo, 2000), and for more basic research, such as that on metabolism (Gatehouse & Markham, 1970), pellet formation (Grimm & Whitehouse, 1963) and vision (Martin & Gordon, 1974a,b). While in the past only a few veterinarians have participated in such research, their involvement now is widespread, either as investigators themselves or as advisors on techniques or on health and welfare.

The part that experienced and motivated veterinarians can play in raptor biology and raptor biomedicine is now well recognised and many names have contributed to these developments, as my reference list testifies. The announcement, rather appropriately at the time of writing this Introduc-

tion, of the establishment in the USA of the Patrick T Redig Professorship in Raptor Medicine and Surgery, illustrates how this subject has now 'come of age' – and is a well deserved tribute to Pat Redig (see Preface).

When the first edition of this book appeared (Cooper, 1978a; 1985b) I pointed out how little scientifically based literature on raptor disease was available with the exception of scattered papers, data in the bibliography by Halloran (1955) and a few articles in falconry books and journals. Indeed, it was largely on account of this dearth of information that the first edition of this book was produced. In the subsequent 20 years, however, the situation has changed dramatically.

Since 1978 many books and scientific papers have appeared that are either directly or indirectly concerned with the health of raptors. Three Proceedings of meetings span that period and together constitute a unique and invaluable series. *Recent Advances in the Study of Raptor Diseases* (Cooper & Greenwood, 1981a) comprised the Proceedings of the First International Symposium on Diseases of Birds of Prey, held in London in 1980 and some of the papers in that volume remain the most up-to-date and authoritative texts on particular subjects. That First Symposium was followed by a Second (*Raptor Biomedicine*) in the USA in 1988 and a Third (*Raptor Biomedicine III*) in South Africa in 1998, both of which have resulted in published Proceedings (Redig *et al.*, 1993; Lumeij *et al.*, 2000). As the subject has evolved so also have new ideas and new findings. However, some topics appear in one of the Proceedings but not the others and as none of them provides basic information on, for example, handling and sample collecting, they need to be used and read both as a set and in conjunction with other works.

Several other books have contributed much to the subject. *Care and Rehabilitation of Injured Owls* by Kay McKeever appeared in 1979: it was a valuable text but had the great disadvantage that it lacked references. This omission was rectified in the fourth edition (McKeever, 1987). Texts on rehabilitation from different countries also provide (and have provided) useful information including (for example) *Caring for Birds of Prey* based on work in Australia

(Olsen, 1990) and the Proceedings and journals of such organisations as the British Wildlife Rehabilitation Council (BWRC) and the International Wildlife Rehabilitation Council (IWRC). A useful, practical, guide to the treatment of raptors for veterinary practitioners is the *Manual of Raptors, Pigeons and Waterfowl* edited by Beynon *et al.* (1996) as is the book *Birds of Prey: Medicine and Management* by Heidenreich, that was first published in German (1996) and subsequently (1997) translated into English.

Sections about raptor diseases are to be found in other books including those by Fowler (1978), Cooper and Eley (1979) and Wallach and Boever (1983). More recently, specific chapters have been produced by Redig (1996a,b; 1997) and by Redig & Ackermann (2000). The second edition of Petrak's (1982) *Diseases of Cage and Aviary Birds* contains a number of references to raptors and is well worth consulting. The appearance in recent years of many comprehensive books on avian medicine has also contributed to a better understanding of diseases of birds of prey (see, for example, Samour, 2000a) although some, such as Ritchie *et al.* (1994) are of less value in terms of raptors because they concentrate primarily on other taxa of birds.

Scientific papers and articles have also appeared with increasing regularity over the past three decades. Review articles range from those by Cooper (1970a, 1976a, 1980a) and Halliwell (1979) to more modern papers, many of them referred to in the body of this book. An encouraging trend over the years has been in-depth studies on morbidity and mortality in individual species – for example, the sparrow-hawk (Cooper, 1980b), goshawk (Cooper, 1982a) and merlin (Cooper & Forbes, 1986). Recent years have also seen research on the welfare and conservation aspects of keeping birds of prey in captivity – for example, the report to the (British) RSPCA by Cromie and Nicholls (1995). Concern over welfare has led to the compilation and use of codes of practice (see Appendix XI) – including, for example, the inclusion of a section on birds of prey in the (British) *Secretary of State's Standards of Modern Zoo Practice* (DETR, 2000a).

Perhaps the most extensive bibliography to date on diseases of birds of prey is that compiled by Poffers and Lumeij (2000) and published in *Raptor Biomedicine III* (Lumeij *et al.*, 2000). A number of other private bibliographies and databases exist, for example those of Professor Helga Gerlach, Dr Murray Fowler and my own. No one list of references can be considered complete as allusions to raptors and their health feature in texts in fields as diverse as archaeology and zoonoses.

Useful additions to the literature written in languages other than English include many theses in German and French – dating back to those by Gerdessen (1956), Stehle (1965), and Bougerol (1967), all of which discussed diseases of birds of prey and supplied a number of references. These have been supplemented by scientific papers on raptor disease – in German, for example, by Kaleta and Drüner (1976) and Kösters (1974). The chapters in *Krankheiten der Wildtiere* (Gabrisch & Zwart, 1987) also provide valuable information. There is sometimes a disturbing tendency for those who publish or lecture to ignore (or to be unaware of) work in languages other than English and this omission can retard the development of the subject as a truly international discipline. There are, for example, many excellent texts in Russian (see Samedov (1978) on parasites of birds of prey), relatively few of which are quoted by 'authorities' in the field.

A useful resumé of the history of raptor medicine, which to a certain extent complements this Introduction, is to be found in the Foreword and Introduction, by Cade and Lumeij respectively, of *Raptor Biomedicine III* (Lumeij *et al.*, 2000).

An important factor in the accumulation and collection of data on diseases of birds of prey over the past quarter of a century has been the willingness of many who keep birds to cooperate with veterinarians. The majority of falconers and aviculturists no longer seek to withhold sensitive information and are generally receptive to modern medical and surgical techniques. This is leading to a situation anticipated by Leslie Brown in his book *British Birds of Prey* (1976a); he was complimentary about falconry and the past and present role of falconers as champions of birds of prey but stated, with regret:

'I could wish that falconers kept better records of such details as moult to adult plumage, the age to which their hawks survive, disease problems, amount of food consumed, and survival rates of captive as opposed to wild hawks, for in these ways they could add considerably to our knowledge of birds of prey . . .'

Similarly, ornithologists and other field workers seem increasingly more amenable to work with veterinarians and to take health and disease into account in their studies on birds of prey. This is, however, a fairly recent trend and not universal. It has been prompted very much by the enthusiasm of some enlightened people, from both disciplines, to work together (Cooper, 1993a) and also by increasing awareness that infectious agents (macroparasites and microparasites) might play a more significant, albeit subtle, role in regulating avian populations than was hitherto realised (see Chapter 14). Even 'popular' books about birds of prey are now more likely to include information about health and diseases – a significant change from even a decade ago

when (for example) one voluminous text devoted only a page to 'Infectious and Parasitic Diseases' (Newton & Olsen, 1990).

The growth and metamorphosis of avian medicine and pathology mean that no book can now cover the whole subject. In my first edition, nearly 30 years ago, I was able to review much of the literature available at that time and to include in my text clinical and pathological data on all the birds of prey that I had personally treated or examined. That material was then probably unique but it is now dwarfed by the volume of literature that has appeared and by the large series of cases seen by colleagues who work predominantly with raptors. Those readers who still require detailed information about my own earlier cases – or, indeed, need access to references and literature that are not included in this new edition – can best be advised with the words of Markham in 1631:

'All which forasmuch as I have shewed the Medicines and cures thereof in the former treatise . . . I will refer you unto the same, and not doubt but it will give you satisfaction.'

Nomenclature

'Hardly a motion could be made by the hawk, hardly a feather shaken, but a special term was applied.'

Gerald Lascelles

The need for a chapter on nomenclature, in essence a glossary, in this book is greater than ever. Even in English, different words can be used for the same thing depending upon whether one uses ornithological, popular or falconry parlance. Terms that are familiar to those who speak British/European/Australasian English may not be recognised by Americans, and vice versa. For that reason alternatives are given in the index and sometimes in the text.

It is hoped that this chapter on nomenclature will therefore help all readers but especially those who are non-Anglophone and who may find the myriad of words used in raptor work confusing and sometimes daunting.

Falconry abounds in unusual terminology, much of which has been in use for centuries and some of which has crept into work with raptors kept for exhibition and breeding. A summary of the more relevant terms was given in an article I wrote over 30 years ago (Cooper, 1968a) while comprehensive lists are to be found in many falconry books. *A Manual of Falconry* by Woodford (1960) is particularly recommended since it reprinted Harting's glossary and vocabulary (1891) and gave the origins of such words. It also provided a list of falconry terms in other languages. A recent publication, *The Encyclopedia of Falconry* (Walker, 1999), is a mine of information and is recommended to all who work with birds of prey.

In this book I have avoided most falconry terms except where they are either commonly used, or pertinent to veterinary work, and in such cases an explanation is given. As was pointed out in Chapter 1, very many diseases of birds of prey were known centuries ago and the terminology was often fascinating – for example, Markham wrote in 1631:

> 'Hawkes have divers infirmities and diseases, as Feavers, Palsey, Imposthumes, Sore eyes, and Nares, Megums, Pantas, casting her Gorge, fouleness of Gorge. Wormes, Fillanders, ill liver, or Goute, Pinne in the foot, breaking the pounce. Bones out of ioynt, Bones broken, Bruises, Lice, Colds, Frounce, Fistulaes, Stone, much gaping, more foundring, privy evill, taint in the feathers, loste of appetite, broken wind, blow on wing, wounds, swellings, eating their owne feet, taking up of veines in Hawkes, Crampe, and a world of others.'

Falconers will still use words such as 'frounce', 'croaks' and 'cramp' and it is important that the veterinary surgeon is aware of their probable meaning.

A knowledge of falconry terms for (external) parts of the hawk's body can also sometimes prove useful; reference should be made to relevant publications including those mentioned above. Internal anatomy is not considered in detail in this book but it is important that anyone dealing with birds of prey has an understanding of it. Paolo Zucca provides an excellent review: standard terminology is important, using *Nomina Anatomica Avium* (NAA) – see Chapter 3.

The birds covered in this book are those in the order Strigiformes, the owls (families Strigidae and Tytonidae), and the order Falconiformes which includes the families Cathartidae (New World vultures), Accipitridae (kites, hawks, eagles and Old World vultures), Falconidae (falcons), Pandionidae (osprey) and Sagittariidae (secretary-bird). Taxonomy of birds is under constant review, partly because of the increased application of DNA techniques, but in this book the names for both orders follow Howard and Moore's *A Complete Checklist of the Birds of the World* (1994).

Heidenreich (1997) discussed the taxonomy of birds of prey in some detail and reviewed some of the controversy that surrounds these species. He drew attention to König's (1982) work which enumerated important differences between New World vultures and other birds of prey. For example, New World vultures have no syrinx nor grasping foot but exhibit a perforated nasal septum: the usual sexual dimorphism (female larger than male) of birds of prey is not a feature of New World vultures and some of their behavioural traits are very different.

Some other terminology relating to birds of prey may be found in ornithological texts, such as *Birds of Prey of the World* (Grossman & Hamlet, 1965) which included an interesting chapter on birds of prey and humans.

The word 'free-living' is used to distinguish raptors in the wild from their captive counterparts: all birds of prey are, strictly, 'wild' birds although after several generations in captivity and selection for certain traits, some are now (probably justifiably) being termed 'domesticated'. The term 'free-ranging', so often used by North Americans, is not to be found in this book except in respect of, say, 'free-range poultry' where the implication is that the birds are essentially captive but remain free to range. 'Captive-bred' is used in its broadest sense of being 'bred in captivity', not the more narrow definition followed in British wildlife and other endangered species legislation.

The terms 'bird of prey' and 'raptor' are used interchangeably in this book to refer to any falconiform or strigiform species. The probable origins of the term 'raptor' have been discussed elsewhere (Cooper, 1996a). Falconers traditionally referred to their birds as 'hawks' and the word is sometimes used in that context. Various falconry words relate to the different species and sexes of birds of prey and these can be confusing to the uninitiated. Thus, for example, the word 'falcon' is used in the ornithological sense to mean a member of the family Falconidae but was traditionally employed in falconry parlance for the female bird alone. The term 'tiercel' meant a male bird. These and other falconry terms will be avoided.

When a specific bird is discussed, the English name will be employed – where necessary in citations, following that given by the author. A list of English and scientific names of all birds of prey mentioned in the text, following the check-list of Howard and Moore (1994), is given in Appendix I.

Other problems of nomenclature concern management since trained hawks are kept rather differently from those in a collection. Some of the terms used by falconers have also crept into captive breeding. The management of trained hawks is discussed in many falconry texts, both ancient and modern, and will not be repeated in detail. Suffice it to say that a trained hawk is kept tethered other than when it is being flown. It has a pair of leather jesses attached to its legs and, except when flying, these are attached by a swivel to a leash. The hawk is carried on a leather glove, or cuff, usually on the falconer's left hand (in Western and Middle Eastern countries).

A trained bird (hawk) may or may not be 'hooded' in order to quieten it. It is flown by reducing its food intake so that it is 'keen' but not starved. During the day it is perched on a 'block', a 'ring perch' or a 'bow perch' (depending on species and size); at night, hawks were traditionally kept indoors on a 'screen perch' but these are rarely used now. It may be carried – for example, to a veterinary surgery – on a portable perch called a 'cadge'. The building in which the bird is housed is called a 'mews' and the droppings of a hawk (which contain both faecal and urate portions) are commonly called 'mutes'. The latter term will be used from time to time in this book. The droppings of 'short-winged' hawks (accipiters) such as goshawks, are called 'slices' since they are shot with considerable force away from the bird's perch. A hawk 'bates' when it tries to fly off the fist or perch, but remains held by its jesses. Other terms are explained elsewhere in the book.

A brief explanation of some scientific terms may also prove useful to those readers who have no veterinary or medical background. Anatomical terminology is covered in Chapter 3; a useful general reference is *Outlines of Avian Anatomy* by King and McLelland (1975). Information on medical words not explained in this chapter can be obtained from standard medical or veterinary dictionaries.

'Health' is a term derived from Old English and can be defined as 'freedom from disease: bodily and mentally vigorous'. The World Health Organization Constitution defines 'health' as 'a state of complete physical, mental, and social well-being, not merely the absence of disease or infirmity' – a reminder that it is a *positive* state – one that can, increasingly, be measured (see Appendix VII). 'Disease' implies that something is wrong – a negative concept – and a useful definition is 'any impairment of normal physiological function affecting all or part of an organism'. Diseases can be infectious (due to or associated with a living organism) or non-infectious.

Insofar as clinical descriptions are concerned, 'clinical signs' can be equated with 'symptoms'; the latter word refers to the subjective feelings of the patient and is now rarely used in veterinary medicine. Some important clinical signs described in the book include 'anorexia' (absence of appetite), 'dyspnoea' (difficult breathing), 'tachypnoea' (rapid breathing), 'dysphagia' (difficulty in swallowing), 'diarrhoea' (loose faeces), 'dysentery' (blood in faeces), 'oedema' ('edema' in American English) (abnormal accumulation of fluid), 'hyperaemia' (increase in blood supply), 'atrophy' (decrease in size of a tissue or organ) and 'hypertrophy' (increase in size of a tissue or organ). Clinical diseases may be described as 'peracute', 'acute', 'subacute' and 'chronic' depending upon their duration while the forecast of the probable course of a disease, regardless of its cause, is the 'prognosis'.

Pathology is 'the study of disease' but usually implies the examination of dead tissues, or of samples taken from clinical cases. The 'aetiology' ('etiology') of a disease is 'the study of the cause' of that disease.

An 'infection' is different from an infectious disease since an infection implies the entry of an organism into a susceptible host, in which it may persist, but detectable clinical or pathological effects may or may not be apparent. Thus, for example, a bird of prey can be *infected* with coccidia but is not necessarily suffering from coccidiosis. In a 'latent infection' there is an inapparent infection in which the pathogen persists within a host, but may be activated to produce clinical disease by such factors as stress or impaired host resistance. A 'pathogen' is an organism capable of producing disease; the term can be used for organisms as diverse as viruses, bacteria and parasites and the adjective describing such agents is 'pathogenic'. The terms 'microparasite' and 'macroparasite' are used by ecologists and are discussed later. A 'lesion' is an abnormality caused by disease of a tissue; usually it is characterised by changes in appearance of that tissue. A 'focus' (plural 'foci') is a small, usually distinct, lesion, such as a micro-abscess in the liver. The word is also used clinically to imply the principal seat of a disease – for example, 'a focus of tuberculosis in the thorax'.

Words with the suffix '-aemia' ('emia' in American English) imply an abnormality, or presence of an obnoxious agent, in the blood. Thus 'toxaemia' is a condition in which a toxin (poison) is present in the blood and the terms 'bacteraemia', 'viraemia' and 'parasitaemia' are self-explanatory. The multiplication of organisms in the blood, usually with pathological effects on organs, is called a 'septicaemia'.

In epidemiological parlance the 'incubation period' is the time between infection and clinical signs. 'Mortality rate' refers to the proportion of deaths during a given time and 'morbidity rate' to the proportion of cases of a particular disease during a given time.

Two terms that are often misused are 'incidence' and 'prevalence'. The former is 'the number of new cases of a particular disease during a stated period of time, in a population under study' whereas 'prevalence' means 'the total number of cases of a particular disease at a given moment of time, in a population under study'.

Both 'veterinary surgeon' and 'veterinarian' are used in this book. The former term, that has interesting historical antecedents, is still in general use in Britain and many Commonwealth countries. In this book it implies one trained in veterinary medicine/science, not a specialist in surgery – in other words, it is synonymous with 'veterinarian'.

In publishing these definitions I realise that I lay myself open to accusations of being too brief and inaccurate and of attempting to make the book readable to the lay person at the expense of the reader who has a veterinary or medical background. Like-wise, my more traditional falconer friends will insist that my description of hawking terms is far from adequate and, in places, open to wider interpretation. Nevertheless, as stressed at the beginning, in a book such as this, which is likely to be used by people from a wide range of disciplines and in different parts of the world, it seems important to include some mention and explanation of technical terms, relating both to the birds and to their diseases.

Anatomy

P. ZUCCA

'Between animal and human medicine there is no dividing line nor should there be. The object is different but the experience obtained constitutes the basis of all medicine.'

Rudolf Virchow

INTRODUCTION

Raptors have always captured man's fancy and imagination; indeed, many ancient civilisations protected them and venerated them as if they were gods. A classic example of this kind of worship, mentioned also in Chapter I, was Horus, an Egyptian god in the form of a falcon (Grossman & Hamlet, 1988).

In the Middle Ages, falconry – which is the art of training falcons for hunting – flourished in Europe and many of these birds were employed in this pursuit. During this period the first text containing detailed descriptions of the anatomy of raptors appeared. This was entitled *De Arte Venandi cum Avibus* and was written by Frederick II of Hohenstaufen (see Chapter 1).

With the passing of time, interest in raptors diminished. A famous text on zoology, written during the second half of the eighteenth century by Figuer and which has been translated into several European languages (Figuer, 1873), stated that 'of all the birds, raptors are the best known amongst the common people but, on account of the few services they render, they do not deserve as much interest as many other birds do'. Furthermore, that work contained numerous incorrect descriptions of their anatomical features. The description of the feet of the raptors is somewhat curious since they are described as having 'four toes, three of which

directed forward and one behind, generally very flexible, with *retractile*, hook-shaped talons'.

The golden age of raptors came to a close but, paradoxically, awareness of these glaring errors led to a systematic study of the anatomy of birds. Although there are more than 9000 different species, very little is known from an anatomical and structural point of view. In fact, most of the studies carried out during the past 200 years, as Harcourt-Brown (2000), shrewdly pointed out, have been directed towards taxonomy. Unfortunately, taxonomists when conducting research for the purposes of classification, mainly take into consideration the differences with regard to muscles and most do not give even an inaccurate description of the whole anatomy of the animal. For this reason, only in the past 30 years or so, thanks to developments in avian medicine, have numerous works on avian anatomy been published adopting a medical approach (Bock, 1974; King & McLelland, 1979, 1984; Petrak, 1982; Rübel *et al.*, 1991; Krautwald *et al.*, 1992; Orosz *et al.*, 1992; Proctor & Lynch, 1993; Harcourt-Brown, 2000a,b).

An important step forward in the field of avian anatomy was made with the publication of the *Handbook of Avian Anatomy: Nomina Anatomica Avium*, now in its second edition (Baumel *et al.*, 1993), which has established an official glossary of avian anatomy terminology. In work with birds of

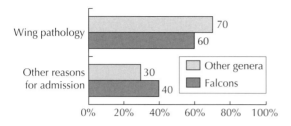

Fig. 3.1 Wing pathology vs other reasons for admission to rehabilitation centres (falcons and other genera).

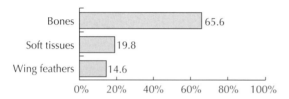

Fig. 3.2 Pathology of feathers, soft tissues and bones of the wing.

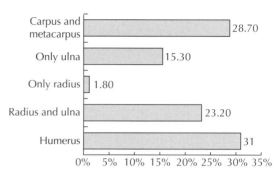

Fig. 3.3 Prevalence of wing bone pathology.

prey especially, where the results are intended for international readership, these terms should be used.

In the light of what has been said, this brief contribution, which purists of anatomy might find reason to criticise, has been written adopting a biological/medical approach, but with a level of precision and detail that would be required by an avian veterinarian. Some special senses, such as sight and hearing, which in this group of animals have reached the highest levels of specialisation to be found in nature, are dealt with in detail. It is of the utmost importance that veterinarians should know the anatomical and physiological features of the animals that they are treating in order to give a correct diagnosis. The prevalence of certain kinds of pathology affecting raptors differs, depending on whether the veterinarian works in a private practice or a rehabilitation centre. The animals brought to a private practice are often raptors used in falconry and one of the areas affected by pathology is the feet, which can be confirmed by my personal observations and by those of colleagues (N. H. Harcourt-Brown, pers. comm.). In contrast, the main problem affecting raptors brought to a rehabilitation centre involves the wings (Delogu, 1993; Zucca, 1995).

In a sample of 413 raptors of the genus *Falco* and of 767 diurnal raptors belonging to other genera present in Italy, which were examined in several Italian rehabilitation centres between 1992–1994, wing pathology represented respectively 70% and 60% of the reasons for admission (see Fig. 3.1).

Figure 3.2 shows how bone pathology of the wing in falcons represents 65.6% of reasons for admission. If we divide the values according to the kinds of wing pathology, we obtain the figures shown in Fig. 3.3. The humerus is the area that is affected most, followed by the carpus and metacarpus, and the radius and ulna. It is rare that either of these is affected individually.

As has already been mentioned, given the purely medical approach of this text, attention has been focused on the areas or the sensory organs that are more frequently affected by pathology and about which the veterinary surgeon should be knowledgeable. The skeletal system and some organs of sense, for example sight and hearing, are dealt with in detail while internal anatomy, such as that of the alimentary, respiratory and reproductive tracts (Figs 3.4, 3.5, and 3.6), is not considered comprehensively in this chapter. However, it is important that anyone dealing with birds should have an understanding of anatomy and therefore reference is made in the appropriate chapters.

If not otherwise stated, most of the data on avian anatomy mentioned below are taken from Proctor and Lynch (1993), Baumel *et al.* (1993), King and McLelland (1979, 1984) and Marshall (1960).

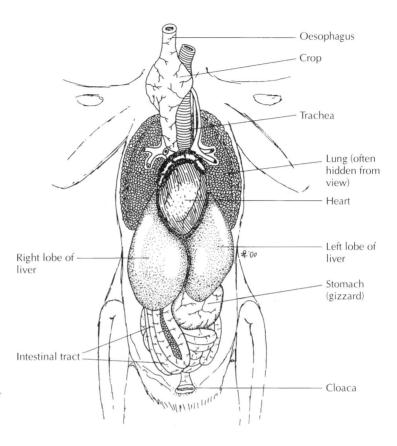

Oesophagus

Crop

Trachea

Lung (often hidden from view)

Heart

Left lobe of liver

Stomach (gizzard)

Right lobe of liver

Intestinal tract

Cloaca

Fig. 3.4 Thoracic and abdominal organs of a falcon, as seen when body is first opened. (Courtesy of Paolo Zucca.)

In order to be able to communicate effectively, vertebrate anatomists have developed a glossary of specialised terms to describe, without margins of doubt, the regions of the body, the localisation of the various structures as well as the main sections used to illustrate the anatomy of vertebrates (Proctor & Lynch, 1993). As the NAA (*Nomina Anatomica Avium*) (Baumel *et al.*, 1993) is *the* reference for anatomical terminology, all the anatomical terms used in this chapter (and elsewhere in this book) adopt the NAA standard.

It is forgone conclusion that the main axis of a bird is always horizontal as when the bird is in flight. Many of the words used can have the same meaning; sometimes lateral and medial have the same meaning as proximal and distal (Proctor & Lynch, 1993). The same can be said for anterior and posterior which mean cranial and caudal. When a bird is in flight we can use the same terms as are used for planes: the three axes (A, B, C) refer to the roll, yaw and pitch hold.

FEATHERS

The most distinguishing feature of a bird is its feathers. All known birds have feathers and no other animals, living or extinct, have this body characteristic. The plumage of nocturnal raptors is soft (Plate 1) and at the same time distinctive in that the wing feathers are slightly emarginated, like a comb, thereby reducing the noise produced by the wings in flight. A silent flight allows the nocturnal raptor to approach close to its prey without being heard. It also allows the raptor to hear better as it is not disturbed by background noises which might be

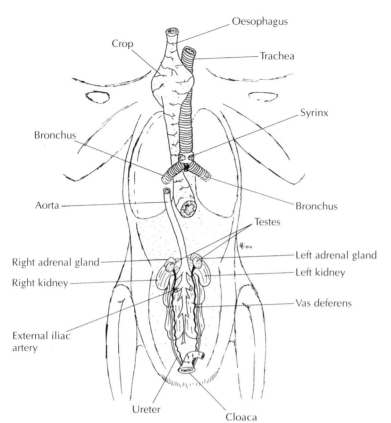

Fig. 3.5 Deeper organs of a falcon, as seen when viscera have been removed. (Courtesy of Paolo Zucca.)

produced were it not for this 'comb'. The plumage of nocturnal raptors that feed on fish and of those with more diurnal habits does not have this morphological characteristic and, instead, is quite similar to that of diurnal raptors.

WING CLAW

The alula (Plate 2) of many species of diurnal and nocturnal raptors bears a wing claw which is not reabsorbed during the first days of its life but, on the contrary, grows in size and can vary in shape and length according to the age of the raptor (the claws of mature common kestrels and peregrine falcons lose their curvature and become straighter). The wing claw is made up of a fixed bony base, a few

millimetres long, on the alula, and is covered by a horny sheath (Zucca & Cooper, 2000).

HEAD

The skull of a bird of prey, an owl, is depicted in Fig. 3.7. Its structure is related to the need for the raptor to see, to hear and to prehend and swallow food. In the place of teeth and heavy mandibles birds have a gizzard (muscular stomach) situated at their centre of gravity. In the first stages of their evolution they had already developed a horny beak which covered the mandibles and, at the same time, lost their teeth. Stephen Jay Gould, with his typical shrewdness, has pointed out that, even though the system for the production of teeth has not been used

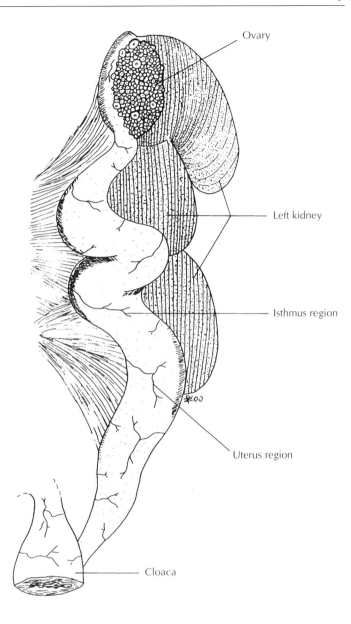

Fig. 3.6 Left ovary and oviduct of a
falcon. (Courtesy of Paolo Zucca.)

in birds for probably about a 100 million generations, the epithelium of chickens is still able to
induce the production of such structures (Gould,
1983). The beaks of birds are very light, much more
so than the teeth and heavy bones that are needed
to keep them in place in other classes of animal
(Proctor & Lynch, 1993).

The beaks of raptors are pointed and hooked but
the shape varies according to the prey eaten (Fig.
3.7). Animals with a non-specialised diet, such as
buzzards, have a moderately hooked beak without
any particularly distinguishing features. Other very
specialised species, as for example falcons (*Falco*
spp.) have a short, strong beak with a notch called

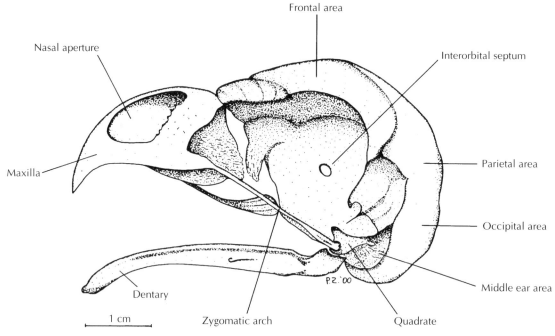

Nasal aperture

Frontal area

Interorbital septum

Maxilla

Parietal area

Occipital area

Dentary

Middle ear area

1 cm

Zygomatic arch

Quadrate

Fig. 3.7 Skull of a barn owl. (Courtesy of Paolo Zucca.)

a 'tooth' which is used for killing prey. Most vultures and certain eagles, the golden eagle for example, have a strong powerful beak for feeding. Many diurnal raptors have a prominent ridge, probably for protecting their delicate organs of sight while diving or pursuing prey in woodlands. This particular conformation of the skull is often perceived by humans as a symbol of pride or authority.

BONES

A characteristic of the bone structures of raptors, common to all birds, is the fusion and reduction in number of bones. The skeleton, with a reduced number of bones fused together, forms a strong, rigid and stable central support to which the flight muscles, limbs and most of the wing quills and tail quills are attached. Both the wing bones and the leg bones exhibit a fusion of distal bone elements, espe-

cially between the carpus, metacarpus and the fingers of the avian 'hand' (Bellairs & Jenkin, 1960; Bock, 1974; Proctor & Lynch, 1993) (Figs 3.8 and 3.9). The axial skeleton, as well, is almost completely fused and the sacral vertebrae are fused with the iliac bones of the pelvis to form a single bone structure called the synsacrum (Plate 3). Furthermore, the body mass is not very high but this is only because the bodies of birds are small. Compared with those of mammals of the same size the bodies of birds are not exceptionally light. The skeleton and the other tissues weigh more or less the same as those of mammals of the same size. Birds, however, have developed compact and centralised body structures (Proctor & Lynch, 1993).

WINGS

The structure of the wings and of the tail vary considerably depending on the hunting methods used

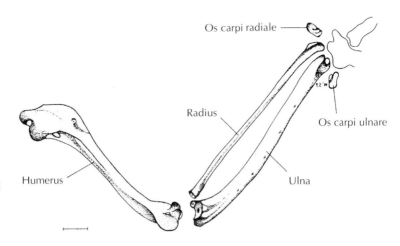

Fig. 3.8 Ventral view of the skeletal anatomy of the proximal part of the left wing of a peregrine. (Courtesy of Paolo Zucca.)

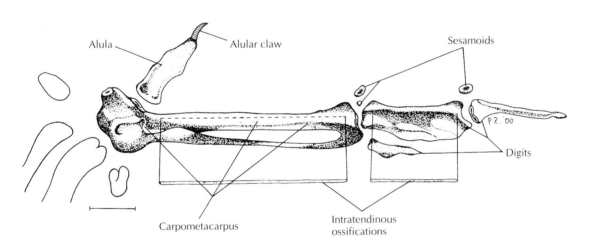

Fig. 3.9 Ventral view of the skeletal anatomy of the distal end of the left wing of a falcon. (Courtesy of Paolo Zucca.)

by the various species (Fig. 3.10): some diurnal raptors pursue their quarry at a great speed for a few minutes while others scan the territory close to the ground or at great height for hours on end. In general, wings of birds of prey can be divided into two categories: those in the first category are pointed, fast-flight wings with high wing-loading typical of those species that swoop down on their prey at great speed while those in the second are soaring wings with low wing-loading and broad tails which enable the raptors to hover for hours with little effort. The wings of hawks and harriers fall into an intermediate group because their wings are quite broad with rounded tips, which allows them to pursue their prey in woodlands (Fig. 3.10).

From an anatomical point of view, most of the wing muscles and leg muscles are situated along the median line of the body and control the limbs by

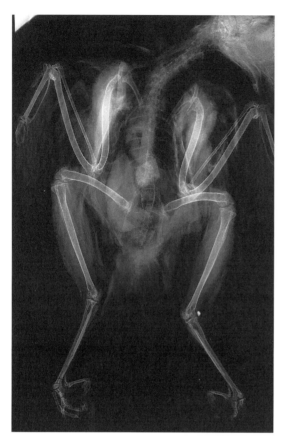

Fig. 3.10 Radiography provides information about the behaviour of birds as well as their health. This Mauritius kestrel, radiographed *post mortem* prior to dissection, shows shortened wing bones and lengthened leg bones – adaptations to its forest habitat.

means of long tendons. Flapping flight would not be possible if most of the flight muscles were on the wings because the excessive weight would weigh them down (Proctor & Lynch, 1993). In order to reduce the weight as much as possible and to maintain a high flight efficiency, many wing bones have undergone fusion (Plate 4).

Furthermore, some species, such as those belonging to the genus *Falco*, have particular bone structures within the tendons called intratendinous ossifications (Vanden Berge & Storer, 1995; Zucca & Cooper, 2000). The veterinary surgeon must always bear in mind the existence of these delicate

yet essential anatomical parts when operating on the distal part of the wing (see Fig. 12.4).

FEET

Raptors use their feet to capture their prey and sometimes to kill it. The shape of the feet and the talons vary as well, depending on the prey and the way the raptor hunts. Raptors that feed upon swift birds captured on the wing, such as sparrow-hawks, have slim toes and sharp talons. Those raptors that capture their prey on the wing such as, for example the peregrine falcon, often have a middle toe that is longer than the others. The short-toed eagle has short thick-toed feet covered with large horny scales to help it grasp snakes on which it feeds, while the thick, powerful feet of the golden eagle are suitable for capturing and holding its prey.

There are raptors with more specialised feet such as the long-legged secretary-bird, which covers many kilometres a day in search of food, or the osprey with its hooked talons and rough spicules on the soles of its feet for gripping live, slippery fish. Vultures do not need to capture live animals and so their talons are blunt and nor are they used for injuring their prey. There are intermediate forms other than the main ones mentioned here.

In almost all species the talon of the middle toe is differently shaped from the others: it is not perfectly conical but it has a groove (Plate 5). This characteristic has a precise functional significance during the capture and killing of prey in that, when the talon penetrates the tissues, the groove allows the blood to flow more quickly and so the prey dies faster. This draws an interesting 'evolutionary analogy' between the talons of most raptors and the teeth of predatory mammals: a section of the canine teeth of a lynx shows identical adaptations.

From an anatomical point of view, the publication used as a reference for the anatomy of the pelvic limb of raptors is the work by Harcourt-Brown (2000a,b), from which further information can be obtained. As was the case with the wing, the veterinary surgeon should remember that intratendinous ossifications are to be found in certain anatomical regions of the feet of various raptors such as the peregrine. Even minor damage to these delicate bones could affect the functioning of this limb.

PEDIGRAMS

Various methods have been developed over the years for identifying an individual bird. External tags and rings (bands), tattoos and microchips are just a few examples of the wide range of artificial markers used on birds. A simple and non-invasive method for the recognition of individual raptors, especially peregrines, has been developed and generally consists of evaluating the scale patterns on the feet and legs (Stauber, 1984). It is usually the middle toes (digit 3) that are examined, taking photographs with a macro lens. The most evident scale patterns of the individual are then drawn on paper using Indian ink.

A simpler system involving photographing the plantar surfaces of the feet and thus producing the characteristic 'fooprint' was used in the 1970s by the Hawk Trust in Britain (J. E. Cooper, pers. comm.). It proved useful in identifying birds that had been lost or stolen. Birds with scars or changed papillae as a result of bumblefoot (see Chapter 8) proved particularly easy to recognise with this technique.

TAIL

The morphology of the tail and its relationship to the uropygial gland are shown in Plate 3.

The tail plays an important part in flight. Those species that are able to change direction suddenly, such as goshawks, often have long tails while soaring species, such as buzzards, have tails with a large load-bearing surface. From an anatomical point of view, in order to make up for the gradual loss of weight in the cranial part of the body, even the number of caudal vertebrae has been reduced and these have undergone partial fusion.

DIGESTIVE SYSTEM

By virtue of the fact that the bodyweight is centralised, the main (and heavier) internal organs

and, above all, the digestive system are suspended between the wings in the body cavity. This allows birds to keep their balance and to maintain their aerodynamic stability without the use of long tails as in reptiles (McGowan, 1991).

From a morphological point of view raptors have a relatively simple muscular stomach. The average pH of the gastric juice in hawks, prior to eating, is lower than in owls (1.7 vs 2.4). The pancreas occupies only half of the duodenal loop in the owls and is even smaller in hawks. Most falconiform species (hawks, eagles and vultures) have relatively small caeca, while they are well developed in owls (Duke, 1987); conversely, falconiforms have a dilatation of the oesophagus, the crop (Fig. 3.11), while owls do not (Fig. 3.12).

Typical features of the digestive physiology of raptors include the production of regurgitated pellets ('casting' using falconry terminology) made up of the indigestible or indigested remains of their prey (teeth, bones, fur, claws, etc.) (see Chapter 4). Owls usually egest a pellet for each meal while hawks may eat more than one meal before casting (Plate 11).

RESPIRATORY SYSTEM

Birds are endothermic animals and generally have a high metabolic rate. Birds, as warm-blooded animals, burn 30 times more metabolic energy than do reptiles of the same size (Gill, 1990). The avian cardiovascular and respiratory systems are extremely efficient, allowing them to withstand great cardiopulmonary stress. Migrating geese, for example, can cross the Himalayas at a height of over 9000m, which in terms of human energetics is equal to riding up Mount Everest on a bike (King & McLelland, 1984). The world altitude record for birds is held by a Ruppell's griffon (vulture) which was sucked into an aeroplane engine at an altitude of about 11000 metres (Burton, 1991). Even though the vulture was soaring, no other mammal of the same size would have been able to breathe enough air so as not to lose consciousness at that altitude (Proctor & Lynch, 1993).

From an anatomical point of view, the respiratory system of birds is unique among all vertebrates on

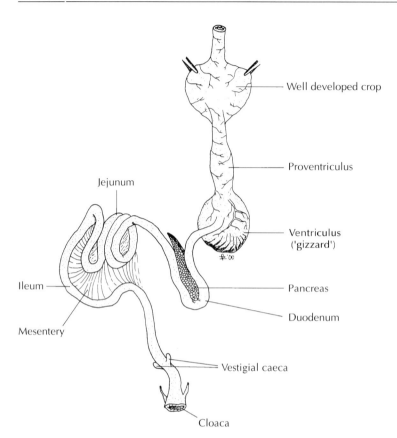

Jejunum

Ileum

Mesentery

Cloaca

Well developed crop

Proventriculus

Ventriculus ('gizzard')

Pancreas

Duodenum

Vestigial caeca

Fig. 3.11 Digestive (gastro-intestinal) system of a falconiform bird. (Courtesy of Paolo Zucca.)

account of its size and capacity (Fig. 3.13). In many birds the main bones of the body as, for example, the humerus, the spinal column and the femur etc. are pneumatised and directly connected with the air sacs and the respiratory system. The air sac system calls for the presence of a large number of apertures called pneumatic holes in the bones. Apertures of this kind can also be found in the bones of larger dinosaurs, which leads one to postulate that they might have had air sacs. The function of these air sacs is not completely clear but it seems that they cause the air in the lungs to flow in one direction and might be used for the dissipation of excess heat (McGowan, 1991).

The respiratory system, as well as the bones, is one of those areas that is often affected by various forms of pathology such as bacterial and viral infections, mycoses or parasitic infestation. Some species of nematodes – for example, *Serratospiculum* spp. – inhabit the air sacs (see also Chapter 7) and can cause respiratory problems when there is a massive infestation (Delogu & Zucca, 1999; Zucca, 2000).

SIGHT, HEARING AND SMELL IN RAPTORS

Even though the morphology of structures of raptors does not differ, in principle, from that of other birds, some groups have developed particular characteristics due to the fact that they are hunters. The range of sensory specialisation is quite vast and

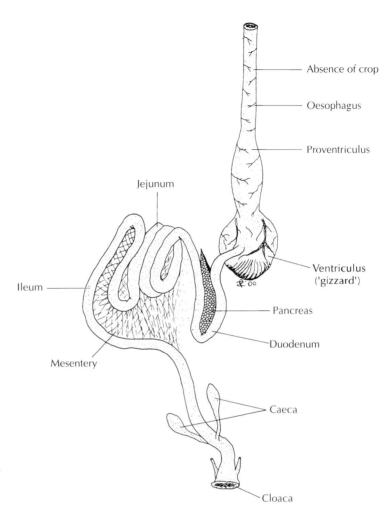

Fig. 3.12 Digestive (gastro-intestinal) system of a strigiform bird. (Courtesy of Paolo Zucca.)

varies from one genus to another but, generally speaking, concerns, above all, sight and hearing – the latter in nocturnal raptors in particular. Most of the information that follows, if not otherwise stated, has been adapted from the following authors: Baumel *et al.* (1993), Bergmann (1987), Brown & Amadon (1989), Burton (1991), Cade (1982), Coles (1997), Cooper (1978a), Cooper & Greenwood (1981a,b), Farner *et al.* (1971–1985), Gensbøl (1992), Grossman & Hamlet (1988), Hume (1991), King & McLelland (1984) and McGowan (1991, 1999).

Sight

The great adaptability of birds to flight has developed at the same rate as the equally complex evolution of the central nervous system which is necessary for controlling their body in a three dimensional world (Proctor & Lynch, 1993).

Balance, coordination and muscular control and the proprioceptive functions of the brain are highly specialised in the class Aves. Furthermore, birds have incredible vision which is necessary for informing the brain about a bird in flight and giving the exact

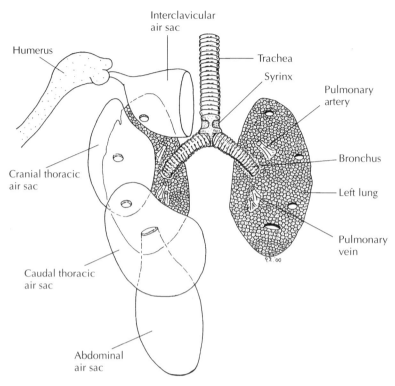

Fig. 3.13 Lower respiratory tract including syrinx, lungs and air sacs. (Courtesy of Paolo Zucca.)

location of objects in the surrounding area. Confirmation of such characteristics, from an anatomical point of view, is shown by the high development both of the cerebellum (Plate 6), which is the part of the central nervous system that controls the balance and the coordination of movements, and the optic lobes (McGowan, 1991).

In general, the eyes of both diurnal and nocturnal raptors are large and specialised. In this group of heterogeneous 'hunting' birds the sense of sight is of vital importance since they have to pick out their prey from afar, even when visibility is poor. Furthermore, the eyes are able to perceive things that humans cannot. For example, diurnal birds can perceive ultraviolet light (Burckardt, 1988).

Visual field

Binocular vision is better developed in nocturnal raptors, whose visual field is 110 degrees, of which

70 degrees is binocular. They therefore have a good binocular visual field with two restricted areas for monocular vision and the rest of the visual field both lateral, backward and upward is a blind spot. For this reason some nocturnal raptors have a second pair of eyes (occipital vision) which is a plumage pattern on the nape that confuses the prey or the predator coming from behind. To compensate for their limited visual field, nocturnal raptors have an extremely mobile neck which they can rotate to 270 degrees making eye movement superfluous. Diurnal raptors have a visual field of about 250 degrees, 50 degrees of which is binocular.

Visual acuity

The visual acuity (ability to discern details sharply) of diurnal raptors is up to eight times that of the human eye. From an anatomical point of view, one square millimetre of the retina of a buzzard has one million nerve cells compared with the 200 000 of the human eye. Furthermore each eye has two foveae, that is to say, two areas of the retina where there is a larger concentration of visual cells which enable the raptor to determine the exact position of its prey. One fovea is used for binocular vision while the other is used for monocular vision.

The raptor's eyes are very large and take up a lot of space in the skull (Fig. 3.7). Since from the outside one can see only the cornea and because all of the eyeball is encased in the skull, the size of the eyes is often underestimated. The eyes of the golden eagle are much bigger than those of humans. From a functional point of view, the bigger the eye, the larger the image on the retina, and the greater are the perceived details – in other words, the greater the resolving power. Nocturnal raptors too have keen sight but since they are active hunters, mostly at dusk or during the night, it is most important that they make the most of the light or, in other words, develop a high sensitivity to light. For this reason the eyes of night-flying species are very large and deep and almost cylindrical. They have large, thick, curved cones and large crystalline lenses with a reduced focal length which allows as much light in as possible. Their retina is mainly composed of rods rather than cones. In fact, rods are receptors that permit better vision in low light conditions while cones are better for detail, good definition and colour – and associated with strong light conditions. Some nocturnal species with diurnal habits, such as for example, the little owl, which is often active during the day, have retinae and eyes similar to those of diurnal raptors; its ability to distinguish colours is reasonably good even though it is of no use at night. This means that many nocturnal raptors are able to see in light conditions that are 100 times lower than the minimum required for vision by human eyes.

Hearing

Even though hearing is very developed in most raptors, it is not always the most important sense for hunting. There are exceptions to the rule such as the harriers that fly close to the ground when hunting, often at dusk; this group of raptors has

a facial disc similar to that of nocturnal raptors. In nocturnal raptors hearing is probably the most developed sense. In fact, it is hearing rather than sight that enables these animals to capture their prey in the dark. Often the auditory meati and the facial discs are asymmetrical. The facial discs are made up of two patches of skin surrounded by rigid plumage that forms an opening which directs sound towards the acoustic meatus and they are structurally similar to the pinnae of mammals. One is larger than the other, as in the long-eared owl. In this species the opening of the right ear is 30% wider than that of the left ear while the posterior patch of the right facial disk is 50% wider for the right ear.

The species of owl which is the most specialised in hunting at night is the barn owl. Detailed studies have been carried out on this animal on account of its exceptional hearing abilities. It is the most nocturnal of the strigiforms and usually only starts hunting well after dusk and terminates before dawn. In unfavourable weather conditions, such as rain or wind, these raptors remain inactive all night long, which goes to show how important hearing is when hunting. It is the only species of nocturnal raptor that is able to hunt in the total darkness of a cage sealed off from light (Payne, 1962). From a structural point of view, the acoustic meati of barn owls are positioned differently on the sides of the head and the sensitivity of each ear to the sound of high and low frequencies is different. These raptors, like human beings, use two different peculiarities of signal stimulus in order to locate its origin: time and intensity. It is clear that when a sound comes from the right it reaches the right ear first and then the left ear; this time lapse, which is limited but at the same time important, is relative to the differences in the intensity of the sound which permits the brain to establish quite accurately the direction from which the sound comes. Due to its anatomical features (asymmetrical acoustic meati) and its functional features (different sensitivities of the two ears to sounds) the barn owl is able to locate its prey not only on two dimensional planes (X and Y) but also in space (Z). In order to calculate the position of the prey on a plane, both time differences and sound intensities are used, while to calculate Z barn owls rely on the differences in intensity, which is possible thanks to the asymmetry of the meati. The differences in intensity and in time are decoded separately using the nerve paths of the mesencephalon (Moiseff & Konishi, 1981). It has been observed that young barn owls do not have this innate ability accurately to locate their prey in space but they tune their system for localising sound sources during the first few months of their life with the aid of sight (Knudsen *et al.*, 1982; Knudsen & Knudsen, 1985).

Smell

Little is still known about this sense in birds, but recent studies seem to attribute more importance to it than in the past, especially in the case of New World vultures. Researchers (Bang & Cobb, 1968) compared the diameter of the olfactory bulb to the diameter of the encephalon of various species of birds belonging to different families and came up with some interesting results: house sparrows (5%), diurnal raptors (14–17%), nocturnal raptors (18%), pigeons (22%), pelicans (37%) and kiwi (*Apteryx* spp) (33%).

BRAIN AND BEHAVIOUR: PECULIARITIES OF THE AVIAN BRAIN

Birds are able to perform problem-solving tasks and other complex cognitive tasks to the same extent as do primates despite their lower brain weight to body weight ratio. Even though the brain of a bird is made up of neurones and glial cells as in mammals, the structure is different (Rogers, 1997) (Plate 6). In mammals, the external part of the telencephalon is 'laminated' (layered), the so-called neocortex, while the neurones in a bird's brain have mostly a non-laminated structure (Vallortigara *et al.*, 2000). For this reason, it was thought that only mammals had a neocortex and that the telencephalon of birds was a hypertrophic development of subcortical nuclei called the striatum. Thanks to the work carried out by Kartner at the University of California, San Diego, USA, it was discovered that only a small part of the avian telencephalon corresponds to the striatum in mammals (subcortical structure) while the remaining regions of the telencephalon correspond to the cortex of mammals. The main difference stands in the different neuronal organisation of the avian neocortex which is structured with nuclei. Thanks to the psychobiological and immunohistochemical work carried out, it has been possible to show that the nucleoneostriatum caudolaterale (NCL) is the same as the mammalian prefrontal cortex (PFC) given its dense dopaminergic innervation, its associated structures and its importance for cognitive tasks (Hartmann & Güntürkün, 1998). Another peculiar feature of avian neurones, compared with those of mammals, is the ability to multiply during the bird's life span. The mammalian brain produces new neurones only when it is growing before birth and for a short time after birth but after this stage of growth it is no longer able to make new neurones, nor is it able to repair lesions of the cerebral tissues (Rogers, 1997). Nobody really knows why birds maintain this ability to generate and regenerate neurones but following the discovery of Fernando Nottebohm (1989) at the Rockfeller University, USA, that the dimensions of the nuclei that control singing behaviour increased in song birds while they were busy defending their territory and singing in spring, Nottebohm came up with an intriguing theory that might explain this peculiarity of the avian brain. The cerebral tissue is relatively heavy and a heavy head would render the body mass of the bird less aerodynamic and less centralised, making flight and manoeuvrability in the air difficult. For this reason, Nottebohm suggested that birds might alter the size of different parts of the brain at different times of the year, as required.

Cognitive abilities of raptors

People do not usually consider birds as intelligent animals and expressions such as 'bird brain', which are to be found in numerous European languages, are a proof of this. There are, however, some birds which are considered to be more intelligent than others. Amongst these are parrots and corvids, thanks to the great deal of research carried out from the 1960s onwards on the cognitive abilities of these animals (Krebs *et al.*, 1996; Pepperberg, 1998; Clayton & Lee, 1999; Heinrich, 1999). Other groups of birds such as galliforms and homing-pigeons are also gaining in the animal intelligence charts as a result of the work of European and Australian researchers (Vallortigara *et al.*, 1990, 1998, 2000; Rogers, 1997; Bingman *et al.*, 1998). However, very few studies on the cognitive abilities of raptors have been carried out. Much detailed research has been performed on the sight and hearing of these birds (see above) but, perhaps on account of their apparently proud and reserved nature, they have not been considered worthy of study from an intellectual point of view. On the other hand, people who work with raptors, such as avian veterinarians, rehabilitors and falconers, know that these animals are able to adapt very quickly to new environmental conditions and critical situations, suggesting great cognitive abilities which still have to be studied from a scientific point of view.

STRENGTH AND PAIN, SOLITUDE AND FEAR

The proud, noble bearing, the infrequent vocalisations and the remarkable physical strength of birds of prey have led veterinarians to underestimate these animals' capacity to feel pain. While frequent reference is made in companion animal medicine to 'pain therapy', in avian medicine sporadic use is made of pain-killers only during surgery, and post-operative pain is rarely taken into account (see Chapter 12). There is a need for pain therapy procedures for birds of prey, especially in wildlife rescue centres which usually deal with animals presenting with serious and painful lesions (such as electrocutions). The adoption of these procedures would constitute a step forward in animal welfare and lead to a rise in the percentage of animals recovered and released into the wild.

No veterinarian with any experience in avian medicine would keep a parrot undergoing therapy in a stimulus-poor environment. It is widely known that for some groups of birds 'behavioural therapy' is just as important as pharmacological therapy. Birds of prey, however, are considered to be 'strong' animals and as such relatively unsocial compared with other species of birds. This means that during hospitalisation they are often kept in stimulus-poor conditions – even in the dark inside cardboard boxes. The most frequent explanation for this type of treatment is that it places them under less stress and that they do not damage their feathers. But birds of prey have no less need of proper behavioural therapy than do other species (see Chapter 13). Although they are less behaviourally social and in this respect more resilient than are psittacine species, the appropriate behavioural approach for these birds needs to be decided on a case-by-case basis. The raptor may be young or adult – needing to be accustomed to humans or requiring imprinting on co-specific models before being released – or it may be a bird kept for falconry, accustomed to close contact with humans, and so on.

In all probability the methodological differences between human medicine and those used with birds of prey are, as suggested by Virchow at the beginning of the chapter, in this respect very slight.

ACKNOWLEDGEMENTS

I would like to thank Prof. J. E. Cooper (D.I.C.E., United Kingdom), Prof. G. Vallortigara (University of Trieste, Italy), Professors G. Kaplan and L. Rogers (University of New England, Australia), Mr Mike Patchett (Trieste, Italy) and Dr Mauro Delogu (Istituto Nazionale per la Fauna Selvatica, Italy) for their suggestions and the bibliography they supplied.

Methods of Investigation and Treatment

'*Declare the past, diagnose the present, foretell the future.*'

Hippocrates

INTRODUCTION

The investigation of raptors can be divided into three main categories:

(1) Clinical work – observation, examination, aids to clinical investigation and laboratory-based tests on live birds.
(2) *Post-mortem* work – macroscopical (gross) examination and laboratory-based tests on dead birds.
(3) Environmental studies – the aviary or enclosure of captive birds, the ecosystem of free-living birds (see Appendix VII).

These each play a part in the detection and identification of diseases and also in *health monitoring* – where the emphasis is not on the diagnosis of disease but on assessing the health status of a bird or group of birds (see Appendix VII). Preventive medicine is discussed in more detail later.

Free-living birds of prey were not covered in any detail in earlier editions of this book although some mention was made where the distinction between free-living and captive birds was not clear-cut (Cooper, 1969b). For example, at a certain stage, raptor casualties ('free-living' birds) become 'captive' – even if they remain so for only a short time. Similarly, some 'captive' birds may be destined for release into the wild – for instance, as part of a reintroduction programme. One cannot therefore easily separate work with captive birds from that with their wild (free-living) counterparts and this is illustrated well in the chapter on pathology in the *Raptor Management Techniques Manual* (Pendleton *et al.*, 1987) where the approach is to birds of prey in general, not just those that are free-living.

The artificiality of differentiating raptors too strictly into categories is further emphasised by the often overlooked point that a falconer's hawk that is being flown is exposed to many of the same hazards as is a free-living bird and also that captive birds may be fed on diets or kept in enclosures that permit the introduction of pathogens from the 'wild'.

The legal situation relating to diagnosis and treatment is also important. In some countries, such as Britain, it is illegal for an unqualified person (i.e. a non-veterinarian) to diagnose or to treat disease in certain animals including birds. This applies whether they are captive or free-living (Cooper, M. E., 1987). In other parts of the world this may not be the case. Similarly, the extent to which availability of certain medicines is restricted to veterinarians varies from country to country.

Even in countries with strict legislation there is usually no objection to emergency or first aid treatment being offered by an unqualified person. Treatment of a bird by its owner is also usually permitted but may lay such an individual open to prosecution under welfare legislation if unnecessary suffering is thereby caused. These and other legal considerations are covered by Margaret Cooper in Appendix XI. As a general rule, those who keep birds of prey in captivity or have to deal with diseases of raptors in the wild should consult a veterinary surgeon (veterinarian). He or she may have limited experience of birds but is likely to have ready access to the medicines, equipment and expertise that are likely to be needed to make an accurate diagnosis and to initiate treatment or control measures. Many local practitioners will develop an interest in the subject and a valuable relationship can ensue between veterinarian and keeper/biologist (Cooper, 1993a). Difficult cases may need to be referred to someone who is particularly experienced in avian medicine, increasing numbers of whom have recognised specialist status – for example, in zoological medicine (UK), avian medicine and surgery (Europe) or avian practice (USA).

Veterinarians in most countries are bound by codes of professional conduct. Thus, for example, if one vet is already dealing with a case, it should not be examined or treated by another without his/her (the first veterinary surgeon's) knowledge and agreement. Such rules may appear tiresome but in the long run they benefit the bird and the client – for example, by reducing the need for investigations to be unnecessarily repeated and by avoiding potentially dangerous interaction of drugs.

Nowadays it is standard for a client to be asked to sign consent forms before examination and treatment of his/her animal. This may also authorise the giving of an anaesthetic and surgical procedures but in no way reduces the professional responsibilities of the veterinary surgeon.

CLINICAL INVESTIGATION

This section covers the investigation of a sick bird of prey with a view to making a diagnosis. The examination of an apparently healthy bird for monitoring purposes follows similar lines but is not discussed in detail here (Appendix VII provides more detail).

Clinical diagnosis is a systematic process involving acumen, as well as method, and the carrying out of supporting tests. The basic steps are depicted in Fig. 4.1.

The timing of the various investigative procedures will depend upon a number of factors, not least of all the physical state of the bird and whether it is captive, relatively accustomed to contact with humans, or free-living and therefore particularly susceptible to stressors. The sequence of events, with comments on timing, is given in Fig. 4.2.

History

The first step in clinical investigation, often long before a live bird is examined, is to obtain as much history as possible. Often this poses few problems but sometimes little is available – perhaps because the bird is a wild 'casualty' or because the owner/keeper is reluctant to divulge information.

Information on history must be recorded, either written down or entered on a computer. An example of a fairly basic examination form that includes spaces for history and other background information is given in Appendix II. Some people prefer to have a 'check-list' of data (for example, length of time in captivity, previous diseases etc.) and to work through this rather than to compile their own history.

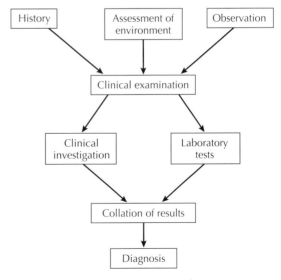

Fig. 4.1 Clinical investigation – principles.

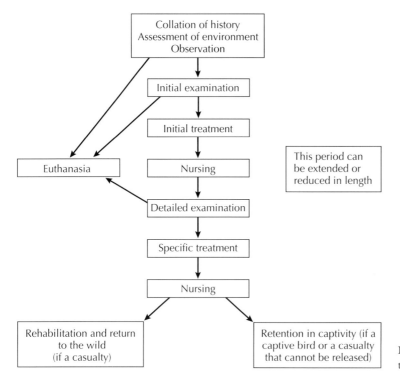

Fig. 4.2 Clinical investigation – timing.

A questionnaire has much to commend it, especially as the owner or finder (if a wild bird) can complete this prior to presentation of the bird, thus saving valuable time. Beynon *et al.* (1996) demonstrated an 'Avian History Form' that is excellent for the purpose. It is useful to ask the owner of the bird to bring a copy of the bird's records. These can be appended to the clinical examination sheet.

As in other branches of veterinary work, regular observation and examination of a captive bird by the owner is very important; some conditions, for example foot lesions, may thus be diagnosed early. Owners and keepers should be encouraged to keep records of such findings.

A full assessment of a captive bird's environment is not easy without visiting the premises from which it came. In the absence of this, data on, for example, size and structure of aviaries, must be sought from the owner. Photos and drawings are of some help. Ecologists can usually provide information about the environment from which a free-living bird originated, sometimes together with samples of, for example, nesting material, soil or water.

Although it is generally true that all raptor patients should receive a full clinical investigation regardless of history or presenting clinical signs, special techniques are often needed or certain procedures bypassed – for instance, when a neurological disorder is suspected (see Chapter 9). The following text refers to general examination.

In the first instance, the bird should be *observed* from a distance, preferably without the observer being seen. This enables an assessment to be made of the bird's general condition, respiration rate and obvious clinical signs of disease before it is unduly disturbed – after which clinical signs may be masked or changed. In the case of captive raptors in breeding condition, especially in 'skylight and seclusion aviaries', further disturbance is often not possible and a provisional diagnosis may have to be made on such an examination alone, coupled with whatever information may be available on food consumption

Table 4.1 Facilities for examination and investigation of birds of prey.

Procedure	Essential requirements	Useful additions	Special precautions	Comments
Clinical examination	Examination table Protective clothing Balance or scales Syringes, needles, bottles, swabs and other equipment for collecting and storing specimens Disinfectants. Handling equipment. Stethoscope	Darkened room Surgical facilities Anaesthetic machine X-ray machine Refrigerator. Hand lens/magnifying loupe Endoscope(s) and light source	Adequate disinfection and ventilation Escape-proof, clean accommodation	Under field conditions clinical sampling is best carried out placing bird on a rubber or plastic sheet. Instruments can be transported on a tray or in closed containers. See Forbes (2000) regarding practice facilities for raptor work
Gross *post-mortem* examination	PM table Instruments Protective clothing Incinerator, macerator, or other means of disposal Disinfectants. Steriliser or autoclave. Bottles for storing specimens. Fixatives	Refrigerator Freezer Balance or scales Protective hood Isolation cabinet X-ray machine. Hand lens/ magnifying loupe or table lamp with magnifier. Measuring equipment – vernier scale calliper and/or ruler with end stop	Adequate drainage, disinfection, and ventilation Escape-proof accommodation	Under field conditions it may be preferable to perform necropsies in the open air, taking hygienic precautions, rather than in a poorly ventilated building
Bacteriology	Laboratory bench Incubator, autoclave Media – solid and liquid Anaerobic and micro-aerophilic atmosphere generators. Sterile swabs and pipettes. Refrigerator Burner – Bunsen or gas Loops – platinum or disposable. Glass slides and cover slips. Simple stains. Light microscope	Anaerobic jar Specialised media Biochemical reagents and/or API system Antimicrobial testing facilities, e.g. disc diffusion, automated systems, E test Laminar flow cabinet	Adequate disinfection and facilities for disposing of cultures	Simple aerobic culture is frequently adequate for initial investigations. Cultures can be forwarded elsewhere for more investigation. Animal inoculation studies may be necessary. These must be carefully planned and every attention paid to the welfare of the animals used and relevant legal controls
Mycology	Same as Bacteriology, but use special media, e.g. Sabouraud's	Ultraviolet light source	See Bacteriology	See Bacteriology
Mycoplasmology	Same as Bacteriology, but use special media		See Bacteriology	See Bacteriology
Isolation of *Chlamydia* (now called *Chlamydophila*)	Same as Bacteriology, but also tissue culture and egg inoculation	Fluorescent antibody techniques PCR	Protective clothing and adequate containment are essential	*Chlamydia* isolation should only be carried out by specialised laboratories
Virology	Laboratory bench Incubator, autoclave Tissue culture Experimental animals	Fluorescent antibody PCR and other techniques Electron microscopy facilities	See *Chlamydia*	See *Chlamydia*
Serology	Various, according to technique used. Simple haemagglutination tests require only serum, antigen, red cells, diluent, and plates	Serum neutralisation tests. Precipitation tests Complement fixation ELISA. Combi tests	Same as Bacteriology and isolation of *Chlamydia*	See *Chlamydia*
Parasitology	Laboratory bench. Hand lens. Low-power microscope. Specimen bottles. Dissection kit Alcohol and formalin Simple stains	McMaster slides Flotation solutions Centrifuge	Adequate disinfection	Adequate parasitological examination can usually be performed with a minimum of equipment. A limited amount of work is possible in the field but laboratory facilities are preferable

Table 4.1 Continued.

Procedure	Essential requirements	Useful additions	Special precautions	Comments
Histology	Laboratory bench. Tissue processing and embedding equipment. Tissue sectioning and staining equipment. Glass slides, cover slips and mounting medium	Cryostat for preparing frozen sections	Adequate ventilation and precautions to prevent fire, explosion, or exposure to hazardous chemicals	Preparations of histological sections can prove an expensive task and small laboratories may find it preferable to forward samples elsewhere for processing
Cytology	Laboratory bench Centrifuge. Slides, methanol. Rapid stains Giemsa (± May and Grunwald). Syringe and needles for aspiration	Papanicolaou and other stains	Adequate disinfection	Preparation of smears – as for haematology. Centrifugation of cell suspensions to concentrate may be necessary
Haematology	Laboratory bench Centrifuge. Capillary tubes Diluents, haemocytometers and counting chambers Glass slides. Methanol Giemsa or other stains	Haemoglobinometer Coulter counter ESR stand	Adequate disinfection	Simple techniques, such as measurement of haematocrit (PCV) and preparation of smears can easily be performed in the field
Clinical chemistry	Laboratory bench Refractometer Automated analyser Centrifuge	Photospectrometer Commercial kits	Adequate disinfection and care when handling chemical reagents	A few simple techniques, such as estimation of plasma or serum protein can be carried out in the field, but the majority require specialised and expensive laboratory facilities. The latter can, however, deal with small quantities
Electronmicroscopy (transmission and/or scanning – TEM/SEM)	Laboratory bench Transmission and/or scanning electron-microscope Ultramicrotome (for transmission): scanning requires critical point drier, and sputter coater	Diamond knives	Care when handling chemicals (e.g. resins, osmium tetroxide) and, especially, glutaraldehyde	Only suitable for fully equipped and well funded laboratories
Radiography	Low kV X-ray machine Film and processing facilities. Protective (lead-lined) gloves and aprons, thyroid protectors, glasses Radiation monitoring badges. Anaesthetic machine	Contrast media	Protective clothing is essential; lead lining of rooms may be advisable; preferable to use chemical rather than manual restraint	A valuable technique for the diagnosis and investigation of skeletal abnormalities and the detection of shot and foreign bodies. National radiation protection regulations must be observed
Chemical analysis/toxicology	Laboratory bench	Full scale analytical equipment		Of immense importance in raptor work, but best performed by specialist laboratories
Photography	Digital camera and computer. Polaroid camera and processing facilities Centimetre scale or rule	More sophisticated camera, where appropriate Camera stand Photomicrography unit. Video	Ensure that photographic equipment does not become contaminated by microorganisms or chemicals	Photographic records are of great value in pathological work and often a vital part of forensic investigations

ELISA = enzyme-linked immunosorbent assay; PCR = polymerase chain reaction.

and other activity and gleaned from, for example, laboratory tests on faeces. Interestingly, this is little different from the situation in the wild where health monitoring (sometimes disease diagnosis) may need to be attempted without handling the bird(s) (see Appendix VIII).

Many people are now emphasising the value of observation. Forbes in Beynon *et al.* (1996) recommended a check-list that could be ticked, of such criteria as 'activity', 'perching', 'tail bobbing' and at Massey University, New Zealand, a standard 'Distant Inspection' form is used for all avian work (Lee, 2000). The use of closed-circuit television, or a video that can be viewed later, permits assessment of birds, especially when they are hospitalised.

During the period of observation various features may be noted. Some useful indicators of health (or lack of it) were given in the chapter on disease that I revised for Jack Mavrogordato's book *A Hawk for the Bush* (Cooper, 1973a). A healthy raptor stands erect, with its wings held up and the hocks (tibiotarsal joints) at a slight angle. Respiration is restricted to the upper part of the body with no sign of tail bobbing or abdominal movement. The normal respiration rate in an undisturbed bird is 10–20 per minute. A full round eye is an important sign; in a bird that is unwell, or perhaps excessively low in condition, it tends to be slightly oval (Plate 7). The colour of the feet and nares is not particularly significant – a yellowish orange colour usually indicates that day-old chicks have been fed – but *pale* coloration on such a diet may be indicative of some metabolic disturbance. Other examples of health include the use of only one leg when at rest and well formed mutes and castings (pellets) (Fig. 4.3). One must not be misled, however, into assuming that a hawk showing these and other 'healthy' signs is necessarily clinically well, since some conditions manifest themselves very subtly. Owners, particularly good falconers and experienced rehabilitators, will often spot early signs of disease; it is then up to the veterinary surgeon to perform a thorough examination.

Some of the more important clinical signs of disease are listed in Appendix V and this may serve as a useful source of information for falconers, rehabilitators and bird keepers. It is not intended to be comprehensive, however; a definitive diagnosis usually needs detailed examination and laboratory tests.

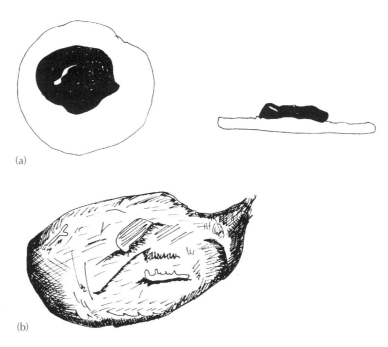

(a)

(b)

Fig. 4.3 Diagrammatic representation of (a) well-formed dropping and (b) normal pellet of a raptor. (Courtesy of Jackie Belle.)

Handling

For a full clinical examination it is necessary for a bird to be handled. In the case of a falconer's bird this poses few problems since the hawk will usually be presented on the fist and is likely to be relatively amenable to contact, especially if it is hooded. A hood prevents the bird from seeing and can also be used on birds which are not trained for falconry. The effect is often spectacular, even on a wild casualty; as a result of being hooded, the bird lies still and may permit minor procedures to be carried out. A similar, though less marked, effect can be obtained by covering the bird's head with a piece of cloth or canvas. It is also useful to carry out handling in a darkened room, using a light source for subsequent examination. The veterinary surgeon who is examining raptors regularly will find it useful to have a 'dimmer' switch to control illumination so that the intensity can be varied.

Handling a raptor in an aviary presents a bigger challenge since the first problem is how to capture it. If circumstances permit it is often best to catch diurnal birds at night, with the aid of a small torch (flashlight), and nocturnal species by day. If a raptor cannot be easily grasped and held it may be necessary to resort to a net or piece of cloth which can be thrown over it. Gloves do not need to be worn for handling birds of prey but may reassure the handler and are often helpful during the act of capturing the bird, even if subsequently discarded. Thin, but strong, industrial gloves which also cover the elbows are ideal for handling a variety of species but all gloves reduce tactile sensitivity.

Whether gloves are worn or not, it is vital to ensure that the bird's wings are held close to the body and not allowed to flap (Plate 8); uncontrolled wing movements can damage the plumage and are distressing to both bird and owner. It should be noted that it is possible to hold a bird firmly (yet gently) in such a position that one cannot be reached by either feet or beak.

Catching large raptors, such as vultures and eagle owls, is often best achieved by grasping the legs, above the feet, and immediately turning the bird upside-down. The wings will then often hang or can be drawn in with a cloth or blanket.

Handling and other procedures have been the subject of research in Britain in order to minimise damage to birds (and handlers!) during statutory inspections under the Wildlife and Countryside Act. The recommendations and specimen forms were given in the Wildlife Inspectors' Seminar Report (DETR, 1997).

Restraint can be stressful (Olsen, 1990). The effect of handling on a ferruginous hawk was investigated by Busch *et al.* (1978), who monitored the bird's heart rate under different conditions. The rate was greatly accelerated when the hawk was restrained but it is noteworthy that hooding resulted in a slowing to 51–66% of the 'maximal' rate. The body temperature may also increase: little information is available on raptors but 'stress (handling) hyperthermia' has been well documented in other species (Maloney & Gray, 1998).

Once the bird has been grasped it should be cast, on its breast, on to a soft towel or blanket. If a hawk is wearing jesses, these should be pulled backwards so that the feet are visible on either side of the tail. I often kneel on the bird's leash which in turn applies tension on the jesses and helps to extend the joints, discouraging flexion of digits. The provision of a soft cloth for the bird to grasp with its talons is often a worthwhile precaution; it helps to calm the bird and reduces the possibility of self-inflicted foot damage. Lay people tend to be wary of the beaks of raptors but it is often the feet which cause the greater damage; in small birds in particular they can be extended at great speed enabling the talons to embed in the hands. Clipping ('coping') the talons of birds received for treatment is, with the possible exception of wild casualties destined for early release, a wise precaution; it serves to protect the handler as well as the bird! Precautions to be taken when clipping talons were discussed by Redig and Ackermann (2000) and are referred to again in Chapter 8. Particular care must be taken when coping falconers' birds.

The handling and restraint of free-living birds will not be discussed here: it resembles in many respects the methods described above, with special techniques developed for, e.g. removing a bird from a net or trap (Clark, 1995). There is a valuable chapter on capturing and handling free-living raptors in the

Raptor Management Techniques Manual (Pendleton *et al.*, 1987). Methods covered under 'capture' include the bal-chatri, bownet, cannon and rocket nets; hand-capture, harnessed pigeon and (for eagles) even helicopter!

Proper examination of a bird of prey that has been cast usually requires two people since one must restrain the patient. In some cases it may be desirable to anaesthetise the bird lightly and this certainly facilitates examination as well as reducing stress for the bird (Plate 9). Alternatively, a self-adhesive wrap can be tried, as originally described by Fuller (1975). This enables one person to secure the bird and then have both hands free. It can prove particularly useful in the field when working with birds of prey that have been captured for examination or study. Fuller used a proprietary bandaging tape that can be cut to different sizes and which will adhere to itself but not to feathers, skin or vegetation.

Single-handed examination of a raptor can also be facilitated by use of an Arab device called a 'Guba' (Cooper & Al-Timimi, 1986). This consists of a cloth jacket which can be tied round the bird's body. Its use permits single-handed swabbing, cleaning of wounds and dosing. 'Restraint jackets' are now available commercially and, although primarily for psittacine birds, can be used for small raptors.

Method for examination

Each person has his/her own method of investigation and it is advisable to adhere to it. I start at the head and work down the body; paying particular attention to any asymmetry between one side and the other. Asymmetry is primarily of importance in detecting a clinical change or lesion (e.g. an eye that is partly closed, in comparison with its fellow, on account of a conjunctivitis or sinusitis) (Plate 10) but morphological asymmetry can also be a sign of inbreeding and may be of value in assessing 'condition' (Brown, 1996). Some important features of clinical examination are given.

Eyes

Examine grossly with light source and with ophthalmoscope.

Head

Palpate and assess calcification by slight (careful) digital pressure on the cranium. Check ears.

Cere and nostrils

Observe for injury, asymmetry or blockage of nares.

Beak

Examine carefully. If overgrown or damaged, difficulty in feeding may result. Examine externally and then open (artery forceps can be used) in order to inspect mucous membranes for colour, lesions, presence of parasites, etc. Most raptors have pink mucous membranes but a blue coloration is normal for a few species, such as merlins. Observe glottis for respiration rate or lesions and trachea for presence of parasites.

A finger can be inserted down the oesophagus to search for foreign bodies or lesions while the use of a small torch (flashlight) or (better) a fibre-optic light will facilitate examination of the trachea. Check tongue for lesions (especially sub-lingual) and for material twisted around base.

Neck

Palpate externally and auscultate trachea and interclavicular air sac with stethoscope. Particularly check crop for evidence of food or air. Use transillumination in smaller birds (see later).

Body

Palpate. The sharpness of the 'keel' (sternum) is an aid to assessment of 'condition' (see later). Use a scoring system to grade this. Disparity in the size of the pectoral muscles can be indicative of muscle atrophy of one side (for example, wing injury) or inflammation (for example, irritant injection) of the area. The keel and overlying skin may have been damaged in a recently imported bird or in one that has been recumbent. Bent keels occasionally occur, sometimes as a result of bone disease.

Auscultate heart in interclavicular space and lungs and air sacs along dorsal and lateral aspects of body.

Gently palpate abdomen for evidence of body fat, food in stomach or space-occupying lesion.

Examine uropygial (preen) gland at base of tail; ensure it is normal in appearance and that the feathers around the external orifice are slightly oily.

Check for (count and collect) ectoparasites.

Palpate cloaca externally but also use lubricated gloved finger to examine interior for calculi, blood or other pathological signs. In addition the cloaca may be examined with a speculum, auroscope or endoscope.

Wings and legs

Palpate all bones and all joints; where possible compare with corresponding member on other side. Assess muscle tone and relative size of muscle masses. Flex and extend joints – feel and listen. Check for areas of feather loss, swelling or deformity. Assess the moult.

Examine legs and feet carefully for lesions; pay particular attention to the plantar surfaces of the feet. Check how sharp are the talons and whether they are damaged: do they show any changes that might assist in ageing (Wyllie, undated)?

Tail

Examine and count feathers, note presence of 'hunger traces' or other feather lesions (consider using transillumination).

The clinical examination of casualty birds prior to release presents legal as well as practical (clinical) challenges (see Appendix XI): some criteria for assessing the health of such birds were given by Cooper *et al.* (1980).

Observations and clinical signs that may assist in diagnosing disease in a raptor patient are listed in Appendix V. The difficulty of accurate diagnosis of internal disease in birds was recognised long ago, as illustrated by the section in the *Boke of St Albans* referring to 'a medicine for a sickness within the body of a hawk' (Fig. 4.4). Modern aids to diagnosis, such as endoscopy, have revolutionised such work in recent years.

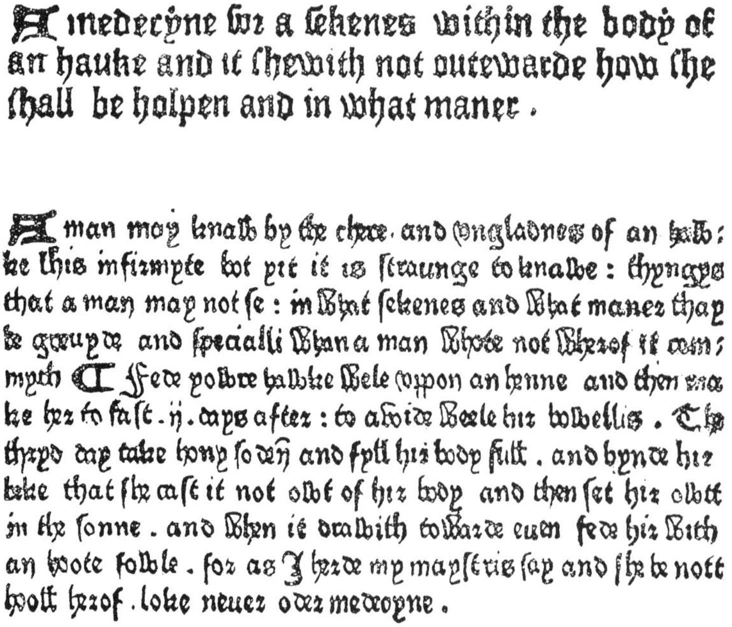
A medecyne for a sekenes within the body of an hauke and it shewith not outewarde how she shall be holpen and in what maner.

A man may knaw by the chere and ungladnes of an hauk: be this infirmyte but yet it is straunge to knawe: thynges that a man may not se: in what sekenes and what maner thay be greved and specialli whan a man whote not wherof it comyth ¶ Fede yowre hawke wele uppon an henne and then make her to fast .ij. days after: to avoide wele hir bowellis. ¶ The thyrd day take hony soden and fyll hir body full. and bynde hir beke that she cast it not owt of hir body and then set hir owt in the sonne. and when it drawith towarde euen fede hir with an hote fowle. for as I herde my maystris say and she be nott hoolt herof. loke neuer oder medecyne.

Fig. 4.4 Internal disorders of hawks were recognised by the early falconers but were generally not differentiated. Here, in the *Boke of St Albans* (1486), a treatment is advocated for 'sickness within the Brashy(??)'.

Weighing and measuring

At some stage of the clinical examination the bird should be weighed. Falconers usually know the weight of their hawk but it is wise to check it; the bird can be made to step on to suitably padded or modified (perch) scales and allowance must be made for the weight of jesses, bells and other equipment. Birds which will not stand on the scales, even if hooded or in subdued light, must be weighed following casting. It may be possible to lay them on the scales for a few seconds, failing which they should be weighed in a cloth bag. Spring balances are ideal for weighing birds that are either free-living or unaccustomed to handling. Electronic balances that use small batteries are available commercially.

Raptors should also be measured – a carpal and possibly other measurements. This and other aspects of morphometrics are overlooked by most veterinarians. It contributes to a better assessment of body 'condition': although defining and measuring this concept are far from easy (Brown, 1996).

Wing injuries (minor)

When searching for *minor* wing injuries, a bird can be held up for a few seconds by its feet; comparison of the positions of the wings will help to reveal any weakness or abnormality. Such a technique should only be used after the legs have been checked and if the bird is not shocked or in low condition.

Heart and lungs

The stethoscope plays an important part in clinical examination – auscultation of heart, lungs, air sacs, gastro-intestinal tract and joints – but some experience is needed of its use with avian patients.

In the case of a falconer's bird with clinical signs suggestive of respiratory disease, examination can resemble that for soundness in a horse in that it is advisable to examine the bird at rest and then following a short flight of about 10–15 m to the fist or lure.

The respiration rate of raptors below 2000 g in weight is usually between 15 and 30 breaths per minute although in very small species, such as merlins, it may reach 50. Larger birds, such as vultures, usually respire 10–15 times per minute. There is, however, often much variation.

Although the stethoscope can be used to monitor heart rate, the latter is likely to increase as a result of examination. In my experience it is almost impossible to count the beats accurately but some colleagues use a pulse oximeter and report good results. Approximate figures for falcons are 200–350 beats per minute.

Heart rate increases significantly during handling. Data on 'normal' heart rate in a captive red-tailed hawk were given by Busch *et al.* (1984): it is surprising that so few other studies have been reported.

AIDS TO CLINICAL INVESTIGATION

In addition to the above standard clinical examination, a number of aids are available. The stethoscope has been mentioned. Other techniques range from the passing of a piece of tubing down the oesophagus or the oral administration of carmine powder (to assess patency and gut transit time) to the use of a clinical thermometer, electrocardiography, ophthalmoscopy and imaging such as radiography or ultrasonography. Most of these examples are discussed elsewhere in the book and attention will be drawn to the role of modern techniques in raptor work.

Transillumination, whereby a strong light is shone through the tissues is not a modern technique but is often overlooked. It was probably first advocated and used by Professor Peer Zwart in Utrecht, The Netherlands. I find it of great value, especially when working in environments where I do not have access to sophisticated equipment as well as when examining raptors in 'developed' countries.

The candling of eggs is a form of transillumination (see Chapter 13).

I do not regularly use a clinical thermometer, except in legal cases and where a bird is suffering from hypothermia, but temperature measurements are advocated by some colleagues as a routine part of examination. The metabolic rate (and hence body temperature) of raptors is inversely proportional to size, and figures for cloacal temperature range from 39.5°C for many of the larger vultures to 41°C for the Eurasian kestrel. However, in my experience, there are variations within a species and even individual birds may give different figures on different occasions. A drop in body temperature at night is a recognised physiological feature of certain owls (Irving, 1955). There is need for more work on the body temperature of birds of prey and its response to disease, physical injury and restraint, as well as on the development of thermoregulation on the young bird.

Radiography

Radiography plays an important part in raptor diagnostic work (Cooper & Kreel, 1976; Harcourt-Brown, 1996a) and also in some aspects of health monitoring of live or dead birds.

Whilst it should be used primarily to confirm or elucidate a diagnosis, radiography frequently has to be employed as a diagnostic tool *per se* (Krautwald & Trinkhaus, 2000). It will help to diagnose fractures, dislocations, foreign bodies and respiratory conditions; it will also reveal lead shot and non-palpable soft tissue lesions and give valuable information on the severity of tissue damage in bumblefoot or joint infections. Contrast media (usually barium preparations) are helpful (Krautwald & Trinkhaus, 2000) and were originally used experimentally – for example, in studies on pellet formation in owls (Grimm & Whitehouse, 1963). The introduction of air plus a small quantity of barium will greatly facilitate examination of the crop and cloaca.

Redig and Ackermann (2000) advocated radiography in all trauma and many medical cases. They urged that both ventro-dorsal and lateral views are taken, the latter with the right side against the cassette, head to the left. I would add to this that limbs should usually be extended, to avoid overlapping of bones. Correct positioning is a key part of good, reliable, technique.

If a raptor is hooded it may be possible to perform limited radiography without further restraint. However, because health and safety regulations increasingly preclude manual restraint, light anaesthesia or sedation is needed (Krautwald & Trinkhaus, 2000).

Most types of X-ray (radiography) machine can be used for avian work although those with a fine focus will give the best results. However, there are many variables, depending upon age, model and design, and the veterinary surgeon who anticipates dealing with birds of prey is advised to try a few test exposures, using a dead bird (a pigeon, if a raptor is not available) before his/her first case arrives on the doorstep.

Good detail is essential for avian radiology and this can be achieved by the use of non-screen film or cassettes that are fitted with detail intensifying screens. For very small areas and for use in the investigation of *post-mortem* material industrial X-ray film is of value, and cassettes designed for mammography (in human patients) provide very fine detail.

Certain features of normal anatomy must be borne in mind when interpreting radiographs of birds, whether alive or dead (Rübel *et al.*, 1991). Thus, for example, bones are frequently seen in the crop and gizzard of raptors, in contrast to poultry and many other non-carnivorous species the gizzards of which contain stones – which should not be confused with foreign bodies! Likewise, urates are radio-opaque and will be visible; in some cases they can hamper interpretation (Fig. 4.5).

Radiography will reveal some conditions that may not be detected during clinical examination – for example, fractures of the coracoid, foreign bodies and soft tissue changes. The radiographical examination of various organs of birds – liver, spleen, heart, urogenital system – was discussed succinctly by Krautwald and Trinkhaus (2000).

For the investigation of respiratory lesions, the lungs are best demonstrated in a lateral view, with the wings folded back above the bird's body. However, for examination of the air sacs the ventro-dorsal view often provides more information because comparisons of the two sides of the patient can be made. Careful positioning is always impor-

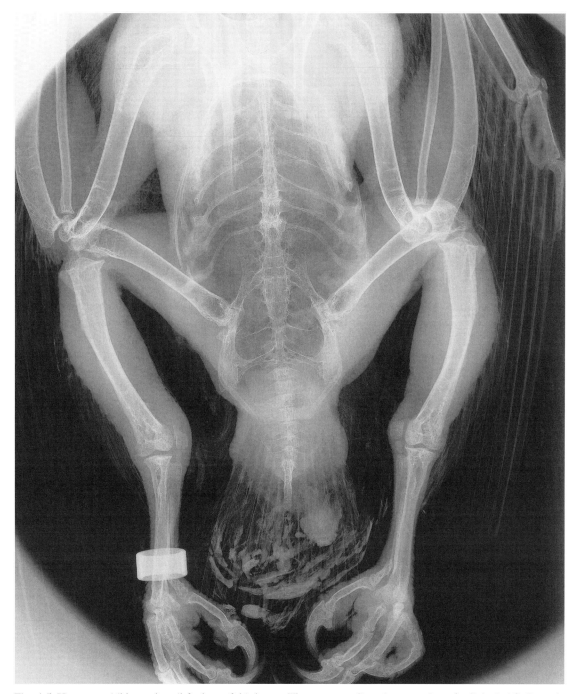

Fig. 4.5 Urates are visible on the tail feathers of this lanner. They can complicate interpretation of radiological findings. A closed ring is also present on the (bird's) right leg. This is a *post-mortem* case and illustrates the value of radiography prior to necropsy. The bird shows evidence of metabolic bone disease.

tant and ideally the radiographs should be taken on inspiration when structures will be most easy to assess.

Prior to *post-mortem* examination a routine whole body radiograph is a valuable diagnostic aid (see later). Not only will this demonstrate major skeletal injuries but it may also help to detect soft tissue lesions and lead shot before the carcass is opened. The usual hurdle is the cost of the examination.

Endoscopy

Various other aids to clinical examination have become almost routine in avian practice in recent years. Endoscopy is an example: rigid endoscopes (e.g. human arthroscopes) can be used to examine the oesophagus, trachea, cloaca and (via a laparoscopy incision) internal organs (Bush, 1981; Böttcher, 1982). Flexible instruments facilitate the examination of alimentary, respiratory and reproductive tracts. Both they and rigid endoscopes permit the taking of biopsies, washings and scrapings. Even if fibre-optic instruments are not available useful results can be obtained, especially of the upper alimentary tract, using an auroscope or the battery-operated 'Focuscope' (Medical Diagnostic Services, USA).

Other imaging techniques

A variety of imaging techniques apart from radiography can be employed. Ultrasonography is a well recognised example (Heidenreich, 1997: Krautwald & Trinkhaus, 2000) and can be particularly useful in diagnosing soft tissue lesions.

Several years ago Furley and Greenwood (1982) described computerised axial tomography (CAT or CT) in birds of prey in the Middle East: using such scanning they were able to demonstrate lesions of aspergillosis. More recently Krautwald-Junghanns *et al.* (1998) reported comparative studies on conventional radiography and CT in evaluating the heads of raptors. Magnetic resonance imaging (MRI) is increasingly being used: in Britain, centres exist where MRI is available and to which cases can be sent.

Assessing body condition

Measurements of body composition can be used to assess 'condition' and also to study, e.g. changes in fat and muscle. Total body electrical conductivity (TOBEC) is a non-invasive method that has proved valuable in studies on raptors (Samour, 2000a; Yamamoto & Santolo, 2000). A valuable review of 'condition' and the various methods of assessing it was given by Brown (1996).

Clinical samples

General information about samples and their value in raptor work is given later (see 'Sampling').

The taking of samples (specimens) for laboratory investigation is an important part of clinical examination. In view of the difficulties inherent in handling a raptor and the stress that prolonged restraint may cause the bird, it is important to ensure that collecting equipment is available *before* the bird is cast.

There is some debate as to which samples and laboratory tests are most important in the initial evaluation of a bird of prey. Redig and Ackermann (2000) listed a 'four-element minimum database' consisting of a total blood count, microbiological evaluation and a parasite examination – together with radiology. My approach, strongly influenced by my involvement in projects overseas where finances and facilities are limited, is to condense this to (a) basic haematology – PCV (packed cell volume) and smears, (b) direct examination and microbiology of buccal and faecal samples.

A variety of other samples may need to be taken, depending upon clinical indications and facilities available. Light anaesthesia is often wise, using isoflurane or sevoflurane if available.

Feathers can be plucked; if primaries or secondaries are to be taken, the bird should be lightly anaesthetised. Removal of feathers may be necessary in order to investigate plumage abnormalities, to search for parasites or to analyse for heavy metals, such as mercury (Berg *et al.*, 1966). Biopsies of skin or feather follicles may be required in some cases.

Skin scrapings can be taken from raptors although

it should be noted that a bird's skin is thin and easily damaged: the application and removal of sticky tape may yield satisfactory results.

Swabs for sampling external lesions should be moistened beforehand in sterile saline and then rolled on the lesion or used to touch a specific lesion. Swabs of pharynx, trachea and cloaca can be taken relatively simply; it is wise to use narrow (human nasopharyngeal) swabs and again they should be moistened.

Biopsies can play an important part in diagnosis and are discussed later in Chapters 6, 8 and 12, as well as in the review by Cooper (1994); small samples can be readily taken from liver, kidney and certain other internal organs as well as skin or feathers. Redig (1977) first advocated biopsy of the lung in respiratory cases, using a 25 gauge needle and 10 ml glass syringe. The needle is thrust through the penultimate intercostal space to a depth of up to two-thirds of the distance to the midline. The material thus obtained is sprayed on to a slide, stained and examined microscopically.

The droppings of a bird can provide valuable information (Lawton, 2000). A bird of prey defaecates and urinates regularly and will often do so when first handled: owls in particular tend to produce large quantities when cast. A 'mute' (faecal/urate) sample can also be removed from the cloaca – and is likely to be voided following a cloacal examination. It is less traumatic for the bird (and often the handler!) if a freshly voided specimen is collected – for example on paper below the perch. It is, of course, the dark portion that is usually required for faecal examination. Ideally two days' pooled samples should be taken and examination for parasites repeated after 7–10 days. When submitting faecal samples for sexing (see Chapter 13) or polymerase chain reaction (PCR) the material should be deep frozen.

Castings (pellets) will not usually be produced during clinical examination; the owner should be asked to bring a fresh (preferably still damp) specimen. 'Normal' droppings and a pellet are shown in Plate 11 and Fig. 4.3. Blaine (1936), the observant and meticulous falconer, provided a useful description of the former:

'Perfect mutes should be pure white of the consistency of thin cream, with a few small lumps of black in the centre.'

Changes in appearance of droppings may be indicative of disease but can also be normal. Thus, for example, green faecal portions occur when a bird has fasted while a tan colour may be associated with feeding day-old chicks (see Appendix V). Castings can also vary in size, colour, appearance and smell. They can be used to provide information about the bird's diet and upper alimentary tract health. Examination of castings (pellets) can be based on methods used by naturalists (Knight, 1968), coupled with routine laboratory investigations.

Samples from buccal cavity, crop, oesophagus, trachea or cloaca may comprise swabs, washings (Brearley *et al.*, 1991), touch preparations, scrapings or biopsies. Deeper samples will usually yield more valuable information than will superficial ones.

Blood samples for haematology, clinical chemistry and other tests are usually best taken from the basilic (brachial) vein, with the bird cast on its back. The vein lies just distal to the elbow joint and is easily exposed if a few feathers are plucked and the area dampened with ethanol or methanol. The vein is best raised by applying pressure on the lateral aspect of the humerus. For small birds (500 g in weight or less) a 25 gauge needle and 1 ml (tuberculin) syringe should be used, though the use of a 'butterfly' attachment will lessen the chance of the needle coming out of the vein when the bird moves. Alternatively, the jugular vein can be used and this appears less likely to result in haematoma formation. Lumeij (1996) recommended taking no more than 1% of a bird's bodyweight for diagnostic purposes: my figure for regular weekly sampling is a maximum of 7 ml/kg bodyweight.

Dresser *et al.* (1999) studied the effects of repeated blood sampling and isoflurane anaesthesia on haematological and biochemical values of American kestrels. They concluded that the combined effect of isoflurane and repeat blood sampling causes more dramatic changes than bleeding alone. Both the method and frequency of blood sampling must be considered when interpreting blood values.

If a bird has to be euthanased, blood can be taken

from the heart – following the same technique as for domestic fowl.

Cutting one or more talons of a bird short may also yield enough blood for PCV and certain other tests, but as a general rule this method should be avoided since not only is it probably painful but it may permit infection to enter the foot and some estimations, such as uric acid, can be adversely influenced by contamination.

For blood smears, only small samples are required, in which case a vein can be pricked (or, if really necessary, one talon cut slightly short, as already mentioned). The method used should be recorded since it can influence results.

Aspiration of fluid (exudate or transudate) or 'pus' (Huchzermeyer & Cooper, 2000) should be preceded by thorough cleansing of the overlying skin. Surgical spirit or a proprietary disinfectant can be used but the latter may persist and destroy organisms on the swab. For foot lesions I usually scrub the area with soap and water, rinse with warm water and dry before inserting a 23 or 25 gauge needle and attempting to aspirate material. Swabs for bacteriology should either be cultured within 6 hours or stored in Stuart's Transport Medium while those for mycoplasmology should be placed immediately in liquid medium.

Table 4.2 provides a breakdown of specimens that may be taken from raptors and lists the site, equipment required and methods of transportation or storage. Adherence to a properly planned protocol helps to ensure consistency and adds credence to results.

Health monitoring and screening

Health monitoring of birds of prey is important and is applicable to both captive and free-living raptors. It provides information on the health status of birds that may appear clinically to be free of disease.

Health monitoring should be a regular procedure in all establishments where birds of prey are maintained in captivity in numbers, particularly if several birds share an aviary or enclosure. It is also the essence of the 'new bird check' and annual 'well bird check' advocated by (amongst others) Forbes (2000).

Health monitoring is also increasingly being recognised as a useful, often essential, prerequisite when raptors are being translocated, especially as a part of introduction or reintroduction programmes. Protocols for monitoring have been developed and these are gaining international acceptance with the encouragement of the IUCN/SSC (International Union for the Conservation of Nature/ Survival Service Commission) Veterinary and Reintroductions Specialist Groups. Lierz and Launay (2000) described procedures for assessing the health of falcons prior to their return to the wild in Arabia and these included a whole range of clinical investigations as well as laboratory analyses and 'stress tests'.

The full protocols for monitoring live birds usually require capture, handling and manipulation. This presents few problems when, for example, capturing and ringing (banding) migrants (Clark, 1995) but under other circumstances is sometimes not practicable nor politically/culturally acceptable, especially when dealing with threatened or endangered species. Even radio-tagging has come under scrutiny (see, for example, Marzluff *et al.*, 1997) and yet this is usually considered a routine technique in raptor biology that can also contribute usefully to health monitoring.

Less invasive techniques of health monitoring are available and others could readily be developed, preferably using captive birds in the first instance. In Appendix VIII non-invasive or minimally invasive techniques are described and their increased use, on an international basis, is strongly advocated. They include the investigation of, for example, faeces, pellets and dropped feathers, and taking full advantage of the information that can be obtained from a rigorous and detailed *post-mortem* examination.

Geographical information systems (GISs) can be used in health studies on free-living birds (Bright, 2000): GISs provide a tool for identifying changes in land usage and for investigating and predicting disease outbreaks. Combined with radio and satellite telemetry, they have great potential.

As mentioned earlier, the taking of samples – whether from live birds, dead birds or the environment – must be carried out proficiently if results are

Table 4.2 Sample collection from raptors.

Specimen	Site	Equipment required	Method of transportation or storage
Blood	Basilic (brachial), tarsal or jugular vein	Syringe, 20–25 gauge needles, bottles, cottonwool, slides and methanol	Bottle containing appropriate anticoagulant, chilled at +4°C. Slides fixed in 100% methanol and/or air-dried.
Serum	See above	See above	Bottle without anticoagulant, usually frozen (but depends upon assay).
Skin biopsy	Body surface	Surgical instruments, general and/or local anaesthetic, skin biopsy punch	In 10% buffered formalin for histopathology, glutaraldehyde for electronmicroscopy. Chilled for other procedures.
Muscle biopsy	Pectoral or leg muscles	See above	As above. Fix at $1\frac{1}{2}$ times length *in vivo* using pins/needles on cork. Snap frozen in liquid nitrogen/isopentane for histochemistry
Liver, kidney, or other internal biopsy	Via laparotomy or laparoscopy incision	Same as above, plus laparoscope and biopsy needle. Ultrasound for guiding endoscope.	See above
Swabs for microbiological examination	Cloacal/buccal cavity or elsewhere	Swabs of different sizes Instruments Alcohol	Transport medium, e.g. Stuart's, chilled
Material for parasitological examination	Buccal cavity or cloaca (or via endoscopy for other sites)	Swabs moistened in sterile saline Transport medium (e.g. for trichomonads)	Ethanol/methanol or methylated spirits Warm saline – rapid transportation to laboratory. Transport medium – ambient temperature of +4°C
Material for cytology	Aspirates or touch preparations	Syringe Needle Swabs	Bottle, chilled or fixed on slide
Material for DNA studies	As above and below	As above and below	Special medium, EDTA (not heparin) and paper (not plastic) bags.
Faeces	Direct from cloaca or freshly voided, from cage or enclosure	Swabs or spatulae Bottle	Sterile bottle, chilled
Feathers	Plucked from site, to include follicle (a biopsy can also be taken)	Forceps Bottle or bag	Sterile bottle or bag, chilled, fixed immediately for histology/EM or in special medium for DNA studies
Cloacal calculi	Removed from cloaca or freshly voided	Forceps Bottle	Sterile bottle, chilled
Semen	Direct from cloaca of male bird (following massage or stimulation) or female after copulation	Syringe Bottle Slides	Sterile bottle, body temperature or chilled (rapid examination is necessary) or fixed on slide
Pellets (castings)	Freshly voided or removed from upper alimentary tract	Dissecting microscope	In sealed plastic bag or sterile bottle.

EDTA = ethylenediaminetetra-acetic acid; EM = electronmicroscopy.

to be reliable and projects reproducible. However, the sample size may need to be very large in order to detect an infectious agent or pathological lesion. Thus, for example, to give 95% confidence limits of finding one positive specimen in a collection of 50 birds, when there is only a 2% incidence, the sample size has to be 46! If the incidence is 10%, 20 birds are adequate. Often it is not possible, on financial or practical grounds, to sample such numbers and therefore interpretation of 'negative' results must be carried out with caution.

Standardisation of procedures is essential if laboratory tests on samples are to provide meaningful results and if repeated studies are to be relevant. Ideally a 'Manual of Standards' for sampling and samples should be produced as is already the case for work with domestic animals (O.I.E., 1996).

Post-mortem examination

This plays an important part in diagnosis and has contributed greatly to our understanding of diseases of birds of prey, both in captivity and in the wild. As Keymer (1977a) pointed out, all those who keep raptors in captivity should be encouraged to submit carcasses for *post-mortem* examination; this should also be routine when working with free-living birds although collection of carcasses can present problems and the type of investigations may vary.

A dead bird should always be assumed to be a potential source of pathogens until proved otherwise. It must be removed promptly from the aviary, mews or place where it was found and placed in one or more clean plastic bags prior to examination. Sometimes it is necessary to examine a raptor *post mortem* in connection with a legal case or insurance claim; under such circumstances it is particularly important that the carcass is received as fresh as possible and that a comprehensive examination is carried out, with full documentation (see 'Forensic examinations').

I originally presented my proposals and methods for *post-mortem* examination of birds of prey, in lay person's terms, in a paper in *The Falconer* (Cooper, 1968b) and that approach was subsequently followed for many years. The method has now been developed and refined (Cooper, 1987b).

As stated earlier, *post-mortem* examination (necropsy) is an integral part of raptor diagnostic medicine and has traditionally been used primarily to determine the cause of death in an individual bird or groups of birds. However, it can be argued that there are diverse reasons for carrying out a necropsy:

(1) To determine the *cause of death* in a bird or birds

(2) To ascertain the *cause of ill-health* in a bird or birds

These are the two traditional purposes and can be conveniently grouped together as 'diagnosis'.

(3) To provide background information on the presence or absence of lesions, macroparasites, microparasites, or of other factors, such as fat reserves or carcass composition as part of assessing 'condition'.

This is 'Health Monitoring' and in addition to its role in evaluating the health status and 'condition' of free-living raptors, helps in the formulation of disease control measures within a collection.

(4) To provide information for a legal case or similar investigation – for instance on the circumstances of death or the possibility that the bird suffered pain or distress while alive.

This can be termed 'Forensic'.

(5) For other investigative purposes, e.g. removal of tissue samples, such as testes, or examination of organs, such as oviducts (Wyllie & Newton, 1999) in order to assist biologists or others.

This can be referred to as 'Investigation'.

The pathologist is not the only person who is interested in, or has possible claim to, a carcass or tissues from a bird of prey. This clash of interests can create friction and, if not properly resolved, may reduce the value of the necropsy or the information that can be gleaned from it. Examples are:

• Bird keepers, falconers and others who may want the bird's carcass returned and, because of this, refuse to have certain organs examined (e.g.

brain) or request a 'whole body' for burial or other purposes.

- Museum curators and taxidermists who require the carcass for mounting or a study skin and therefore put restrictions on how much 'damage' can be carried out during the course of the necropsy. Reference collections may also ask for the body, but may be more accommodating in their requirements.
- Scientists from other disciplines who require samples for certain investigations, e.g., a toxicologist may want brains for a particular analysis, an anatomist adrenal gland for histological study, an archaeologist skeletal material for comparison with ancient bones, an avian biologist the whole body for carcass composition in order do assess condition.
- In legal and insurance cases not only individual tissues but also the whole carcass may need to be available for investigation by the police, by other pathologists (called by the prosecution/defence) or by forensic scientists.
- Cultural considerations may have to be taken into account: for example, the Maori of New Zealand have strong beliefs about certain species of bird and how the bodies and organs of these should be handled, examined and used.

Biologists frequently bemoan the apparent lack of interest amongst veterinarians in contributing to scientific knowledge. They allege, for instance, that many avian veterinary pathologists miss opportunities to record information that could be of use to field ornithology by (for example):

- Not weighing birds.
- Not taking measurements – or, when these are done, not recording data that are compatible with those used by ornithologists.
- Not keeping records of (or in some cases, not even examining) such structures as the preen gland, or not documenting the moult patterns.
- Not quantifying, collecting or submitting for identification ectoparasites and endoparasites.
- Not recording details of crop or gizzard contents of wild birds.
- Not saving material, frozen or in appropriate media, for DNA studies.

- Not consulting and collaborating with ornithologists when, for instance, a rare or interesting bird is received for examination.

It should be clear from all the above points that *post-mortem* examination of a bird of prey is often no longer a simple matter of opening the carcass and making a diagnosis. The following guidelines can help in ensuring that the necropsy is of maximum value:

(1) Before carrying out any necropsy, ascertain:

  (a) What is requested – a diagnosis (cause of death or ill-health)? Health monitoring? Forensic investigations? Other investigations?

  (b) Whether the carcass or parts of it are required by the owner, local ethnic communities, a museum, a reference collection, or by scientists for other investigations.

  (c) Whether the species or individual is of sufficient importance to warrant discussion beforehand with aviculturists, zoo/museum personnel or ornithologists in order to ensure that maximum use is made of the carcass.

One should then agree the availability or otherwise of bodies or body parts before commencing the examination. The latter may well need to be restricted if the body is needed for other purposes: 'keyhole' necropsy is possible, especially if an endoscope is used.

(2) During the necropsy remember to do the following:

  (a) As a routine, perform standard morphometrics and *always* weigh the bird.

  (b) When time permits, examine and record information on structures and tissues that might not be of immediate relevance to the necropsy, but which may provide data for others. Where possible, photograph or draw these.

  (c) Record parasites and make an attempt to count them. At the very least, save (preserve) a selection of those parasites found. Whenever possible have them identified.

(d) Quite apart from the requirements of others, retain *post-mortem* material for a period after carrying out the examination, in case there is a need to repeat sampling or to embark on new tests. As an adjunct to this, relevant material from free-living raptors should be submitted for toxicological examination.

(3) Following a *post-mortem* examination, be prepared to discuss the findings, so long as this is compatible with professional confidentiality. Data should be made available to those who may be able to use them in their research, in field work or in programmes of captive breeding. Findings should be published.

Post-mortem examinations (necropsies) of raptors may be carried out by a range of people: practising veterinarians, specialist pathologists or by non-veterinary personnel such as raptor biologists (see, for example, Newton *et al.*, 1999b). Some necropsies, especially of free-living birds, will need to be performed in the field, far from a well equipped laboratory (see Appendix X). In all cases it is important that adequate facilities are available – of necessity, these may be simple in the field – and that basic protocols are followed, relating to both technique and health and safety. A useful resumé of these was presented by Waine (1996). The facilities needed for gross *post-mortem* examination are given in Table 4.1.

Post-mortem methods for raptors differ little from those used for other species of bird. Extra features may, however, include a whole-body radiograph in order to check for presence of lead shot, undiagnosed fractures or skeletal disease – or to provide baseline data. My earlier work on *post-mortem* techniques, when I was working for the UK's Medical Research Council (MRC), showed the value of radiographic examination of dead birds prior to examination. A small, relatively inexpensive dental unit was found to give good results, with excellent contrast. A fixed voltage of 55 kV and fixed film–focal distance (FFD) of 75 cm were used with a variable exposure time, depending

upon the size of the bird, from 5–10 seconds. Such a long period of exposure would preclude its use with live birds but for *post-mortem* investigation the method was ideal. There are often financial constraints on the *post-mortem* examination of birds but radiography should always be considered, especially when dealing with young birds, forensic cases or threatened species (Cooper & West, 1988).

During the *post-mortem* examination itself, initial attention should be paid to the exterior of the bird for evidence of skin, feather or foot lesions or the presence of ectoparasites. If the carcass was submitted or stored in a plastic bag this should be carefully examined for dropped feathers, regurgitated food or parasites: occasionally the diagnosis is to be made on the basis of what is found in the bag rather than on *post-mortem* lesions!

The techniques used for external structures are very similar to those described earlier for clinical examination. Some, such as investigation of the preen gland, or transillumination of feathers, can often be carried out in more detail or with more ease on the dead bird. Careful note should be made of jesses, ring transmitters and tattoos, and a search made for transponder 'chips'. Where feasible, the bird should be aged: criteria used for barn owls were described by Newton *et al.* (1997), and Wyllie (undated) used talon features: some of their methods are applicable to other species.

The bird should be weighed at an early stage. There is usually weight loss following death, especially if a delay has elapsed before *post-mortem* examination or the carcass is not properly wrapped. For example, a kestrel weighing 180 g at death may weigh only 155 g when examined 36 hours later.

As mentioned earlier, the measuring of birds (morphometrics) is a much neglected part of *post-mortem* examinations, especially by vets, and yet it is a vital part of data collection. A bodyweight alone means little: a barn owl weighing 200 g may be an overweight nestling or an emaciated adult. Standard ornithological measurements should be used (Fig. 4.6a,b), carpal length being the first choice. Measurements should be made when birds are freshly dead as shrinkage can occur *post mortem*, especially once drying commences (Eastham *et al.*, 2001).

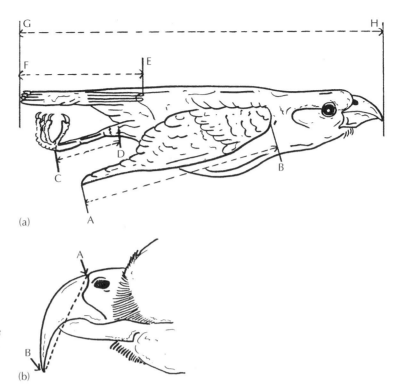

Fig. 4.6 Important measurements:
(a) carpus, tarsus, tail and whole
body (A–B Carpus; C–D Tarsus; E–F
Tail; G–H Whole body). (b) Base of
beak to tip of beak (A–B Base of
beak to tip of beak).

Data on bodyweight *and* morphometries help in the assessment of a bird's condition but it is argued by some that measurement of body composition, in a live bird using total body electrical conductivity (Samour, 2000a; Yamamoto & Santolo, 2000), is more sensitive and relates better to the animal's health status. A comprehensive review of assessment of condition of birds was provided by Brown (1996) who emphasised that carcass analysis, which is sometimes possible after necropsy, provides the most complete information about body condition.

As in clinical examination, careful note should be taken of any asymmetry. This may reflect clinical disease but can be an example of fluctuating asymmetry (FA), sometimes an indicator of inbreeding and, perhaps, of poor condition (Brown, 1996).

It is important that a record is kept of *post-mortem* findings. An assistant can record findings during the examination or a tape-recorder (preferably voice-activated) may be used. All findings should be inserted on to a form. My own is shown in Appendix III. Forensic (legal) cases may require special paperwork as different questions may need to be asked and answered (see Legal aspects and also Forensic examinations).

Post-mortem findings should, whenever possible, be stored on an appropriate database. MedARKS (Teare *et al.*, 1999) is popular and widely used and can be applied to pathological data but perhaps a more suitable system, already in use in Germany and a source of information on thousands of samples and records collected since 1955 is PARS (Pathological Anatomical References), established at IZW (Institut für Zoo- und Wildtierforschung) (Wisser & Jewgenow, 1997).

An internal examination is usually carried out with the bird on its back. Feathers can be plucked from the breast or, if the body is likely to be required for taxidermy, the bird should be skinned. Subcutaneous fat should be noted and 'scored' and its colour recorded.

Once the sternum is lifted the main internal organs can be seen (Fig. 3.4) but these will need to be displaced, removed and opened. Viscera must be examined and any abnormalities recorded and sampled. When time and facilities permit, individual organ weight and organ : bodyweight ratios should be calculated. The work by Barton and Houston (1996) illustrates the value of such information. Body fat should be assessed.

Depending upon the findings it may be necessary to dissect pathological lesions such as abscesses, adhesions or skeletal abnormalities.

It is important to observe and to record the appearance of the gonads, not only of captive birds used for captive-breeding but also of free-living raptors. Wyllie and Newton (1999) were able to differentiate female sparrow-hawks and common kestrels that had laid eggs from those that had not on the basis of the appearance of their oviducts – 'wide and convoluted' in the former category – 'thin and straight' in the latter.

It is always advisable, but not always practicable, to examine the brain although, as will be discussed in Chapter 9, *post-mortem* autolysis is rapid and subsequent histopathological examination may be hampered by fixation artefacts. If a nervous disease is suspected, full examination of the nervous system is essential and this also is discussed in Chapter 9. If a bird has to be killed on humanitarian grounds it can, once unconscious, be perfused with formalin or glutaraldehyde via either the carotid artery or the heart. This renders microbiology useless but very much improves fixation and subsequent laboratory examination of the brain.

My own technique for brain examination is to remove the head and to skin the cranium. At this stage intraosseous haemorrhages may be seen in the skull. The skull is opened longitudinally using a scalpel blade (for small specimens) or a hack saw (for larger). Once an incision has been made, the skull can usually be split in half by inserting the points of a pair of scissors into the crack and opening them slowly. The skull and brain are then bisected; one half can be placed immediately in formalin for histopathology, while the other can be dissected and examined. Both the brain and meninges must be carefully inspected, and a low-power stereo-microscope or dissecting loupe is useful in this context. The brain should be sliced and each portion examined.

Some tissues may need to be examined in particular detail because of the clinical history or because a specific research project is underway. Thus Krone *et al.* (2000) detected *Sarcocystis* in the breast muscles of a long-eared owl but such a parasite could easily be missed during routine examination.

A number of methods – for example, chemical, use of *Dermestes* beetles – are available for preparing bone or skeletal specimens.

When examining small birds, chicks, embryos or eggs (see Eggs), there is merit in carrying out a 'mini necropsy' – a term that I have borrowed from human paediatric pathology. This requires the use of small instruments (ophthalmological are ideal) and a dissecting microscope, magnifying loupe or a table lamp with magnifier.

Young birds can present particular problems on account of their size and also because they are often partly autolysed. Nevertheless, the basic *post-mortem* examination differs little from that described above. Whenever possible, radiography should be carried out in order to assess skeletal growth. It is important that the yolk sac is examined carefully. Note should be taken of the presence or absence of the 'egg tooth' on the beak and the size and appearance of the bursa of Fabricius must be recorded. Careful inspection for developmental abnormalities, both external (e.g. syndactyly, hydrocephalus) and internal (e.g. heart defects) is vital. There is interest in the growth and differentiation of the brain in birds – differences were reported nearly 50 years ago between nidifugous and nidicolous birds – and therefore the brain of nestlings should, whenever possible, be weighed. This is one of the many fields in which the pathologist can provide data of value to colleagues who are involved in avian biology and ethology (Cooper, 1993a).

Eggs

The pathological examination of raptor eggs that have failed to hatch has become standard in recent years. I started to examine eggs of captive birds in the 1970s and published proposed 'Request',

'Examination' and 'Summary of Findings' forms for eggs and embryos some years later (Cooper, 1987b; 1993b). Two of the latter are reproduced, with modifications, in Appendix III.

Eggs for examination should be submitted promptly. If there is any delay they should be separately wrapped in tissue paper and kept in a fridge (*not* a freezer) until they can be despatched. As a general rule no more than 14 days should elapse between placing an egg in the fridge and its examination. As with necropsies, any delay in examination must be recorded.

Eggs should be carefully wrapped (separate, as above, even if in one box) and well insulated. If posted (mailed) they – like carcasses – must conform with relevant postal regulations. A full history should accompany the samples and this must be wrapped separately – for example, in a plastic bag – in order to prevent contamination and soiling by egg contents.

As can be seen from Appendix III, in my examinations I place considerable emphasis on description of the egg and adequate clinical history. My approach is as below:

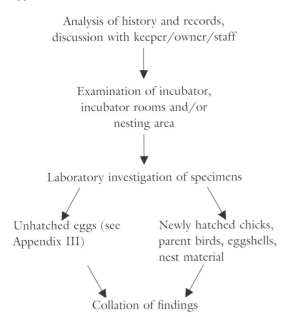

Analysis of history and records, discussion with keeper/owner/staff

↓

Examination of incubator, incubator rooms and/or nesting area

↓

Laboratory investigation of specimens

Unhatched eggs (see Appendix III)

Newly hatched chicks, parent birds, eggshells, nest material

Collation of findings

Additional action: retention of material, especially from rare species, as part of a Reference Collection (see Appendix VII).

The important external features are the size, shape and integrity of the egg. It should be measured, its shape recorded (or drawn) and any cracks or other external abnormalities noted. Candling is a key part, before the egg is opened. Candling is discussed in more detail in Chapter 13. White light candling remains the standard method of assessing *in-ovo* development but for thick, deeply pigmented, eggs infrared and ultraviolet candling – or even magnetic resonance imaging (MRI) – can be employed.

It is obviously of importance to ascertain whether the egg is fertile or not – if in doubt it should be described as 'probably fertile' or 'probably infertile'. If the egg *is* fertile, the age of the embryo at death should be assessed on the basis of its size. The embryo should be examined for evidence of physical abnormalities or infection. Bacteriological and mycological culture of the yolk sac, albumen and embryonic liver should be carried out. Histopathological examination of embryonic tissue may prove useful.

Apparently infertile eggs must also be examined carefully. Some will be infected (contaminated), and culture should be performed in this instance too.

Eggshells should always be retained, dried, after examination. Their thickness should be calculated as eggshell thinning is a feature of chlorinated hydrocarbon toxicity and certain other pathological conditions. A micrometer can be employed to measure directly but the alternative is to obtain an index of thickness based on the weight, length and breadth of a blown egg. Various indices can be used: these were assessed by Green (2000). There is also interest in the structure of avian eggshells and some interesting work on this subject has been published (Tyler, 1966; Board *et al.*, 1977); Hussong (1996) used pore structure to distinguish falcon hybrids.

Egg contents can be preserved and deep-frozen for subsequent chemical analysis and this should be routine when dealing with threatened or endangered species.

Before a carcass or egg is discarded, note must be made of the samples removed and the laboratory tests proposed. It is clearly bad practice to dispose of material and then later to regret that certain samples were not removed. Unfortunately the method of preservation will influence the tests that can subsequently be performed so that, for example, freezing will make histology difficult while fixation will kill organisms. If in doubt, it is best to keep the whole carcass chilled (+4°C) for 5–7 days and then to deep-freeze it. If this is not possible, a selection of tissues should be taken and duplicates fixed and frozen for subsequent study.

Sampling

A 'sample' can be defined as 'a specimen . . . collected for analysis on the assumption that it represents the composition of the whole' (Blood & Studdert, 1988). The definition emphasises the importance of good sampling technique.

Samples (sometimes called 'specimens' in this chapter) play an important part in the diagnosis of disease in raptors and the health monitoring of supposedly 'normal' birds of prey. Samples may be taken from live birds, from dead birds or from the environment. Correct sampling will help to yield reliable results and facilitate accurate interpretation and appropriate action. In legal cases such precision can be even more important (see Forensic examinations).

Mistakes can occur at any of the following stages:

- Selection
- Taking
- Packing
- Transportation
- Reception
- Processing.

An error or inconsistency introduced early in the sequence above can adversely affect subsequent actions and easily prejudice results.

Samples are of different types, depending upon (a) their source, (b) their purpose and (c) how they are presented, handled and transported.

Therefore, when working with raptors, one has to plan carefully the samples to be taken and how this is to be done. Sometimes it is permissible and ethically acceptable to kill a bird for the collection of specimens. Often, however, this is not possible and

use has to be made of opportunistic examination and sampling of carcasses that are found dead or of live birds that are being handled for another purpose, or of minimally invasive techniques, such as collection and examination of voided faeces, dropped feathers or regurgitated pellets (Cooper, 1998).

Consistency in sampling methods is vital if results are to be reliable and if different studies are to be comparable. Examples of where methods are important include:

- Swabs for microbiology – should they be cotton wool or alginate coated? large or small? dry or in transport medium (which type?)?
- Faeces for parasitology – does one take a whole faecal sample or only a portion? (in the case of the latter, peripheral or from the centre?), kept at room temperature or chilled?

Protocols and the use of standard equipment will help to minimise variation. In some cases standard equipment is vital – for example, the need to use special syringes and sample vials when taking blood for zinc analysis.

The time that elapses between taking a sample and processing it is also a fundamental consideration in assessing and interpreting results. Thus, for example, a delay in processing one set of swabs may result in the culture of fewer bacteria, or perhaps an overgrowth of one species (such as *Proteus*) so that the findings cannot reliably be compared with those from another set of swabs.

The taking and transportation of samples in the field, especially in relatively inaccessible or isolated areas, can present particular problems (Pendleton *et al.*, 1987). Special equipment may be required and improvisation is often essential (Cooper & Samour, 1997). The key to consistency and standardisation is to develop and to use protocols, whereby the method to be used is clearly defined and followed. It is also important to include details of the protocol in any published 'Materials and methods' so that other investigators can (preferably) employ the same techniques or at least be aware of where discrepancies may have occurred that might have influenced the results. In this regard, reference should be made to the publication *Manual of Standards for Diagnostic Tests and Vaccines* (O.I.E., 1996): some of the section on birds is relevant to raptors but more importantly the whole concept of GLP (good laboratory practice) and both quality control and validation of techniques is one that needs to be applied to bird of prey work.

Legal aspects

The collection, transportation and processing of samples are likely to be covered by legislation including Post Office regulations, health and safety and the Convention on International Trade in Endangered Species (CITES) (Cooper, M. E., 1987) (see Appendix XI). Even tiny samples may require CITES permits if they originate from species of animals that are listed on the Appendices of CITES or (in the European Union) the relevant Annexes and are 'recognizable derivatives' (Cooper, 1995). A resolution at the CITES Conference of the Parties (COP) in Nairobi, Kenya, in April 2000 failed to alter this ruling and, as a result, wildlife biologists and veterinarians who are sending specimens from one country to another need to continue to be aware of the legislation and to be vigilant in their adherence to it (Cooper, M. E., 1993). Sample collection from raptors is summarised in Table 4.2.

The emphasis here is on sampling *post mortem*. Clinical sampling was discussed earlier. Removal of *post-mortem* specimens for laboratory investigations may appear straightforward but care needs to be taken. In the case of external material, the technique resembles that described for clinical samples. When dealing with internal tissues care must be taken not to contaminate material unnecessarily. For example, if the lung is to be examined bacteriologically, it should be handled with clean forceps *before* the intestinal tract (which in raptors almost always harbours *Escherichia coli*) is opened. Specific lesions may be swabbed or removed for further investigations. If a blood-borne infection is suspected, a swab of heart blood should be taken; the heart should be removed and incised with sterile instruments before a fine nasopharyngeal swab is inserted into a ventri-

cle. At the same time blood smears can be taken. Alternatively, blood can be aspirated from a ventricle, using a needle and syringe.

The tissues chosen for histopathology will depend upon the lesions found and the degree of autolysis present in the carcass, but whenever possible a full selection should be taken. The minimum should be lung, liver and kidney plus any abnormalities. Careful dissection of the cranial part of the kidney will usually permit kidney, adrenal and gonad to be included in one section. Two pieces of heart – a transverse and a longitudinal section (LS) – should be taken from larger specimens; the former should be through the great vessels at the base of the heart. In the case of smaller hearts such sectioning may prove impossible and instead an LS of the whole heart must be taken. Fixation and processing are discussed later in this chapter.

Samples for electronmicroscopy depend upon whether scanning electronmicroscopy (SEM) or transmission electronmicroscopy (TEM) is to be used. Material submitted for SEM – for example, feathers showing lesions in the shaft, barbs or barbules – should be clean (i.e. feathers taken from a live bird or freshly moulted rather than from the floor of a cage or aviary) and dry. They should be handled with care, preferably without touching the barbs or any lesion and packed in a crush-proof container before being sent to the laboratory.

Material for TEM – for example, tissue biopsies, feather follicles – must be fixed rapidly in 2% glutaraldehyde, following the protocol above. In the case of plumage samples, the important component will be the follicular epithelial cells rather than the feather itself. Ideally, a biopsy of the feather follicle should be taken: a less satisfactory alternative is a freshly plucked feather, with some epithelial cells attached to the base which is immediately fixed in 2% glutaraldehyde for 4 hours. The specimen should be transferred to buffer and packaged as outlined above.

The material to be taken for toxicological examination is entirely dependent upon the poison suspected and the tests to be performed. The sampling of feathers for mercury was mentioned earlier. Maschek (1997) and Maschek *et al.* (1998) reported multi-element analysis of feathers for heavy metals using neutron activation. Liver, brain and body fat may be needed for organochlorine analysis. If there is any doubt over the tissues to be submitted for toxicology it is best to deep-freeze the carcass, carefully wrapped in a plastic bag, with a few specimens taken beforehand for histology/microbiology until instructions from the laboratory are received.

Laboratory investigation of clinical and post-mortem *samples*

Space does not permit detailed description of all laboratory techniques and therefore reference will be made to a number of relevant publications. Subsequent chapters will also cover some procedures.

Recent years have seen great advances in clinical investigative techniques for birds. Lumeij (1987) made particularly important contributions to our understanding of avian clinical pathology. He drew attention to such important considerations as the volume of blood that might be taken, how the treatment of samples might affect results and, in a separate chapter, the influence of dehydration (in pigeons) on plasma urea, creatinine and uric acid. One of the first texts of the new millennium, a book edited by Alan Fudge (2000), has provided up-to-date information on the selection and interpretation of laboratory diagnostic tests in exotic species, and this includes some information on birds of prey. There can be no doubt that the taking and examination of samples is an integral part of modern raptor medicine.

It is debatable whether samples for laboratory examination should be dealt with 'in-house' (in the veterinary practice, for instance) or submitted to a competent laboratory elsewhere. The former is often rapid and convenient but the latter may be more reliable. Some tests can only be performed in laboratories that have the required facilities and so there is no dilemma in such cases. If a practice wants to do its own tests it needs the correct facilities and equipment. A summary of requirements is given in Table 4.1.

Inexpensive, rapid, techniques such as cytology will often yield immediate results and can readily be carried out in a practice or even in the field. For example, smears of caseous material from the mouth of a bird, stained with Gram, Giemsa or a rapid stain such as 'Diff-Quik', may reveal bacteria, yeasts, protozoa or worm eggs as well as normal and abnormal host cells. Cytological techniques are discussed in more detail later.

Although the main aim of laboratory investigations is to aid diagnosis and prognosis, one must not forget how little is still known about the normal biology (the gut flora, for example) of most species. Every effort should, therefore, be made to collect specimens for examination and to submit them to an appropriate laboratory or authority. The results may not directly benefit the bird in question but will often yield useful scientific (baseline) data.

Samples that may be taken from birds of prey include faeces, castings (pellets), feathers, blood, swabs, washings, touch preparations and biopsies. Table 4.2 lists samples, sites, equipment required and recommended methods of transportation.

Laboratory techniques used in raptor work are listed, in a summarised form, in Table 4.3.

Microbiological (bacteriological and mycological) methods are similar to those used for other species. It does not appear to be advantageous to incubate bacterial cultures at temperatures of more than 37°C despite the higher body temperature of most birds. Aerobic and anaerobic culture should always be performed.

Microbiological techniques are not only of use in diagnosis of disease. They can also play a part in the maintenance of hygiene in mews and aviaries. Many organisms, such as *Staphylococcus aureus* and *Aspergillus* spp., can be spread by air currents, and it is possible to monitor airborne contamination by employing bacteriological 'settle plates' (Cooper, 1978a,b) or a volumetric impaction method (Dykstra *et al.*, 1997).

Once isolates of bacteria have been obtained, they need to be identified. A useful early guide was the book produced by the American Association of Avian Pathologists (Hitchner *et al.*, 1975). The next step is usually testing for sensitivity to antimicrobial agents. This is accomplished using standard agar plates and paper discs impregnated with the agents or the new E tests (AB BIODISK, Solna, Sweden). Tests for mycoplasmas, chlamydiae (chlamydophi-

Table 4.3 Laboratory techniques in raptor work.

Technique	Recommended methods		Comments
Aerobic bacteriology heart blood, skin or visceral lesions	Blood agar plates and MacConkey's – incubated at 37°C for 24 hours (72 hours if no growth)		Special media for certain organisms (e.g. Lowenstein–Jensen for *Mycobacterium* spp. [incubated for 10 weeks at 37°C]). Identification of bacteria is based upon (1) colonial morphology, (2) staining reactions (especially Gram), (3) biochemical tests, (4) (where necessary) phage typing, (5) molecular biology methods, e.g. PCR, (6) serotyping
intestinal samples	Blood agar plate MacConkey's plate Deoxycholate plate Citrate agar (DCA) plate Selenite F broth plate Wilkins–Chalgron anaerobe agar	Incubated as above; After 24 hours, Selenite subcultured on to MacConkey's and DCA. Many labs prefer Rappaport–Vassiliadis (MSRVC) medium	
Anaerobic bacteriology tissue samples	Same as above, but incubated anaerobically at 37°C for 48 hours		See above
Mycology	Sabouraud dextrose agar plates – one at 37°C for 7 days, the other at 22°C for up to 21 days. Direct microscopy of fresh or prepared material ('cooked' in 10% KOH) to detect hyphae and spores in samples		Other media may also be needed. Identification based upon tests similar to those above, plus special investigations (e.g. fluorescence)
Mycoplasmology tissue samples	Mycoplasma growth medium		See Furr *et al.* (1977) and Heidenreich (1997)
Isolation of *Chlamydia* (now called *Chlamydophila*) tissue samples	PCR, ELISA and fluorescent antibody techniques can be used to detect the organism. Alternatively, *Chlamydia* can be grown in tissue culture, eggs or experimental animals		See Heidenreich (1997)
Virology tissue samples	Tissue culture Egg inoculation Animal inoculation Fluorescent antibody technique		Methods depend upon sample and presumptive diagnosis
Serology serum samples	Serum neutralisation Gel diffusion precipitation Complement fixation ELISA Fluorescent antibody		Preferred method varies Poultry laboratories can often assist with serological investigations
Parasitology skin scrapings and/or feathers faeces/intestinal contents pellets (castings) blood	Direct microscopy plus treatment of sample with 10% KOH prior to examination. Wet preparations in physiological saline plus salt or sugar flotation using McMaster counting chamber. Lugol's iodine: identification of cysts ZnSO₄ flotation: amoebae, cysts *Trichomonas* medium Thin smears fixed in methanol and stained with Giemsa or air-dried and stained with a rapid stain		Protozoa (e.g. *Trichomonas*) can be detected in fresh wet preparations, but are killed – and thus difficult to identify – in concentrated salt or sugar Other stains can also be used. Careful examination is necessary in order to detect a low-grade parasitaemia

Table 4.3 Continued.

Technique	Recommended methods	Comments
Histology tissue samples	Tissues dehydrated in alcohol. Embedded in paraffin wax, and sectioned at 6μ or less. Stained routinely with haematoxylin and eosin. Frozen sections may be rapidly prepared using cryostat. A freezing microtome has the advantage of using carbon dioxide and thus can be used when there is no electricity	Many staining techniques available. Some (e.g. detection of fat) cannot be carried out on paraffin sections and either fresh or fixed tissues must be examined frozen Biopsies taken using thermo/electrocautery or cryosurgery often produce artefacts that can prove confusing in sections

Cytology
  touch preparations
  washings,
  brushings and
  aspirates
	Air-dried for Romanowsky. Certain rapid stains. Fixed in methanol for other methods	Fresh material should be used. See basic protocols and guidelines to cell identification and evaluation by Campbell (1984) and Cooper (1985a) and further developments by Campbell (1993)

Haematology
  smears
  blood in EDTA or lithium
  heparin
	See 'Parasitology' – blood. Examination of smears for abnormalities, differential counts. PCV (haematocrit) estimation using standard techniques. Haemoglobin needs modified method. Total counts using special diluents. Coulter counters can be used for RBC counts	

Clinical chemistry
  blood in lithium
  heparin (depends on the
  tests required)
	Standard procedures for electrolytes and enzymes (colour reaction systems and atomic absorption or flame spectrophotometer methods)
	Automatic analysers
		Advisable to submit samples to a reputable laboratory and to use it routinely. Check requirements beforehand

Electronmicroscopy tissue samples	Standard TEM and SEM procedures	Rapid fixation of very small fresh specimens is essential

Chemical analysis/toxicology
  tissue samples
  calculi
  blood
	Standard gas-liquid chromatographic and other procedures	

DNA studies	Various – depend on samples	
Feather examination	Direct microscopy with or without KOH treatment Culture (bacteriological or mycological) Virology/PCR DNA techniques Histology Electronmicroscopy	
Semen examination	Direct microscopy – wet or fixed (stained) preparations Bacteriology	An under-utilised source of information
Bone examination	Culture, usually following grinding Histology, usually following decalcification DNA techniques	Even fossil material may yield DNA (Fleischer *et al.*, 2000)

EDTA = ethylenediaminetetra-acetic acid; KOH = potassium hydroxide; PCV = packed cell volume; RBC = red blood cell; SEM = scanning electronmicroscopy; TEM = transmission electronmicroscopy.

lae), viruses and humoral antibodies (serology) usually require special equipment and facilities.

Parasitological examinations are again similar to those used in other species and can usually be easily carried out in a veterinary practice or even in the field (see Appendix X). Wet preparations should always precede flotation methods. It is essential that a representative sample is obtained and a useful guide to this, in a range of species, was given by Needham (1977). The time of sampling may be important: the excretion of coccidial oocysts in some birds follows a 'circaduodian rhythm' (Boughton, 1988). Examination of the faecal sample may reveal features other than parasites; feather, fur and vegetable matter are common, and excess numbers of erythrocytes and cellular debris may be seen. The person carrying out the examination should record what he/she sees, not merely report 'No parasites detected' or 'No abnormalities observed'.

Eggs of *Eucoleus* (formerly *Capillaria*) and certain other parasites may also be detected in scrapings from buccal cavity, crop or gut, in regurgitated food and in castings (pellets). Castings should always first be examined carefully with a hand lens or dissecting microscope and then soaked in a small quantity of normal saline before parasitological or microbiological investigation. They can be radiographed in order to detect metallic shot; lead and steel shot are then readily differentiated with a magnet (Miller *et al.*, 2000).

Material for histological examination should be fixed promptly in at least ten times its own volume of 10% formalin, or, preferably, 10% neutral buffered formalin. The latter has the advantage that tissues can be stored in it for longer periods and there are fewer artefacts. This and other aspects are discussed in standard textbooks such as *Histological Laboratory Methods* (Disbrey & Rack, 1970). Where applicable, the specimen should be incised to permit penetration and when there is much blood present a change of fixative after 24 hours is advisable. After fixation the material should be trimmed and processed. Decalcification is often necessary; for example, when investigating foot lesions it is far preferable to cut a transverse section of the whole digit, and to decalcify it before embedding, than to take the affected soft tissues only.

Paraffin wax sections are usually adequate although frozen sections may be necessary in emergency cases or where fat stains are required. The routine stain of choice is haematoxylin and eosin though others, especially Gram, Periodic acid Schiff (PAS), Grocott and Ziehl–Neelsen may be necessary.

Autolytic changes can make interpretation difficult; an example is pyknotic erythrocytic nuclei which can easily be mistaken for chronic inflammatory cells. The rate of autolysis varies according to the type of tissue involved; thus, brain and liver will deteriorate very rapidly (Fig. 4.7). Unfortunately, *post-mortem* change in various organs is often the norm rather than the exception, especially when a carcass is despatched by post or has been collected in the field. The avian pathologist will find the papers on sequential *post-mortem* changes in the chicken (*Gallus domesticus*) and mallard duck (*Anas platyrhynchos*) by Munger and McGavin (1972a,b) and Morrow and Glover (undated) respectively of help in deciphering such changes.

Much remains to be learned of the normal histology of birds of prey. From time to time structures are seen which appear to be unreported or the significance of which is unclear: for example, Borst *et al.* (1976) reported ectopic bone in the lungs of birds, including the Eurasian kestrel, and I have frequently seen this in sections with no evidence of a pathological response.

There appear to be no comprehensive texts available that deal specifically with the normal histology or histopathology of birds of prey and the pathologist involved in such work must usually refer to standard poultry books, such as *Diseases of Poultry* (Calnek *et al.*, 1991 and other editions) and *The Histology of the Fowl* (Hodges, 1974) as well as more modern works that include some material on raptors, such as Randall and Reece (1996). Supplementary texts include those on comparative histology such as the books by Patt and Patt (1969), Andrew and Hickman (1974) or Leake (1975). More information is needed on the histopathological changes that occur in diseases of raptors: even our understanding of the pathogenesis of 'frounce' (trichomoniasis) is based largely on studies made 40 years ago in pigeons (Mesa *et al.*, 1961).

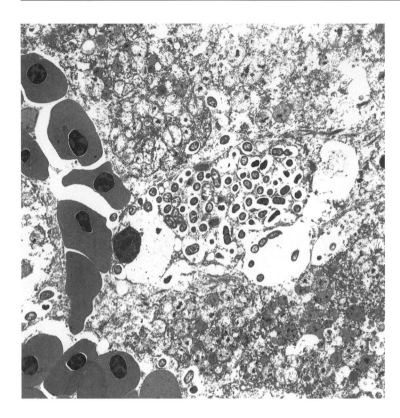

Fig. 4.7 *Post-mortem* examination affects some tissues more rapidly than others. Here red blood cells (left) are still well preserved, but liver cells (centre and right) are showing marked degeneration (TEM × 1500).

Electronmicroscopy plays an increasingly important role in diagnosis and research and the techniques used are similar to those in poultry. Both transmission electronmicroscopy (TEM) and scanning electronmicroscopy (SEM) are used. Consultation with the electronmicroscopist is important and he/she will give guidance on the type of fixative that should be used. There is increasing interest in the use of one fixative for both light and electronmicroscopy – a mixture of formaldehyde and glutaraldehyde is an example – and a useful review article on this subject was by McDowell and Trump (1977).

The taking and examination of blood is now a routine part of raptor medicine and provides serological, haematological, biochemical and parasitological information. Properly taken blood samples can be used for haematology, biochemistry and for the production of serum and for the preparation of smears. Each of these can be used in different ways (see Table 4.3). In addition to its role in diagnosis,

blood analysis can be used as one indicator of a bird's health or even, perhaps, to assess a free-living bird's physiological response to its environment (Brown, 1996).

For serological tests either clotted blood or serum is needed. My own technique for serum removal is to collect the blood in a tall narrow glass bottle, such as a 'Universal' container, and to loosen the clot from around the edge with a sterile needle. The bottle is kept at room temperature for 24 hours to encourage contraction of the clot and the serum removed from the surface with a syringe and needle, if necessary after gentle centrifuging. Serological testing cannot be discussed here; suffice it to say that screening of serum samples for evidence of exposure to organisms or disease plays an important part in diagnosis and health monitoring of both captive and free-living raptors – as has been done, for instance, in Chile in studies on condors (Toro *et al.*, 1997).

The history of blood studies in raptors is an interesting one and illustrates the advances that have been made in approximately 30 years. In my early studies in the 1970s I was able routinely to measure only packed cell volume (PCV), red cell count and haemoglobin. PCV (haematocrit or HCT) was assayed using a standard micro-haematocrit centrifuge and red cells by the method described by Leonard (1969). Natt and Herrick's solution was used for the red cell techniques (Cooper, 1972c; 1975b).

The later 1970s and the 1980s saw an upsurge of interest in, and publications on, the haematology of raptors and other non-domesticated birds: examples included the work of Gerlach (1978), Smith and Bush (1978), Kirkwood *et al.* (1979), Gee *et al.* (1981), Lepoutre (1982), Rehder *et al.* (1982), Rehder and Bird (1983) and Bini *et al.* (1989). The paper by Gerlach contained coloured photographs of leucocytes of raptors, which supplemented well the extensive monograph on avian haematology by Lucas and Jamroz (1961). A section in the *Raptor Management Techniques Manual* (Pendleton *et al.*, 1987) provided a useful summary of techniques and some baseline data. All authors during that period emphasised the importance of establishing baseline data, preferably over a long period of time in view of possible variations.

Recognition of avian blood cells and interpretation of changes require knowledge and experience. Useful reference books are those by Hawkey and Dennett (1989) and Campbell (1984) and the chapter by Jennings (1996). The thesis (in French) by Fromont (1993) includes excellent line drawings of cell types. Christine Hawkey, arguably the pioneer in the field of comparative haematology, provided an overview of the subject in her 1991 paper and included discussion of the effects of stress and infection on blood parameters. Hauska and Redig (1997) provided information on cells and cell changes on the basis of examination of approximately 400 smears from both healthy and diseased birds of prey and pointed out that (a) raptors show a predominantly heterophilic leucogram and (b) the morphology of the leucocytes generally resembles that seen in other avian species.

Examples of haematological values for a number of genera are given in Table 4.4. These are based on a combination of my own data over several years

with some modifications made in line with the values listed by Beynon *et al.* (1996) and Heidenreich (1997). As the subject develops it will become more and more important to have reference values for individual species (and perhaps even for birds of different sexes, different ages and from different localities), in both health and disease. Some such data are already published; see, for example Smith and Bush (1978), Gerlach (1979), Gee *et al.* (1981), Kösters and Meister (1982), Cooper *et al.* (1986), Ferrer *et al.* (1987), Gylstorff and Grimm (1987), Lavin *et al.* (1992), Redig (1993a), Döttlinger (1995), Beynon *et al.* (1996), Samour and D'Aloia (1996), Toro *et al.* (1997), Boal *et al.* (1998a) and der Pilar Lanzarot *et al.* (2001). ISIS (International Species Information System) data are also available and applicable (Anon, 1997) as is the LYNX programme (Bennett *et al.*, 1991) which provides quantitative and qualitative data on a range of species. Information from several sources was collated by Samour (2000a) and by Carpenter *et al.* (2001). It is important that laboratories collaborate in pooling information in order to expand and improve the database.

Interpretation of haematological changes follows very much the approach in other species but some caution is needed, PCV (haematocrit) values being an example. Low PCV values have long been considered a feature of debilitated and anaemic birds while elevated values indicate haemoconcentration, sometimes on account of dehydration – for example in birds that have been transported. However, PCV is not necessarily a useful indicator of condition in birds of prey. Dawson and Bartolotti (1997) discussed this in the context of their research on American kestrels. Amongst other things they reported a decline in PCV with the time of day and an increase with the 'level of infection' of *Haemoproteus*. Boal *et al.* (1998a), however, reported no change in PCV with haematozoan infections.

Examples of haematological changes that may be associated with infectious diseases include leucopenia, leucocytosis, heterophilia, lymphocytosis, monocytosis, eosinophilia, 'toxic' cells (i.e. degranulated heterophils, toxic granulation in heterophils and cytoplasmic basophilia in heterophils) and 'reactive' lymphocytes and monocytes. A brief, but very,

Table 4.4 Some haematological data for birds of prey.

	Falco spp.	*Aquila* spp.	*Buteo* spp.	*Accipiter* spp.	*Gyps* spp.	*Bubo* spp.
PCV/HCT (haematocrit) (l/l)	0.30–0.45	0.30–0.50	0.35–0.45	0.30–0.50	0.30–0.50	0.30–0.55
Haemoglobin (g/l)	100–180	110–170	120–180	150–200	120–160	100–186
Red cells (erythrocytes) ($\times 10^{12}$/l)	2.0–3.5	2.0–3.0	1.65–2.5	1.5–3.0	2.0–3.0	1.5–2.5
White cells (leucocytes) ($\times 10^{9}$/l)	7.0–20.0	10.0–20.0	5.0–22.0	10.0–20.0	10.0–20.0	4.0–20.0
Heterophils ($\times 10^{9}$/l)	5.0–15.0	5.0–15.0	5.0–15.0	5.0–20.0	5.0–15.0	2.0–12.0
Lymphocytes ($\times 10^{9}$/l)	3.0–15.0	4.0–15.0	3.5–15.0	5.0–15.0	4.0–15.0	1.5–7.0
Monocytes ($\times 10^{9}$/l)	0.0–1.0	0.0–1.5	0.0–1.2	0.0–1.0	0.0–1.5	0.0–0.7
Eosinophils ($\times 10^{9}$/l)	0.1–0.7	0.1–2.0	0.1–1.5	0.1–2.0	0.1–1.8	0.0–0.5
Basophils ($\times 10^{9}$/l)	0.0–0.85	0.0–0.5	0.0–0.5	0.0–1.0	0.0–0.6	0.0–0.5
Thrombocytes ($\times 10^{9}$/l)	5.0–50.0	10.0–50.0	5.0–45.0	5.0–50.0	10.0–50.0	5.0–35.0
Fibrinogen (g/l)	<5.0	<5.0	<5.0	<5.0	<5.0	<5.0

helpful review of leucocyte changes in raptors was provided by Victoria Joseph in Fudge's *Laboratory Medicine* (2000).

Careful interpretation is needed by an experienced haematologist, coupled with an analysis of history, clinical findings and other laboratory tests. Where reference values for a species are not available, (careful) use can be made of those for related species.

Falconiform species have relatively large erythrocytes – up to $16 \times 8\,\mu m$ – and while such figures are usually not of diagnostic importance, measurements are worth recording for future reference; the possible significance of erythrocyte size was discussed by Palomeque and Planas (1977). Balasch *et al.* (1976) reported sedimentation rates for a number of birds of prey and it is possible that these too might prove useful in diagnosis. Haemoglobin components of raptors were studied by Inge Hiebl *et al.* (1987a,b; 1989), and similar work by Bauer (1985) threw new light on the possible relationship of New World vultures to hawks and storks.

Blood smears provide valuable information and should always be prepared, even if only a little blood is available. In the field, where samples may be limited in size and often impossible to repeat, I take two smears and sufficient blood for a PCV estimation. Smears should be air-dried, fixed with 100% methanol and stained. If staining is to be carried out later the smears can be transported air-dried (subject to any relevant legislation if being moved out of the country – see Appendix XI) and only fixed prior to staining. Insofar as staining is concerned, my own long-term preference is Giemsa which should be used at a strength of 10% at pH 7.2 (for parasites), 6.8 (for blood cells) for 1 hour; Leishman sometimes shows eosinophilic granules and rods better and rapid stains such as 'Diff-Quik' are now very popular. The latter are easily carried out and produce nice preparations but the colours tend to fade.

Good blood smears produce reliable results and the importance of preparation was emphasised recently by Cooper and Anwar (2001) who pointed out that the failure to detect blood parasites in birds (often reported in papers – see, for example, Blanco *et al.* (1998)) may reflect the quality of the smears rather than whether or not the parasites are present.

Assessment of pathogenicity to raptors of haematozoa is not easy and, in the absence of controlled experimental studies, is often circumstantial. Thus, for example, Munoz *et al.* (1999), on the basis of the high parasitaemia (45%) and marked anaemia (PCV 0.22), concluded that a *Babesia shortti* infection in a common kestrel might have caused death.

Careful and often prolonged examination, using oil immersion, is necessary to detect blood protozoa. Microfilariae can usually be seen readily under low magnification and this should always be the first part of microscopical examination of smears. Subsequent high magnification and oil immersion work must be thorough and systematic. Parasites may predominate in certain areas of a smear and there may be preponderance of white cells. Quantification is important (Godfrey *et al.*, 1987).

Smears are used for differential counts as well as for detecting parasites and cellular abnormalities. If a bird is anaemic there are usually lowered PCV and/or haemoglobin levels, but another clue in some cases is an increase in immature erythrocytes including those that have basophilic staining to their cytoplasm (Markus & Oosthuizen, 1972). Damaged white cells ('smudge' and 'basket' cells) should be counted since not only will this ensure a more reliable differential count but it is also possible that increased numbers of such cells may be correlated with disease. Only an experienced person should attempt to distinguish a 'smudged' monocyte from a 'smudged' lymphocyte: my own approach is to put all smudged cells into one category.

Examination of the buffy coat, following PCV estimations, can prove useful and may readily detect microfilariae (see Chapter 7).

Our knowledge of the blood biochemistry of raptors has increased exponentially since Halliwell (1981) and Gee *et al.* (1981) provided a useful introduction to the subject. The subject was discussed succinctly in the *Raptor Management Techniques Manual* (Pendleton *et al.*, 1987). More recently, Lumeij (1996) provided a useful review and emphasised some of the pitfalls when sampling: he also discussed raptors in a general paper on clinical chemistry (Lumeij, 1997).

Some examples of biochemical values are given in Table 4.5. Again, these are based on a combination of my own results together with some amalgamation of figures from Beynon *et al.* (1996) and Heidenreich (1997). The points made earlier about haematological values are relevant also to biochemical data. More detailed figures are to be found in Gerlach (1978, 1979), O'Donnell *et al.* (1978), Cooper *et al.* (1986), Gee *et al.* (1981), Ferrer *et al.* (1987), Garcia-Rodriguez *et al.* (1987), Gylstorff and Grimm (1987), Lavin *et al.* (1992), Döttlinger (1995), Samour and D'Aloia (1996) and Toro *et al.* (1997). Carpenter *et al.* (2001) collated data from a number of sources for four species of bird of prey. The paper by del Pilar Lanzarot *et al.* (2001) is important because it provides data on free-living nestling peregrines, possibly the first study of its kind. Gascoyne *et al.* (1994) presented guidelines for the interpretation of plasma biochemistry values in birds (and mammals) with unknown reference ranges and their database included both the Falconiformes and the Strigiformes. That paper is a valuable contribution to a better understanding of

Table 4.5 Some blood biochemistry data for birds of prey.

Measurement	Range	Comments
Total protein (g/l)	25.0–50.0	A useful indicator of health: hypoproteinaemia is a sign of malnutrition or certain diseases
Glucose (mmol/l)	10.0–25.0	Lowered when bird is hypoglycaemic (secondary to starvation or certain diseases) Normal values are considerably higher than those for mammals. See text
Uric acid (μmol/l)	400–1200	Raised values in birds that are dehydrated, have just eaten or have severe renal disease (or can be artefactual – urate contamination of sample)
Urea (mmol/l)	0.3–2.0	Of limited value (cf uric acid)
Albumin (g/l)	10.0–20.0	An indicator of nutritional status
Globulin (g/l)	15.0–30.0	Raised values can be indicative of infectious disease
Creatinine (μmol/l)	30.0–60.0	May be raised in renal disease but not invariably so
ALT (μ/l)	10–60	Raised values may indicate organ damage
ALP (μ/l)	25.0–500	Raised values may indicate osteoblastic activity. Seasonal changes can occur (Gerlach, 1978)
GGT (μ/l)	0.0–6.0	Raised values in hepatic (biliary) disorders
AST (SGOT) (μ/l)	100–250	Raised values with organ or tissue damage
CK (μ/l)	100–800	Elevated following exercise and various diseases
LDH (μ/l)	100–750	Elevations can indicate hepatic disease but may not be significant (short half-life)
Cholesterol (mmol/l)	5.0–10.0	Raised following a meal or if diet is high in fat
Calcium (mmol/l)	2.0–3.0	Raised in egg-laying females, lowered in metabolic bone disease. Lowered in renal disease (see below)
Phosphate (mmol/l)	1.0–2.0	Raised in certain renal diseases, lowered if intestinal absorption impaired. Reversed Ca:P values can be a feature of renal disease before uric acid elevation is apparent
Potassium (mmol/l)	1.5–3.5	Low values may be artefactual. Raised in renal and intestinal disease
Chloride (mmol/l)	100–150	
Sodium (mmol/l)	150–175	Raised in renal disease/dehydration
Iron (μmol/l)	2.0–20.0	Figures at top of range may be associated with high dietary iron intake

the meaning of biochemical results and how best to use them, especially in veterinary practice.

The correct use and interpretation of units is important. For over 20 years the SI (Système International d'Unités) has been recommended for use by the medical professions and is currently followed by the majority of countries in the world. Unfortunately many publications in the USA still use the older 'conventional' units, which often leads to confusion and difficulty in translating results. In this book SI is used throughout. When conversion is necessary, reference should be made to an appropriate publication such as that published by the Royal Society of Medicine Services (Anon, 1988).

In the past veterinary practices have tended to use 'dry' methods for blood analysis while diagnostic laboratories have employed 'wet' techniques. The latter have many advantages in terms of accuracy and reliability as well as cost but require high standards of staff training. Various analysers are available. Portable instruments, suitable for use in the field (see Appendix X) can be used for certain tests, e.g. hand-held refractometers for protein estimation.

Although many of those working with raptors submit blood for haematology and clinical chemistry, there is still a dearth of information on 'normal' values of many species. A similar situation applies to enzymes, although as long ago as 1977 Redig was able to report encouraging results for the former in red-tailed hawks, including one bird in which liver function had been impaired by treatment with carbon tetrachloride. Research on other species may not be relevant to raptors.

There is increasing interest in the use of plasma biochemistry as a means of assessing the condition of free-living birds but there are many variables and careful interpretation is needed (Brown, 1996).

The earliest reference I have been able to trace to the use of blood gas studies in birds of prey is that of Calder and Schmidt-Nielsen (1968), who investigated panting and blood carbon dioxide levels in a number of species of bird, including the turkey vulture. Results for this bird when it was resting at 22–25°C were blood pH 7.51 and pCO_2 27.5. During panting, at an air temperature of 44.5°C, these figures changed to 7.56 and 19.0, respectively. Now blood gas analyses are frequently measured as a routine during long-term surgery.

Histochemistry is proving of increasing value in veterinary medicine in a wide range of species, including birds of prey. Tissues such as muscle may need to be snap frozen (see Table 4.2).

Carcasses and tissues that remain after processing should not be discarded as they may be needed at a later date. They can form part of a reference collection (Cooper & Jones, 1986; Cooper *et al.*, 1998) and thus be made available to others for study. Formalin fixation is not good for DNA extraction and such tests as PCR (polymerase chain reaction) can be adversely affected. However, work on *Entamoeba histolytica* suggests that the deleterious effects of formalin are both time- and concentration-dependent (Ramos *et al.*, 1999) and so, if formalin has to be used for fixation, it should be as dilute as possible.

The veterinary clinician or pathologist may be asked to examine semen samples from birds of prey (see also Chapter 13). These will usually have been taken from the cloaca of the male following massage or natural copulation and should not contain urates or faeces. Semen samples should be kept cool (+ 4°C) but not frozen. If mixed with a diluent or saline, the latter should be at the same temperature as the semen to reduce damage to spermatozoa. Various tests can be performed on semen. Fixed samples can be stained and examined for abnormal

spermatozoa or cells indicative of infection. Some variation in sperm size is normal and can be ignored. Fresh semen is used to assess motility and concentration of sperm. It must be remembered that the sperm concentration of some falcons is low compared with that of domestic birds (Boyd, 1977). Tests used in mammals, amongst them enzyme analyses to monitor cellular damage following freezing, are increasingly playing a role in raptor work. Bacteriological culture of semen may be carried out and this does not differ from other microbiological techniques: it is important because of evidence from work in other species of the possibility of sexual spread of pathogens (Poiani & Wilks, 2000), including salmonellae (Reiber *et al.*, 1995).

Toxicological (chemical) examination cannot be covered here. This is a specialised field and there are many publications on it. It is also discussed, particularly in the context of free-living birds, elsewhere in this book (see Chapters 10 and 11). As was mentioned earlier, the laboratory will specify how it requires material to be submitted and it is vital that its instructions are followed. A laboratory cannot look for 'poisons' in general; some idea must be given of the toxic agent suspected. It is, therefore, most important that a full clinical history is obtained, and appropriate pathology carried out (to eliminate non-toxic causes of death) before tissues are submitted.

Sampling for DNA ('genetic analysis') will also not be discussed in detail. Suffice it to say that tissues, such as muscle, are the best source but DNA can also be retrieved from blood (EDTA, not heparin, should be used as anticoagulant), from feather follicles and from faeces. Samples for DNA studies should be frozen or stored in ethanol: formalin is not generally satisfactory. Freezing of blood will cause a loss of DNA and so the taking and storage of large samples (1 ml or more) is advisable.

Feather samples should be kept in sealed plastic bags and examined initially with a hand-lens or stereo-microscope (Cooper, 1972a; 1989). In either case the specimen should be viewed with both reflected and transmitted light. Following this, feathers can be soaked in 40% sodium hydroxide which renders them transparent and permits more careful examination for parasites or other abnormalities. A range of other tests can then be performed. Scanning electronmicroscopy has proved very useful in the differentiation of lesions of barbs and barbules and has been used in forensic cases.

While plastic bags are usually best for storing feathers, they should not be used when the objective is to examine follicles for DNA. In this case paper envelopes are preferable.

The use of experimental animals has proved necessary in some fields of raptor medicine. Rodents may, rarely, be used in the diagnosis of microbial disease or detection of toxins. More often embryonated eggs or chickens are employed for such work. Other birds may be of use in experimental studies – for example, starlings (*Sturnus vulgaris*) or pigeons (*Columba livia*) as models for bumblefoot (Cooper & Needham, 1981; Cooper, 1987a). Raptors themselves have been used for toxicological and microbiological research and it is probable that they will play a more important role in future – for example, in assessing the safety and efficacy of vaccines (Remple, 2001). It is even possible that germ-free (or at least gnotobiotic) birds may be produced in due course. Experimental animals must be used humanely and in Britain, the European Union (EU) and certain other countries, the appropriate licences and/or certificates must be held (see Appendix XI).

Making a diagnosis

The accurate diagnosis of disease or cause of death requires a careful analysis of *all* findings, coupled with history and, sometimes, circumstantial evidence. In a proportion of cases no diagnosis can be made or there are findings that may or may not have contributed to death. Alternatively, there may be a number of lesions that together may have proved fatal but it is impossible to implicate any one as the prime cause.

Analysis of cause of death in free-living birds is particularly difficult because of bias: thus, for example, raptors hit by cars are more likely to be found than those that die in woodland. Kenward *et al.* (1993) pointed out that birds wearing trans-

mitters yielded carcasses that were fresher and thus more likely to provide useful data. Biologists doing studies on free-living raptors are inclined to be rather simplistic in their 'diagnoses', often determining the presence of infectious disease on gross findings alone – see, for example, Newton *et al.* (1997) – and there is merit in having the input of a veterinary pathologist, who can carry out supporting laboratory tests, in such work.

Improvements in diagnosis will follow when more data are available on the prevalence of various conditions. There is a particular need for information on free-living raptors and retrospective studies of *post-mortem* findings, such as those in red-tailed hawks over 18 years by Franson *et al.* (1996) and (over a comparable period) in great horned owls by Franson and Little (1996), are therefore very much needed.

Sudden death

A bird that dies suddenly, especially unexpectedly, can prove to be the cause of controversy, of dispute and sometimes of legal action. Very great care must therefore be taken in dealing with such cases. There is merit in having a *post-mortem* examination carried out by an experienced pathologist.

Forbes (in Beynon *et al.*, 1996) provided a useful Table of 'Causes of sudden death' and listed 13 such causes, ranging from hypocalcaemia and trauma to acute viral infections and tick toxicity. In some cases a careful gross *post-mortem* examination is usually adequate *per se* in order to reach a diagnosis – for instance, respiratory obstruction, egg-binding and gut prolapse – while in others, e.g. acute bacterial and *Caryospora* infections and cardiovascular disorders, supporting laboratory tests are needed. Identification of a few conditions, such as hypoglycaemia, are based largely on circumstantial evidence. Background history, especially if coupled with inspection of the location where death occurred, can prove invaluable – for example, in determining the likely cause of 'night fright'.

Species susceptibility may have to be taken into account when diagnosing the cause of death and may be relevant to legal proceedings. Thus, Northern goshawks appear to be particularly prone to hypocalcaemia, they and other accipiters to hypo-glycaemia and merlins to *Caryospora* infection.

Forensic examinations

Litigation involving birds of prey is becoming com-monplace and the veterinary clinician needs to be vigilant in order to reduce the risk of legal action or allegations of malpractice. Some advice on how this might be done was included in a special issue, on forensic veterinary medicine, of *Seminars in Avian and Exotic Medicine* (Cooper & Cooper, 1998). The veterinarian may also be involved in legal cases as an expert witness, on account of his/her specialist knowledge of birds of prey. In such cases it is particularly important that samples (from live or dead birds) are carefully selected, taken, trans-ported and stored. A 'chain of custody' is essential, perhaps particularly so where DNA evidence is concerned.

Whenever there is any suggestion that a case might go to court or be the subject of dispute, mate-rial should be stored and detailed contemporaneous notes compiled. Such notes may be required by the court in their original form.

Heidenreich (1997) provided a useful chapter on 'Forensics' which included data on age determina-tion and identification of birds of prey.

TREATMENT

Although treatment of particular conditions will be discussed in subsequent chapters, principles will be dealt with here. Throughout this book, the scien-tific names of drugs are used in preference to trade-names, which usually mean little to those working in other countries. Reference is only made to trade-names when no suitable chemical name is available or when a particular preparation is being recom-mended. Dosages of some drugs are given as a formulary in Appendix IX.

There are very few drugs licensed for birds and this means that one has usually to use an agent that has been developed primarily for the treatment of humans or domestic animals. In some countries, including the UK, a consent form may then be used,

by which the owner of the bird signs to say that he/she is aware of the situation and, in giving permission for the use of the unlicensed drug, accepts any attendant risks.

As with other species, treatment of raptors can be either (a) specific, or (b) non-specific (supportive or palliative). Specific treatment may be medical (by the use of medicinal agents ('drugs')) or surgical.

Only limited research has been performed on the metabolism of therapeutic agents in raptorial birds but this situation is changing as more studies emerge. There are still unanswered questions, many of which relate to the specialised anatomy and phys-iology of birds. For example, the metabolic rate of birds usually increases as bodyweight declines and this will influence (accelerate) the absorption, metabolism and elimination of many agents. This feature is particularly noticeable when using injectable anaesthetic agents such as ketamine: induction is far more rapid in an accipiter weighing 200 g than in an eagle of 3 kg.

Since body size can affect the rate at which drugs are absorbed, metabolised and excreted it is not strictly correct to give drug dosages for birds of prey in general in terms of mg/kg bodyweight. Kirkwood (1983) therefore recommended the use of the formula bodyweight$^{0.75}$ for the estimation of dose rate. The principle here is that smaller birds need relatively higher doses of drugs than their larger counterparts or the same dose repeated more frequently. Allometric scaling was discussed in more detail by Pokras *et al.* (1993) and the whole ques-tion of 'levels of metabolism' and how these influ-ence therapy by Dorrestein (1996) who pointed out that the formula reflects the relationship between metabolism and mass in the context of the surface area from which heat is lost.

Some drugs appear to be contra-indicated or excessively toxic in birds of prey. Research on the toxicity of gentamicin in great horned owls (Bauck & Haigh, 1984) showed that the response varies greatly, even within the one species. Reactions in owls receiving gentamicin ranged from death within 3 days to no clinical signs at any stage.

The high body temperature of small birds may influence the fate and efficacy of drugs; indeed, even in mammals, the question of the effect of a fever on drug absorption has been investigated (van Miert *et al.*, 1976). On the other hand, research on reptiles has indicated that they tend to maintain themselves at a higher temperature when infected with bacteria and this has led to suggestions that the development of a fever may play a beneficial role in recovery of mammals from infection. This subject was discussed in an editorial in *The Lancet* (Anon, 1977); although birds were not specifically mentioned, it is tempting to postulate that the higher body temperature of many species may be advantageous – as originally postulated nearly a century ago by Strouse (1909).

Administering medication

Oral administration of agents to raptors is commonly practised and in some cases can be efficacious. However, especially in smaller birds with a rapid gut passage time, absorption of, for example, antibiotics can be less than satisfactory. Early work by Williams Smith (1954) showed this to be the case in poultry – only low serum values were present following oral antibiotics – and subsequent work in other species has confirmed this.

When medication *is* to be given to birds of prey by mouth it must either be administered *per se* or be secreted in food. As a general rule birds of prey drink very little and therefore incorporation of a drug 'in the drinking water' is impracticable. Some falconers' birds will, especially if hooded, permit their beak to be opened and a tablet or capsule put in their mouth. Alternatively the drug can be hidden in a piece of meat or inside a dead chick or mouse – although it is possible that absorption may be impaired in the latter case. Certain liquid preparations can be injected into the prey while medical paediatric drops can be dropped into the bird's mouth while it is on the fist or if it is cast. Some of the latter preparations appear highly palatable and are readily taken by individual birds. Other agents may, however, prompt regurgitation (see Appendix IX).

Appendix IX provides a list (formulary) of medicinal agents that can be, or have been, used in birds of prey. Other examples and further information is to be found in Beynon *et al.* (1996), Heidenreich (1997), Huckabee (2000) and in earlier editions of this book. The appearance of more and more papers on pharmacokinetics – see, for example, the work by Robbins *et al.* (2000) on piperacillin and by Harrenstien *et al.* (1998) on enrofloxacin, in red-tailed hawks and great horned owls – makes the use of such agents less problematic.

From time to time it may be necessary to medicate a raptor without handling it – those in breeding aviaries or at hack in the case of 'captive' raptors, or even occasionally free-living birds – and here there are often problems of diagnosis as well as treatment. In such cases the appropriate drug is usually best hidden in an item of food and this offered to the bird after 24–48 hours' starvation. Careful observation may be advisable in case it is subsequently regurgitated.

If oral treatment has to be given forcibly the bird should be cast and the beak opened; the capsule should be pushed with a finger over the back of the tongue and down the oesophagus. Alternatively, for solutions and suspensions, a piece of rubber tubing (suitably lubricated) can be used as a stomach tube and passed down to the crop or (owls) lower oesophagus (Plate 12). Tiny raptors, such as pigmy falcons and little owls can be dosed with curved metal needles of the type used for psittacine birds or rodents, but care must always be taken.

Oral medication is generally given on an empty crop and stomach. However, some drugs are readily regurgitated in which case they should be administered after a *small* meal of lean meat.

The administration of drugs by injection is now standard but this was not always the case. Falconers were traditionally apprehensive about the use of injections and in the 1960s and early 1970s would still recount horrific stories of birds collapsing and dying after an injection. In other cases the hawk did not die but showed clinical signs of 'cramp'. Such effects were attributable, in my view, to the (now rare) administration of unsuitable drugs by this route – for example, use of procaine penicillin can result in tremors, incoordination and collapse. Nowadays there is far less concern about the use of the parenteral routes but the veterinary surgeon should still be careful to ensure that injections are given correctly, with the minimum of discomfort or tissue damage to the bird. As small a needle as possible should be used – if practicable, 25 or 26 gauge – and a small volume of drug. In the case of the latter, one must balance the need for a small volume with the dangers of inadvertent overdosage or local tissue damage if too concentrated a solution is used. Hygiene is important and the use of ethanol or methanol to dampen the feathers helps visibility as well as (probably) reducing numbers of pathogenic organisms.

The most frequently used injection routes remain the intramuscular, intravenous and subcutaneous. Intraperitoneal injections can pose problems and should usually be reserved for euthanasia; if they are to be given the needle should enter through the midline midway between the sternum and the cloaca to reduce the risk of entering an airsac.

Intraosseous injections have found favour in recent years for the administration of fluids (Dorrestein, 2000). The method is ideal for young birds, where there is ready access to the bone cavity but in older birds the technique is not always easy, and infection (osteomyelitis) can follow if the needle remains in place for too long. At least one company now sells specifically manufactured intraosseous needles for use in avian patients. Long-term administration of fluids or other agents may require the insertion of a cannula or, preferably, a 'vascular access port' (VAP) – a technique that has long been used in research but only recently applied to clinical cases (Orcutt, 2000).

For the intramuscular injection either the pectoral or leg (thigh) muscles should be used. I tend to favour the latter since the injections are often easier to give and do not present a hazard of impairing flight or of accidentally damaging delicate abdominal organs (Fig. 3.4). A hooded hawk on the fist can sometimes be given a small intramuscular injection into the leg without restraint, so long as only a 25 or 26 gauge needle is used.

It is always advisable to withdraw the plunger slightly before giving an intramuscular injection in order to help avoid inadvertently hitting a blood vessel.

Intravenous injections are best given into the basilic (brachial) vein and instructions for locating this vein were given earlier in this chapter. It is important to ensure that air is not given intravenously, although a few small bubbles appear to do no harm. In addition it must be remembered that, following removal of the needle, a subcutaneous haematoma will form; this can be minimised by applying moderate pressure with a swab immediately. Blood under the skin will gradually break down (during which time the area will become green in colour) and it should be possible to use the vein again after 72 hours.

Subcutaneous injections are used primarily for vaccines and fluid replacement. Any area of exposed skin can be used but suitable sites are the nape and the skin overlying the medial surfaces of the legs. Moistening of the skin with an alcoholic agent will greatly facilitate the technique as it clears the skin and permits visualisation of the injection – and of any immediate sequelae, such as haemorrhage.

Other routes of administration are intratracheal and nebulisation (Dorrestein, 2000), both of which are of value in the treatment of aspergillosis and other respiratory infections, and topical application of agents to skin, buccal cavity, cloaca or conjunctiva. Rees Davies (2000a) reviewed nebulisation and emphasised its value, using nebulised saline, as a means of rehydration.

Various so-called 'complementary and alternative' medicines and techniques are widely available in human medicine (The Royal Society, 1999) and some have been advocated for use in captive raptors. At least one osteopath treats birds in Britain and homeopathy has been reported to be useful in some cases by a number of bird keepers and rehabilitators and a few veterinarians (Roberts, 2000). Aviculturists also report using aromatherapy, herbalism, propolis, royal jelly, colloidal silver and Bach therapy with success in cage birds and some of these have been applied to raptors. I have no personal experience of these or other 'alternative' techniques – and must confess, with my conventional medical background, to being unclear as to why some of them might work – but I retain an open mind. The important point is that birds should not suffer unnecessarily: recourse to 'conventional' treatment should always be an option if there is no response. One has to remember that for centuries before the advent of modern techniques falconers' birds were treated using methods that included herbalism and there is anecdotal ('non evidence-based'!) indication that some of these proved successful. Arab falconers still follow such practices. One traditional method of treatment of infected wounds that I have tried, with apparent success, in birds is the application of honey – as used for centuries in humans and recently the subject of scientific study (Cooper, R. A. *et al.*, 1999).

Arab falconers have for long used traditional medicines to treat their birds (Allen, 1980) but in very few cases have these been scientifically assessed. Some can be dangerous – for example, ammonium chloride (Samour *et al.*, 1995) – while others, such as 'moomian' which I saw administered to many hawks in Qatar in 1981, appear to be harmless and may even have some beneficial effects.

Non-specific therapy consists of stabilisation (when the patient is first presented), the palliative (symptomatic) treatment of wounds and clinical signs, and nursing. Nursing is a key part of all treatment and goes hand-in-hand with specific (medical or surgical) therapy. It is discussed in more detail later in this chapter.

Stabilisation is a standard treatment regime for all incoming raptors. Forbes, in Beynon *et al.* (1996), advocated fluids, dexamethasone, iron dextran, B-vitamin complex, high calorific enteral preparation and enrofloxacin (or another antibiotic).

Emergency care

Emergency situations necessitate emergency treatment and Redig and Ackermann (2000) put forward four principal problems that occur frequently in raptors and warrant urgent attention: anorexia; low condition/anorexia; respiratory disease with dyspnoea; and nervous diseases. To these might be added life-threatening haemorrhage. A thorough clinical investigation of such cases is often contra-indicated because of the risk of jeopardising the patient's survival.

'Emergency care' is now a well developed disci-

pline in veterinary medicine and many of its features – body system evaluation, acute fluid therapy, pre-surgical stabilisation and respiratory support – are applicable also to birds of prey. A recent issue of *The Veterinary Clinics of North America* (Rupley, 1998) covered the subject in some detail. The critically sick raptor may be treated while conscious but sometimes light isoflurane anaesthesia can be beneficial, so long as this is administered with caution (and with nitrous oxide if available) since it minimises stress during evaluation and therapy.

Dyspnoea can be life-threatening and needs prompt attention. Handling should be minimised and the bird should never be placed on its back. Oxygen can be given by mask, in an anaesthetic chamber or via an air sac. Haemorrhage must be stopped by direct pressure or, in severe cases, by use of a tourniquet which must be released every 30 minutes.

Nursing

Nursing of birds is a practical subject that has made many advances in recent years. It is of the greatest importance in work with raptors, especially wild bird casualties. Basic guidance was given in *First Aid and Care of Wild Birds* (Cooper & Eley, 1979) and increasingly specific advice, as knowledge advanced, appeared in a number of papers or chapters of books – see for example, Cooper (1979a), Coles (1984), Redig (1996a) and Dorrestein (2000).

Nursing can be divided into five main areas, these being: (a) provision of warmth, (b) minimising stressors, (c) metabolic management, (d) analgesics and (e) monitoring. Each will be discussed briefly.

Provision of warmth

Provision of warmth is vital whenever a bird of prey is being treated. Being endothermic, a raptor will attempt to maintain its body temperature and if the ambient temperature is low it will expend a considerable amount of energy in so doing. As a result the bird may become hypoglycaemic and die. In addition, a low temperature may act as a stressor and precipitate shock. Methods of keeping a bird warm range from bringing it indoors from an outside aviary to wrapping it in a towel or the provision of heating in the form of a 'hospital cage' or a suitably wrapped hotwater bottle.

Heat loss can be significant during and after surgery and the maintenance of the bird's temperature at such time is crucial; this is discussed in Chapter 12.

Minimising stressors

Minimising stressors is an adjunct to any treatment and is particularly important when treating casualties. A bird that is regularly disturbed by noise or movement will be stressed and may also damage itself in attempts to move. With diurnal species it is often wiser to keep the patient hooded, or in a closed box or dark cupboard, except when treatment is being carried out. Cardboard boxes are very useful. A balance has to be maintained between reducing stressors and regular monitoring.

Metabolic management

Metabolic management can be further divided under the headings of fluids, electrolytes and nutrients.

Maintenance of fluid balance is important to counteract shock and should be considered particularly when a bird has suffered blood loss or shows clinical signs of diarrhoea or vomiting. Dehydration cannot be assessed clinically as easily in birds as it can in mammals – 'skin tenting', for example, is often not a reliable sign. Venous refill time (following compression) is often a better indicator; usually veins refill within 2 seconds. More marked dehydration will be indicated by dry mucous membranes and increased PCV.

Dextrose-saline (5% dextrose, 0.85% NaCl) probably remains the most straightforward method of replacing fluid. Preferably it should be used orally but it can be administered subcutaneously, intravenously or intraosseously at a dosage of up to 4% bodyweight daily. If used by injection, dextrose-saline *must* be sterile. In order to improve renal function and to help counter acidosis 2–4% lactated Ringer's solution can be given intravenously or subcutaneously. Other compounds can also be used in

fluid replacement and many of these may confer additional benefits as they contain amino acids or other nutrients.

An alternative technique under field conditions is to use an oral electrolyte mixture – a technique which has been found of value in human cholera patients and in domestic animals with 'scours'.

Rehydration can also be accomplished using nebulisation (Rees Davies, 2000a).

We still know relatively little about electrolytes and water balance in birds of prey with the exception of some experimental work – for example, on the red-tailed hawk by Johnson (1969). It is of interest to note that the nasal glands of raptors appear to play only a minor role in electrolyte balance, in contrast to the situation in some other species of bird.

Provision of nutrients is important for the same reasons described earlier, under provision of warmth. The sick raptor that does not feed will lose condition and a small bird, such as a sparrowhawk or merlin, may quickly reach a critical level at which it will die of hypoglycaemia or starvation. If a bird refuses to feed voluntarily then it may need to be tempted or forcefed. Tempting a bird to feed needs patience and experience and can include ruses such as a change of diet, offering attractive morsels of fresh meat or viscera and taunting the bird with the food so it opens its beak; the food can then be put inside and, with luck, will be swallowed.

Forcefeeding is usually not difficult. The bird's beak should be opened and a small moistened bolus of meat pushed over the tongue and down the oesophagus. It is always best to forcefeed 'little and often'; any attempt to fill a sick bird's crop with food in one session is likely to result in regurgitation. Birds with 'sour crop' should not be forcefed. Liquid food can be administered by oesophageal tube (Plate 12).

Analgesics

Analgesia is discussed in Chapter 12. In Chapter 3 Paolo Zucca urges that more attention should be paid to pain relief, especially when dealing with wild bird casualties. Apart from welfare considerations, a bird that is in pain will generally not fare well on account of anorexia, reluctance to move or secondary complications.

Monitoring

Monitoring of the sick raptor must be as unobtrusive as possible. As implied earlier, casualties in particular will react adversely to frequent disturbance. In such cases monitoring may need to be restricted to observation of behaviour and respiration rate.

Rehabilitation

Hand-in-hand with nursing is the emergency/first aid treatment of raptors that was covered earlier. Often, it is most important to nurse the bird, with supportive treatment, for the first 24–72 hours and to delay a definitive diagnosis until it has improved in condition.

Rehabilitation of sick/injured/displaced birds of prey is part of raptor medicine but has also developed into a discipline of its own in many parts of the world, (Cooper, 1987a) (Plate 13). It involves a wide range of people, apart from veterinarians, and can be very emotive. It, above all, raises the question of how much time and money should be devoted to care of the individual bird as opposed to the management of the species. Sometimes there is a conflict of interests – 'welfare versus conservation'. Euthanasia can be an important contribution to the cessation of suffering in a raptor but may not be acceptable to some people. Some people state that a casualty raptor should be treated only if it has a realistic opportunity of return to the wild (a legal obligation in some countries – see Appendix XI): others argue that retention of handicapped birds in captivity is justifiable for educational or research purposes. Each case has to be judged on its merits and various points need to be taken into consideration.

The majority of raptor casualties have traumatic injuries, mainly fractures. These are discussed in Chapters 3 and 5.

The second largest category of casualties are 'orphans' but a good proportion of these are not in specific need of human intervention and should probably either be left where they were found or be given some supportive care in the wild – for example, by placing them in a more secure site away from domestic predators or, possibly, by temporarily supplementing their diet.

Some casualties may be oiled (see Chapter 13), others poisoned (see Chapters 10 and 11) and some have an infectious disease (see Chapter 6). The last of these can pose a threat to other birds in a rescue/rehabilitation centre and may even present a zoonotic hazard if (for example) infected with *Mycobacterium avium*. Very careful thought has to be given to the desirability and wisdom of admitting and attempting to treat such birds: there are legal as well as practical considerations.

Literature on rehabilitation often provides sound advice to those who tend raptors and many of the techniques used, especially in terms of nursing, supporting care and rehabilitation (see below) are applicable to other birds of prey as well as to casualties.

Many apparently hopeless cases – both captive and free-living – recover because of dedicated care and attention by people who can devote time and patience to the bird. Under this heading are many veterinary nurses, falconers, aviculturists and zoo personnel. The staff of the better 'wild bird hospitals' and similar rehabilitation establishments are usually extremely proficient in the nursing care of wild birds and achieve impressive results in treatment. More birds could be saved and given the chance of a reasonable life in the wild or in captivity if supportive treatment was improved and this point will be emphasised in succeeding chapters.

Physiotherapy

Physiotherapy (usually termed 'physical therapy' in North America) can play a key part in treatment, especially the rehabilitation of injured wild birds. Martin *et al.* (1993) discussed the principles insofar as raptors are concerned (see also Chapter 5).

Therapeutic ultrasound is widely used in the physiotherapy of humans and, increasingly, of domestic mammals. Its role in birds needs careful evaluation, but Wimsatt *et al.* (2000) reported encouraging results when it was employed to prevent and to correct contractures associated with wing bandaging in pigeons.

Prevention of disease

The maxim that 'prevention is better than cure' is very true of diseases of captive birds of prey (Cooper, 1985c) and is immortalised in the words of Richard Blome (1686) – see Appendix VII. Prevention of non-infectious diseases is usually managemental. Thus, for example, careful mixing of birds of different sexes will minimise the risk of trauma in aviaries while not hooding a bird that is due to cast may prevent respiratory blockage. Measures can even be taken to protect free-living birds, for example, from injury by careful construction of power lines, from poisoning by correct disposal of chemicals.

Hygiene remains a key part of the prevention of most infectious disease and is discussed in more detail in Chapter 6. Redig and Ackermann (2000) emphasised the importance of using materials for mews and other accommodation that can be easily cleaned. Disinfectants are often forgotten in this age of potent antimicrobial agents (Payne *et al.*, 1998) but they – and hot water – still play a vital role in reducing numbers of pathogens (see Chapter 6). Autoclaving is the method of choice for sterilising surgical equipment but some items, such as endoscopes, must be disinfected using, for example, glutaraldehyde.

Exclusion of arthropod vectors is probably the best available way of preventing infection with blood parasites (Mutlow & Forbes, 2000) but presents practical problems, not least of all because netting designed to exclude *Culicoides* will also reduce air flow.

Zoonoses are, strictly, 'diseases and infections that can be naturally transmitted between vertebrate animals and man' (Cooper, 1990) but the term can be broadly used to cover any danger presented to humans from organisms or their products (e.g. toxins). The risks from raptors are probably rela-

tively few but prevention is prudent. As Redig and Ackermann (2000) stated, in the context of *Salmonella*: 'Proper sanitation and hygiene precautions are generally sufficient to prevent these and other infections with zoonotic potential.' I would expand this slightly, bearing in mind the increasing need to be wary of litigation, and argue that those keeping raptors in captivity or dealing with them in the wild should (a) be aware of the potential of zoonoses and the risks that these may present to themselves, staff and visitors, (b) always practise good hygiene and reduce unnecessary contact between humans and birds, especially if the former may be immunocompromised and/or the latter known or suspected to be infected (even if clinically normal) with potentially dangerous organisms, (c) encourage prophylactic measures for those who handle birds or their products e.g. immunisation against tetanus, and (d) develop professional links with the medical and veterinary professions and public health authorities so that appropriate protocols can be developed and followed. Kirkwood *et al.* (1994) pointed out that a zoonotic organism such as *Salmonella enteritidis* can easily proliferate and spread within a zoo or aviary environment and that 'cacheing' of food by birds of prey may contribute to such a build-up.

Concern over the excessive use of antibiotics, coupled with the fact that they do not always effectively eliminate pathogenic bacteria from the intestinal tract, has led to interest in the use of 'probiotics' in domestic animals and, to an increasing extent, in so-called exotic species. Probiotics usually contain species of lactobacilli and streptococci and are often recommended for young raptors (see Chapter 6). 'Competitive exclusion' is used in poultry in many countries of the world in order to control salmonellae. The principle is to provide newly hatched chicks with adult-type intestinal microflora *per os*, and these appear to prevent or to hinder colonisation by pathogenic bacteria: the technique is now being extended to the control of *Escherichia coli* 0157 and *Campylobacter jejuni* (Mead, 2000).

Vaccination (immunisation) of birds of prey has long been advocated as a means of preventing infectious disease (Cooper, 1975d) but is still only used for a very small number of conditions, sometimes with doubtful efficacy. Other approaches are discussed elsewhere in this book, including the use of sera and immunostimulants. Forbes and Fox (2000) working with *Caryospora* in merlins, suggested that allowing or creating infection in young birds and then treating them during the pre-patent period, might have promise as a means of producing uninfected but immune birds.

Non-infectious Diseases

'Violence done to parts is one of the causes of suppuration but . . . it must be a violence attended with . . . death in a part, such as in many bruises, mortification, sloughs . . .'

John Hunter

INTRODUCTION

The quotation above is a reminder that there is not always a clear-cut distinction between non-infectious and infectious causes of disease: one can lead to the other or the two may co-exist. It is, however, convenient to divide them and they are therefore covered here and in the next chapter.

Many non-infectious factors may cause or contribute to disease or death in birds of prey both in captivity and the wild. The most important categories are trauma, hypothermia, hyperthermia (including burns), electrocution and drowning. A review of such factors in wildlife, including birds, was included in my chapter (Cooper, 1996b) in *Non-infectious Diseases of Wildlife*. In that account I divided physical insults into (a) injuries caused by accidents, and (b) injuries caused by temperature changes, and emphasised the importance of investigating such incidents in a systematic way, including (in the case of free-living animals) standard procedures in terms of collecting population data, defining environmental variables, collecting samples and keeping records. Wobeser (1994) provided valuable background information on carrying out such techniques.

Genetic and developmental abnormalities and poisoning are other examples of non-infectious diseases: they are covered in Chapters 10 and 13.

TRAUMA

Traumatic injuries are a very common cause of disability or death in raptors (Samour, 2000a), and was well known to early falconers, for example Berners (1486) who recommended methods of treatment for hawks that have been wounded (Fig. 5.1). Trauma is characterised by local tissue damage followed by an inflammatory reaction. Systemic responses may include water and electrolyte disturbances, metabolic and endocrinological effects, thrombosis, embolism and infection.

Free-living birds may be shot, damaged by traps, struck by cars or fly into powerlines, buildings or windows. Such trauma was the reason for presentation of 63.1% of casualty birds in a 1-year study in Germany (Lierz, 2000). Physical injury, sometimes resulting in death, can also occur in free-living raptors as a result of their becoming entangled in materials such as wire or plastic containers. Ellis and Lish (1999) reported mortality in young birds of prey in Mongolia that was the result of the parents bringing rubbish ('trash') to build nests.

Some birds that survive these various accidents find their way into captivity as casualties, and trauma is generally considered to be the most common reason for free-living raptors to be found dead or submitted alive for treatment.

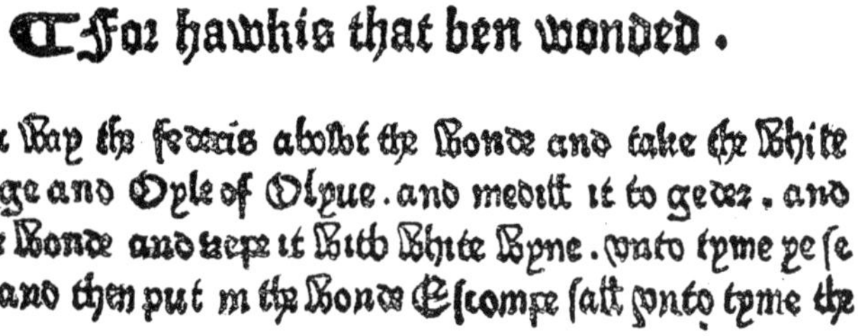

⟨Ⅎoɹ hawkis that ben wonded .

Ᵹake a Ꝑap the fᶜᵃᵗⁱˢ aboᵘt the Ꝃonde and take the ᵂhite of an ᶜgge and Ꝅple of Ꝅlyue . and medilt it to geᵗᵉᶻ . and anoynt the Ꝃonde and ᵏᵉᵖᶻ it ᵂith ᵂhite Ꝃyne . vnto tyme ye ſe ᵗᵉᶻ fleſh . and then put m the Ꝃonde ᶜ ſcompe ſalt ᵖⁿᵗⁱ tyme the

Fig. 5.1 Trauma was well recognised by early falconers as a cause of illness and death. Here a recipe is given for treating a hawk that is 'wonded' (wounded). From the *Boke of St Albans* (1486).

Road traffic accidents

Motor vehicles are an important cause of death in free-living raptors – for example, in a *post-mortem* survey of 67 barn owls in Britain, Cooper (1993b) found that 28 were either killed by, or had injuries associated with, such collisions. A comparable survey of barn owls in Hawaii showed trauma, mainly vehicular, to be the most common cause of death (Work & Hale, 1996). It should be stressed, however, that some birds may be struck by cars because, for example, they have an underlying infectious disease or are in poor condition or have deficient eyesight: the collision is the 'presumed' cause of death. Such birds are also more likely to be found and submitted for examination by the public than, for example, those that die in a forest following predation or a parasitic disease. At the time of writing, the Hawk and Owl Trust and the Mammal Society, both based in the UK, are co-ordinating a national survey of road casualties (Anon, 2000a).

Captive bird injuries

Captive raptors are also prone to injuries. Falconers' birds that are being flown can suffer a similar fate to their free-living counterparts: they may also damage their wings or keel when bating on to a hard surface, especially if they are in poor condition and can become tangled in jesses or leashes. Too long a leash can contribute to trauma as the bird may generate too much force when bating and thereby damage a limb. Young Harris' hawks in particular commonly fracture a tarsometatarsus. Twisted jesses can sometimes cause constrictions and ischaemia.

In zoological collections birds may hit or damage themselves on wire; alternatively, fighting may break out, with resultant injuries or death to a smaller or less aggressive individual (see Chapter 13). In breeding aviaries a number of physical mishaps can befall a raptor. Birds may strike a badly positioned perch or even become entangled in vegetation that is part of the 'natural' flora of the enclosure. The latter can be a particular danger to birds that already have an injury, such as a healed wing fracture, and are thus not easily able to extricate themselves. Captive raptors sometimes suffer 'night fright' due to disturbance by, for example, cats or fireworks and can fatally injure themselves as a result.

The distance *between* perches can be important. If perches are close the bird just jumps from one to another. If far apart the bird can fly between the two but has distance available to 'brake' before landing. If a medium distance apart the perches may not permit adequate 'braking' and so there is a hard landing that can cause damage, including bumblefoot (see Chapter 8).

Every effort should be made to prevent conflict between birds that are kept in captivity. Arent and Martell (1996) provided a useful table of raptor species that can be safely housed together and this was reproduced in Redig and Ackermann (2000). Commonsense must also prevail; a female goshawk that is hungry is very likely to kill a mate or a smaller bird of another species. Aggression between captive birds is not always fatal, however: puncture wounds and lacerations are common sequelae and these may become infected (see Chapters 6 and 8).

Predation

Predation is usually a cause of death but may result in injury if the prey escapes. Free-living birds of prey can be predated by a number of species, including other raptors. A bizarre example of predation reported in *The Daily Telegraph* 9 June 1999 was the osprey, ringed as a rare bird in Scotland, that was later swallowed by a crocodile in the Gambia – the ring was recovered from the stomach of its predator by a local fisherman.

Predation is an important cause of injury or death in both free-living and captive birds. The 'predators' involved can range from other raptors of the same or other species, such as the great horned owl in North America, to voracious social insects, such as safari ants (*Dorylus* sp.) in the tropics. Dogs and cats can injure birds of prey (although sometimes the role is reversed!) and humans can inflict similar damage intentionally or by accident. Falconers' and free-living birds may be injured or bitten by their quarry. Secondary infections following bites are common (Chapter 6). Snakebite is mentioned in Chapter 10.

Capture and transportation injuries

Damage to falconers' birds and wildlife casualties can also be inflicted during capture and in transit. The cere and talons are particularly vulnerable. Damage to the head may lead to epithelial proliferation and the result can be a hypertrophied cere and partly or totally occluded nares. Obstruction of the nares leads to respiratory embarrassment and there is distension of the soft tissues around the eyes as the bird breathes. The nares can be widened surgically (and this has been done traditionally by some Arabs 'to improve performance') but the nostrils may become obstructed again within a few weeks. Skeletal preparations have confirmed that birds with severe cere damage often also have underlying lesions (exostoses) in the skull.

Injuries during capture can be minimised by careful design and use of traps and nets: Clark (1981) described modifications to the Dho-Gaza that reduced entanglement (and thus the danger of damage) of birds caught by it.

Useful general advice on transporting casualty raptors was given by Olsen (1990) who emphasised (a) keeping the bird cool and quiet, and (b) preventing feather damage. Injuries associated with transportation may be markedly reduced by careful handling and packing by using well-designed carrying boxes. International Air Transport Association (IATA) Regulations (published annually) have helped to standardise containers for birds transported by air (see Appendix XI). Not all aspects of the IATA Regulations are universally accepted as desirable for raptors – for example, few falconers favour the provision of perches – but in general they are an important contribution to the welfare of birds in transit. The excellent chapter on transport in Mavrogordato's book *A Falcon in the Field* (1966) is still relevant today. Mavrogordato emphasised the advisability of not having perches nor absorbent material in a travelling box and recommended airholes low down and a hole in the roof for the insertion of food. Like him I remain a great believer in cardboard boxes for short journeys although I usually put newspaper on the floor: layers of this can be removed to reduce soiling (and examined for signs of abnormal mutes or castings!). For longer journeys, or as a permanent travelling container, a wooden box should be constructed. It is encouraging to note the quality of design of many of the carrying boxes that are now being produced commercially.

Transportation of an injured bird to a veterinary practice needs careful thought. In the case of a fractured wing there is merit in providing support, by using a cohesive bandage or by binding the wing to the bird, even (temporarily) in a stocking. When a leg is damaged, the bird should not be restrained: instead, it should be transported in a darkened box with a non-slippery floor.

Subdued light and hooding are useful aids to handling captive birds (see Chapter 4) and will reduce damage. Falconers' birds which are of nervous temperament need particularly careful management, and the use of padded perches, such as a rubber tyre, as a portable 'cadge', will help to reduce damage to wings.

Treatment of traumatic injuries

Traumatic injuries can involve soft tissues or the skeleton or a combination of both. Investigation and treatment are basically similar to that for other avian species but special care must be taken when restraining the patient in order to reduce injury to it or the handler. Light anaesthesia, with isoflurane for example, will prove invaluable. The patient must be stabilised and haemorrhage must be controlled (Dorrestein, 2000). Fresh wounds must be cleaned, irrigated and disinfected. Wound closure may or may not be necessary as is the application of dressings and bandages. Degernes and Redig (1993) reviewed wound healing in raptors and described in detail methods of assessment and treatment of wounds in birds. A useful flow chart depicting wound management was provided by Redig (1996b). An understanding of how wounds heal is important to both diagnosis and prognosis. As in mammals, wound healing may be retarded by various endogenous and exogenous factors, including protein and other deficiencies, hormonal disorders, infection and the development of chronic inflammation.

Treatment of injuries is but one part of attention to diseases, non-infectious or infectious, that affect the limbs. This work requires a sound knowledge of anatomy and also an understanding of how tissues heal and the factors that may enhance or retard such important processes as epithelialisation, callus formation, axonal regeneration and the proliferation of muscle fibres, blood vessels and serous membranes.

A scientific and systematic approach characterises the CD-ROM produced by Nigel Harcourt-Brown (2000). It is an excellent aid to surgery and management of pelvic limb ('leg and foot') diseases. The work is based on dissections of peregrines and goshawks and as a result provides a typographical illustration of every region for the two species. Orthopaedic and integumentary disease are described, as are conditions involving (for example) displacement of tendons. Other valuable texts providing information on radiographic and surgical anatomy are the books by Krautwald *et al.* (1992), Orosz *et al.* (1992) and Smith and Smith (1992). Kostka (1992) carried out a comparative radiographic study of four species of bird, one the common buzzard and related this to anatomy, physiology and pathology.

Feather damage is covered in Chapter 13 and the treatment of maggot-infested wounds in Chapter 6. 'Night fright', due to disturbance in the dark, can

be a differential diagnosis for sudden death (see Chapter 4).

Gunshot wounds can pose problems. Radiography is important in ascertaining where shot is lodged and one must usually give a guarded prognosis initially in view of the possibility of internal damage. Shot wounds should be thoroughly cleaned but it is not usually necessary to remove the shot pellet or bullet unless this is likely to hamper healing or, by virtue of its position (e.g. in the skull) produce specific clinical signs.

If a talon is torn out it is usually best to dress the wound for 2 weeks as well as applying a disinfecting agent. Plastic nail covering, produced for dogs and cats, can be applied: this either falls off when the talon has healed or can be removed. Skin wounds can be sutured using a variety of materials or allowed to heal by second intention (granulation), in which case care must be taken to avoid secondary infection. Dressings for wounds on the body can, if necessary, be sutured into place.

Injured birds should be kept warm, should receive fluids and electrolytes (see Chapter 4) and be forcefed if necessary. Careful monitoring is vital: as pointed out at the beginning of this section, local trauma may be followed by a variety of systemic disturbances.

Soft tissue injuries

Soft tissue injuries can be superficial – erosions or ulcerations – or deep, involving connective tissue, muscles, tendons, nerves or internal organs (viscera). The effect of such injuries is related to the site, not just the severity, of the wound. Thus, damage to the patagium may be only superficial in terms of tissue damage but serious insofar as flight is concerned. Similarly, a relatively minor fracture near a joint may affect flexion or extension, and thus be the cause of traumatic injury elsewhere (Fig. 5.2a,b).

Subcutaneous emphysema is sometimes seen, both in free-living birds and in young captive-bred falcons. Studies on pigeons, in which the condition is common, confirm that air in such cases originates from a damaged air sac. It can be removed, aseptically, with a needle and syringe, repeating the

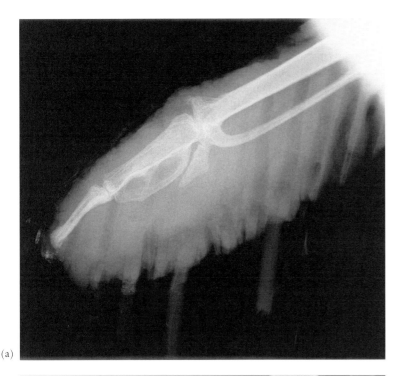

(a)

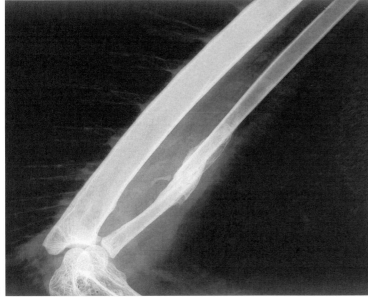

(b)

Fig. 5.2 Radiographs of the wing of a golden eagle: (a) pronounced soft tissue reaction and carpal damage due to trauma; (b) the cause of the above – a fracture near the joint which was associated with inflammation that restricted flexion and thus permitted the wing to droop. Radio-opaque urates are also visible in (a) at the tip of the wing. Some of the feathers are 'in blood': vascular sheaths are visible.

procedure as necessary or using a small radiosurgical incision that will remain open for longer. Many cases resolve naturally, if left alone (and so long as the emphysema is not causing interference to the bird).

Superficial injuries may be associated with haemorrhage and bruising. The presence of green-coloured tissue around a wound is usually indicative of bruising – at least 72 hours beforehand – but the possibility of infection (for example with a *Pseudomonas* sp.) must not be ignored.

Any injury is liable to become infected, as Hunter's quotation reminds us: a breach in the integument serves as a portal of entry for bacteria and occasionally other micro-organisms (see Chapter 6), as well as dipterous larvae (myiasis).

Skeletal injuries

Skeletal damage of various types can occur as a result of trauma. Fractures are particularly common and can occur in both free-living and captive raptors, although those in the latter category usually involve falconers' birds that are either being flown or are newly tethered – fractured tibiotarsi are prevalent in the latter, especially if the owner is inexperienced in the management of a trained bird or, perhaps, are associated with a calcium deficiency.

Most fractures of birds of prey involve the wings (thoracic limbs) or legs (pelvic limb). The long bones that make up these limbs are strong but light-weight with thin cortices. Some limb bones may be pneumatised (Fig. 5.3). Wing injuries of raptors were reviewed by Simpson (1996) and foot and leg injuries by Harcourt-Brown (1996b).

Fractures in raptors can be classified as in other animals: simple, greenstick, comminuted or compound. Most are traumatic in origin – and thus form the basis of this chapter – but it must be remembered that metabolic bone disease, infection and neoplasia can also be causes.

In some cases of fracture, euthanasia is the preferred or only option. In many others repair can be considered, but much depends upon the species of bird, its status (free-living or captive) and the likelihood of full recovery. Each case should be judged on its merits, with strong emphasis on the welfare of the individual bird.

Many factors have to be taken into account when assessing fractures of raptors. Often they are comminuted or compound. Those in casualty wild birds may have occurred several days earlier and as a result there are already complications – infection, dead or dying bone, a dehydrated and malnourished patient. In some cases bone healing may already have commenced, often with incorrect alignment. Callus formation is rapid in birds, especially those that are small and have a high metabolic rate and in this context it is worthy of note that in 1855 Salvin and Brodrick discussed the treatment of fractures in hawks and stated that a splint may be removed 'after

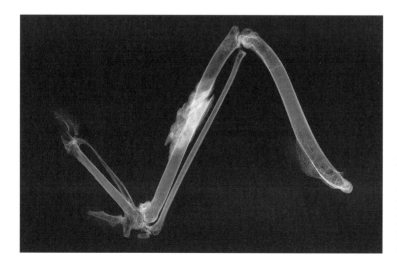

Fig. 5.3 In legal cases it is often wise to prepare bones and to radiograph them. This sparrow-hawk shows a healing fracture of the radius which has been effectively splinted by the intact ulna. The pneumatisation of the humerus can be seen.

about three weeks' time . . . when the limb will be found straight and sound again'.

Assessment of birds with fractures must be thorough. Often it is wise to delay detailed investigations (and certainly surgery) until the bird has been stabilised. Support of injured limbs may or may not be feasible. Subdued lighting and confined space will often help, especially with casualties. First aid attention may be needed, such as control of haemorrhage, and supportive therapy, including antibiotics if infection is suspected, can be important.

Fractures are common in raptors. A useful review of fractures seen in Europe was by Baumgartner *et al.* (1994). Studies by Schuster (1996) on frequency, localisation and type of fractures in birds showed that of fractures of the pectoral girdle those involving the coracoid were the most prevalent.

Fractures may be treated by external or internal methods or by a combination of these. As Patrick Redig pointed out in 2000, most techniques used in mammals have been tried in birds. Redig stressed that the goals in raptor orthopaedics are to utilise fixation so that (a) it does not rely on coaption, (b) undue morbidity is avoided – especially impairment of joint integrity, and (c) the fixation device can be totally removed after clinical union. He added the need for the technique to be 'relatively inexpensive' – particularly important when working with casualties or in poorer parts of the world.

External methods can be divided into (a) external coaptation (bandages and splints), and (b) external fixation (fixation pins). Bandages and splints are simple and cheap and much favoured by rehabilitors and by those working in poorer locations. They work well where the adjacent bone is intact and acts as a natural splint, e.g. in midshaft radius or ulna. They also provide temporary support when, for example, the bird is being transported. In the context of pelvic limb fractures, however, Harcourt-Brown (1996b) described the splint as 'usually the most inappropriate method of repair', giving as exceptions tarso-metatarsal fractures and those of the phalanges. Like bandaging, splints can cause contractures, reduced joint mobility and even bone loss. External fixators are far preferable in most cases; the principles were listed by Simpson (1996b).

Internal fixation has for long been a popular method of fracture repair in birds, and good results by pinning, wiring and sometimes (larger birds) plating have been reported by many authors. The use of such techniques in raptors is similar to that in other species and will not be discussed in detail; Harcourt-Brown (1996b) and Simpson (1996) describe them well.

Patrick Redig has made a particular study of the repair of fractures in birds of prey, and over 20 years ago, at the Conference on Bird of Prey Management, presented preliminary results (Redig, 1977). In that early paper he drew attention to the different prognosis (in terms of complete recovery) for fractures, depending upon (a) their position (for example a proximal radial fracture carries a good prognosis if treated within 5 days, while the prognosis for a distal fracture of the same bone is only fair), and (b) the bones involved (metacarpal fractures carry a poor prognosis whereas humeral fractures are usually excellent or good). These points remain valid.

Redig also emphasised that surgical treatment of fractures *must* be carried out early (within 5 days) if optimum results are to be obtained. This in no way contradicts my own point (earlier) that heroic surgery should not be embarked upon before the bird's condition has stabilised (Cooper, 1975a). An initial delay of 36–72 hours, during which time the bird is stabilised and nursed, is invaluable; thereafter surgery should be undertaken promptly.

Specific fractures need specific treatment and again these cannot be covered in detail here. In the case of the wings the categories are straightforward – fractures of the humerus, radius–ulna and carpometatarsus. Harcourt-Brown listed those of the pelvic limb as pelvis and synsacrum, femur, tibiotarsus (and fibula), tarso-metatarsus and digits. Some fractures present particular problems: for example, Grifols (2000) described the successful repair of a mandibular fracture with a 3.9 cm defect in a bearded vulture using a bone graft and external fixation device.

Bone repair is a combination of vascular and cellular processes, leading to the formation of bone and cartilage. For union to be satisfactory, positioning of bone ends must be adequate but, in addition, the bird needs to be in good metabolic and nutritional health.

If a bird is to be released or to be flown for falconry, it should be able to use its feet or wings properly but in captive-breeding establishments and zoological collections this may not be so important and therefore partial success in treatment may be acceptable. Indeed, in some cases, it may be considered best to amputate the distal portion of a limb, especially if a wing hangs down and becomes soiled or if a foot is only an encumbrance. Amputation can be justifiable; some birds treated thus can live for many years in captivity, appear to thrive and sometimes breed. They can be important as educational aids, especially if the original injury was caused by humans. Thus, one tawny eagle that I treated in Tanzania lived in a zoological collection for nearly 20 years with only one foot.

The amputation of a whole limb can prove successful – an early account of such an operation on a wing was given by Holt (1977) but restriction of activity can result. The use of prosthetic limbs may prove of practical use, especially to aid mobility or copulation of valuable breeding birds. Such techniques are not new; the fitting of an artificial limb to a sea eagle was recorded in *The Times* of 17 May 1965 and as long ago as 1664 John Evelyn, the diarist, recorded seeing in London a captive crane 'having hadd one of his leggs broken, and cut off above the knee, had a wooden or boxen leg and thigh with a joint so accurately made that the creature could walke as if it had been natural.'!

The whole question of amputation has to be judged on a case-by-case basis. As a general rule, amputation of the foot is likely to prove less of a problem in a (captive) accipiter than a falcon – where bumblefoot of the other foot often supervenes.

Severely damaged digits or talons can be amputated: even falconers' birds can thrive surprisingly well with such a handicap but loss of digit I can produce problems because of the need to grip. Amputation may also be necessary on account of frostbite (see later) or because a constriction on the leg (for example, injury by a trap or aviary netting) severely damages the tissues and results in a swollen, insensitive, foot that gradually becomes ischaemic and develops dry gangrene. A more cautious approach has to be taken with casualty birds intended for release: a full assessment is needed before committing such cases to a life in the wild (Cooper *et al.*, 1980).

As an alternative to amputation, the trailing tip of a wing may be remedied by surgical patagiectomy (Robinson, 1975). This technique involves the removal of a piece of patagial membrane and is described in Chapter 10. The patagium (propatagium) itself may be easily injured and this can affect flight. Simpson (1996) provided valuable advice on how to treat these and stressed that they should always be corrected with the wing in an extended position.

All of the above procedures carry responsibilities for the welfare of the bird and there are occasions when it is clearly unethical to amputate, and euthanasia must be the preferred option.

Whilst a number of cases of lameness or impaired use of the wing are attributable to a fracture or luxation, a percentage show no skeletal abnormalities on radiography, and soft tissue damage either can be diagnosed or must be assumed. In some instances there is history of an injury, for example a falconer's bird bating or being damaged by its quarry, and the clinical picture may resemble a 'sprain'. The affected area is swollen, warm and painful. It usually heals spontaneously within 14 days and treatment, other than rest and possibly analgesia, is of little value. Nerve damage also occurs from time to time, again usually following trauma. In some cases one can elicit pain on palpation but in others nothing can be detected and treatment must be palliative, with good feeding and rest in a suitable cage or room. It may be necessary to bind an affected wing to the body to prevent it from hanging. Such conditions usually recover spontaneously within 3 weeks.

In the case of nerve damage to the legs, use of the limb or digit is impaired and there is usually flaccidity. Sometimes the foot 'knuckles over' and the dorsal surfaces of the digits become abraded. There is sometimes, but not always, lack of sensation. My approach to such cases (see Chapter 9) has in the past been to provide supportive treatment (for example, by protecting the digits or padding the perch) and to wait 3 weeks; if after this time there is no improvement I assume the condition is irreversible. Now surgery to tendons may be feasible.

Another situation that can give rise to lameness or incapacity of the feet is 'surgery' of bumblefoot by lay persons. A common sequel to this is damage to the nerves (or the tendons themselves) supplying the digital flexors; as a result the bird cannot flex the digit or digits. The talon on a paralysed digit usually does not become worn and must be clipped frequently. Tendon repair here and elsewhere is possible (Harcourt-Brown, 2000a,b) but in some cases another muscle may duplicate the action and therefore minor flexor or intrinsic muscle tendons can usually be treated conservatively. Harcourt-Brown pointed out that lack of surgical access to the plantar canal can prevent tendon repair at the metatarsophalangeal junction – a common site of injury.

Birds of prey may dislocate a phalanx. These cases are usually due to trauma, especially in the early stages of training a hawk. If there is no ligament damage the luxation can be corrected under light anaesthesia. Torn ligaments can be sutured.

Dislocation of other joints may also occur. That of the vertebral synsacral joint will cause paralysis (see Chapter 9). Luxations of hip, femorotibial and intertarsal joints can be repaired surgically (Harcourt-Brown, 1996b,c) as can those of shoulder and elbow. Some cases recover spontaneously but most require reduction, often together with immobilisation of the joint by plastering or bandaging. Reduction of a dislocation should be carried out within 72 hours; if there is delay, irreversible damage may occur.

Anaesthesia appropriate for the surgical repair of fractures and other orthopaedic procedures is discussed in more detail in Chapter 10.

Arthritis

Arthritis may follow a traumatic injury or infection. Investigation of possible cases of arthritis should include tests of function. The joint must be fully flexed and extended and the angle of extension compared with the 'normal' limb. The degree of freedom of movement of the joint is also important. Chronic arthritis may result in a thickened joint but often no other abnormalities are visible. In acute cases, however, the swollen joint is usually also painful and warm to the touch. Pus can sometimes be aspirated but bacteriological culture may prove negative.

Early cases of arthritis appear to respond to appropriate antibiotics and to non-steroidal anti-inflammatory agents but when longstanding, for example following chronic 'bumblefoot' (see Chapter 8), when there is likely to be lysis of bone, they are usually incurable. In one instance, concerning a lagger, arthritis and ankylosis of the distal phalangeal joint had resulted in a 'fixed digit' with the permanently erect talon an encumbrance to both bird and handler. The talon was amputated with good results and the bird was subsequently used successfully for falconry.

Skeletal deformities may be attributable to mycoplasmosis, as postulated by Erdélyi *et al.* (1999) – see Chapter 6. Other infectious causes, such as mycobacteriosis, may also need to be considered in differential diagnosis.

Other skeletal conditions

Other orthopaedic conditions that may be encountered from time to time include non-union of fractures with 'false joint' formation, and osteomyelitis (Cooper & Kreel, 1976). In neither case is the prognosis good and the latter in particular may necessitate amputation. John Hunter (1728–1793), who is quoted at the beginning of this chapter, reported non-union of a fracture in a golden eagle, and the specimen is held in the Hunterian Museum of the Royal College of Surgeons of England. I have also encountered a case of bilateral degenerative disease of the heads of the humeri in a kestrel; clinically both wings drooped and if the bird fell on to its back it could not right itself. The aetiology was not determined.

Articular gout, which should be distinguished from visceral gout (Siller, 1981), can cause painful swellings, especially on the feet. Urate deposits can be removed surgically.

Rehabilitation and release

When a bird is recovering from an injury exercise is important (see also 'Physiotherapy' in Chapter 4). Holz and Naisbitt (2000) compared the weights of Australian goshawks that had and had not been exercised prior to release. They suggested that exercise is an important part of any rehabilitation programme. Judicious design of an aviary, with perches at different heights and variable distances apart, will help to achieve this, as will 'flying lessons' with the bird flown to a lure or tethered on a line. Many such techniques are used in the pre-release conditioning of casualty birds and reference can usefully be made to papers such as that by Snelling (1975) and to those mentioned below.

If captive or casualty birds are intended for release it is important to ensure that a skeletal or soft tissue injury has healed satisfactorily. Originally my approach with wing injuries was to insist that there should be no impairment of function nor change in anatomy before a bird could be returned to the wild. However, a number of veterinarians and rehabilitors have records of birds surviving (and in some cases breeding) in the wild following release with healed fractures where either the alignment was poor or the movement of the joint was impaired. Much, of course, depends upon the species and the locality into which it is released but the belief of some colleagues, such as Brian Coles (pers. comm), is that most birds probably have 'reserve powers' and are able to compensate for any relatively minor deficiency in wing (or leg) function. Coles substantiates this by reference to free-living birds (including some raptors) found with badly healed fractures which had apparently been able both to recover and, subsequently, to survive in the wild. However, a recent paper on American kestrels (Murza *et al.*, 2000) showed that handicapped (male) birds may be less inclined to attack potentially dangerous prey, suggesting that even minor residual injuries may have an adverse effect on success in the wild. Injuries to the eyes and to digits may have an even more significant effect on survival.

Rehabilitation of casualty birds of prey is now a subject in its own right and is practised in many parts of the world (Plate 13). A whole volume of literature is available, some of which is complementary to work on captive or free-living raptors. Csermely (2000) and Martell *et al.* (2000) drew attention to the paucity of literature on the release and survival of birds of prey and presented data. It is encouraging to note studies on the ability of released birds to hunt and to survive, as there are important welfare considerations in rehabilitation (Bennett & Routh, 2000).

Assessment of the health of birds prior to release has attracted much attention in recent years. Guidelines were propounded by Cooper *et al.* (1980) and these have since been refined and improved.

HYPOTHERMIA AND HYPERTHERMIA

The response of birds of prey to changes in temperature is of considerable ecological interest; a useful early review was that by Mosher (1976). In temperate climates birds are more likely to be exposed to low temperatures than to high.

It is probable that species differ in their tolerance to cold; this was shown many years ago in snowy owls which have a lower critical temperature than other owls (Scholander *et al.*, 1950). Birds from warmer climates seem to be more susceptible to wing tip oedema (WTO) (Simpson, 1996) (see Chapter 13).

It must also be remembered that a young raptor is usually less able to maintain its body temperature than is an adult, and that certain drugs, particularly anaesthetic agents, will lower a bird's temperature and render it susceptible to the effects of cold.

Hypothermia

A drop in temperature *per se* need not prove dangerous to a bird of prey but it can serve as a stressor and may potentiate hypoglycaemia. Young (nestling) birds are particularly susceptible (see Chapter 13) and may die following fairly non-specific signs of lethargy, fluffed-up plumage and reduction in food intake. An unacclimatised tropical bird can react adversely to low temperature and may develop clinical signs as a sequel. Heidenreich

(1997) provided temperature tolerance guidelines while Redig and Ackermann (2000) listed species that, in their experience, should have supplemental heat when the ambient temperature drops below 0°C. Some birds of prey, however, such as the snowy owl, which shows anatomical and physiological adaptations to cold, is likely to be more adversely affected by hot sunshine than by a drop in temperature.

Cold weather can have an adverse effect on free-living birds. It can kill them directly but is more likely to affect feeding – and, indeed, to result in a need for more food more often. Cold weather can also influence reproductive success (Dawson & Bartolotti, 2000) and, perhaps, have a similar effect to that of wearing radiotransmitters, as suggested from work on eagles (Marzluff *et al.*, 1997).

Any bird that has become chilled should be warmed gradually to a temperature of 35°C. It should be given fluids and nutrients. Frostbite damage needs topical treatment and may necessitate amputation.

Although the importance of good ventilation has been emphasised elsewhere, it should not be forgotten that exposure to wind can be deleterious, especially to a falconer's bird on a block or ring-perch. Birds show obvious dislike of a strong wind and exposure to it may predispose to disease – air sacculitis, for example. It will also result in heat loss and a subsequent increase in food consumption and this must be borne in mind when small birds that are being kept for falconry are exposed to such weather. Very often a slight change in management will help to reduce the risk – for example, the provision of better shelter around a weathering ground.

Frostbite has been reported in many avian species. Affected birds show ischaemia and necrosis of digits, which may later slough: some cases develop heart lesions. Frostbite can occur in captive raptors when exposed to very low temperatures or when there is a 'chill factor' such as a cold prevailing wind (see below). Wing tip oedema (WTO) may be a manifestation of frostbite (see Chapter 13).

A combination of wet and cold can rapidly prove fatal to a captive bird of prey. A falconer's bird in particular may become soaked if exposed on a perch in heavy rain or if it plunges into a pond or river during a flight. As a result the plumage becomes water-logged and the bird's insulation disappears. The bird appears hunched and stiff and may even show signs of incoordination. The cloacal temperature drops to 35°C or less. Treatment is entirely palliative; the bird should be warmed and the plumage dried with a towel, fan heater or hair drier. Under no circumstances should the bird be exposed to low temperatures again until it has fully recovered – preferably not for 24 hours. Wing tip oedema appears to be related to low temperatures and is discussed in Chapter 13.

Hyperthermia

Although many birds of prey can withstand high temperatures for short periods, they do not in general like excessive heat and will try to avoid it. Overheating can occur in the tropics and, occasionally, in temperate climates. Birds being flown for falconry are especially susceptible. In confinement a raptor may become overheated on account of poor design of an aviary, because it comes into too close contact with an infra-red heater or light bulb in a 'hospital cage' or if it is left in a car on a hot day without adequate ventilation or cooling. Eggs and nestlings can easily become overheated and die if an aviary is poorly designed, especially if plastic or PVC sheeting is used. The provision of shade is always important but especially so for such species as gyrfalcons and snowy owls, that are heat-sensitive.

The response of birds of prey to hot environments was discussed by Mosher (1976) who drew attention to the efficiency of panting as a method of heat dissipation so long as the bird can replace its lost water and maintain blood gas concentrations. Mosher also referred to the work of Bartholomew and Cade (1957) who demonstrated a countercurrent system in the tarsus of American kestrels which presumably plays a part in withstanding high ambient temperatures. Calder and Schmidt-Nielsen (1968) investigated panting and blood carbon dioxide values in birds, amongst them a turkey vulture, and discussed the subject of heat stress.

An overheated bird will pant, let its wings hang loosely and partly close its eyes. It will tend to seek a cool or sheltered place. In more severe cases there is prostration and a degree of hyperthermia detectable to the touch, dehydration may be apparent and the tongue and buccal mucous membranes are usually dry and discoloured (yellowish-brown) in appearance. Cutaneous erythema and other skin lesions may be present if burning has occurred and cardiovascular failure ('shock') can be a sequel.

Treatment of the affected bird must be prompt. It should be moved to a sheltered place and slowly cooled, if necessary using a cool damp cloth on the head, feet and underside of the wings. Fluids can be given and skin lesions should be treated topically. I have personally treated only a few cases of overheating, mainly in the tropics. Most cases have responded quickly to a cool environment and oral and parenteral saline.

Heat stress has been shown to cause eggshell thinning in poultry (Premovich & Chiasson, 1976) and should be considered in differential diagnosis when birds in aviaries in hot areas – or perhaps free-living birds in disturbed habitats – produce abnormally thin eggs.

BURNING AND ELECTROCUTION

Both captive and free-living raptors may become burned or electrocuted. In the case of captive birds this usually occurs if they come into contact with electric heaters or, if being flown, powerlines. Free-living birds may be burnt in vegetation fires, especially if nesting. Burning may be accompanied by the inhalation of toxic fumes (see Chapter 10). Electrocution of raptors on high voltage powerlines is common in some parts of the world, including Europe and Africa. Haas (1993) described treatment methods and ways of minimising such threats.

Often the only clinical signs visible are charred feathers but close examination will reveal skin burns of varying severity and haemorrhages. These lesions will be painful and the bird may show dehydration; shock is a common sequel. As Dorrestein (2000) stressed, birds with extensive or severe burns need emergency attention. Treatment consists of nursing, especially the maintenance of body temperature and administration of fluids, and the topical treatment of the burns. Antibiotics and corticosteroids will help

to prevent infection and counteract shock. If more than 50% of the body surface is burned, the prognosis is usually poor.

Post-mortem examination of birds that have been burned or electrocuted will show internal lesions in addition to those described above. There may be free blood in the internal organs and this may be dark and unclotted in appearance. Petechial haemorrhages and discoloration are seen in muscles. Inhaled particles may be found in the respiratory tract. In the case of electrocution the distribution of lesions depends upon the path the current took; careful dissection is necessary and the bird should be skinned.

Characteristic changes have been detected using scanning electronmicroscopy in the feathers of birds

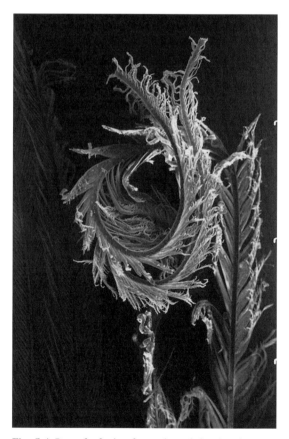

Fig. 5.4 Part of a feather from a kestrel showing damage due to burning. There is twisting and contraction of barbs and barbules (SEM × 105).

that have been burned or electrocuted (Cooper *et al.*, 1989). The former, for example, produces a curling and distortion of barbs and barbules (Fig. 5.4).

Current concern over vegetation fires (WHO 2000a,b) may result in a decrease in burning incidents in birds as well as in other animals and humans. An important step in the reduction of electrocution deaths in free-living birds, which will also apply to those flown by falconers, is the modification of design of powerlines to minimise the chances of a bird electrocuting itself.

DROWNING

Raptors may drown in the wild in water troughs, less frequently in reservoirs and lakes. In captivity drowning occurs if an aviary has an unsuitable waterbowl or if, due to some disability or entanglement in a leash, a bird is unable to extricate itself.

Free-living birds of prey may be attracted to water by potential prey species (Craig & Powers, 1976). In other instances the underlying cause for a high prevalence of drowning incidents is less clear (Shawyer, 1987; Cooper, 1993b).

In most cases the bird is dead before it is found – at *post-mortem* examination the plumage is waterlogged (or matted, if it has dried) and there is fluid and inhaled debris in lungs and air sacs. Petechial haemorrhages may be seen.

In the unlikely event of a bird being found that is still alive, it should be treated by physically removing fluid from the respiratory tract – by holding it upside down, with beak open – and artificial respiration should be applied. The administration of oxygen may help.

IRRADIATION

I have no specific information on the effects of ionising radiation on birds of prey. It is reasonable to assume that excess exposure is undesirable and therefore use of radiography or radiotherapy should be restricted whenever possible. It is of interest to note that in work on total body X-ray irradiation in the budgerigar (*Melopsittacus undulatus*) – one of the few publications not dealing with poultry – birds that died following irradiation were found to have a luxuriant growth of an *Aspergillus* sp. in the lungs (Schlumberger & Henschke, 1956).

Information on effects of radiation on free-living raptors may result from studies in Chernobyl, scene of the world's worst civil nuclear power accident (in 1986), where scientists at the International Radioecology Laboratory are studying the effects of the radioactivity release on the environment. Amongst the 180 species of bird living and breeding in the Chernobyl exclusion zone are common kestrels (Bonham *et al.*, 2000).

ELECTRIC AND MAGNETIC FIELDS (EMFs)

Again, little information is available, but Fernie (1998) studied the effects of electric and magnetic fields on selected physiological and reproductive parameters of American kestrels and was able to show suppression of plasma melatonin in some birds and some changes in behaviour as well as reproductive success. Fernie concluded that American kestrels perceive EMFs as light and therefore alter their photoperiod: males may be more sensitive than females. The findings may be relevant to birds that nest under transmission lines that generate EMFs.

Infectious Diseases, excluding Macroparasites

'When meditating over a disease, I never think of finding a remedy for it, but, instead, a means of preventing it.'

Louis Pasteur

INTRODUCTION

Under this heading are those diseases of raptors caused by, or associated with, such infectious agents as viruses, chlamydiae (chlamydophilae), mycoplasmas, bacteria and fungi. Biologists now tend to call these (together with protozoa) 'microparasites' (see Appendix VII) and that term will sometimes be used in this chapter. Protozoan and metazoan parasites ('macroparasites') are, however, covered in Chapter 7 and some specific aspects of infectious disease elsewhere – for example, arthritis in Chapter 5, pododermatitis (bumblefoot) in Chapter 8 and 'emerging' diseases in Chapter 13.

Host–parasite relations are an all-important consideration in studies on the health of birds (see Chapter 14 and Appendix VII) and there has been much published on this in recent years (May & Anderson, 1978; Hamilton & Zuk, 1982; Cooper, 1989a,b). Although this has largely been orientated towards free-living birds, the findings are relevant also to captivity and can often help to explain the appearance/disappearance of infectious agents and the phenomenon of 'emerging diseases' and may even assist in formulating control measures. An important practical point, not always recognised by lay people, is that the presence of an organism in or on a bird, even if it is a potential pathogen, does not necessarily equate with disease. Nor does the presence of antibody.

In the case of 'microparasites', the host reaction includes the ability of the bird to mount an immune response, which may have both a humoral and a cellular component: this in turn can be influenced by such factors as intercurrent disease and nutritional status (Appleby *et al.*, 1999). Immune responses are discussed in more detail in Chapter 13. The apparent ability of birds to resist infection is commented upon in various places in this book. The (usually) high body temperature may play a part, as might the tendency of birds (and reptiles) to prevent the spread of pathogens by entrapping them in fibrin (Huchzermeyer & Cooper, 2000).

Infectious diseases are common causes of disease and death in raptors (Cooper, 1993e; Samour, 2000a) and a few authors have ranked them as being even more important than trauma. In an evaluation of 917 autopsies Villforth (1995) stated that 52.8% of falconiform and 60.4% of strigiform birds died from infectious causes. In 'wild' falconiforms the figure was 28.7% and 'wild' owls 40.4%.

In this chapter the main groups of infectious agent are first discussed, followed by a breakdown on the basis of organs affected and with more detailed information on some particular diseases.

Several viral diseases have been reported from birds of prey (Ritchie, 1995; Forbes & Simpson, 1997a) amongst them avian pox, Newcastle disease, adenovirus infection and herpesvirus infections;

these will be described later. Isolation of viruses requires sophisticated equipment and many avian pathologists are not able to include virology as a routine part of clinical or *post-mortem* work. Nevertheless, the situation is changing and every opportunity should be taken to submit material to appropriate laboratories for virological examination.

Chlamydia psittaci occurs as an organism or can be detected serologically in a range of avian hosts: Taday (1998) recorded positive results in 376 species from 29 orders. Gerbermann *et al.* (1990) studied the incidence of *Chlamydia* in a raptor collection and Gerbermann and Korbel (1992) reported findings in free-living raptors. Schettler *et al.* (2001) detected antibody titres in 267 out of 422 birds of prey in Germany. Chlamydiosis (*Chlamydia psittaci* infection) was reported from a number of birds of prey – both Falconiformes and Strigiformes – by Keymer (1974).

The treatment of chlamydiosis – or, indeed whether or not action should be taken over the carriage of *Chlamydia* in raptors – has tended to be extrapolated from work with psittacine birds. However, there are public health considerations which have prompted debate on this issue. Recently, for example, there has been interest in the use of azithromycin, a macrolide antibiotic, in birds of prey. Verwoerd (2000), working in the United Arab Emirates (UAE), suggested the use of azithromycin by tablet or oral suspension (not capsule), once a day with food, to treat chlamydiosis in falcons. In view of the likelihood of a carrier state, a 28-day period of treatment was advised.

A serological survey of 71 captive and free-living raptors by Riemann *et al.* (1977) showed 30% to be positive for Q fever (*Coxiella burnetii*) antibodies (and, incidentally, 8% positive for *Toxoplasma* and one bird only positive for infectious bursal disease virus).

Mycoplasmas (Mycoplasmata) were first reported from birds of prey 25 years ago (Furr *et al.*, 1977). Subsequent to that work those colleagues and I isolated mycoplasmas from tracheal swabs of seven healthy peregrines at an establishment in Britain where there was a history of respiratory disease. One isolate hydrolysed arginine and the others glucose; they were all negative when typing was attempted

using antisera against seven species of mycoplasma, amongst them poultry pathogens. Mycoplasmas have subsequently been isolated by other workers from birds of prey – from buzzards (Bölske & Mörner, 1981), from a prairie falcon (Halliwell & Graham, 1978a) and from a saker falcon with a skeletal deformity (Erdélyi *et al.*, 1999). A useful review of current thinking was by Lierz *et al.* (2000) who isolated various species of *Mycoplasma*, including *M. meleagridis*, from tracheal swabs and/or air sac biopsies from different raptors that had been found injured or debilitated in Germany. The birds did not show clinical signs nor histological lesions. A further report (Lierz *et al.*, 2000), from the UAE, confirmed a high prevalence of *Mycoplasma* on culture but no clinical signs, suggesting that the organisms might be normal flora. The role of mycoplasmas in raptor disease is still little understood and more work is needed, including more extensive microbiological and serological surveys and (probably) experimental inoculation of birds.

Many species of bacteria are involved in raptor disease and considerable attention is paid to them later in this chapter. Laboratory examination plays an important part in diagnosis of bacterial diseases and properly conducted antibiotic sensitivity tests are important if therapy is to be successful (Fudge, 2001).

Much still remains to be learned of the 'normal' bacterial flora of raptors. Many organisms can be isolated from the feet, pharynx and cloaca of apparently healthy birds and some such organisms can prove pathogenic (Needham *et al.*, 1979; Cooper *et al.*, 1980). Some indication of the range of bacteria that has been associated with disease in non-domesticated birds is to be found in the relevant parts of Alan Fudge's (2000) excellent book *Laboratory Medicine: Avian and Exotic Pets.*

Relatively few species of fungi have been incriminated as a cause of disease in raptors. However, aspergillosis due to *Aspergillus fumigatus* is probably one of the commonest causes of death in captive birds. Candidiasis, due to the yeast *Candida albicans*, occurs in raptors (Beaulieu, 1992; Velasco, 2000); and can be a significant cause of morbidity and mortality (Redig, 1986). Both aspergillosis and candidiasis are discussed in detail later.

Blastomycosis was reported from two birds of prey by Kaleta and Drüner (1976); the infection involved the beak but no details were given. It is possible that other mycotic infections may occur from time to time, especially of skin lesions. Keratinophilic fungi can often be isolated from the feathers of birds (Pugh, 1966) and from time to time are associated with feather loss, feather damage and folliculitis.

Birds of prey can be a source of zoonoses (see Chapter 4). In addition, birds can inflict wounds with their talons and beaks which may be infected with *Staphylococcus aureus* or other organisms, including *Clostridium tetani*. Occasionally, if a falconer or aviculturist becomes ill his doctor, or a hospital, may request information on the health of his birds on the grounds that a zoonosis might be involved. I have been asked for such assistance on a number of occasions but never has the bird been implicated. Moreover, I have been unable to trace any evidence that birds of prey cause or contribute to the allergic disease 'bird-fancier's lung' in humans. This does not mean, however, that raptors cannot be involved in such conditions.

Hygiene is of great importance when birds of prey are kept in captivity (see Chapter 4). There is substantial evidence that poor hygiene, coupled with the 'intensification' of birds, can lead to a build-up of organisms, such as enteric bacteria, as well as parasites (e.g. *Caryospora*). Personal hygiene will protect birds and the handler. It should also be practised when working with free-living raptors in the field. Detailed data on hygiene, including recommended disinfectants, were first given in a chapter on preventive medicine in birds of prey in *Zoo and Wild Animal Medicine* (Cooper, 1978c) and the principles remain unchanged. It is impossible to sterilise a raptor's surroundings, with the possible exception of small items such as water containers, and the aim should therefore be to reduce the number of organisms by destroying and/or diluting them. A surface must be clean before it is disinfected. Hot water alone is a remarkably good disinfectant and scrubbing with soap and hot water is strongly recommended. If a chemical disinfectant *is* to be used, it should be chosen carefully; some guidelines were given by Cooper (1978a,b) and

examples are listed in Appendix IX. Probably the safest disinfectant is a surface-acting compound, such as cetrimide, but the efficacy of such chemicals against viruses is doubtful and they may be inactivated by soap. Phenolic compounds and formalin are both effective against bacteria but the former are now difficult to obtain in many countries and only the latter has any virucidal activity (care must be taken because of its toxicity to humans and birds). Following adequate exposure of a surface to a phenol or formalin the disinfectant must be washed off. Washing soda, when still available, is cheap and effective against viruses but rinsing is again necessary. Disinfectants approved and tested for use against certain pathogens of farm animals, including poultry, are often useful. Fumigation of a mews or enclosed quarters, using formaldehyde and potassium permanganate, can be an effective way of reducing the numbers of organisms in a building but must be carried out with care.

It is virtually impossible to disinfect adequately an enclosure that contains vegetation. Hurrell (1973) and others subsequently suggested that exposure to rain and sun reduces the numbers of pathogens and this is clearly partly so. Nevertheless, breeding aviaries should be examined in the autumn and such items as feeding platforms and water containers cleaned. Replaceable materials, such as logs and bark, can be removed and burned. If such an enclosure becomes contaminated (for example, with avian tuberculosis organisms) the only long-term solution is probably to remove the birds and to leave the aviary to 'rest'; removal of the vegetation and, if possible, the top few centimetres of soil will probably help. *Aspergillus* and other fungi can multiply in damp soil and in leaves that may cover parts of an aviary in winter in temperate countries.

The management of a large collection of captive birds of prey necessitates an appropriate health programme (see 'Health monitoring and screening' – Chapter 4 and Appendix VII) and one important aspect of this is monitoring of the environment as well as of the birds themselves. A number of techniques can be employed to monitor ventilation while the use of bacteriological settle plates, as mentioned in Chapter 4, can help in assessing the contamination of the building. The different numbers of bacterial and fungal colonies that grow on each plate give an indication of the relative contamination. For example, when investigating respiratory disease of hawks in one falconer's mews, I obtained a count of 1160 colonies in one ('dirty') corner, 56 in a 'clean' area and only four in the owner's domestic living room. Results such as these are subject to many variables – and some colleagues are doubtful of the value of using settle plates – but in my experience they can give a guide as to where changes in management or design might be advantageous.

In the succeeding part of this chapter some of the more important infectious diseases will be discussed. In many cases they will be grouped together under a clinical heading, such as 'Respiratory conditions', regardless of the aetiological agent involved. Some organisms, however, will be listed separately and not related to specific pathogenesis or clinical signs. Certain infections are included in Chapter 13.

INFECTIONS OF THE SKIN (INTEGUMENT) AND OTHER SUPERFICIAL TISSUES

Infectious conditions of the feet ('bumblefoot') are discussed in Chapter 8 and other skin diseases in Chapter 13. A useful general reference is the chapter by Malley and Whitbread in the *Manual of Raptors, Pigeons and Waterfowl* (1996). The beak and talons are particularly susceptible to traumatic damage (see Chapter 5) but may also become infected. Secondary bacterial infections of the cere and digits may follow injury and a variety of organisms are isolated, including *Staphylococcus aureus*, *Escherichia coli* and *Proteus* spp. Falconers often speak of 'fungus' infections of these sites. Confirmation of such diagnoses is not frequent although yeasts may be isolated and I have had a single isolation of *Mucor hiemalis* from sloughed material from the talons of a golden eagle. Local infections of the cere may result in partial obstruction of the nares, with clinical signs of noisy respiration. The nares should be cleaned with a small swab and topical treatment applied daily for 7–10 days.

Skin infections *per se* are relatively uncommon in birds of prey but may occur following injuries,

including abrasion by jesses and rings. Falconers' birds and those that are free-living may also be infected by a bite from a prey item: grey squirrels (*Sciurus carolinensis*), for example, are frequently the cause of such infections in trained hawks in Britain. In such cases a variety of bacteria, including anaerobes, can usually be isolated. Treatment of minor wounds is often successful using a disinfectant, such as cetrimide or povidone–iodine, rather than sulphonamides or antibiotics but the danger of a more extensive, sometimes blood-borne, infection must be considered. A differential diagnosis in cases of chronic dermatitis should be neoplasia, especially squamous cell carcinoma (see Chapter 13).

Skin granulomas are seen from time to time and are commonly associated with *Staphylococcus aureus* although sometimes no organisms can be isolated. Surgical excision and/or antibiotics should be employed in treatment. In a paper on cutaneous diseases of wild birds Blackmore and Keymer (1969) described tumour-like masses on one wing of a kestrel; these proved to be due to tuberculosis. Similar tuberculous lesions were reported in a barn owl by Bucke and Mawdesley-Thomas (1974) and I have diagnosed them in two buzzards. Infection with a *Mycobacterium* sp. should therefore always be considered in differential diagnosis of cutaneous lesions and at the very least a Ziehl-Neelsen stain (touch preparation or impression smear) of the tissue should be prepared.

Drying and cracking of the skin of the feet is common in large captive birds, especially eagles (Harcourt-Brown, 1996b) and these lesions may give rise to dermatitis, involving various genera and species of aerobic bacteria. Occasionally, gangrene can supervene, with anaerobic organisms predominating. Prompt attention to such breaches in the integument is important.

Conjunctivitis and keratoconjunctivitis occur, again often following trauma. Bacteria are usually involved; frequent isolates are *S. aureus* and *E. coli*. Arnall and Keymer (1975) reported *Mycoplasma* infections of the eyes of birds of prey but gave no details. If treatment is not prompt, excoriation of surrounding skin and purulent dermatitis may occur and this feature was reported in 1619 by Bert who described a 'hot humour that runneth out of the eye, and scaldeth all the feathers from that part under the eye, and maketh it bare'. Bert went on to describe clinical signs of 'wiping of the eye against the wing' and this is often a feature of such infections.

Antibiotic therapy, using an ophthalmic preparation, is usually satisfactory and vitamin A may be a useful adjunct in case a deficiency is involved. If severe ulceration and photophobia are present suturing the eyelids together will help to prevent further damage. Generalised ophthalmitis may respond to parenteral antibiotics but often the sequel is a non-functional eye and/or enucleation.

Otitis externa is seen occasionally; it may progress to otitis media and otitis interna. Clinically, cases of otitis externa show damp feathers in the region of the auditory meatus. If the inner ear is involved the bird's head may be held on one side and nervous signs may result (see Chapter 9). Treatment should be with systemic antibiotics.

Bursitis can occur on both the wing and the leg. 'Blain', which has long been recognised by falconers, is probably bursitis of the carpus. The 'watery blister' on the joint frequently becomes damaged so that fluid seeps out giving the feathers a wet appearance. The condition probably follows trauma; two cases that I examined were in birds that had repeatedly struck their wings against the walls of the mews. The lesion can be drained, taking sterile precautions, and antibiotic applied topically. If the fluid is cloudy, suggestive of infection, a suitable intramuscular antibiotic should be used, preferably following culture. One of my cases developed myiasis (maggot infestation) but made a complete recovery following topical application of an antibiotic and insecticidal product. Writing in 1855 Salvin and Brodrick discussed the treatment of blain and mentioned that 'it is very difficult to cure, and . . . if of long standing, will generally produce a stiff joint'. Such arthritic complications are still often seen if treatment is delayed or antibiotics are not used. Another sequel, which can also follow other infections or traumatic insults to the end of the wing, is that the part of the wing distal to the carpus may be sloughed.

I have seen only one case of bursitis on the leg – a buzzard which suddenly, and inexplicably, developed a soft, painful, well circumscribed swelling over its patella. The lesion showed up well radiographically. It was drained under anaesthesia but subsequently became infected; it was later operated upon and its wall was cauterised. It recurred after several months and the bird finally contracted aspergillosis and a cloacal calculus. In recent years 'wing tip oedema' (WTO) has been increasingly reported and there has been uncertainty as to the relationship, if any, of this to bursitis (see Chapter 13).

Bursitis may be confused with septic arthritis which is discussed in Chapter 5 and with wing tip oedema which, because of its uncertain aetiology, is included in Chapter 13.

Cloacitis is frequently associated with calculus formation (see Chapter 13). Cloacitis *per se* can occur, however, and is commonly accompanied by excoriation and inflammation of the skin round the vent and soiling of the area with urates. Clinical signs vary but usually the bird shows discomfort when defaecating and may ruffle its feathers and attempt to peck at the cloacal region. Diagnosis is based on visual inspection and examination; the presence of cloacal calculi should be excluded by palpation or radiography. *E. coli* appears to be the usual cause of the infection but bacteriological culture is always advisable; I have isolated *S. aureus* from one case and this necessitated (and appeared to respond to) cloxacillin treatment. Oxytetracycline *per cloacam*, parenterally or orally, is frequently effective in treatment when *E. coli* is involved. The administration of oral liquid paraffin (mineral oil) or a surgical lubricant will ease discomfort and local treatment of the vent area is advisable. Following recovery the mutes may appear unusual in that faecal and urate portions are mixed; this I attribute to damage to the cloacal chamber.

A variety of other organisms can be isolated from the cloaca of healthy birds – for example *Proteus* spp. and *Streptococcus* spp. – and could presumably be a cause of cloacitis. These and other microparasites may be transmitted during copulation (Poiani & Wilks, 2000). Studies on the bacterial flora of the cloaca were carried out by Cooper *et al.* (1980) and of the nasal mucosa by Richter and Gerlach (1981).

Cloacitis may follow the use of instruments, such

as specula, during artificial insemination. Care must be taken whenever such equipment is used and they should be disinfected between birds. The risk of venereal spread of organisms is discussed in more detail later: it is another reason for practising strict hygiene during artificial insemination.

RESPIRATORY CONDITIONS

Respiratory diseases have long been recognised in captive birds of prey (Latham, 1615; Bert, 1619). Forbes (1996a) reviewed the subject and drew attention to the ease with which upper respiratory tract (URT) conditions could be differentiated from lower respiratory tract (LRT) conditions. Infectious diseases include rhinitis, sinusitis, tracheitis, pneumonia and air sacculitis. In the series of cases discussed in the first edition of this book respiratory infections, including aspergillosis, were responsible for 62 out of 208 deaths. Although bacteria, fungi and viruses are particularly important, the role of metazoan (macro) parasites in respiratory disease should not be overlooked (see Chapter 7): Lavoie *et al.* (1999) emphasised the importance of always looking for nematodes in raptors with respiratory problems. Non-infectious causes must also, of course, be considered but are not covered specifically here. Sometimes they predispose to infectious disease.

Stressors (see Chapter 13) appear to play an important role in the onset of respiratory diseases; they often follow a change of environment (especially in recently imported birds), other infections, or traumatic injuries. It is also possible that a vitamin deficiency, particularly vitamin A, can predispose to respiratory infections. Short-term breathlessness occurs in so-called 'asthma' (Chapter 13).

Laboratory examination plays an important role in investigation. Swabs, biopsies and washings can be used to make a diagnosis in a live raptor and if a bird dies or has to be killed it should be submitted for full *post-mortem* examination in order to ascertain which of the many respiratory conditions is involved. It should be noted, however, that some raptors with respiratory signs including so-called 'asthma', show only minor lesions (such as interstitial oedema or pulmonary congestion) and no sig-

nificant organisms can be isolated; the diagnosis in such cases is obscure.

Rhinitis was traditionally known to falconers as 'cold' or 'snurt' and is still readily recognised. It is characterised by unilateral or bilateral nasal discharge, sneezing and, sometimes, anorexia. Affected birds should be kept warm and unless a secondary infection supersedes, will usually recover spontaneously. Some cases become chronic; the nares are blocked and there may be intermittent bouts of noisy respiration and sneezing. The nares should be cleaned with a small human nasopharyngeal swab dampened in saline and the bird kept under careful observation. This syndrome may possibly be associated with sinusitis and air sacculitis.

Cases of rhinitis (and sinusitis) may sometimes be diagnosed using radiography or (better) computerised tomography (CT) (Krautwald-Junghanns *et al.*, 1998). Sinusitis is common in captive falconiform birds but less so in owls. Swollen sinuses can be associated with infectious agents (bacteria, *Trichomonas* (Samour, 2000b), probably mycoplasmas) or, occasionally, with other factors such as *Cyathostoma* worms (Simpson & Harris, 1992) or neoplasms (see Chapter 13).

Birds with sinusitis are often anorectic, may show a nasal discharge and usually have a swollen face, especially around the eyes. Other conditions of the head should be considered in differential diagnosis – for example, bee sting and inflammatory lesions of the buccal cavity. There is considerable overlap between sinusitis and rhinitis on the one hand and sinusitis and air sacculitis on the other and it is quite possible that all three conditions are closely related.

Medical treatment of infective sinusitis has been achieved with a number of anti-microbial agents (see Appendix IX). In some cases the causal organisms are probably not completely eliminated, as the condition recurs. On other occasions the characteristic facial swellings disappear but the bird may continue to show respiratory signs and blocked nares. Surgical removal (lancing and removal, followed by flushing) of pus can prove valuable in particularly resilient cases, especially if accompanied by systemic antibiotic therapy. The operative technique recommended is similar to that used in poultry (Roberts, 2000) and described succinctly by Dorrestein (2000). The earliest written record that I have been able to trace of surgically draining the sinuses in raptors is that of Campbell, in Canada, who reported in 1934 that he had 'operated on several eagles and vultures for mycotic sinusitis, removing the fungus growth that collects and painting the cavities with iodin'. I have little doubt that the 'fungus growth' was necrotic debris and that the cases were not mycotic in origin.

Occasionally a subcutaneous soft tissue swelling of the head region may be seen following sinusitis. Such swellings contain caseous pus and may be pedunculated. They appear to arise as a result of extension of infection from the sinus and can be removed surgically.

The causal organisms in sinusitis are not known but it is tempting to incriminate a *Mycoplasma* spp.; the rapid clinical response to spiramycin in some cases might support this. Although usually only single birds are affected, in Kenya I was consulted (by telephone only!) concerning an 'epizootic' that killed seven birds of prey (Cooper, 1973c), suggesting either a common source of infection or transmission from one bird to another.

Tracheitis (including syringitis) can be due to parasites (mainly *Syngamus*), bacteria or fungi (usually *Aspergillus*). A lesion in the trachea of a peregrine that died of pericarditis and perihepatitis yielded *S. aureus* and it was suggested that the respiratory tract had served as the portal of entry (Anon, 2001). Investigation of tracheitis/syringitis must therefore include examination of faeces or washings for worm eggs, of swabs or washings for micro-organisms and direct observation of the respiratory tract itself, using an endoscope, for pathological lesions that can then be sampled.

Birds with pneumonia usually show signs of dyspnoea, especially on exertion. Most cases are probably bacterial in origin although predisposing factors can include chilling and transportation. Organisms isolated from cases *post mortem* have included *E. coli*, *S. aureus* and a *Pasteurella* sp. Affected birds usually respond to an appropriate course of antibiotics. As with so many avian diseases, careful nursing, particularly warmth, fluids and feeding by hand (see Chapter 4), can be an invaluable aid to recovery.

Greenwood (1973) described bronchitis as a rare condition of hawks: it too will respond to appropri-

ate antibiotic therapy. It must be distinguished from syngamiasis and physical obstructions of the upper respiratory tract, which can produce similar clinical signs.

Air sacculitis of hawks is a condition that I first recognised over 30 years ago but which was not described elsewhere for a considerable period, other than mycotic air sacculitis associated with *Aspergillus fumigatus* (Stehle, 1965) and inflammatory lesions of the air sacs due to *Serratospiculum* worms. Subsequently, however, colleagues reported a similar clinical syndrome. Redig (1978) associated air sacculitis with *E. coli* infection and other causes include *Serratospiculum* (air sac) worms, bacteria, *Chlamydia* and *Aspergillus* (Samour & Naldo, 2001). My original cases were in the cold autumn of 1968 when many birds of prey were being imported into Britain from tropical countries; a number of these showed a clinical disease which, on *post-mortem* examination, proved to be an air sac infection.

Clinical signs of air sacculitis may be slight but affected birds are usually anorectic and often regurgitate food. Respiratory signs are variable. Regurgitation usually occurs within 5 minutes of ingestion but may be delayed for up to an hour. The respiratory rate is often accelerated (up to 60 per minute) but dyspnoea is often not apparent unless the bird is either exerted or *in extremis*. Radiological examination of chronic cases may reveal a narrowing and opacity of the air sacs.

The lesions seen at autopsy are a thickening and opacity of the air sac walls (Plate 14) and, often, the serosae. Usually some yellowish debris is present on the air sac walls. On histological examination the air sacs are inflamed and often adherent to other tissues. The debris from the air sacs may yield *Escherichia coli* or other organisms. Mycoplasmas have also been identified from hawks with clinical signs of respiratory disease (Furr *et al.*, 1977). However, as was mentioned earlier, there is as yet only limited evidence that these organisms are responsible for disease.

Treatment of air sacculitis necessitates an early diagnosis since once the condition is severe the tissues are damaged and complete resolution is unlikely. *Serratospiculum* worms can be killed with an appropriate anthelmintic (see Appendix IX) and then removed by surgery or endoscopy.

Air sac infection may also be a feature of other respiratory diseases of birds of prey, including rhinitis and sinusitis; clinical examination of some such cases would certainly suggest so. Birds that have recovered from such infections often seem prone to further respiratory disease. In some instances, even after apparently recovering from air sacculitis, a bird will show slight persistent dyspnoea or tachypnoea and the soft tissues cranial (anterior) to the eye may become distended as the bird breathes. The latter is a useful clinical feature that is quickly noted by conscientious owners and well recognised by Arab falconers. Although the old falconer's terms 'kecks', 'croaks' and 'pantas' probably covered a variety of respiratory conditions, I suspect that Bert's description of 'a Hawke that bloweth, and is short or thicke-winded' referred to a chronic case of air sacculitis.

Aspergillosis has been recognised in birds of prey for many years. The earliest specific reference I have found to it was a communication to the Pathological Society of London (Crisp, 1854). The subject was a captive peregrine falcon and the description of the lesions is sufficiently accurate and similar to those seen today to be worth repeating:

> 'The pericardium was studded with small round
> elevated tubercles; and the spleen and liver were
> also tuberculated. The peritoneum, in some
> places, was covered with patches of thick lymph
> of old standing, which had a mouldy
> appearance; and on microscopical examination
> the sporules of mould were very apparent.'

Aspergillosis was traditionally considered to be the commonest infectious cause of death in captive raptors in Britain (Cooper, 1969b; Keymer, 1972) and continues to be one of the most important diseases of captive raptors in many parts of the world (Aguilar & Redig, 1995; Redig, 1996a). There is strong evidence of increased susceptibility of some species – the gyr falcon is the most oft-quoted example but Joseph (1996, 2000) also lists the golden eagle, osprey, goshawk, rough-legged buzzard and red-tailed hawk as being particularly at risk from the disease. Aspergillosis appears to be less common in owls than in diurnal birds of prey, although this is not necessarily the case; an early record in strigiform

birds dates back to 1935, when Hamerton described two affected eagle owls at the London Zoo.

Free-living raptors are also exposed to *Aspergillus* and susceptible to aspergillosis, but work on prairie falcons suggests that it is predominantly a disease of captive birds (Morishita *et al.*, 1998). The role of stressors in precipitating aspergillosis in free-living goshawks was emphasised by Redig *et al.* (1980a).

Aspergillosis has been investigated in detail by Patrick Redig who reported some of his earlier findings at the International Symposium in 1980 (Redig, 1981). Redig emphasised at that time the role in diagnosis of serology, air sac lavage or laparoscopy. More recently (Aguilar & Redig, 1995; Jones & Orosz, 2000; Redig & Ackermann, 2000) similar techniques were still being advocated, with the addition of an ELISA (enzyme-linked immunosorbent assay) test for antibodies, and the promise that antigen detection tests and serum electrophoresis might soon be added to the armoury. A useful diagnostic aid is haematology where a leucocytosis and heterophilia are often a feature. Other changes may also be helpful: Hawkey *et al.* (1984) described morphologically abnormal heterophils in the circulating blood of a king shag (*Phalacrorax albivenier*) with aspergillosis.

Diagnosis of aspergillosis therefore must involve a combination of techniques. Endoscopy plays a particularly important role in diagnosis (or confirmation of diagnosis). Rigid instruments can be used to view the air sacs, flexible ones to investigate the respiratory tract.

Radiography can be of value in diagnosis, as described originally by Ward *et al.* (1970) but often only when lesions are fairly extensive. Both lateral and ventro-dorsal views should be taken. Usually distinct nodular lesions are seen and there may be a reduction in size of the air sacs. Pneumatised bones may contain distinct densities. Opacity of the air sac fields is more likely to be indicative of air sacculitis or of large numbers of *Serratospiculum* worms.

Microbiology is of value in diagnosis but should be linked with cytology since tracheal swabs and air sac aspirates (or lavage) from both affected and non-affected birds may yield *Aspergillus* on culture.

Aspergillus fumigatus is recognised in human medicine as 'opportunistic' and the same situation appears to apply in avian work, since aspergillosis is usually a sequel to some other factor, especially low condition or intercurrent disease. It is also a common cause of death in recently imported birds; in a letter to Mr J. G. Mavrogordato in 1940, now in my possession, the Pathologist at the London Zoo, Colonel A. E. Hamerton, drew attention to this when he wrote 'it is a comparatively rare disease among hawks at the Zoo and only occurs amongst new arrivals that have been kept in unsuitable conditions. . . .' There is also increasing evidence that long-standing deficiencies, especially of vitamins A and B1, are involved in predisposition to aspergillosis. As with domesticated birds, it seems probable that a spore-laden environment will enhance the chances of the disease developing and for this reason falconers and aviculturists are well advised to avoid musty hay lofts and other poorly ventilated buildings for their birds. The use of bacteriological settle plates can help to monitor the air-borne contamination of an enclosure, as suggested earlier. There is little sound evidence that aspergillosis can be transmitted from one bird to another; more than one affected bird on the same premises is probably indicative of an infected environment. Work on passerine birds has shown that the majority of nests harbour *A. fumigatus* and, often, other fungi (Apinis & Pugh, 1967) and this should be borne in mind when cleaning and disinfecting breeding quarters at the end of the season.

Acute aspergillosis can occur, usually following the inhalation of large numbers of spores (Joseph, 1996). Subacute disease may take up to 6 weeks until clinical signs are seen while 'chronic' aspergillosis can develop over months.

The onset of aspergillosis is often insidious, with loss of weight and lethargy common early signs. Dyspnoea is often only observed when the lungs are involved or the bird is subjected to exercise; *post-mortem* cases with extensive fungal lesions in all air sacs have been seen when no respiratory signs were evident in life. Some birds may appear relatively unaffected when at rest, on a perch, but can develop severe dyspnoea and cyanosis when cast on their back for examination. A few cases develop signs associated with the presence of *Aspergillus* lesions. The pathology – gross and microscopical – also

varies. Many cases are chronic, with extensive fungal lesions: one goshawk examined *post mortem* had an aspergilloma forming a complete cast of the left abdominal air sac. Others appear more acute, with active lesions (more acute, fewer chronic, inflammatory cells) in the lungs as well as air sacs. Occasionally *post-mortem* examination of a raptor reveals small granuloma-like lesions on the air sacs which, when examined histologically, are found to contain fungal hyphae but death is due to some other cause such as trauma. Such instances suggest that *Aspergillus* lesions may not prove fatal but become 'walled-off' – possibly to initiate an infection later? Aspergillosis is often diagnosed *post mortem*. Affected birds are thin and there are nodular yellow lesions in the air sacs and other internal organs. Distinct fungal growth is often visible in lung lesions. On histological examination septate fungal hyphae are seen in the affected tissues; the stains of choice are PAS or Grocott.

Treatment of aspergillosis also is not easy. In earlier days the only agents available were amphotericin B, pimaricin, 5-fluorocytosine and nystatin. Fuller *et al.* (1974) used amphotericin B by both the intravenous and aerosol routes and this was also recommended by Ward *et al.* (1970). I tried a variety of drugs in the 1970s and 1980s with some apparent success (and described this in earlier editions of this book).

In recent years the triazoles have become available and Joseph (2000) discussed the various combinations that can be used in therapy. Redig and Ackermann (2000) described oral itraconazole and nebulisation with clotrimazole and intratracheal amphotericin B – if respiratory tract lesions are seen – as 'the currently recommended treatment'. Only amphotericin B is fungicidal: the others are fungistatic so prolonged treatment may be necessary, combined with supportive care and attempts to promote the bird's immunocompetence. Some cases, with extensive (or inaccessible lesions) fail to respond to any treatment. Surgical removal of lesions blocking the syrinx may be helpful. The product 'F10', based on a quaternary ammonium compound, a new biguanide complex, has found favour for the treatment of aspergillosis in birds of prey in Arabia (Verwoerd, 2001) and in Britain (J. R. Best, J.

Chitty & K. Eatwell, pers. comm.). Controlled clinical trials are needed on this and some other promising antimycotic agents.

Goshawks, gyrs and snowy owls appear to be particularly susceptible to aspergillosis and some veterinarians routinely give such birds itraconazole 'prophylactically' (see Appendix IX), with no apparent hepato- or nephrotoxicity. The continued, confident, use of this agent has been facilitated by studies on its pharmacokinetic disposition in red-tailed hawks (Jones *et al.*, 2000).

It is prudent to avoid corticosteroids in cases were aspergillosis is suspected since there is substantial evidence from both mammalian and avian work that immunosuppression can result in active infection.

Although *A. fumigatus* is the usual isolate in cases of mycotic air sacculitis and pneumonia, occasionally other *Aspergillus* spp. may be involved. *Aspergillus niger* has been associated with pneumonia and oxalosis in a great horned owl (Wobeser & Saunders, 1975). Weigand-Lommel (1999) established polymerase chain reactions for the differentiation of *A. fumigatus* and *A. flavus*. A *Mucor* sp. was isolated from a case of air sacculitis in a kestrel by Kaleta and Drüner (1976). *Geotrichum candidum* was identified by the Commonwealth Mycological Institute from a buzzard in which the gross and histopathological lesions were identical to those in *A. fumigatus* infection.

Prevention of aspergillosis in captive raptors is based upon ensuring that birds are in good health and condition and not exposed to excess numbers of spores. The latter means reducing access to damp, especially mouldy, vegetation where *Aspergillus* may flourish. Colleagues working in New Zealand on some of the world's rarest birds (non-raptors) pay particular attention to ensuring that aviaries are not too low and deprived of sunlight. They argue that such conditions are stressful and expose birds to large numbers of spores. Excessive iron intake ('iron overload') with haemosiderosis and/or haemochromatosis (deposition of iron-containing pigment in the tissues) may also predispose to aspergillosis and other infectious diseases (Plate 15).

As mentioned earlier, prophylaxis with itraconazole is often valuable and was recommended by

Redig (1996c) for captive raptors undergoing a change in management and for high-risk species. Some authors advocate concurrent clotrimazole by nebulisation (Joseph, 2000). The product 'F10', as already mentioned, has been recommended for prophylaxis, coupled with reduction of spore counts by hygiene and improved management.

Vaccination would be of inestimable value and is a field in which research might prove fruitful. In 1972 encouraging work was reported in London on vaccination of mice (Cooper, 1972b) but did not develop further. The prospects of vaccination against aspergillosis improved following work by Redig and, in turkeys, by Richard *et al.* (1982). Most recently, Joseph (2000) suggested an autogenous vaccine but stressed: 'Further studies are necessary to evaluate fully the benefits.'

Respiratory diseases are seen in free-living birds of prey but there is a need for more data on their prevalence and distribution. Studies on migrating birds (Clark, 1995) and casualties (Cooper, 1987a) could contribute substantially to knowledge.

GASTRO-INTESTINAL (GI) CONDITIONS

In this section a number of conditions of the gastro-intestinal tract will be mentioned, including a few that are not due to infectious agents. Nevertheless, they are included here since they must be considered in differential diagnosis.

Forbes (1996b) provided a useful review of conditions causing chronic weight loss, vomiting and dysphagia, amongst them infectious diseases of the GI tract.

Many different bacteria may be isolated from the alimentary tract of apparently healthy raptors. In the case of the lower intestine, or a 'clean' faecal sample, the usual isolates are *Escherichia coli* and *Proteus* spp. Many other organisms can be cultured from the pharynx including *S. aureus*, *Bacillus* spp. and *Corynebacterium* spp. The role of these is not always clear but it is not unreasonable to assume that they might assume a pathogenic role under certain circumstances. Studies on the gut flora of raptors were carried out some years ago by a number of investigators – for example Needham *et al.* (1979) and Cooper *et al.* (1980).

Viruses can be involved in enteritis and this is discussed later.

Stomatitis is also discussed in more detail later. Although often caused by *Trichomonas* or *Eucoleus* (*Capillaria*) (see Chapter 7), it can also be due to bacteria and other organisms. Oesophagitis, especially affecting the crop, can be due to these and other macro- and microparasites.

Enteritis is common in birds of prey, in some cases associated with gastritis, and often the aetiology is uncertain. Affected birds show discoloured (dark) mutes which are often foetid; in addition there may be regurgitation of food. Occasionally fresh blood is seen in the mutes and while this is probably a manifestation of intestinal damage it should be noted that haemorrhagic enteritis has been described as a sign of 'shock' in birds (personal communication with Keymer, 1972). Often in enteritis the mutes are voided with less force than is usual though it should be noted that this can also be a feature of other debilitating diseases. Loose faeces/mutes are not necessarily indicative of enteritis (see Appendix V).

Laboratory examination of mutes and regurgitated material from cases of enteritis/gastritis may suggest that a parasite is involved, for example coccidia or *Capillaria* worms. Alternatively, in severe cases of enteritis, ascarid worms may be 'flushed out' by the passage of ingesta and mislead the owner or veterinary surgeon into thinking that they are the cause. Often, however, the only significant laboratory finding is a profuse pure growth of *E. coli*. It is my belief that these bacteria can be the cause of enteritis/gastritis and both clinical and *post-mortem* observations support this. For example, an African goshawk developed diarrhoea and presumed enteritis shortly after being moved to a new (colder) locality and only oxytetracycline-sensitive *E. coli* could be isolated from faeces; it recovered rapidly after oxytetracycline therapy. A peregrine examined *post mortem* showed enteritis together with hyperaemia and oedema of the proventriculus and gizzard; a profuse growth of *E. coli* was isolated in pure culture from the affected areas and no parasites were found. These and many other cases help to substantiate a role for *E. coli* in some gastro-

intestinal conditions. Clinical diagnosis of *E. coli* infection must be based upon the isolation of *E. coli* (usually β-haemolytic) in pure culture from mutes and upper alimentary tract and clinical signs of alimentary disease. Typing of the *E. coli* can help in determining its origin. Treatment consists of antibiotic therapy and nursing, including fluid replacement and small meals at frequent intervals.

Coliform organisms can also be involved in other infections. Other bacterial causes of enteritis are *Salmonella* spp. (*S. enteritidis* and *S. typhimurium*), *Proteus* and *Pseudomonas* spp. Young raptors are particularly sensitive to GI infections and Forbes (1996b) and Forbes and Rees Davies (2000) recommended a probiotic for 14 days to help protect hand-reared chicks. Brisbin and Wagner (1970) described an outbreak of 'coli bacillosis' in a captive collection of American kestrels, which was treated successfully with oral furazolidone.

A secretary-bird I examined in Kenya died of acute pancreatitis from which only *E. coli* could be isolated and I have obtained the same isolate from cases of pneumonia, pericarditis and nephritis. Hamerton (1939) isolated *E. coli* from a case of purulent pericarditis and Fiennes from a hepatic abscess (personal communication with Keymer, 1972), both in falconiform birds. The role of the organism in septicaemia is discussed later.

Falconers sometimes speak of their hawk having a 'chill'. The condition is not a clearcut clinical entity but commonly follows a stressor, such as a drop in temperature or heavy rain. The affected bird flies poorly, often shows a reduced appetite and may be hunched or 'fluffed-up' in appearance. Occasionally it regurgitates or may pass loose faeces. There is usually spontaneous recovery within 48 hours – my advice is to bring the bird indoors and to keep it warm. Such 'chills' are possibly due to a low grade *E. coli* infection, perhaps an upset of the normal bacterial flora. *E. coli* has been isolated from the faeces of some such cases – which is not unusual – and also, in profusion, from pharyngeal swabs.

E. coli can pose problems when it is isolated from organs at *post-mortem* examination. It is a normal part of the gut flora and if examination of a carcass is delayed, the organisms can be detected in the liver, kidneys and lungs. Isolation in pure culture from the heart blood or bone marrow is more significant although caution must still be taken in incriminating the organism as the cause of death. Interpretation of the role of *E. coli* depends upon a number of factors, particularly the clinical history, gross *post-mortem* findings, and degree of autolysis of the carcass. One must also take into consideration whether the organism was isolated in pure culture and how profuse or scant was the growth. In some cases histopathological examination will help to support or refute a diagnosis of *E. coli* infection.

A pseudomembranous gastritis compatible with a *Clostridium* infection was reported by Enderson and Berthrong (1980).

Stomatitis is sufficiently important to warrant a section of its own. It can be associated with trauma, vitamin A deficiency, capillariasis, candidiasis and viral infections (Cooper, 1985b). To these Samour (2000c) added pseudomoniasis – a sequel to trichomoniasis – and there is no doubt that *Pseudomonas*, an opportunist, commonly multiplies where the oral mucosa is already damaged. Oral (and oesophageal) abscesses in *Buteo* spp. can be a feature of pasteurellosis (Morishita *et al.*, 1997). Severe cases of stomatitis, regardless of the aetiology, can readily lead to secondary infection, and there may be involvement of bone (Fig. 6.1).

'Inflammation of the crop' was recognised by falconers for many centuries. It was characterised by regurgitation of food a short time after swallowing. Most of the nineteenth and twentieth century authors discussed it in some detail but Mavrogordato, in the first edition of *A Hawk for the Bush* (1960), reported having never seen the condition. In my view 'inflammation of the crop' may be due to bacterial or parasitic oesophagitis, adverse reactions to oral medication, gastritis or certain other non-alimentary disorders, particularly air sacculitis.

A number of cases of 'inflammation of the crop' recover without specific treatment; others appear to respond to oral tetracyclines plus careful feeding with fluids or, as Woodford (1960) suggested, protein hydrolysate. Greenwood (1973) discussed crop infections in young birds and described clinical signs of immediate regurgitation and flicking of food. He recommended treatment by infusion

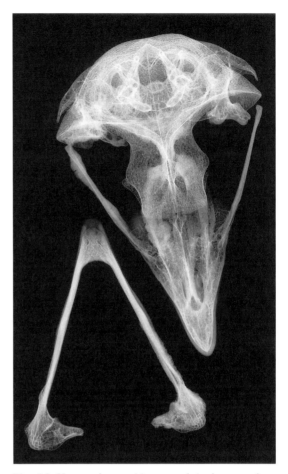

Fig. 6.1 Untreated stomatitis can result in deep-seated lesions, sometimes involving bone. In this eagle owl there are exostoses on the maxillae and rami of the jaw.

of antibiotic into the crop. The response to antibiotics in such cases would suggest a bacterial aetiology.

The only bacteria that I have isolated from swabs of regurgitated food from affected birds are *E. coli* and other members of the Enterobacteriaceae and it is again probable that these may be involved. On one falconer's premises cases of regurgitation occurred on a number of occasions in trained hawks. Some cases showed clinical signs of air sacculitis and appeared to respond to tylosin. When throat swabs were taken after an outbreak a number of bacteria were isolated, amongst them *Staphylococcus aureus* and a *Corynebacterium* sp. The significance of these organisms is uncertain but it is possible that they played a part in the syndrome.

Oesophageal capillariasis, due to *Eucoleus* (*Capillaria*) worms in the upper alimentary tract, was described in detail in the previous editions (Cooper, 1978a, 1985b) and is discussed in Chapter 7; it is one important cause of 'inflammation of the crop'. Severe crop infections, especially those due to *Trichomonas*, can lead to ulceration and even, in a few cases, fistulation. Free-living vultures in Tanzania were found to have crop lesions associated with botfly (*Gasterophilus pecorum*) larvae, probably acquired by feeding on infected zebra (*Equus burchelli*) (Cooper & Houston, 1972).

'Sour crop', probably first described in Germany by Stehle (1965), is very different from 'inflammation of the crop'. It is a toxaemia and follows the retention of food in the crop rather than its being passed to the proventriculus. The meat putrefies and toxins are released. Death can occur within a day. Forbes (1996b) recommended that birds that have taken over 4 hours to empty their crop should receive emergency treatment. Fluids should be given by tube to encourage passage of food. If this fails regurgitation should be stimulated: if the food remains in the crop it must be milked out manually into the mouth and removed. The crop can then be flushed with warm saline and the bird given fluids and antibiotics.

Difficulty in 'casting' (production of pellets) can also occur because of increased pressure within the body or abnormal consistency of food, especially an excess of dry skin, hair or feathers.

Regurgitation of food is also a common clinical sign in birds suffering from other diseases, especially air sacculitis, and, in some cases, aspergillosis. Such birds may show crop lesions at *post-mortem* examination but these are usually only areas of hyperaemia or inflammation which are secondary to the repeated regurgitation of food. In my view the primary cause of the regurgitation is inflammation of the air sacs (particularly the interclavicular?) and serosal surfaces. Medication – for example, large tablets or capsules of antibiotic – can also cause regurgitation.

Regurgitation in birds of prey need not be pathological. Most species normally regurgitate indigestible material (such as bone and fur) as a 'casting' or 'pellet' and observant owners will get some guide as to the health of their bird by examining this pellet. In a healthy bird, it is well formed and once voided, dries quickly; in a sick bird it is misshapen, wet and may contain undigested food. Persistently misshapen pellets occur in some raptors and are sometimes associated with difficulty in casting; a lesion of the stomach or crop may be responsible or increased pressure in the body cavity because of egg-laying (Forbes & Flint, 2000). In other birds the production of pellets is intermittent – a bird will, for example, cast every 2–3 days instead of at its usual 24-hourly intervals. Although delay in casting can be a sign of disease, some such birds appear quite healthy and the pellets they produce are normal. The reason for this is unknown; much work is needed on the 'meal to pellet interval' (MPI) as emphasised by Duke *et al.* (1975).

Occasionally a trained bird may regurgitate or vomit due to 'motion sickness'. This was described some years ago by Lorant de Bastyai (1968) and I have known other cases, including a kestrel which, when transported hooded in a car, would bring up its previous meal (from the stomach) unless allowed to face the front of the vehicle! Forbes and Rees Davies (2000) warned against letting a bird travel with food in its upper alimentary tract unless it was known not to be liable to 'motion sickness'. Birds of prey may also regurgitate when handled, injected or given certain drugs (see Appendix IX).

Candida albicans can often be isolated from the alimentary tract of apparently healthy raptors but it may also cause clinical disease (Beaulieu, 1992). Velasco (2000) differentiated between a more common form of disease, characterised by pseudomembranous areas of necrosis of the upper alimentary tract – often a differential diagnosis for trichomoniasis and capillariasis (see 'Inflammation of the crop' – and distal gastro-intestinal lesions that may cause inappetence, vomiting and dehydration. Diagnosis of candidiasis is based on a combination of cytology (Gram or rapid stain) or culture of material from the affected area. Velasco advocated treatment with anti-fungals such as nystatin or azoles (Velasco, 2000 see Table I). *Candida* can be transmitted venereally in some species of bird (Poini & Wilks, 2000) and this may be relevant to raptors.

There is little published information on disease of the gall bladder in birds of prey although scattered reports exist – for example, cholecystitis in a Javan fish owl at the London Zoo (Hamerton, 1935) and bile duct carcinomata (see review by Forbes *et al.*, 2000a). An enlarged gall bladder, full of bile, is commonly seen in birds that have died of inanition or been chilled.

Infectious disease of the liver (hepatitis) is discussed elsewhere: bacteria and viruses are most frequently implicated. Forbes (1996b) described a hepatopathy, possibly due to an infectious agent, that was a feature of falcons and associated with hypoglycaemia on exertion.

Much of the foregoing is based on work on captive birds. GI diseases are seen in free-living raptors but little has been published on them. Data on conditions diagnosed in birds caught on migration or recently submitted as casualties could throw more light on the importance of these and other diseases (Cooper *et al.*, 1993; Clark, 1995).

More information on GI conditions is given in Chapter 10. Neoplasms are discussed in Chapter 13.

PERITONITIS AND SEPTICAEMIA

Peritonitis and septicaemia have been reported in both captive and free-living birds of prey: often the lesions follow trauma, such as fractures or shot wounds. *E. coli* is commonly the cause but I have isolated other organisms from such cases including *Pseudomonas* and *Staphylococcus aureus*. *S. aureus* was reported as a cause of pericarditis, perihepatitis and other inflammatory lesions in a peregrine (Anon, 2001).

Birds with acute peritonitis usually die quickly, with few clinical signs other than anorexia and depression. Occasionally the patient shows diarrhoea and regurgitation for 24 hours before death. Treatment with antibiotics has not, in my experience, proved successful. More chronic peritonitis,

often localised, is detected sometimes on laparoscopy or during *post-mortem* examination.

Diagnosis of a septicaemia is also not always easy. Clinically affected birds show severe lethargy and pyrexia may be detectable. Bacteria can be cultured from the blood or, at *post-mortem* examination, from the heart. The failure to isolate organisms from the heart blood of cases that show a typical septicaemia at autopsy is often attributable to the administration of antibiotics before death. Prompt use of an appropriate antibiotic may prove effective in treating a bird with a blood-borne infection and for this purpose the intravenous or intraosseous route is recommended.

TUBERCULOSIS

Avian tuberculosis (mycobacteriosis), usually due to *Mycobacterium avium*, now usually called *M. avium* subspecies *avium*, is frequently diagnosed in both captive and free-living birds of prey although there appear to be geographical variations: Redig and Ackermann (2000), for instance, describe it as 'uncommon in raptors in North America'.

Typical cases of tuberculosis (TB) in birds of prey show clinical signs of a chronic loss of weight over several weeks. The appetite usually remains good but water may be drunk to excess and there can be diarrhoea. There are few other clinical signs although some birds show a tendency to close their eyes as if sleeping: this may be a non-specific feature. The infection primarily involves the liver, intestinal tract and bone although interesting atypical cases of my own have included an African fish eagle with concurrent aspergillosis (Kaliner & Cooper, 1973) and a (free-living) buzzard with a large cystic tuberculous lesion on its leg (Cooper, 1968c). In view of these cases, and those reported by others (Blackmore & Keymer, 1969; Bucke & Mawdesley-Thomas, 1974) elsewhere, mycobacteria should always be borne in mind when dealing with an unusual case. The causal organisms may take a long time to culture but a direct smear of a lesion, if stained with Ziehl-Neelsen stain, may reveal them.

Clinical diagnosis of tuberculosis is not always easy. Laparoscopy, with liver (or intestinal) biopsy is a valuable technique. Radiology can be helpful, especially in demonstrating 'punched-out' lesions in the long bones – characteristic of tuberculosis, according to Redig and Ackermann (2000). Useful review papers on tuberculosis in raptors were those by van Nie *et al.* (1982) and Lumeij and van Nie (1982) and in the latter the value in diagnosis of laparoscopy – if necessary followed by liver biopsy – was strongly emphasised.

A tuberculin test was recommended by Stehle (1965) and subsequently advocated by Heidenreich (1997) but has never proved successful in my hands, even in proven cases of tuberculosis. The staining of a faecal smear with Ziehl-Neelsen stain has been useful in some cases, primarily those in which intestinal lesions have subsequently been detected by laparoscopy or *post mortem*. However, care must be taken not to mistake small numbers of saprophytic acid-fast organisms for pathogens. Haematology can also aid diagnosis.

The successful use of a polymerase chain reaction to detect *M. a.avium* in faeces (Thornton *et al.*, 1999) and formalin-fixed:paraffin-embedded tissues (Gyimesi *et al.*, 1999) opens up some new possibilities for definitive diagnosis.

In my view raptors with tuberculosis should be killed (euthanased). The disease is a danger to other raptors and to humans. Nearly 40 years ago Marks and Birn (1963) reported only ten cases of avian tuberculosis in humans in Britain but there has been an increase there and elsewhere – partly associated with immunosuppression due to HIV and other factors but also, interestingly, in immunocompetent people, especially children (Cowan *et al.*, 2000).

Other veterinarians have recommended therapy; for example, Greenwood (1973) advocated the use of rifampicin in raptors and reported two instances where treatment appeared to be successful. A definitive diagnosis of tuberculosis could not, however, be made in the birds involved. Whether or not one should attempt to treat avian tuberculosis is debatable. Some authors, including myself, feel that the zoonotic risk of *Mycobacterium avium*, especially in locations where human contacts may be immuno-compromised, make therapy unwise. Others recom-

mend treatment where birds are valuable and where appropriate hygiene can be practised. Beynon *et al.* (1996) listed agents that can be used, usually in combination with enrofloxacin, cycloserine and ethambutol, for example clofazimine and cycloserine.

Prevention of tuberculosis is not easy, though care should be taken to check any birds used as food items for internal lesions of the disease before they are eaten. In the case of European wood pigeons (*Columba palumbus*), the tendency for pigeons infected with TB to have a darker plumage may be a useful clue (McDiarmid, 1948).

Vaccination of birds against tuberculosis would be of great benefit and was discussed in an earlier paper (Cooper, 1975c) but is unfortunately not yet feasible in raptors. Host resistance is probably an important feature as is the size of the challenge, in terms of number of organisms. It must be assumed, however, that not every free-living raptor that ingests a tuberculous bird contracts the disease despite being exposed to vast numbers of mycobacteria. Kenward (1976) added some weight to this view when he reported that a captive (trained) goshawk ate at least one pigeon in which TB was diagnosed without contracting the disease.

In view of the resistant nature of the mycobacteria all steps should be taken to prevent their being introduced to a collection. Other infected birds of prey and free-living pigeons, possibly also sparrows (*Passer domesticus*), are probably the main hazard but mammalian species may harbour and presumably disseminate the organism including deer and the European hedgehog (*Erinaceus europaeus*) (Matthews & McDiarmid, 1977). Once a case has been diagnosed, thorough and repeated disinfection is recommended.

OTHER BACTERIAL INFECTIONS

Many species of bacteria can be isolated from birds of prey. Some are normal (possibly beneficial) flora and some contaminants or transient flora and some of exogenous origin involved in infection and/or disease. There is often no clear-cut distinction: opportunists can take advantage of an immuno-compromised host and (as I say in my lectures)

'Today's commensal is tomorrow's pathogen'. Thus, for example, the culture of *Pseudomonas* from infected wounds is common and *Staphylococcus epidermidis* may or may not be the cause of a lesion. Other organisms can be isolated from (and often are the cause of) lesions in a variety of sites – for instance, *Corynebacterium* from the uveal tract and bone marrow of a case of endophthalmitis (MacLaren *et al.*, 1995). Keymer (1972) listed anthrax, erysipelas, listeriosis, pasteurellosis and salmonellosis as bacterial diseases that could be contracted by birds of prey from infected food.

I have diagnosed pasteurellosis in both captive and free-living strigiform and falconiform birds and have also isolated a *Pasteurella* sp. from birds that showed no clinical or *post-mortem* evidence of pasteurellosis. Subacute pasteurellosis was reported in a captive goshawk by Woodford and Glasier (1955) and in a peregrine by Bougerol (1967). The *Pasteurella* that has mainly been isolated from raptors, both falconiforms and strigiforms, is *P. multocida* serotype 1. Aye *et al.* (1998) were able to demonstrate the virulence of isolates from birds of prey to domestic fowl. Morishita *et al.* (1997) described 22 'avian cholera' cases in raptors and described the lesions in detail.

Anthrax is relatively rare in captive birds although there are a few reports; for example, Hamerton (1943) reported two fatal cases in eagles fed infected meat at the London Zoo. The disease must, therefore, be taken seriously and care taken to ensure that infected food is not given to captive birds. Any mammal that dies unexpectedly should be checked for anthrax. The situation in the wild is of interest since raptors, especially vultures, seem rarely affected clinically but possibly play a significant role in the dissemination of the organism. Studies on this aspect have usually involved the use of captive experimental birds (Urbain & Nouvel, 1946); David Houston and I used a white-backed vulture in our work on anthrax in Kenya (Houston & Cooper, 1975).

I have been able to trace only one record of erysipelas infection in a captive falconiform bird – a bald eagle (Franson *et al.*, 1996) although there are reports of it in free-living raptors and recent casualties (Keymer, 1972; Redig, 1978; Simpson *et al.*,

1997). However, there are at least three records of the disease in captive owls and therefore this infection, which like the others being discussed under this heading is a zoonosis, must be considered in diagnosis. The series of cases described by Blackmore and Gallagher (1964) included a little owl and that bird, in common with most of the others affected, showed no specific signs of disease. This point emphasises that many of the generalised bacterial infections do not produce typical clinical signs and a definitive diagnosis in such cases must usually be based on microbiology and other laboratory tests.

Listeriosis does not appear to be prevalent in either captive or free-living birds of prey; however, in view of the difficulty in culturing the organism, cases may have been missed. Keymer (1972) could locate only one record of a case in a captive bird.

Salmonellae have been isolated from cloacal swabs of healthy raptors (Wernery & Joseph, 1997) but have also been reported as a cause of disease (Forbes, 1996b). However, there are relatively few records of clinical salmonellosis in captive birds of prey (Keymer, 1972; Smith, 1993a) despite the numbers of suspect wild animals that must be fed to them. I have encountered no clinical or *post-mortem* cases of salmonellosis in raptors and have only rarely cultured a *Salmonella* sp. from faeces, despite routine microbiological examination of large numbers of birds in both Western Europe and East Africa. Sykes *et al.* (1981), however, suggested that salmonellosis could pose a threat to birds in large breeding facilities. It could also be significant in free-living birds, especially if nesting ledges or boxes become contaminated. *Salmonella* spp. can be transmitted sexually and have been identified in the semen of chickens (Poiani & Wilks, 2000).

Although pseudotuberculosis, caused by *Yersinia pseudotuberculosis*, is a relatively common and important disease in cage and aviary birds, it does not appear to be so prevalent in birds of prey. I have never encountered a case. It is possible that some cases have been misdiagnosed since 'typical' caseous lesions on the gut, liver and spleen are often a feature of tuberculosis and aspergillosis. In the letter to J. G. Mavrogordato to which I referred earlier,

Hamerton drew attention to this confusion when he wrote, 'I think by pseudotuberculosis you probably mean *Mycosis* – a disease of the air sacs which produces lesions resembling those of tuberculosis'.

Clostridial enterotoxaemia, cased by toxins of *Clostridium* spp., has been reported in birds of prey. For example, Köhler and Baumgart (1970) recorded fatal cases in three captive hawks due to the feeding of meat contaminated with *Clostridium perfringens* type A. More recently Wernery and colleagues (2000) reported enterotoxaemia caused by *C. perfringens* type A/B and *C. histolyticum* in falcons in the United Arab Emirates. Affected birds may be incoordinated and show diarrhoea and haemorrhages. Routine pathology and toxicology often fail to detect any cause of death in such cases, and diagnosis must be based on clinical history unless facilities permit the toxins to be demonstrated. Specific antitoxins would almost certainly be effective in treatment but are usually not available; antibiotics and adsorbents should be tried.

While certain species of vulture appear to be resistant to the toxins of *Clostridium botulinum* Types A, B and C by both oral and injectable routes (Kalmbach, 1939a) this is not true of all birds of prey. Botulism has been reported from a variety of free-living birds (Lloyd *et al.*, 1976) but is probably unlikely to present a significant threat to captive raptors. However, the feeding of infected maggots could possibly pose a hazard to small species that are kept for aviculture, as reported some years ago from the London Zoo (Smith *et al.*, 1975).

VIRAL INFECTIONS

Newcastle disease (PMV-1)

Newcastle disease in raptors was recently reviewed by Manvell *et al.* (2000). It has been known for some time in birds of prey; for example, Keymer and Dawson (1971) recorded it in a free-living Eurasian kestrel and in three young captive barn owls. Clinical signs were minimal. Serological surveys have also shown evidence of infection; for example, a positive titre in the serum of a red-tailed hawk in a survey

by Kocan *et al.* (1977a) and in 28 out of 432 samples from birds of prey in Germany by Kaleta and Drüner (1976). Pierson and Pfow (1975) reported eight cases of the disease in 'Shaheen hawks' and seven out of the eight died. There were no clinical signs suggestive of the disease but the virus could be isolated in the laboratory. Schneeganß (1990) demonstrated PMV-1 in bearded vultures (lammergeiers).

Chu *et al.* (1976) isolated Newcastle disease virus from 11 out of 14 birds of prey that died in captivity. In each case the virus isolated was of the velogenic (highly fatal) type. Some of the birds showed clinical signs of inappetence, head twisting and incoordination but in the majority the only common feature was death. Experimental inoculation of birds by Winteröll (1976) resulted in clinical signs of convulsions and paralysis and significant histological lesions were described.

It is wise, therefore, to consider Newcastle disease a significant threat to captive raptors. It is possibly also a danger to free-living birds of prey especially if these are in contact with infected pigeons or even domestic fowl (*Gallus domesticus*) – a scenario that can occur very easily, even in African national parks (Cooper & Mbassa, 1994) or village communities in poorer countries.

There is as yet no specific therapy for Newcastle disease and the aim should be to prevent entry and establishment of infection (Forbes, 1997a). Hygiene is all important and is discussed below. Vaccination can also be considered. I first used inactivated (beta-propiolactone) vaccine in several captive East African species with no ill effects and at that time suggested its use in the face of an outbreak, although, as discussed elsewhere (Cooper, 1975c), I had reservations about the protection it confers. Attenuated vaccines may be preferable; Chu *et al.* (1976) reported the safe use of live Hitchner B1 vaccine, and Winteröll (1976) successfully protected falconiform and strigiform species with both LaSota and Galivac live vaccines. Winteröll's birds resisted experimental infection but the antibody titres obtained were low. It is probably best *not* to use live vaccines in birds intended for release: Lierz and Launay (2000) reported the safe use of inactivated vaccines, a mixture of two products, in falcons prior to their return to the wild in Arabia.

There are steps other than vaccination that can be taken to help to prevent or exclude Newcastle disease. The use of poultry and pigeons as food for captive birds of prey can be hazardous (Chapter 10) and, as a general rule, contact between raptors and other species of bird should be avoided. In the case of aviaries, free-living wild birds may prove a threat – not only of Newcastle disease but also of other avian pathogens. Even mammals such as house mice (*Mus musculus*), may occasionally harbour Newcastle disease (Johnson *et al.*, 1974).

Avian pox

Pox has been recorded in both captive and free-living birds of prey, primarily falconiforms (Ritchie *et al.*, 1994). Early reports included cases in peregrines imported into Britain (Cooper, 1969c; Greenwood & Blakemore, 1973) and a red-tailed hawk in the USA (Halliwell, 1972). The host range of avipoxviruses is relatively wide: Bolte *et al.* (1999) reported that, of the approximately 9000 species of bird, about 232 species in 23 orders have been reported with a natural infection. Essentially poxviruses are species-specific but can cross to other species of bird and, generally, cause a less severe disease (Heidenreich, 1997). An excellent historical survey of avian pox, with a bibliography of 677 references is to be found in the dissertation by Meurer (1991).

Clinically, avian pox produces classical pock lesions, especially around the eyes and beak and on the feet. The pocks are slightly raised plaques which are brownish in colour. Occasionally they may be seen on the mucous membranes. Affected birds usually retain their appetite and appear in good health although extensive scabbing may result in closure of the eyes and inability to feed. In addition, the lesions may be pruritic and secondary infection can follow scratching by the bird's feet or beak.

Diagnosis of pox infection can usually be made on the basis of the clinical signs (Samour & Cooper, 1993). Confirmation can be by direct electronmicroscopy of scab material (Cooper, 1969c) or histological examination, using haematoxylin and eosin or Lendrum's (phloxine–tartrazine) stain, of a skin biopsy when characteristic ballooning of epithelial cells and intracytoplasmic inclusion (Bollinger) bodies are seen.

Treatment of pox is at present non-specific and may include the use of antibiotics to control secondary bacterial infection and vitamin A to aid healing. Surgical removal or ablation (cautery or cryoprobe) of larger lesions may help the affected bird to see or to feed. Hand-feeding is essential if the patient is unable to take food for itself. Carefully nursed birds usually recover but scars may remain. Prevention of the disease depends upon the exclusion of the virus from collections; recently imported birds are a particular threat and a quarantine period for incoming birds (whether statutory or voluntary) will help to reduce this risk. Hygiene will minimise the risk of the (relatively resistant) virus being spread mechanically, and control of biting insects is also desirable. Prophylactic vaccination, which can be useful and has been used extensively in the Middle East, is possible (Samour & Cooper, 1998).

OTHER VIRAL INFECTIONS

A viral hepatitis (hepatosplenitis) was first described many years ago in owls in the USA (Green & Shillinger, 1935) and Europe (Burtscher, 1965) and a similar disease of falconiform birds was reported in North America (Graham *et al.*, 1975).

The causal agents of these diseases are sometimes referred to as owl herpesvirus (OHV) and falcon herpesvirus (FHV) respectively. A useful early review of the host spectrum of OHV was given in a paper by Burtscher and Sibalin (1975); it is interesting to note that both the tawny owl and barn owl proved resistant to a massive experimental infection. More recent reviews by Kaleta (1990), Wheler (1993) and Gough *et al.* (2000) are valuable for reference, while both Schröder (1992) and Sander (1995) carried out specific studies on raptor herpesviruses. A serological survey by Schettler *et al.* (2001) revealed antibodies to FHV in an osprey in Germany, possibly for the first time.

Heinrichs (1992) published a literature survey of herpesvirus infections of non-domesticated birds. Herpesvirus isolates from various species of bird, including raptors, were studied on the basis of their restriction endonuclease patterns (Günther, 1995).

Herpesvirus disease is usually peracute and often fatal. In subacute cases clinical signs are restricted to lethargy, anorexia and diarrhoea. Blood samples show a progressive leucopenia. Affected birds may live a few days: most die but some recover. At *post-mortem* (or laparoscopic) examination, the liver and spleen are swollen and owls in particular may show pharyngeal and intestinal lesions. On histopathological examination there are characteristic lesions of necrosis in the liver and intra-nuclear inclusion bodies may be seen. A detailed description of lesions and diagnostic techniques was given by Peckham (1975).

A diagnosis is usually based on gross lesions, and demonstration of inclusion bodies (Heidenreich, 1997) can be confirmed by inoculation of fertile eggs, tissue culture or susceptible birds. Both OHV and FHV are pathogenic for owls, ring-necked doves (*Streptopelia* sp.) and kestrels (Eurasian and American) and, additionally, FHV for other species of falcon. An alternative approach to confirming diagnosis is direct electronmicroscopy (EM) of tissues (Sileo *et al.*, 1975; Kocan *et al.*, 1977b).

There is no specific treatment for viral hepatitis; affected birds should be isolated or, possibly, killed to reduce the risk of spread. The source of the virus is usually infected pigeons. The sensitivity of avian herpesviruses to different chemical disinfectants was investigated by Wagner (1993) and it is interesting to note that strigid herpesviruses were more resistant than psittacid.

Remple (2000, 2001) discussed the requirements for a safe and efficacious vaccine and stressed the need for clinical research on the subject, using experimental birds. Wernery *et al.* (1999) reported the successful use of an attenuated herpesvirus vaccine in common kestrels. They were unable to isolate herpesvirus from cloacal swabs during their experiment, suggesting that there is little danger to other birds from use of the vaccine. However, as mentioned earlier, caution is required in the use of live attenuated virus vaccines and it is an important precaution, in my view, never to use such vaccines in birds that are intended for release.

Herpesvirus infections are a potential hazard to captive birds of prey throughout the world. The diagnosis of the disease in free-living raptors – for example, eagles in Spain (Ramis *et al.*, 1994) – and its presence in racing pigeons, certainly in Europe (Forbes *et al.*, 2000b) – suggests that both captive and free-living raptors are at risk. A particular concern is always that herpesviruses may get into captive-breeding programmes where birds – some of them threatened species – are intended for release. Restrictions on importation were originally envisaged as ways of protecting birds – and, indeed, countries. In the context of the UK, Greenwood (1977) suggested that selective import controls on prairie falcons and European eagle owls might be desirable until more was known about the ability of recovered birds to carry the virus. Herpesvirus infection was not for some time reported in Britain: an account of the disease in a group of falcons was probably the first formal record (Greenwood & Cooper, 1982) followed by cases in an imported great horned owl and a captive merlin. Now, as Forbes *et al.* (2000b) point out, the virus must be considered a real danger to captive raptors, especially as some birds may be latent carriers.

Liver and intestinal lesions in raptors may also be associated with an adenovirus (Sileo *et al.*, 1983; Forbes, 1997b). The cases reported by Forbes were in Mauritius kestrels, indicating how vulnerable this and other threatened, isolated, species might be to introduced infectious agents (Dutton *et al.*, 2000). Affected falcons showed minimal signs: diagnosis was *post mortem*.

Many other viruses are likely to prove pathogenic to raptors, especially if host resistance is reduced or the bird is susceptible to infection because it has not previously been exposed to the agent (Forbes & Simpson, 1997a). West Nile virus was reported in the USA, where it killed or caused clinical disease in both strigiform and falconiform birds of prey, as well as in a small number of humans (Steele *et al.*, 2000). Other viruses may follow suit.

Avian influenza virus was recently isolated from a saker falcon (a falconer's bird) in Italy; Magnino and colleagues made the interesting comment that

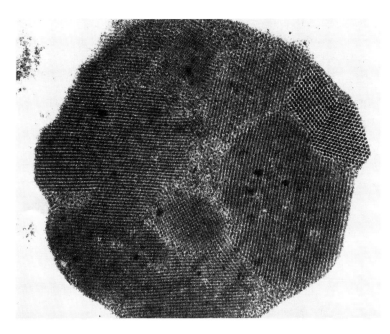

Fig. 6.2 Viral particles from a case of PBFD (psittacine beak and feather disease) in a cockatoo. This disease has not yet been reported in raptors but viral infections affecting the feathers are likely to be discovered in due course (TEM × 150 000).

awareness of the susceptibility of falcons to influenza virus may date back to experimental studies, also in Italy, nearly 100 years ago (Magnino *et al.*, 2000). A particularly worrying report may be that of avian polyomavirus (APV) infection detected in buzzards and a kestrel found dead in Europe (Johne & Müller, 1998): the virus causes fatal disease in many psittacine species and its presence in raptors could be relevant to the spread and effect of the virus in a wide range of species. Psittacine beak and feather disease (PBFD) has not been reported yet from birds of prey but is prevalent in parrots; examination of feather follicle material should be routine in order to detect this or similar infections (Fig. 6.2).

Arthropods can be vectors of viruses that may or may not cause clinical disease (Manilla, 1985). Thus, Hoogstraal (1972), summarising his previous studies, drew attention to the isolation of Manawa virus from *Argas* ticks that infested vulture nests in Pakistan. More research is needed on such host–parasite relationships, especially in view of current concerns about vulture populations in the Indian sub-continent (see Chapter 13). The spread of parasitic arthropods by migrating birds has to be considered, especially if there are climatic changes

that may favour their survival (Cooper & Mellau, 1992).

Whether neoplasms of viral origin, such as Marek's disease or leucosis occur in raptors is debatable (Forbes & Simpson, 1997a; Forbes *et al.*, 2000a). Early reports in falconry and other journals were based on gross or histological examination – for example, Woodford and Glasier (1955) recorded the former in three sparrow-hawks while Halliwell (1971) described lesions indicative of the disease in a great horned owl and Jennings (1969) in a little owl. Another report described lesions indistinguishable from Marek's disease in a free-living tawny owl (Baker, 1977) but as the author pointed out, in none of the reports listed was virus isolated. In a virological and serological survey of zoo birds in the USA (Cho & Kenzy, 1975) ten raptors were examined but all were negative for Marek's disease as were the other non-galliform species. Neoplasia is discussed in more detail in Chapter 13.

Brief mention should be made of the transmissible spongiform encephalopathies (TSEs). These are neurological disorders that appear to be caused by prions – proteinaceous agents that lack nucleic acids. Mammals are the prime hosts – for example, bovine spongiform encephalopathy (BSE) in domestic cattle and certain other ungulates, scrapie in sheep – but there has also been one report of a similar disease in ostriches (*Struthio camelus*) (Schoon *et al.*, 1991). It is not known whether birds of prey might be susceptible, as a result of ingesting 'infected' carcasses, but mechanical spread of such material is possible and vulture release programmes in Europe have now ceased using ruminant species as food, as a precaution. Those working with raptors should be vigilant.

As this chapter shows, microparasites can be responsible for a wide range of diseases in birds of prey. However, they can also be harboured (often, apparently, as part of the 'normal flora/fauna') on skin surfaces or within respiratory or alimentary tracts. Such organisms can spread from bird to bird in a variety of ways: by direct contact, by aerosol, via vectors, by contact with faeces or other contaminated material, possibly even venereally. Whether or not organisms transmitted from one bird to another cause disease depends upon a number of factors, as mentioned earlier in this chapter and discussed again later in the text.

Parasitic Diseases

O. KRONE and J. E. COOPER

'No more intimate relationship exists between one species and another than the bond linking parasites with their hosts.'

John T Cloudsley-Thompson

INTRODUCTION

Parasites can always be found in association with raptors, regardless of whether the birds are free-living or kept in captivity. The traditional opinion is that parasites often cause no severe harm to their host but the pathogenicity of parasites to birds of prey is insufficiently studied. Case reports describe death in birds of prey due to parasitic infections. It is known that parasites can reduce the physical condition of a falconer's bird resulting in poor hunting performance. In most cases a parasitosis (parasitic disease) occurs as 'condition disease', i.e. another underlying factor enhances a parasitic infection. These factors can be emaciation, infectious diseases, intoxications and everything else with a weakening effect on the bird's immune system. Medical treatment against parasites is usually only required when a parasitosis becomes apparent. This is the case when parasites occur in large numbers, in young or immunologically weakened birds. On a population scale, only very little work has been carried out on the effect of parasites on birds of prey. In general, it is known that parasites can have a significant selective effect on their hosts (Goater & Holmes, 1997). They can regulate the population size of their hosts (Anderson & May, 1979a,b; Tompkins & Begon, 1999) and may be responsible for population cycles

(Hudson *et al.*, 1998). They can influence the demographic structure (Freeland, 1976) and the geographic distribution of their host populations (Markus, 1974).

Modern classification separates the pathogens into microparasites (viruses, fungi, bacteria, protozoa) and macroparasites (helminths, arthropods). The former, the microparasites, are covered primarily in Chapter 6. The parasites here will be discussed under the two main headings *ectoparasites* (arthropods) and *endoparasites* (protozoa, helminths). Each paragraph contains basic information about the general biology of the parasite, when possible the prevalence with which the parasite is found in or on the raptor species, information on pathogenicity and the treatment.

ECOLOGY

The majority of the *ectoparasites* of raptors are transmitted from bird to bird and in some cases via an intermediate host e.g. a hippoboscid fly (Plate 16d). Infections with ectoparasites in free-living birds of prey often occur when raptors that are usually solitary live in a family or group structure. Close contact between birds in captivity is likely to favour a build-up of ectoparasites, especially if it is coupled with poor hygiene. Some ectoparasites, such as chewing lice and mites, live permanently on their host while others (ticks, fleas, flies) only temporarily. A wide variety of arthropods called nidicoles feed on organic material and detritus in the nests of birds. Occasionally they can be parasites of the birds themselves.

Most of the *endoparasites* of birds of prey have complex life-cycles, containing one or more intermediate hosts. These parasites are highly reproductive, to ensure that some stages reach the next host. The eggs are often produced non-continuously, depending on the season or time of day. Some protozoan parasites have an indirect life-cycle (*Sarcocystis*), while others (*Trichomonas*) have a direct development cycle. Only a few helminths have a direct development, such as some threadworms of the subfamily Capillariinae, which can accumulate in a paratenic host. From the standpoint of development and life-history, the trematodes not only possess by far the most complex developmental cycles among the parasites, but also among all members of the animal kingdom (Cheng, 1986). The most complicated life-cycle of a trematode from a raptor includes up to four obligate hosts. The majority of helminths use the food of the bird of prey to infect them. In some cases the last intermediate host is manipulated by the parasite to become more easily a victim of the final host, the bird of prey. This behaviour increases the probability that the parasite reaches the definitive host where it matures. Only a few nematodes (for example, *Cardofilaria*) of raptors are transmitted by biting arthropods.

ECTOPARASITES

All ectoparasites of raptors belong to the phylum Arthropoda, the classes Arachnida (ticks and mites) and Insecta (fleas, flies, hippoboscids, chewing lice). They all have an exoskeleton and are heterosexual, but some are parthenogenetic, too. The most common ectoparasites of raptors are shown in Table 7.1. The former order Mallophaga has changed its name to Phthiraptera (Lyal, 1985).

Table 7.1 Common and scientific names of important ectoparasites.

Common name	Scientific name
Ticks and mites	Acarina
Fleas	Siphonaptera
Flies (hippoboscids)	Diptera (Pupipara)
Chewing lice or Mallophaga	Phthiraptera (Amblycera and Ischnocera)

Ticks

Ticks develop from eggs through larvae and two nymph stages into adult parasites. They suck blood and can possibly act as vectors of microparasites. Ticks are occasionally found on birds of prey, especially on less feathered parts of the head (cere, eyelids, angle of bill). Raptors in Europe that are unable to fly due to trauma may survive for some days by feeding on earthworms. They walk around in the bush or grassland and often become infested with larvae, nymphs or adults of ticks (e.g. *Ixodes ricinus*). If left alone the ticks will, after engorging themselves on blood, drop off. Parsons (1974) reported a case in which a newly imported lanner falcon was parasitised by ticks. The bird had a massive infestation of larval ticks (*Argas* sp.), approximately 300 being counted. The areas of attachment (under the thighs) showed gross lesions of excoriation, haemorrhage and necrosis and these changes were confirmed histologically. In addition, the bird had a heavy louse burden, damage to beak, cere and feet, and stomatitis (probably trichomoniasis). Cooper *et al.* (1993a) found ticks (*Amblyomma lepidum* and *Rhipicephalus turanicum*) on migrating birds of prey in Israel. Schilling *et al.* (1981) reported heavy infections with *Ixodes arboricola* in nestlings of peregrine falcons in Baden-Württemberg, Germany, in the 1970s. In 1979 23% of the chicks were infected and most of them died. A single nestling carried a maximum of 320 ticks. Successful treatment of chicks and nest sites with Antorgan® (Shell-Chemie GmbH), an insecticide, was performed. Antorgan® is no longer on the market. Ivomec® (MSD AGVET, Haar, Germany) can be used as a 'spot on' application in a 10% dilution for the birds, and Ardap® (WDT, Garbsen, Germany) for treating nesting material. Forbes and Simpson (1993) described severe effects of *I. ricinus* in captive birds of prey. They found subcutaneous haemorrhage and oedema of the head which was most pronounced around the site of attachment of the tick on the head of a peregrine falcon which died in an aviary. Three falconers' birds infested with *I. ricinus* showed similar signs, including closure of the eye and the auditory canal and unilaterally swollen oral cavity. Treatment consists of methylprednisolone, fluid therapy and amoxicillin. Single ticks are best removed with forceps, making sure not to leave the mouthparts embedded in the tissue. Chastel *et al.* (1991) tested *I. pari* from birds as potential vectors for arboviruses and concluded that these ticks play no important role in transmission or dissemination of this virus.

Mites

The larva which hatches from the egg undergoes two moults to become an adult. Mites sometimes cause trouble in birds of prey. The red mite (*Dermanyssus gallinae*) lives in buildings and attacks birds at night, causing irritability, skin lesions and, possibly, anaemia. It may be difficult to detect unless the mews or aviary is examined with a torch (flashlight) at night; the parasites may then be seen. Infestation with the Northern mite (*Ornithonyssus sylviarum*) is much easier to diagnose. It lives on the host and also sucks blood; as Salvin and Brodrick (1855) stated in *Falconry in the British Isles*: '. . . it is a species of *Acarus*, and makes its first appearance in the nares of the Hawk, burrowing in these parts, as also into the eyelids'.

Trained hawks often become infected from affected prey, especially rooks (*Corvus frugilegus*). Heidenreich (1997) found a *Knemidocoptes* sp. in the cere and in the horn of the bill in a hybrid falcon and treated the lesions with liquid paraffin. Bougerol (1967) recorded a *Knemidocoptes* sp. on accipiters but gave no details. A captive juvenile great horned owl infected with *K. mutans* had bilateral proliferative papillary hyperkeratosis on the feet. The owl was successfully treated with ivermectin at a dose of 200 mg/kg body weight (Schulz *et al.*, 1989).

Mumcuoglu and Müller (1974) recorded the death of a free-living eagle owl from aspergillosis and a *Pseudomonas aeruginosa* infection; these authors suggested that feather mite damage predisposed to the dual infection. A nasal mite (*Boydaia falconis*) was recorded from an American kestrel from Texas (Pence & Casto, 1976). Fain and Smiley (1989) recovered a lung mite (*Pneumophagus bubonis*), parasitic in a great horned owl. Ospreys frequently carry the feather mite *Bonnetella fusca* (Plate 16c), especially on the under wing coverts of the secondaries, with no obvious effect on the feather structure. In addition to the specific mite, Miller *et al.* (1997) recorded another mite species, *Analloptes* sp., and the chewing lice *Kurodaia haliaeeti* on ospreys from Ontario, Canada. A comprehensive checklist of parasitic mites of Falconiformes and Strigiformes was provided by Philips (2000), containing 86 species of parasitic feather, quill, respiratory, skin, and nest mites (Acarina). Mites can be killed with insecticides but great care should be taken in view of the apparent high susceptibility of predatory birds to chlorinated hydrocarbons (Cooper, 1965; Bougerol, 1967). Following removal of the bird, the aviary can be dusted with 2% malathion or fumigated with formaldehyde and potassium permanganate. Either of these techniques will help to eliminate red mites. In the case of *O. sylviarum*, a pyrethrum, derris or piperonyl butoxide product can be used to dust the bird but none of these is completely effective. Alternatively, the bird can be sprayed with a 0.5% solution of trichlorphon which kills the mites readily (Cooper, 1974b). Malley and Whitbread (1996) suggested treatment with piperonyl butoxide blended with pyrethrin (Ridmite Powder™, Johnson).

Light dusting of the bird with pyrethrin (0.5–2.0%) or its derivates, malathion (5%) or carbaryl (0.5%), and repeated in 10 to 14 days, was recommended by Smith (1996). Ivermectin (0.2 mg/kg = 200 µg/kg body weight) can be applied locally diluted 1 : 10 with water.

Fleas

Metamorphosis in fleas is holometabolic ('complete'); i.e. the stages look completely different. The larva which hatches out of an egg undergoes two moults. The third-stage larva spins a cocoon and pupates. The only parasitic stage is the adult, which develops in the cocoon. Fleas are generally rare on birds of prey other than as temporary visitors derived from the prey or, occasionally, on nestlings. A possible exception is the stickfast flea *Echidnophaga gallinacea*, essentially a tropical species, but increasingly being reported elsewhere, which attaches itself to the skin of the host. Cooper (unpublished data) found large numbers of this flea on the feet of a free-living black-shouldered kite in Kenya, and Cooper and Mellau (1992) suggested that it might be spread by migrating birds. A number of species of flea are found in the nests of both falconiform and strigiform birds; examples of British species were listed by Smit (1957). Control of these parasites is not easy since the life cycle is completed off the host; nesting material and casting, which may harbour ova, larvae or pupae, should be removed.

Flies

Eggs and larvae of the flies *Lucilia* and *Calliphora* spp. are frequently found in wounds, where they feed on necrotic and living tissue, causing additive damage or even death. When the larvae are fully grown, they drop off. They bury themselves in loose soil or debris and undergo a pupa stage, before the adults hatch. Crocoll and Parker (1981) found *Protocalliphora* larvae causing bleeding and swellings around the ears in nestlings of broad-winged hawks. Cooper (pers. comm.) stated that myiasis is a potential problem in the rare Mauritius kestrel, in which he found larvae of *Passeromyia heterochaeta* in the nares. Death of a bird from myiasis is believed to be due to toxaemia or septicaemia (Soulsby, 1974). Such flies lay their eggs in the damaged tissue of handicapped birds and the larvae (maggots) hatch within 8–24 hours, depending on the temperature.

Flies tend to prove troublesome in hot weather; and especially under tropical conditions. Wounds must be examined carefully – at least once a day – and the prophylactic use of a safe insecticidal product may be desirable. Wounds in general should be disinfected and covered with bandage or dressing to prevent myiasis (see Chapter 4). Treatment

of myiasis consists of the cleaning of the wounds, preferably by irrigation with warm water containing soap or a quaternary ammonium disinfectant. As many maggots as possible should be removed manually. The exposed larvae can be sprayed with a pyrethrum-based product; maggots in the wound should be flushed out (Butynski, 1995). Necrotic tissue should be removed and a suitable insecticidal/antibiotic product applied. If the larvae have entered the body orifices and are feeding on internal organs, euthanasia should be considered. If myiasis occurs in young birds in breeding aviaries, nesting material should be removed. Malley and Whitbread (1996) suggested spraying the bird with 0.0005% ivermectin (i.e. 0.5 ml Ivomec 1% injection for cattle in 1 l of water) prior to removing the maggots. Using ivermectin in a raptor, the critical dosage of 0.2–0.4 mg/kg should not be exceeded, especially in young or debilitated birds.

The fly species *Carnus hemapterus* has so far been found on nestlings only. Blackish faeces of the flies are often detectable under the wings of chicks. The fly itself is very small (2 mm long) and loses its wings when it reaches the host. It feeds on blood. The abdomen of the female can greatly enlarge due to the development of her ovaries and the eggs. The eggs are deposed in the nesting material. In the same year the larvae hatch, feed on organic nest material and overwinter as puparia. Infestations in nestlings from Germany starts in mid May and lasts until the end of June (Walter & Hudde, 1987). In southwestern New Jersey, USA 88% ($n = 103$) of young barn owls were infested with *C. hemapterus* (Kirkpatrick & Colvin, 1989). Lacina (1999) found reduced mass growth in nestlings of Eurasian kestrels infected with *C. hemapterus* in Eastern Bohemia.

Black flies of the family Simuliidae feed on the blood of their hosts. They generally can be found near rivers and streams. The eggs are laid beneath the surface of water. The larva spends its life under water and pupates in a cone-shaped cocoon after which the adult fly leaves the aquatic habitat. Black flies are vectors for the blood parasites *Leucocytozoon* spp. Attacks by *Prosimulium* have been reported as a common cause of death in young red-tailed hawks in rainy seasons in California, USA (Brown &

Amadon, 1968). Smith *et al.* (1998) documented parasitic blackflies at 42 red-tailed hawk nests in Wyoming, USA. A total of 13 chicks (*n* = 87) died as a result of blackfly infestation. Flies can be killed by pyrethroids.

Hippoboscids

Development in hippoboscid or 'louse' flies is very rapid. The females are pupipar; i.e. the stage of a larva is missing. Gravid females produce a single pupa within a few days and deposit this in the nesting material or between the feathers of the birds. The adult flies suck blood, and can transmit *Haemoproteus* and other protozoan parasites (Keymer, 1969).

Hippoboscids such as *Ornithomyia avicularia* (Plate 16b) are common on birds of prey. *Pseudolynchia canariensis* and *Icosta* sp. were collected from migrating raptors (mainly Steppe buzzards) in Israel (Cooper *et al.*, 1993a). Young *et al.* (1993) found a prevalence of 17% (*n* = 382) for *Icosta americana* and *Ornithomya anchineuria* on northern spotted owls (*Strix occidentalis caurina*) in north-western California, USA. They fly off during handling of the bird. Bird ringers (banders) often report hippoboscids on nestling birds of prey. If they occur on captive birds, they can be removed manually or the raptor can be dusted lightly with pyrethrin (0.5–2.0%) or its derivates, malathion (5%) or carbaryl (0.5%). The treatment should be repeated in 10–14 days (Smith, 1996).

Mosquitoes

Most mosquito species lay their eggs in water. The larva is free-living and undergoes four moult stages before transforming into a pupa. The pupae are very active and sensitive to disturbances. The imago hatches from the pupa and grows into the adult stage. Only the adult females are haematophagous. They feed on vertebrates, including birds of prey, and can transmit blood parasites such as *Haemoproteus*, *Plasmodium* and, probably, avian pox. Unexplained swellings on the head may also be attributable to such bites (see Chapter 13): they usually resolve spontaneously.

Chewing (biting) lice

Chewing lice of the order Phthiraptera – formerly called Mallophaga – are common on birds of prey. They spend their entire life-cycle on the bird. The eggs are attached to the feathers. The first nymph undergoes three moults before becoming adult. The suborders Ischnocera and Amblycera feed on feathers, skin debris and blood. Representatives of both families can cause damage to feathers, irritation and increased preening activity. They often multiply when raptors are stressed, debilitated or sick, possibly because such birds do not preen properly. The eggs are deposited on the specific regions where the chewing lice live. *Craspedorrhynchus* and *Aegypoecus* are mainly found on the feathers of the head, whereas *Laemobothrion* (Plate 16a) and *Colpocephalum* inhabit the body and wings, and *Degeeriella* and *Falcolipeurus* live on the wings of falconiform birds (Pérez *et al.*, 1996). Mey (1997) described two new subspecies (*Degeeriella discocephala stelleri* and *Kelerinirmus rufus camtschaticus*) from the Steller's sea eagle (*Haliaeetus pelagicus*) and a new *Craspedorrhynchus* species from the wedge-tailed eagle (*Aquila audax*) (Mey, 2001). An annotated checklist of chewing lice parasitising caracaras including a new species (*Caracaricola chimangophilus*) is provided by Mey (2000). Mey (1998) listed 12 genera of ambyloceric and eight genera of ischnoceric chewing lice of Falconiformes. In this classification he did not list the ambyloceric genus *Pterophilus* (Clay & Price, 1970), which is monotypic with *P. sudanensis* (Clay & Price 1970) and only found on the African swallow-tailed kite (*Chelictinia riocourii*) (Mey, pers. comm.). Lice of the genus *Strigiphilus* are confined to the owls (Strigiformes). Treatment with insecticides such as a pyrethrum spray is relatively safe and, if given repeatedly, effective. Trichlorphon has been shown to be effective against poultry lice and, in view of its apparent safety, is recommended. Treatment suggested by Smith and Smith (1988) is either dusting or fumigating the bird with 0.5% carbaryl dust (every 10–14 days; 5% for perches and nest boxes), 4–5% malathion dust, 0.5–2% pyrethrin dust, rotenone dust, ether or chloroform. A good method of collecting and counting lice from living

Table 7.2 Common and scientific names of endoparasites.

Common name	Scientific name
Unicellular parasites	Protozoa
Tapeworms	Cestoda
Flukes	Trematoda
Spiny-headed worms	Acanthocephala
Roundworms	Nematoda

birds is the use of a plastic bag containing cotton wool soaked in ether or chloroform; the bird is placed into the bag, with its head outside, for about 5 minutes. The lice are anaesthetised or killed and drop off into the bag.

ENDOPARASITES

In raptors, endoparasites of particular importance are protozoa, tapeworms, flukes, roundworms and spiny-headed worms. The different groups are shown in Table 7.2. Depending on the life-cycle of the parasite, habitat, region, climate and foraging behaviour of the raptor, some endoparasites are relatively common whereas others are rarely found in raptors. Some examples of the eggs of these parasites are shown in Fig. 7.1.

Prophylaxis

Most raptors become infected by endoparasites due to feeding on prey. In general, one should avoid feeding carcasses of prey species, found dead in the wild, to captive raptors since this is a natural source of infection for birds of prey. Pigeons and other birds can act as a source of *Trichomonas*, rodents are a source of coccidia or cestodes, other birds of coccidia and nematodes, and a variety of vertebrates (amphibians, reptiles, birds, mammals) of trematodes. For some nematodes, insects (beetles, flies) may serve as intermediate hosts and earthworms as paratenic hosts. For raptors in aviaries access to earthworms and insects should therefore be minimised. It is sensible to select grit or sand as material to cover the ground.

In many collections birds are treated regularly for intestinal parasites. The use of anti-parasitic drugs in general is only useful if there is evidence of a parasitosis, i.e. clinical or subclinical signs of disease. Piperazine and thiabendazole can be used but neither drug is particularly effective against threadworms; ivermectin or fenbendazole is more suitable in such cases. Praziquantel is safe and effective against trematodes and cestodes (see Appendix IX). Predatory birds will usually take oral anthelmintics if the latter are crushed in a piece of meat, or, in the case of large hawks, placed inside a dead mouse which can be swallowed whole. Often birds of prey can be observed tearing small pieces of meat out of their prey, leaving the drug behind. To ensure that the bird gets its medication, force-feeding is sometimes necessary (see Chapter 4). A parasitological examination a few days later should help to ascertain whether the treatment was successful. However, it must be remembered that strict hygiene will go a long way towards the control of parasites and this must always be practised. Routine faecal examinations (at 2–3 month intervals) can serve as an indicator for the presence of endoparasites and such investigations form an important part of health monitoring of supposedly normal birds (see Chapter 4). Recently imported raptors should always have faeces examined. It is also wise to check faeces of all birds which are to be put in an aviary for breeding, since some parasites with a direct life-cycle can easily multiply in these small, yet intensive, surroundings and it is useful to know which parasites are likely to be introduced into the enclosure. If faecal samples show that worm eggs are still present, the treatment is repeated. In general, worm egg counts can give only a very rough indication of the parasite infestation. The number of eggs found only rarely represents the true infective status with endoparasites. Some trematodes produce eggs in cycles, depending on the season and sometimes even on the time of day.

Protozoa

Trichomonas gallinae is one of the most significant protozoan parasites of birds of prey and is responsible for the disease that has long been known to English-speaking falconers as 'frounce'; it occurs typically in falcons and sometimes in hawks and

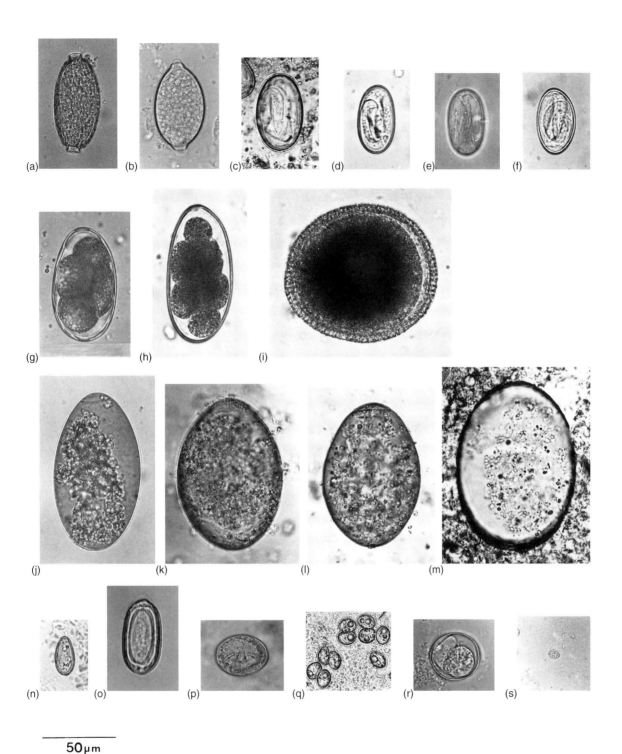

50 μm

Fig. 7.1 Reproductive stages of the most common endoparasites: (a–o) eggs of helminths, (p–r) protozoa.
(a) *Capillaria tenuissima* with typical net-like surface; (b) *Eucoleus dispar* with dotted surface; (c) *Serratospiculum tendo*;
(d) *Physaloptera alata*; (e) *Synhimantus laticeps*, (f) *Microtetrameres cloacitectus*; (g) *Syngamus trachea*; (h) *Hovorkonema variegatum*; (i) *Porrocaecum* sp.; (j) *Neodiplostomum attenuatum*; (k) *Nematostrigea serpens*; (l) *Strigea falconispalumbi*;
(m) *Paracenogonimus* sp.; (n) *Metorchis* sp.; (o) *Cladotaenia globifera*; (p) oocysts of *Sarcocystis* sp.; (q) oocyst of
Caryospora sp.; (r) *Trichomonas gallinae*. (Courtesy of Oliver Krone.)

owls. The life-cycle is simple, in that the trophozoite doubles by binary fission, without forming cysts. Pigeons (*Columba livia*) are the natural hosts of *T. gallinae* and in them the infection is maintained by passing the parasite with the crop milk to the youngsters. Cooper and Petty (1988) suggested that *T. gallinae* was a significant mortality factor, which might influence the reproductive potential of the British goshawk population. Pepler and Oettlé (1992) reported an outbreak of trichomoniasis on the Cape Peninsula in South Africa and surroundings in seven species of birds of prey in 1990 and 1991. Boal *et al.* (1998b) documented a greater prevalence of *T. gallinae* among urban nestlings (85%) than exurban nestlings (9%) of Cooper's hawk in southeastern Arizona. They also found a higher nestling mortality among urban (50%) than exurban nests (5%) (Boal & Mannan, 1999). Real *et al.* (2000) diagnosed high prevalences of *T. gallinae* in nestlings of Bonelli's eagle in Spain, but only a small proportion developed clinical signs or died.

Trichomoniasis is basically a stomatitis but the early signs may be only mild – the 'flicking away' of food or difficulty in swallowing. On clinical examination one may see yellow caseous material in and around the mouth, pharynx and oesophagus (Plate 17a). Later the bird loses its appetite and may become dehydrated. Eventually the lesions can involve the ears, larynx, respiratory tract, and other internal organs. In cases of intranasal or intrasinal trichomoniasis, clinical signs can be oedema of the lower eyelid, fluttering of the skin above the infraorbital sinuses or dyspnoea. Caseous lesions within the lumen of the trachea result in severe dyspnoea and abdominal–thoracic breathing (Samour *et al.*, 1995). Occasionally mouth lesions are associated with a foetid smell. Definitive diagnosis is not difficult so long as therapy has not yet started. A moist swab of the exudate should, if expressed into warm isotonic saline, reveal motile flagellate organisms with an undulating membrane.

The danger of trichomoniasis is a reason for ensuring that care is taken when freshly killed pigeons are used for food or, perhaps, for not using them at all (see Chapter 10). Even healthy pigeons can harbour *T. gallinae*. A useful precaution is to freeze and thaw pigeons before using them as food; this appears to kill or incapacitate the parasites. Nev-

ertheless, one must bear in mind that *T. gallinae* can probably also be transmitted directly from one bird to another, as reported in an American kestrel (*Falco sparverius*) by Stone and Janes (1969).

Other conditions may simulate 'frounce', in particular oesophageal capillariasis and various types of stomatitis. Stehle (1965) listed eight possible causes of stomatitis in captive birds of prey including vitamin A deficiency, pox and fungal infections. It is important, therefore, to ensure that any cases of stomatitis are examined clinically and swabs or scrapings taken for examination and/or culture before treatment is instigated. Metronidazole, at a dose of 30–65 mg/kg body weight orally, should be given for 5–7 days (Smith, 1996). Heidenreich (1997) recommended karnidazole 1 tablet/500 g body weight once as a safe and effective medication.

Various blood protozoa have been recorded from raptors. Blood parasites frequently detected in blood smears belong to the genera *Haemoproteus*, *Leucocytozoon*, *Plasmodium* and *Trypanosoma*. Transmission is usually by biting arthropods, such as hippoboscids, simulids and mosquitoes. Bennett *et al.* (1965) differentiated between the genera *Parahaemoproteus* transmitted by ceratopogonids and *Haemoproteus* transmitted by hippoboscid flies. Because gametocytes of both genera are indistinguishable morphologically in thin blood smears, they are reduced to subgeneric rank (Levine & Campbell, 1971). The sexual development occurs in the arthropods, whereas the parasite multiplicates asexually in different tissues and, in the case of *Plasmodium*, in the blood of the birds too. Schizonts can be found, depending on the parasite, in the liver, brain, muscle or in endothelium cells and in *Plasmodium* infections in the blood. The gametocytes, which inhabit the blood cells, can therefore be detected in the blood smear. *H. tinnunculus* and *H. brachiatus* are the valid species found in birds of the family Falconidae and *H. elani*, *H. nisi* and *H. janovyi* are the valid species found in birds of the family Accipitridae (Peirce *et al.*, 1990). For the osprey *H. elani* is listed (Bishop & Bennett, 1992). *Haemoproteus* spp. are most frequently encountered in the Falconiformes (53.1%, *n* = 333), followed by the Strigiformes (22.6%, *n* = 178) than in other orders of birds examined in Central Europe (Kučera, 1981b). *Leucocytozoon toddi* is the only parasite of this genus reported to date from birds of the order Falconiformes (Greiner & Kocan, 1977), whereas *L. ziemanni* is the only species in birds of the order Strigiformes. In his literature survey of birds from Central Europe, Kučera (1981a,b) stated that Strigiformes are found to be infected with *Plasmodium* in 2.3% of cases (*n* = 178) and with *Leucocytozoon* in 9.9% (*n* = 162), but Falconiformes in not a single case (*n* = 333) infected with *Plasmodium* and only 1.3% with *Leucocytozoon* (*n* = 334). Bennett *et al.* (1993a) listed six species of *Plasmodium*: *P. elongatum*, *P. fallax*, *P. circumflexum*, *P. lophurae*, *P. relictum* and *P. vaughani*, for birds of the family Accipitridae and three species of *Plasmodium* for birds of the family Falconidae: *P. relictum*, *P. circumflexum* and *P. polare*, in their checklist of the avian species of *Plasmodium*.

Furthermore, the same authors mentioned eight different species of *Trypanosoma* found in falconiform and seven different species in strigiform birds, but *Trypanosoma avium* is probably the only species of this genus occurring in owls and hawks (Bennett, 1970; Krone, 1996). The life-cycle of *Trypanosoma* includes biting arthropods (black-flies, mosquitoes, ceratopogonids) in which multiplication by binary fission occurs. With the next blood meal of the arthropod the parasite is transmitted to the new host. *Trypanosoma* was detected in 4.5% of strigiform and 1.2% of falconiform birds examined in Central Europe (Kučera, 1982). Other blood parasites of raptors include *Hepatozoon neophrontis* (Bishop & Bennett, 1992), *Babesia shortti* (Samour & Peirce, 1996) and *Atoxoplasma* (Greiner & Mundy, 1979). In a study on blood parasites in raptors from Florida, USA, Forrester *et al.* (1994) found the Strigiformes to be most often infected (63%, *n* = 54) followed by the Falconiformes (33%, *n* = 94). Among the infections with haemoparasites, *Haemoproteus* spp. were most common (67%), followed by *Plasmodium* (22%), *Leucocytozoon* (9%), *Trypanosoma* (1%) and microfilariae (1%). Peirce *et al.* (1983) diagnosed infections of blood parasites in 20.3% of raptors from Britain, 14.2% from Spain and 24.1% in the United Arab Emirates.

The effect of blood parasites on their hosts is poorly understood. In general, the pathogenicity of blood parasites in most birds of prey is relatively low (Peirce, 1981). The degree to which parasites are pathogenic is difficult to assess, since sick or dying birds in the wild rapidly fall victim to predators or their carcasses go undetected (Peirce, 1989). A rise in parasite numbers in blood may be associated with stress during breeding time, migration or debilitation due to starvation, or concurrent diseases. Gyr falcons appear very susceptible to diseases caused by *Plasmodium relictum* (Remple, 1981). Valentin *et al.* (1994) reported the death of five of seven nestlings of snowy owls infected with *Parahaemoproteus* in a zoological garden near Berlin, Germany. Death in nestlings of great horned owls was attributed to *Leucocytozoon* infections (Hunter *et al.* 1997). Clinical signs can be depression, weakness and emesis. Therapy consists of chloroquine 25 mg/kg bodyweight orally in four dosages over 48 hours, starting with 10 mg initially (Remple, 1981). Heidenreich (1997) suggested chloroquine initially 25 mg/kg bodyweight orally and repeated application of 15 mg/kg after 12, 24 and 48 hours. In addition primaquine 0.75 mg/kg bodyweight can be administered orally.

Coccidia of the genera *Eimeria*, *Sarcocystis* and *Caryospora* are frequently reported from birds of prey. A differentiation on the basis of oocysts is not possible for *Frenkelia* and *Sarcocystis* spp. In the intermediate host the cysts of *Frenkelia* develop in the brain, while cysts of *Sarcocystis* are found in the muscles.

Most coccidia of raptors have an indirect life-cycle, including an intermediate host. Mice and birds are the intermediate hosts for *Sarcocystis*. Odening (1998) listed 12 species of *Sarcocystis* (including *Frenkelia*) for which raptors are the definitive hosts. Coccidia of the genus *Caryospora* have a direct or alternatively an indirect life-cycle, with a rodent as intermediate host. The coccidia multiply in the epithelial cells of the small intestine of the definitive host and are excreted with the faeces. The typical oocysts – sporulated in *Sarcocystis* and non-sporulated in *Caryospora* – are visible in the faeces. Raptors often act as definitive hosts, but cysts of *Sarcocystis* in other tissues than the intestine, mainly skeletal musculature and heart, are also found in some birds of prey (Munday, 1977; Crawley *et al.*, 1982; Krone *et al.*, 2000). These tissue cysts are often hard to differentiate from megaloschizonts of haematozoa. Two cases were reported in which raptors had a *Sarcocystis* encephalitis (see Chapter 9). A Northern goshawk and a golden eagle had neurological signs such as unilateral debilitation, paralysis and a slight head tilt (Aguilar *et al.*, 1991; Dubey *et al.*, 1991).

The pathogenicity of genera regularly infecting the intestine varies, with *Caryospora* being most pathogenic in captive birds of prey, especially in young birds. The pathogenicity of *Sarcocystis* is discussed controversially, often recording no pathogenic effect, but several cases of coccidiosis caused by *Sarcocystis* in raptors with severe intestinal damage have been reported (Cooper & Forbes, 1986; Gylstorff & Grimm, 1987). Upton *et al.* (1990) described 14 species of *Caryospora* and 18 species of *Eimeria* affecting birds of prey. Clinical signs often comprise weight loss, inappetence, depression, vomiting, haemorrhagic faeces, diarrhoea or acute death (Forbes & Simpson, 1997b). Young merlins are especially susceptible to infections with *Caryospora*, showing severe diarrhoea or acute death (Forbes & Fox, 2000). It is preferable to control reinfection by hygiene and routine parasitological examination of faeces. Infections with *Sarcocystis* or *Eimeria* can be treated with sulphadimethoxine 25–55 mg/kg bodyweight orally for 5–7 days (Cawthorn, 1993). A safe and effective treatment is clazuril 5–10 mg/kg bodyweight orally on 2 consecutive days (Heidenreich, 1997). Toltrazuril 25 mg/kg bodyweight given once weekly by mouth for 3 weeks is currently the most effective treatment for *Caryospora* infections (Forbes & Simpson, 1997b) (see Appendix IX).

Raptors probably act as an intermediate host of *Toxoplasma gondii* (Cawthorn, 1993). Experimental studies have indicated that the heart and breast muscles often become infected with *T. gondii*. Until now detection of *T. gondii* in raptors was only possible by measuring antibody titres (Lindsay *et al.* 1991; Dubey *et al.* 1992; Lindsay *et al.* 1993).

Giardia has been reported from turkey vultures (Meyer & Jarrell, 1982) but little is known of its significance in this and other birds nor of its relevance to public health.

Flukes

Trematodes are mainly found in the intestinal tract of birds of prey. The adult worms can be identified by their typical appearance: they have an oral and a ventral sucker, a digestive system consisting of a prepharynx, pharynx, oesophagus and one or two intestinal caeca. All trematodes of raptors are hermaphroditic. The eggs have a shell with an operculum, a lid-like cap at one end. The typical life-cycle contains three hosts, with a snail as first and a vertebrate as second intermediate host. The most common fluke species found in birds of prey are *Strigea* (Plate 17c) and *Neodiplostomum* (Plate 17b) (Sitko, 1998). *Nematostrigea serpens* is a specific trematode of the osprey. The development cycle of *Strigea falconispalumbi* is one of the most complex life-cycles among parasites. The adult trematodes deposit their eggs in the intestine of their host. The eggs leave the raptor with its faeces and need to fall into water where water snails (*Planorbis* spp.) live. The ciliated miracidium, the first stage of the trematode, actively penetrates the water snail. Within the snail the parasite multiplies by passing two sporocyst generations. The newly developed cercaria leaves the snail. As a free-swimming stage the cercaria penetrates tadpoles. In parallel to the developing tadpole the parasite transforms into the mesocercaria. The tadpole or frog must be eaten by a vertebrate, which is the third intermediate host. Within the vertebrate the trematode transforms into the metacercaria. The third intermediate host can be a mammal, bird, reptile or amphibian, but not a fish. When the third intermediate host is ingested by the definitive host, the raptor becomes infected. The cycle is completed: the fluke matures and produces eggs (Fig. 7.2).

In general, trematodes are rarely pathogenic. However, there are a few descriptions of parasitosis caused by flukes. Dedrick (1965) reported a fatal disease characterised by low condition and diarrhoea associated with *Strigea* sp. in a captive prairie falcon, and Greenwood *et al.* (1984) described severe enteritis in an infected saker falcon due to a trematodosis. Despite their only partly known pathogenicity, flukes are of interest from an ecological perspective: differences in the abundance of *Strigea falconispalumi* in Eurasian buzzards from various areas can indicate diversity of intermediate hosts in the habitat of the Eurasian buzzard (Krone & Streich, 2000). Liver flukes (*Metorchis*) of fish-eating birds can cause cholangitis, cholangiectasis, icterus and hepatitis.

Fluke eggs are commonly seen in faecal samples

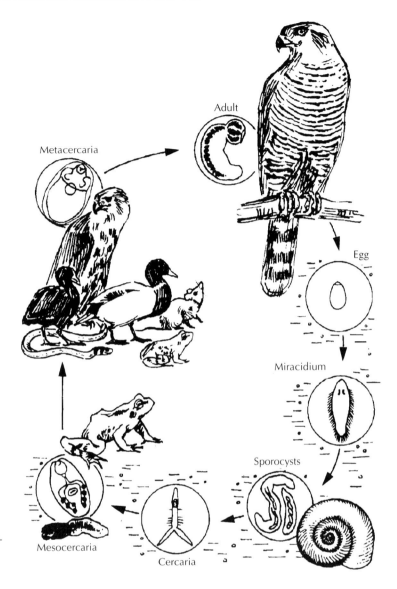

Fig. 7.2 Life-cycle of *Strigea falconis-palumbi* consisting of four obligate hosts. (Courtesy of Odening, 1967.)

where their numbers undergo daily fluctuations. Eggs are often produced seasonally. If treatment is required, praziquantel can be given in a concentration of 50 mg/kg bodyweight orally or subcutaneously (Smith, 1996). In captivity there is little chance of flukes completing their life-cycle, since suitable intermediate hosts are unlikely to be present.

Tapeworms

Cestodes inhabit the small intestine of birds of prey. They can be identified by their scolex (the hold-fast organ), narrow neck and the segmented strobila consisting of single proglottids. *Cladotaenia globifera* is the most often diagnosed tapeworm in Europe. The life-cycle is indirect, using mice as intermediate host. After the egg is ingested by the intermediate host, the oncosphere hatches and penetrates the intestine, forming a cysticercus in internal organs. The life-cycle is completed when the definitive host feeds on infected mice (Wetzel & Enigk, 1937). Other tapeworms found in birds of prey are *Mesocestoides, Anomotaenia, Matabelea, Lingula, Idiogenes, Choanotaenia, Hymenolepis,*

115

Oligorchis, *Paracladotaenia* and *Raillietina* spp. There are few reports of cestodes being pathogenic to their definitive host, the raptor. They are usually diagnosed when proglottids or eggs are seen in the faeces; large numbers appear to be correlated with poor condition. Pathological alterations can be enteritis and thickening of the intestinal mucous membrane. Clinical signs can range from general debilitation, diarrhoea, weakness to death (Bogue, 1980). Wetzel and Enigk (1937) stated that metabolic products of the tapeworm can provoke irritation and inflammation of the mucosal layer of the intestine, resulting in maldigestion and malabsorption. In large numbers, tapeworms can cluster and cause obstruction. Appropriate drugs for treatment include praziquantel 50 mg/kg bodyweight orally or subcutaneously (Smith, 1996) or niclosamide 125 mg/kg bodyweight orally (Lierz & Remple, 1997). Care should be taken, however, as some birds react adversely to the medication and may regurgitate or vomit.

Roundworms

Nematodes can be found in nearly every organ of raptors, but are most common in the digestive and respiratory system. Identification is based on the elongated, cylindrical body which is tapered at both ends. Infections do not necessarily cause clinical signs, depending largely upon the species and the number of parasites, their locality and the health status of the host. Life-cycles of only few nematode species are known completely. Threadworms of the subfamily Capillariinae are the most often diagnosed helminths in birds of prey (Frey & Kutzer, 1982; Smith, 1993a; Krone, 2000). The upper alimentary tract is often infected with *Eucoleus dispar*, a synonym of *Capillaria contorta* (Barus & Sergejeva, 1989b; Krone & Cooper, 1999). The development of *E. dispar* is direct, but can be expanded by involving earthworms as paratenic hosts. This threadworm can cause disease of varying severity (Trainer *et al.*, 1968; Cooper, 1969a), and sometimes this is a differential diagnosis for trichomoniasis, candidiasis and vitamin A deficiency. Affected birds show white diphtheritic membranes in the oesophagus and crop and, in some cases, buccal cavity and pharynx (Plate

17d). A scraping of this material will, if examined under the microscope, show the characteristic eggs with a dotted surface. In birds that die there is usually a severely inflamed upper alimentary tract on the surface of which adult worms can be demonstrated. On histological examination, worms are seen embedded in the mucous membrane. Often oedema and varying degrees of inflammatory reaction are present. The worms and eggs may also be occasionally detected in sections of the buccal cavity or pharynx of apparently healthy birds of prey during histological examination. Gyr falcons in particular seem to be susceptible to oesophageal capillariasis (Clausen & Gudmundsson, 1981). Diluted ivermectin 0.2 mg/kg bodyweight (1:9 with lactated Ringer's solution) intramuscularly is an effective treatment (Smith, 1996).

Baruscapillaria falconis and *Capillaria tenuissima* inhabit the intestine of hawks and owls (Barus & Sergejeva, 1989a, 1990). The surface of the eggs of these threadworms has a netlike structure and their life-cycles are unknown. At low densities affected birds do not show clinical signs. In heavy infections signs can be diarrhoea, anorexia and weight loss. During normal necropsy threadworms are often difficult to find unless the material is very fresh but they and large numbers of eggs are usually visible in smears or histological sections of the gut. The examination of the digestive system under low-power magnification is a more reliable technique for the detection of these fine worms.

Intestinal ascarids cause little trouble in small numbers in a healthy host but can be pathogenic in large numbers. Nematodes of the genus *Porrocaecum* are common in birds of prey (both captive and free-living) which have died of inanition; in such cases the worms may block the lumen of the intestine (Plate 17f) and tens of thousands of eggs per g are present in the faeces. The life-cycle of *Porrocaecum angusticolle* is indirect, with Insectivora as the intermediate hosts. The eggs of the adult worms are passed out in the faeces of the bird. The intermediate host becomes infected by ingesting these eggs. The parasite hatches and differentiates within the intermediate host and can be found finally in capsules surrounded by connective tissue of the mesentery. When a raptor feeds on this intermediate host it becomes infected itself and the worm can reach maturity (Osche, 1955). The pathogenicity derives from the metabolic toxins of the worms. Perforations of the intestine are also reported. Bougerol (1967) recorded six adult *Ascaridia* in the lung of a peregrine. Recommended treatment consists of levamisole 10–20 mg/kg bodyweight orally for 2 consecutive days (Smith, 1996) or flubendazole or fenbendazole 25 mg/kg bodyweight orally every day for 5 consecutive days (Lierz & Remple, 1997). These and other treatments are listed in Appendix IX with some variations in dose rates.

Only a few species of nematode of the order Strongylida live in raptors. *Syngamus trachea*, also known as the 'gapeworm', may be found in the respiratory tract of hawks. Care should be taken, because not every red worm found in the trachea or bronchi belongs to the genus *Syngamus*. In a study of more than 2000 birds of prey examined at a Canadian bird clinic, not a single *Syngamus* was diagnosed (Lavoie *et al.*, 1999). A species belonging to the genus *Cyathostoma* was found in the air sacs of one goshawk (Cooper, 1985b) and in the orbital sinuses of a Eurasian kestrel (Anon, 1983). Three species of *Cyathostoma* are known to occur in raptors: *C. americanum*, *C. brodskii* and *C. lari*. Lavoie *et al.* (1999) found 11% of hawks and owls (*n* = 107) from Quebec, Canada infected with *Cyathostoma* spp. *Hovorkonema variegatum* has been detected in Eurasian sparrow-hawks (Krone, 1998) and Northern goshawks (Lierz *et al.*, 1998). *Syngamus* and *Cyathostoma* can infect their hosts directly, when the definitive host is ingesting eggs or third-stage larvae, or indirectly via transport hosts (earthworms, insects). Within the definitive host the larvae enter the intestinal blood vessels and migrate with the blood stream via liver and heart into the lungs. Some larvae penetrate the intestine and migrate directly into the lungs. Following their last exsheathings, the worms can be found permanently in copulation (y-shaped appearance) in the bronchi and trachea. The females feed exclusively on blood while the males feed mainly on the mucous membrane and additionally on blood (Hartwich, 1994). *Hovorkonema* uses earthworms for its development. After the eggs are ingested by earthworms, the parasite develops until the third larval stage is reached,

which is infective for the definitive host. Within the definitive host the larva migrates through the peritoneal cavity into the lungs. Here it undergoes the last exsheathings to become subadult. Later the worms migrate into the bronchi and air sacs where they copulate. Their typical eggs contain a cluster of 8–16 blastomeres.

Syngamus can cause open-mouth breathing, mild gurgling sounds, or severe dyspnoea, obstruction of the trachea and pneumonia, even in small numbers. A small lesion may appear at the site of attachment, and blood clots and an abundance of mucus are usually found in the trachea. The gradual inability of the bird to breathe causes it to gape in an attempt to take in more air. Infected birds often jerk their heads as if trying to dislodge an obstruction (Bogue, 1980).

Clinical signs of *Cyathostoma* infections comprise emaciation and dyspnoea. Severe diffuse pyogranulomatous air sacculitis is the major pathological alteration in clinically infected birds (Lavoie *et al.*, 1999). *Hovorkonema* is found in the trachea (Plate 17g) and more often in the air sacs where inflammation and thickening of the air sac walls can be detected (Plate 17h). These worms can be treated successfully with thiabendazole (100 mg/kg bodyweight) or mebendazole (50 mg/kg bodyweight) orally. Treatment should be repeated after 10–14 days. Bogue (1980) suggested thiabendazole 500 mg/kg bodyweight orally, once a day for 7–10 days.

A wide variety of parasites of the order Spirurida lives in raptors. *Serratospiculum* inhabits the air sacs of falcons (Plate 17i). The life-cycle is partly known due to laboratory experiments by Bain and Vassiliades (1969) and by Samour (1999). The adult worms deposit their eggs within the air sacs. These embryonated eggs are coughed up and swallowed and either find their way out with the faeces or the regurgitated pellets. When the eggs are ingested by insects, the larvae hatch and develop to the third infective stages which are encapsulated in the body fat. Up to now it is unclear if the falcons become infected by feeding on these arthropods directly or if other birds, on which the falcons feed, serve as transport hosts for the parasite, as Bigland *et al.* (1964) speculated. Wehr (1938) for the first time described *Serratospiculum amaculata* from peregrine and prairie falcons from North America, a species which later was reclassified in the genus *Serratospiculoides* by Sonin (1968). Two species of the genus *Serratospiculoides* (Sonin, 1968) and seven species of *Serratospiculum* (Bain & Mawson, 1981) parasitise the respiratory system of birds of prey. Generally serratospiculiasis is a disease of falcons, but Sterner and Espinosa (1988) diagnosed *S. amaculata* from a Cooper's hawk and Ackerman *et al.* (1992) from a bald eagle in North America. Ward and Fairchild (1972) observed clinical signs of regurgitation and plaque-like lesions in the mouth within which typical *S. amaculata* eggs could be seen, in a peregrine. A prairie falcon died due to an infection with hundreds of *S. amaculata* in its thoracic and abdominal air sacs. Samour (1999) described histopathological findings such as haemorrhages and necrosis in the lungs, hyperplasia of the air sacs and dilatation of the glandular complex in the proventriculus associated with *Serratospiculum seurati* in falcons from the Middle East. There is usually a considerable inflammatory reaction, including squamous metaplasia in the air sac walls around the worm. The cause of death in a prairie falcon following anaesthesia was attributed to *S. amaculata* (Kocan & Gordon, 1976). Eggs of *S. amaculata* are found in the lymphatics of the lung and hepatic veins of the liver and living larvae in a chronic lesion involving the proventriculus of prairie falcons from North America (Bigland *et al.*, 1964). *Serratospiculum* worms and eggs are sometimes seen in association with lesions of aspergillosis (Crisp, 1854), but this seems to be more an exception than the rule. Several authors (Cooper, 1985b; Heidenreich, 1997) described *Serratospiculum* as a parasite of the tropics, which has proved to be incorrect. Jefferies and Prestt (1966) observed *Serratospiculum* spp. in peregrines found dead in Britain; they did not ascertain whether the peregrines were native or escaped birds. Heavy worm infections should be reduced manually with endoscopic instruments. For treatment Smith (1996) recommended levamisole 10–20 mg/kg bodyweight orally for 2 consecutive days or thiabendazole 100 mg/kg bodyweight orally initially and repeated in 10–12 days.

Microfilariae have been recorded from a variety of birds of prey, but their prevalence in blood smears is very low. Bennett *et al.* (1982) listed microfilariae of *Cardofilaria*, *Chandlerella*, *Splendofilaria* and *Singhfilaria* spp. for the Falconiformes and *Cardofilaria* and *Aproctella* spp. for the Strigiformes. These larvae are transmitted by Diptera as intermediate hosts. Kučera (1982) summed up the literature on blood parasites in birds of prey and found microfilariae in 2.6% of the strigiform birds examined ($n = 113$) and in 0.6% of the falconiform birds examined ($n = 173$) in Central Europe. Adult stages of *Cardofilaria pavlovskyi* are located in the body cavity of sparrow-hawks in Germany (Krone, 1998). A better technique than blood smears for a reliable diagnosis of microfilariae is the examination of the 'buffy coat' from the haematocrit centrifugation (see Chapter 4).

Physaloptera spp. are found in the oesophagus and proventriculus. They are often sucked on to the mucous membrane in the upper alimentary tract. In heavy infections they may cause irritation and inflammation of the mucous membrane. The life-cycle is unknown. Insects are believed to act as intermediate hosts.

Synhimantus spp. can infect the upper alimentary tract of a variety of hawks and owls. This genus of nematode has specific halt-fast organs, called cordons, on its anterior end. Occasionally the parasites are visible in the pharynx of the birds (Plate 17e). The irritation provoked by these parasites can cause problems in the feeding behaviour of raptors. Seventeen specimens of *S. laticeps* were found to be the causative agents of an ulcer in the mucous membrane of the proventriculus in a common buzzard (Krone, 1998). The life-cycle is unknown. Insects are supposed to be intermediate hosts.

Mictrotetrameres spp. inhabit the proventriculus; the females live in the glandular tissue and the much smaller males in the lumen of the proventriculus. After fertilisation the females produce eggs which leave the host via its faeces. Insects or isopods, acting as intermediate hosts, ingest the eggs. The larvae hatch within the intermediate host and penetrate the gut, enter the haemocoel and develop to the third infective stage. When a bird of prey is feeding on such an intermediate host, it becomes infected (Schell, 1953; Mawson, 1977). Inflammatory reactions from females embedded in the glandular tissue of the proventriculus do not appear to have been reported.

Cyrnea spp. are mainly detectable in the lumen of the proventriculus of birds of prey. In large numbers they may cause similar problems to those associated with *Synhimantus* spp.

Raptors infected with nematodes and trematodes were treated successfully, using fenbendazole 25 mg/kg bodyweight orally for 3 days, by Stehle (1977). A concentration of 100 mg/kg bodyweight orally of fenbendazole initially and a repeated treatment after 3 weeks (where faecal samples are still positive) with 25–30 mg/kg bodyweight orally daily for 7 days for oral capillariasis and intestinal nematodes was used by Lawrence (1983) and Santiago *et al.* (1985). Fenbendazole can also be administered at a dosage of 25 mg/kg bodyweight for 3–5 consecutive days (Smith, 1993a; Lierz & Remple, 1997). These and other anthelmintics are listed with comments in Appendix IX.

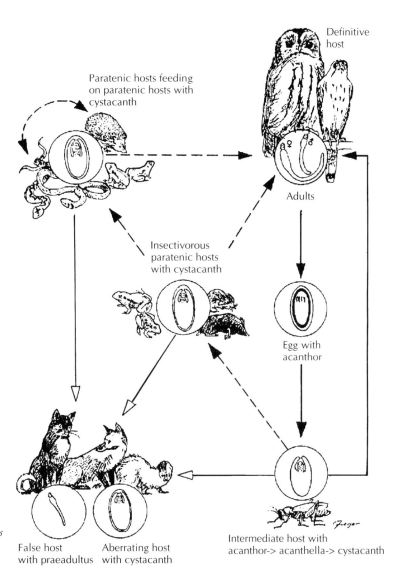

Fig. 7.3 Life-cycle of *Centrorhynchus aluconis*, an acanthocephalan worm. (Courtesy of Odening, 1969.)

Acanthocephala

Acanthocephalan ('spiny-headed') worms (e.g. *Centrorhynchus aluconis*) are characterised by a bisectioned body. The proboscis, a halt-fast organ, is armed with rows of thorns. The neck divides the proboscis from the trunk. The life-cycle of the spiny-headed worms contains two hosts. An arthropod is the intermediate host which has to ingest the acanthocephalan egg, containing the partially developed acanthor. Within the intermediate host the acanthor penetrates the intestine and settles in the haemocoele. Differentiation turns the acanthor into the acanthella, an elongated form. After enclosing itself with a sheath, the stage is known as cystacanth. The cycle can be enlarged due to paratenic hosts, increasing the probability of infecting the definitive host, the raptor (Fig. 7.3).

Of the helminths the Acanthocephala have the lowest prevalence in birds of prey. *Centrorhynchus* is the most commonly diagnosed genus in Europe. Furmaga (1957) reported a high prevalence of acanthocephalans (4.1%) in birds of prey from Poland compared with Krone (1998) who found a prevalence of 1.1% in Falconiformes from Germany. Gomez *et al.* (1993) described a higher prevalence (15%) of Acanthocephala in Spanish Falconiformes. A possible explanation could be the fact that intermediate hosts, such as grasshoppers and paratenic hosts such as lizards and snakes, are more abundant in the Mediterranean region of Europe. Little is known about the pathogenicity of thorny-headed worms. Smith (1996) pointed out that in extremely heavy infections the parasites may penetrate the intestinal wall and cause generalised peritonitis resulting in the death of the raptor. At present no effective treatment is known.

Acknowledgements

We are grateful to M. Rudolph for the electronmicrographs of the ectoparasites and to E. Mey for the specimen of *Laemobothrion tinnunculi*. We are indebted also to H. Hofer and E. Mey for their helpful comments on the manuscript. Furthermore, we should like to thank K. Ernst for her technical assistance and H. Hofer for reading an earlier version of the manuscript.

Foot Conditions

'When your hawkes fete be swollen she hath the podagre.'

Dame Juliana Berners

INTRODUCTION

Various conditions may affect the feet or legs of captive birds of prey. The subject is discussed in a separate chapter in this book in view of its practical importance. There are also accounts of 'bumblefoot' and other afflictions of the feet and legs in free-living birds of prey but these are not common in comparison with the plethora of references to captive raptors.

The structure and function of the foot and leg ('pelvic limb') of birds of prey were described in a scholarly study by Harcourt-Brown (1996b,c) and the importance of an understanding of relevant anatomy is stressed by Paolo Zucca (Chapter 3).

Traumatic injuries of the legs and feet occur in both free-living and captive birds. In free-living birds such injuries of the legs are usually traumatic: fractures and other conditions are covered in Chapter 5. Injuries involving the feet are associated with bites from predators, ill-fitting rings (bands) or trap wounds. Self-mutilation (see Chapter 13) can result in damage to and infection of the digits.

Pedal diseases of captive birds may, in addition, be due to trauma. A condition that is frequently seen in falconers' birds is a swelling of the 'ankle' (metatarsophalangeal) region associated with excess bating. This occurs particularly in accipiters. The provision of better fitting jesses of softer leather is usually adequate for resolution of the problem,

together with changes in management in order to reduce trauma.

Swollen feet can also result from hard landings on perches: the question of how far apart perches should be sited was discussed in Chapter 5.

Poorly fitted jesses may also result in infection: the skin of the leg becomes abraded and fails to heal due to continuous chronic irritation. Bacteria may enter and a dermatitis can result. The offending jesses should be removed and the bird released in a suitable large enclosure. Topical treatment of the wound is advisable and, in severe cases, debridement and a course of antibiotic may be desirable. Similar infections may result when birds are trapped, while birds in collections may damage their feet or legs on the wire of the cage.

Metatarsal and digital constrictions can occur if jesses (especially the thin Arabian variety) become twisted or tangled for too long around the feet.

Lesions caused by closed rings on the legs of captive-bred birds are generally rare but can occur when a jess is also applied to the leg and the two rub together. There was concern about the possible effects of rings and 'cable ties' on birds' legs (and eggs) when new legislation was introduced in the UK (Cooper & Gibson, 1983) but problems are rare. Illegally taken birds sometimes have had rings forced on their legs and these not infrequently cause damage, often resulting in infection.

Contact dermatitis, which can involve the feet and

legs, is well recognised in poultry (see, for example, Bruce *et al.*, 1990) and some lesions seen in birds of prey, especially those (usually casualties) that have been recumbent in contact with various substrates or dressings, may have a similar aetiology and/or pathogenesis.

Offending items such as rings and jesses will need to be removed in order to treat wounds. Ring (band) cutters are available commercially and a variety of other methods can be used. Anaesthesia will facilitate ring removal.

Other infectious lesions of the legs that occur in birds of prey are described in Chapter 6. Arthritis and osteitis are not uncommon; they will be discussed later in connection with 'bumblefoot' but it must be remembered that they can occur independently. Metabolic and other generalised diseases which may produce leg or foot lesions – for example, articular gout – are discussed in Chapter 13. A special form of 'bumblefoot' (see below) was described by Heidenreich (1997): it occurs in birds used for hunting and is characterised by oedema and swelling, at the end of the hunting season when the bird is inactive. The condition is probably cardiovascular in origin and related to physiological changes but is important as it can progress and become an infectious lesion.

'BUMBLEFOOT'

The term 'bumblefoot' is not a scientific one but is used here to cover the range of inflammatory and/or degenerative conditions that can affect the feet of birds of prey, especially but not exclusively in captivity. Conditions of the foot are amongst the most important and prevalent clinical problems seen in captive hawks. In falconry literature they were recognised and recorded as long ago as the fifteenth century when it was referred to as 'podagre' (Fig. 8.1). The Arabs, who have practised falconry for centuries, list foot problems as one of the most significant diseases of their trained falcons – an observation borne out by my own experience and that of other colleagues who have worked in the Middle East (Cooper, 1976a).

There have been many publications on the clinical features, prevention and cure of bumblefoot. An early paper was by Halliwell (1967), who presented a review of foot conditions seen in falconers' birds in America and included discussion of their aetiology. In Germany the term 'dicken Hände' is used for foot diseases and in a paper by Kösters (1974) the relevance of this description and the importance of healthy feet to a falconer's bird were emphasised.

Foot conditions also occur in birds in zoological collections (Hamerton, 1935). They are, however, more frequently seen in the Falconiformes than in owls.

Important advances have been made in our understanding of the pathogenesis of bumblefoot (Cooper, 1980a, 1987b; Cooper & Needham, 1981) but for a relatively long period the methods of treatment remained virtually unchanged (Cooper, 1980b). Research is needed on the value

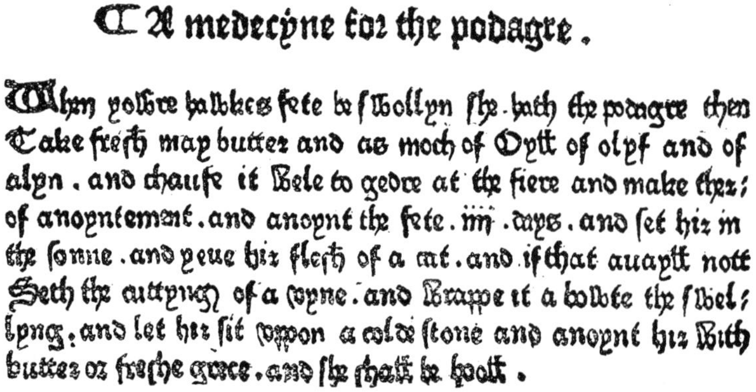
A medecyne for the podagre.

When yowre hawkes fete be swollyn she hath the podagre then
Take fresh may butter and as moch of Oyll of olyf and of
alyn. and chause it wele to gedre at the fiere and make ther;
of anoyntement. and anoynt the fete. iiii. days. and set hir in
the sonne. and yeue hir flesh of a cat. and if that auaylt nott
Seth the cuttyng of a vyne. and wrappe it a bowte the swel;
lyng. and let hir sit uppon a colde stone and anoynt hir with
butter or freshe grece. and she shall be hoole.

Fig. 8.1 In the fifteenth century the term 'podagre' was used to describe conditions that caused swelling of the feet of hawks. From the *Boke of St Albans* (1486).

of vaccination and immunomodulation (Satterfield & O'Rourke, 1981).

Bumblefoot *does* occur in free-living birds but is rare. Most pedal lesions seen in such birds are minor, unless complicated by, for example, pox or other intercurrent diseases. The Arab tradition of releasing back to the wild trained hawks with bad feet is generally sound: ringing (banding) and recapture returns have shown that some such lesions heal. Müller *et al.* (2000) demonstrated that wild-caught birds respond well to free flight (and to a quail-free diet) in terms of a reduction in bumblefoot morbidity, but that this did not apply to captive-bred falcons.

As implied above, terminology of foot conditions in birds of prey (and, indeed, other birds) is confused; falconers refer to both 'corns' and 'bumblefoot' (Moore & Ronniger, 1966) but the distinction is often not clear. 'Corns' have long been recognised on the feet of many species of bird: perhaps one of the earliest preserved examples is in the Museum of John Hunter (1728–93): 'The toe of a fowl, with a corn upon its margin.'

Clinicians and pathologists often like to use the word 'pododermatitis' (Redig & Ackermann, 2000) but there are those who disapprove of this term. I am happy to call foot lesions in raptors 'pododermatitis' because, in virtually every case, there is some inflammation present – albeit sometimes only diffuse infiltrates or aggregates of chronic inflammatory cells in the dermis. I am also in favour of scientific terminology that is comprehensible to all, not just Anglophones!

In this chapter a variety of lesions is referred to as 'bumblefoot' but only in certain cases is the clinical picture identical to that described for classical 'bumblefoot' in chickens (Roberts, 2000). My own approach is to consider each case of foot disease as a separate entity. The classification given later is a useful guide but no two cases are identical and the surest approach to treatment is to carry out as full an investigation as possible and to commence therapy early before chronic changes occur.

Some general points should be covered before the different types of bumblefoot are discussed in any detail.

It is important to understand the anatomy of a raptor's feet before debating the cause, treatment and prevention of bumblefoot (Harcourt-Brown, 1996b,c). The foot is protected by a thick layer of stratified squamous epithelium over which lies a layer of keratin. On the plantar surface there are hard papillae which assist in grasping. Underlying tissues consist of connective tissue, muscle, bone, nerves and blood vessels. In the succeeding few pages I shall describe the different types of bumblefoot and shall discuss their natural history. In virtually all, however, the initial pathology is related to damage of the epithelium and, in some cases, the entry of pathogenic organisms (Ellis, 1986; Gentz, 1996).

The tendency for foot lesions to become infected is interesting since birds appear to be relatively resistant to infection of wounds, whether natural or surgical – an observation that goes back to the work of Strouse (1909). The lower skin temperature of the feet might, therefore, be contributory and it is possible that the digits may have a relatively poor blood supply. There is also, of course, the important point that the feet are more likely to become contaminated by bacteria than are other parts of the body although this does not necessarily explain why *Staphylococcus aureus* (which is uncommon in raptor faeces) is so often the predominant organism rather than enteric bacteria such as *Escherichia coli* or *Proteus* spp.

The source of the infection may be organisms which live on the surface of the feet themselves and routine swabbing of the feet of healthy raptors has shown that many species of bacteria can be present. Often these are indicative of faecal contamination – *E. coli* and *Proteus* are common isolates – while the occasional culture (anaerobically) of *Clostridium tetani* would suggest that soil may have contaminated the area. More often, however, the bacteria cultured are staphylococci and it is these that are most commonly involved in foot infections. In one early survey (Cooper & Needham, 1976) 10.8% of 37 birds of 12 species yielded *S. aureus* and 62.1% *S. epidermidis*. *S. aureus* can also sometimes be isolated from other sites, such as from throat swabs of apparently healthy birds, suggesting that such sites too may serve as a focus of infection. Bacteriological examination plays an important part in the diagnosis and treatment of bumblefoot and, together with antibiotic sensitivity tests, is advisable whenever a case is being investigated. An important point here is to remember that anaerobic culture may yield organisms not detected aerobically.

Histology plays an important part in the investigation of bumblefoot, both for diagnosis and research. If surgery, however minor, is carried out the material that has been removed should not only be cultured bacteriologically but also examined histologically. Fixed samples can, if necessary, be retained until funding is available to process them; would that such samples had been stored in the past as they could have helped to throw light on what may be a changing pattern of foot disease! Histological examination will help to ascertain whether bacteria are still present – pockets of *S. aureus* in particular are frequently seen – and will also enable the degree of fibrosis and other reaction to be assessed. Biopsy of foot lesions can also prove useful, especially when they are proliferative, and histology should again be performed. Bumblefoot rarely kills a bird directly but any foot lesion seen at *post-mortem* examination should also be examined.

Partly as a result of the difficulty in obtaining material from cases, especially early in the course of the disease, other species have been used to study the pathogenesis of *S. aureus,* in particular, the European starling (*Sturnus vulgaris*) and domestic pigeon (*Columba palumbus*) (Cooper, 1987b; Cooper & Needham, 1981).

I have particularly emphasised the role of microbiology and histopathology in the investigation of bumblefoot because they are still not always utilised to the full. However, it must be remembered that these and other laboratory techniques should be used to back up clinical observations, not to replace them. Careful examination of foot lesions is vital, if necessary under light anaesthesia, and in many cases radiography is desirable.

Prevention of the different types of bumblefoot will be discussed later but a general point should be made here. There are three main aspects of preventing foot lesions in captive birds, these being: reduction of trauma to the foot; hygiene; and ensuring that the bird is in healthy condition and receiving an adequate diet. Vaccination might play a part in prevention but little work has been done. This is another aspect which could justifiably and usefully be investigated in, say, a colony of European or American kestrels or perhaps an experimental 'model' in starlings or other species.

Treatment of bumblefoot may be managemental, medical or surgical and is often a combination of all three. These aspects are discussed in detail later.

Types of bumblefoot

My own classification of foot lesions, first put forward for consideration and comment by colleagues 30 years ago, does not meet with everyone's approval but continues to be a useful guide and has helped to ensure some consistency in terminology. Oaks (1993) divided cases into five rather than three categories and related these to the severity and prognosis. His category (class) I is a non-disrupting hyperaemia or hyperkeratotic devitalisation of the plantar epithelium that carries a good prognosis while category V, at the other end of the scale, is characterised by deep infection including bone lesions and the severity of the lesion often warrants euthanasia.

In this chapter I shall follow my own classification, from 1–3 but the descriptions broadly match the progression plotted by Oaks (and others) using different scoring systems.

Type 1 bumblefoot

Here there is a mild localised lesion, often of only one digit. The lesion may be proliferative (a raised 'corn') or degenerative with a flattening and thinning of the epithelium or, in some cases, hyperaemia leading to erosion or ulceration. Both proliferative and degenerative lesions may progress to a scab. Such cases are often benign and frequently no organisms may be cultured or seen in histological sections. They are commonly associated with poorly designed perches or abrasive surfaces and changing these will often result in spontaneous recovery although some proliferative lesions may never disappear completely. Redig and Ackermann (2000) also advocated the use of 'skin tougheners' – preparations that can be sprayed on the skin to protect it and to encourage healing.

Amputation of a bird's foot will result in increased use of the other limb, and a swollen foot, often progressing to bumblefoot, is a common sequel, particularly in falcons. Impaired use of one leg – for instance, on account of a poorly healed fracture – can have the same effect.

Clinical signs associated with Type 1 bumblefoot vary. Some affected birds show a tendency to favour one leg: the affected foot may be slightly swollen or warm to the touch. Sometimes the lesions can be seen without any accompanying clinical signs.

Ulcerated lesions should be treated with antisepsis or antibiotic while a light dressing will, so long as it is left in place by the bird, discourage the entry of infection. I have used adhesive drapes e.g. 'Op-Site' (Smith and Nephew, UK) or 'Tegaderm' (3M Medical Surgical Division, St Paul, USA), which both protect the wound and permit visual inspection.

Some proliferative lesions prove on histological examination to be benign papillomata. They can be removed surgically; cryotherapy is an excellent technique but damages the tissues, making histological examination of the mass less easy. It is possible that some such lesions are of viral origin, as is the case with some papillomata of other birds (Ritchie, 1995). The recent report on virus-like particles in a case of pododermatis in a Northern gannet (*Monus bassanus*) illustrates the value of examining such lesions both histologically and electronmicroscopically (Daoust *et al.*, 2000).

The majority of proliferative lesions of raptors, however, are composed not of papillomatous tissue but of thickened epithelium and scab which sometimes overlie a small focus of infection and will respond to a suitable antibiotic or, as Salvin and Brodrick described in *Falconry in the British Isles* in 1855 '. . . the contents may be easily removed by merely cutting down upon them with a sharp knife, and squeezing the matter out'.

The presence of a scab on a foot or digit may indicate a Type 1 bumblefoot lesion, but often is a sign that infection is, or has been, present. In this respect, scabs may represent an intermediary between Type 1 and Type 2 bumblefoot. It is therefore important to ascertain whether they are traumatic or infectious in origin and to take appropriate action before the condition deteriorates. Bilaterally identical scabs usually indicate a poor perching surface.

Type 2 bumblefoot

This is more extensive and characterised by swelling of the foot (Plate 18). Type 2 bumblefoot is almost invariably associated with pathogenic bacteria; essentially there is an acute (heterophilic) inflammatory lesion although histological examination (Cooper, 1987a) usually shows the presence of chronic reaction, such as fibrous tissue and mononuclear cells, as well as 'abscessation'. The latter contains a central mass of caseous material – histologically a mixture of fibrin, blood cells and bacteria (Huchzermeyer & Cooper, 2000).

Some cases of Type 2 bumblefoot result from a deterioration or infection of Type 1 but others appear to arise spontaneously. A sharp talon (in the case of falcons, usually the hind one) can easily pierce the sole of the foot and introduce infection. Some birds tend to 'clench' their feet as a part of normal behaviour and the majority will do so during recovery from anaesthesia or restraint. Care must always be taken when handling a bird to minimise the risk of self-puncture of the sole: my own approach to examining the plantar surfaces, by drawing back the bird's feet using the leash and jesses, will discourage flexing of digits (see Chapter 4). The use of 'perches which are too slender' may also cause the ball of the foot to be pierced by the talons, according to Keymer (1977a). Poorly designed perches readily predispose to traumatic injuries, and sharp edges in particular may be responsible for the establishment of, first, Type 1 bumblefoot which may progress to a Type 2 foot infection.

Some cases of Type 2 bumblefoot are attributable to infection following the entry of a foreign body. A common cause in tropical areas, and occasionally in temperate areas, is a sharp thorn entering the sole of a digit and this can occur in free-living as well as captive raptors. The area becomes swollen, hot and painful but often there is little or no overlying scab. The thorn may be visible, as is a splinter in a human finger, and should be removed. Local antiseptic or antibiotic will usually control the infection.

Recently captured birds sometimes show infected foot lesions, especially of the digits, which are probably attributable to trapping or wire-netting damage. If heavy birds are kept on concrete or a similar rough surface they may abrade their feet and infection can enter, as described earlier in tawny and steppe eagles (Cooper, 1976b); a change of substrate will accelerate healing.

The characteristic clinical features of this type of swelling (usually of the sole but sometimes of one or more digits) are heat and pain. Affected birds often lie down or stand in their waterbath in order to reduce the pain. A hard scab usually overlies the swollen area. The swollen tissues contain 'pus' which may either be caseous in appearance or consist of a clear serous exudate. Culture will normally reveal bacteria, and cytology reveals bacteria and inflammatory cells, mainly heterophils and macrophages. In early cases the bacterial isolates are often coagulase-positive *S. aureus* but other organisms can also be isolated. Radiography of such cases will usually reveal soft tissue swelling (Fig. 8.2) but no involvement of bones.

The presence of *Escherichia coli* or other Gram-negative enteric bacilli from foot lesions is probably an indication of subsequent infection with faecal organisms and can make treatment difficult. Moore and Ronniger (1966) suggested that *E. coli* in one of their cases might have originated from dog (*Canis familiaris*) faeces that contaminated the lawn where the hawk sat but, in the absence of typing of the organism, it seems more probable that this organism came from the bird's own faeces.

Other bacteria may establish themselves as a result of unhygienic surgery or following extensive antibiotic therapy; examples include *Pseudomonas* spp., which are notoriously difficult to eliminate. I have often attempted to isolate mycoplasmas from foot lesions but this has never proved successful. I have seen yeasts in direct smears but never cultured them. Kösters (1974) warned against the long-term use of antibiotics to treat bumblefoot on the grounds that 'a fungus infection can develop'.

Histological examination of material removed surgically from Type 2 bumblefoot cases has confirmed that bacteria (especially staphylococci) are present in large numbers in the scab, as well as in

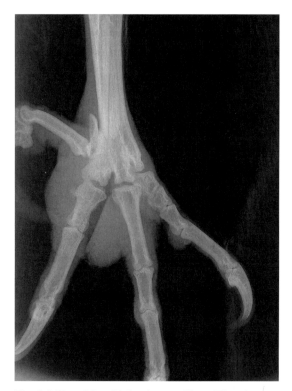

Fig. 8.2 Type 2 bumblefoot in a gyrfalcon. There is a pronounced soft tissue swelling.

the underlying soft tissues. Histologically, the scab closely resembles the human clavus ('corn') in that there is an area of excessive hyperkeratosis which exerts considerable pressure (and hence damage) on the underlying tissues. It is therefore not surprising that such cases often recur.

Type 2 bumblefoot can be treated initially with an appropriate antibiotic following a sensitivity test on an aspirate from the lesion. Early treatment is important. Fibroplasia in birds begins to occur as early as 3–5 days after tissue damage (Nair, 1973) and antimicrobial therapy is far less likely to prove successful once fibrosis is extensive.

Cloxacillin, flucloxacillin and lincomycin have for long proved valuable in the treatment of *S. aureus* infections but other agents have also been used successfully, including cephalosporins and fluoroquinolones (Redig & Ackermann, 2000) or clindamycin or gentamicin coupled with a steroid applied topically in dimethyl sulphoxide (DMSO). Current interest in the use of antibiotic-impregnated polymethyl methacrylate beads (AIPMMA) was summarised by Remple and Forbes (2000) who reported encouraging results, using a variety of antibiotics, in cases of bumblefoot that ranged in severity from Class II–Class IV in an overall range from I–V.

If antibiosis alone is going to be effective the clinical response is usually fairly rapid – a reduction in swelling within 5 days. If this fails, surgical debridement is probably needed and is discussed later.

Some practitioners administer vitamin A routinely (orally or by injection) to bumblefoot cases (Types 1, 2 and 3) since a number of people have suggested an association between bumblefoot and nutritional deficiencies, especially vitamin A (Graham, 1970). This theory could be correct in view of work on bumblefoot in poultry, for example by Jaksch (1960), but it should be noted that foot diseases still occur in hawks fed on day-old chicks, which are a rich source of the vitamin. Interestingly, the only severe case of bumblefoot in both feet that I have encountered in an owl was a young bird which also showed swollen eyelids and ocular lesions suggestive of a vitamin A deficiency.

Roberts (2000) reported that homeopathic remedies (sulphur and silicea) were 'useful' in the therapy of bumblefoot in poultry and some owners and vets have used similar substances to treat birds of prey (see Chapter 4).

Therapy must be accompanied by husbandry measures. The possible role of the perching surface in initiating Type I lesions was mentioned earlier. There is dispute as to whether hard or soft surfaces on perches are more likely to predispose to bumblefoot. What does seem certain is that once a bird has Type 2 bumblefoot it should have a padded perch in order to reduce trauma to the feet and pain. In some cases a change from a block to a padded ring perch alone will result in improvement and even recovery. An affected bird should also be given every opportunity to rest the foot by lying down, should be fed well (on a mixed diet) and not be flown. There is no doubt that a captive bird stands for longer each day than it would in the wild and this may predispose to foot conditions but flying a bird to the fist or lure when it has Type 2 or 3 bumblefoot will only exacerbate the condition. Heavy inactive birds, especially eagles, gyrs and sakers, seem particularly prone to bumblefoot and it is probable that in such cases the prolonged pressure on the feet is deleterious and permits damage to the epithelium through which bacteria may enter. The fact that cases of both Type 1 and Type 2 bumblefoot will heal spontaneously if the bird is released or given the freedom of a large aviary adds support to this theory. Even partial reduction of pressure on a foot – for instance, using the now commercially produced 'bumblefoot recovery pads' – will reduce pain (see later) and may encourage resolution of lesions.

Hygiene is probably also important in order to reduce further bacterial infection of the lesion. In particular, the perches on which the bird stands should be cleaned and disinfected. I have cultured many species of potentially pathogenic bacteria from such perches and also from falconers' gloves. Attempts to clean gloves are advisable: particularly ancient gloves and other equipment should be destroyed! As was mentioned earlier, *S. aureus* can be cultured from the feet of healthy birds and it is possible that it may be acquired from human carriers, as Jeffrey Needham and I first postulated in 1976 (Cooper & Needham, 1976). More recent work on the bacteriological flora of feathers by Pérez *et al.* (1994) would appear to support this claim. Personal hygiene, such as hand washing, is therefore also advisable. It should not be forgotten that *S. aureus* can cause other diseases in birds of prey – for instance, peritonitis, pericarditis and perihepatitis (Anon, 2001).

Some years ago it was shown (Devriese & Devos, 1975) that certain antibiotics, administered orally, will suppress skin populations of *S. aureus* in poultry. The concept opens up possibilities for using competitive inhibition as a means of reducing numbers of *S. aureus* and other potentially pathogenic bacteria.

Prevention of Type 2 bumblefoot *per se* is not easy. Where it follows Type I lesions, the measures mentioned earlier, relating to perch surfaces and hyperaemic/ulcerated changes, are relevant. A means of minimising the risk of self-inoculation is to cut ('cope') the talons of birds when they first come into captivity or whenever handling is necessary. Such a procedure is not new; as Kösters (1974) pointed out, it was routinely practised in falconers' birds in Germany in the Middle Ages.

Care of the talons is an important part of routine management of captive raptors as well as playing a part in prevention of bumblefoot. Redig and Ackermann (2000) listed four aspects and advised against interfering with the sharp edge on the medial side of the talon of the third digit as this plays a part in grooming feathers. In addition, it is important to ensure that injuries to the feet are treated early in order to prevent infection.

Attention to the general health of the bird, including regular examination of the feet, can enable early recognition of lesions. The plantar surfaces should *always* be checked when a bird is being examined, in captivity or in the wild.

If medical treatment fails or is only partly successful, surgery of Type 2 bumblefoot is necessary and this will be discussed later.

Type 3 bumblefoot

This is essentially a chronic state and usually follows Type 2. There is often still some infection present but this has usually been walled off by fibrous tissue, producing one or several pus-filled sacs. In severe long-standing cases the locomotory system may be affected, with damaged tendons and arthritis of the phalanges or tibiotarsal joint. It is important that such cases are radiographed in order to assess the degree of bone involvement: arthritic changes are usually destructive and can extend into the shafts of long bones (Fig. 8.3).

Chronic lesions of bumblefoot are often only hot and painful intermittently but the bird is usually unable to use the foot (or feet) satisfactorily. The measures outlined later, relating to analgesia and other palliative care, are relevant here.

Medical treatment of Type 3 bumblefoot is rarely successful, partly because systemic agents are unable to reach the affected parts and also on account of irreversible damage to the tissues. Antibiotics may ameliorate the situation initially but the swelling returns within a few days of cessation of treatment. Local preparations are sometimes advocated for Type 3 (and Type 2) bumblefoot but their value is doubtful. I have used staphylococcus toxoid sys-

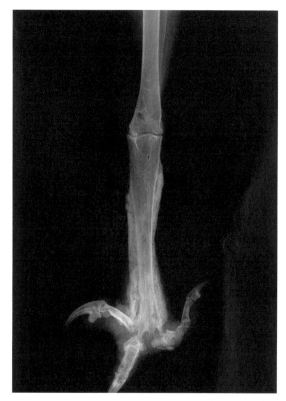

Fig. 8.3 Severe osteitis in a buzzard – a sequel to a long-standing, untreated foot infection.

temically but with no apparent success; an autogenous vaccine might be more successful. Radiotherapy (employing X-rays and five doses of 150 rads) was used in Canada (Bird & Lague, 1975): there was some initial success but David Bird subsequently told me that the birds thus treated had shown remissions later. In most cases of Type 3 bumblefoot, therefore, the only course of action is either surgery or euthanasia.

Surgery for bumblefoot

Surgery, ranging from simple debridement and flushing to radical excision of damaged tissues has a part to play in all types of bumblefoot.

A surgical approach to foot infections is not novel. The earliest detailed reference that I have found to such a technique was Latham (1615) who wrote:

'You must have your Hawke well and easily cast, and with a sharp knife search and pare out the pinne, or core . . . the which if it have not planted it selfe too deep amongst the sinews, whereby to annoy and hurt them, it will easily be amended . . . and so dresse it thrice in the week, and withall let her sit very soft and warme, and this will cure her out of all doubt.'

This is a magnificent description and cannot be improved upon to any great extent. A more scientific description of an essentially identical technique was given by Kost and described in 1962 in the first edition of *A Manual of Falconry* (Woodford, 1960). In Kost's day anaesthesia was not advocated; nowadays anaesthetic agents for birds are far safer and should always be used. I first described my surgical technique (designed to promote healing by first intention) in detail in the earlier edition of this book (Cooper, 1978a, 1985b) and further refined it in a paper in the *Annals of the Royal College of Surgeons of England* (Cooper, 1980c).

Prior to surgery, radiographs should be taken to assess whether or not there is bone involvement; the presence of arthritis or osteitis will drastically reduce the chances of success. It is also wise, now that reference values are available for many raptors, to carry out pre-operative haematology (see Chapter 4).

The rationale of surgery is to open the affected area to remove all infected or necrotic tissue and to prevent re-infection before healing has taken place (Plate 19). Care must be taken to ensure that all necrotic material is removed whilst leaving tendons and nerves intact. Irrigation with the enzyme trypsin may assist in this respect but others use saline or 0.5% chlorhexidine. Redig and Ackermann (2000) emphasised that iodine-containing solutions should *not* be used. I use a 10 ml syringe and a 26 gauge needle and find that the force of the spray helps to dislodge dead tissue as well as moistening the area. An appropriate antibiotic can be included in the trypsin solution. The skin wound is closed using mattress sutures, taking care to ensure apposition of healthy epithelium without destroying the normal architecture of the sole too drastically. A vital part of the operation is the dressing of the wound with a pad of gauze which can be sutured to the skin or

held in place with adhesive plaster. This protects the wound and is usually left in place until the tissues are healing, although it can be removed after a few days to permit inspection of the foot. Redig & Ackermann (2000) recommended using a seton (of sterile gauze or umbilical tape) and placing the foot in a 'ball bandage'. The latter is changed daily, with continued irrigation and replacement of the seton for 10–20 days.

Immediate post-operative care consists of oral or systemic antibiotics, possibly supplemented with systemic vitamin A and good nursing including feeding by hand. Analgesics and other means of reducing pain are strongly recommended. Longer-term care may involve regular anaesthesia – sometimes once or twice a week for several months – in order to check lesions and to change dressings, and this may bring with it the possibility of adverse responses to isoflurane (see Chapter 12). Such birds are likely also to be fed chopped food, to avoid unnecessary use of the feet, in which case the beak may overgrow and need coping.

The sutures can be removed at any time after 10 days but may be left in place for up to a month. Surgery may need to be repeated later but often (approximately 60% of cases) a successful cure results on the first occasion. If both feet need surgery there is merit, largely on welfare grounds, to operate on the second one 7 days after the first but occasionally it proves necessary to perform both operations at one time. In such cases the bird may tend to lie down for 3–4 days until healing commences and analgesics may be indicated (see Chapter 12).

Sometimes it is impossible to close the wound, especially if large quantities of tissue have been removed. Dressings will help but healing can be very slow. Chitty (2000a) described the use of a small intestine submucosa graft in order to close defects and suggested that the method might reduce healing time.

Remple (1993) described a method of foot casting that protects the plantar surface from trauma that can retard healing. The cast is kept in place for 14–21 days.

Bumblefoot occurs in other birds, as well as in raptors, and work on these species may yield information of value. For example, Reidarson *et al.* (1999) described a 'novel approach to the treatment of bumblefoot in penguins'.

I first gave a lecture on the surgical treatment of bumblefoot in Abu Dhabi (Cooper, 1976a); in that paper I emphasised the need for strict asepsis and correct surgical technique if the results are to be successful. Those golden rules still apply. Surgery should therefore be carried out by a qualified veterinary surgeon. There are still owners of birds who attempt to open bumblefoot lesions without anaesthesia and with minimal hygienic techniques; the results are usually poor, the bird can be subjected to pain and there may be secondary infection or damage to nerves or tendons (see Chapter 8).

That birds of prey with bumblefoot are in pain cannot be doubted from the clinical signs that they show and their apparent response, in terms of behaviour and often appetite, when they receive analgesics. Studies on poultry have demonstrated nociceptors in the legs (Gentle & Tiltson, 2000) and similar work, on the feet as well as the legs, would be of value in birds of prey. The assumption at present should be that pain follows surgery and that everything possible should be done to reduce this. Analgesics are a key part (see Chapter 12) but additional measures, especially in long-term cases, include the use of polystyrene 'shoes' and/or foam-padded perches to reduce pressure on the feet and the provision of chopped food (or hand-feeding) to minimise painful or difficult movement.

Prevention of Type 3 bumblefoot consists primarily of prompt attention to milder foot lesions (themselves usually Type I or Type 2 bumblefoot, sometimes incidental lesions) in order to prevent their becoming chronic. Chronicity is characterised by a proliferation of mononuclear cells (Fig. 8.4) and fibrosis. Milder lesions in turn are less likely to occur if one follows the five important elements put forward by Pat Redig and summarised in Redig & Ackermann (2000):

(1) An appropriate diet
(2) Suitably sized, shaped and covered perches
(3) Adequate space for untethered birds to land normally
(4) Avoidance of obesity
(5) Adequate exercise and observation of the feet.

To these I would add 'coping' of the talons.

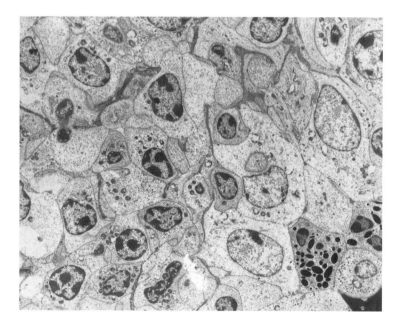

Fig. 8.4 Transmission electronmicroscopy (TEM) of material from a foot infection showing a preponderance of (mononuclear) cells, which helps to explain the chronicity of the condition (TEM ×3000).

Other conditions of the foot

Broken talons can be associated with pain and extensive bleeding, especially if the germinal epithelium is exposed. Cautery or haemostatic chemicals can be used to control simple haemorrhage – using, for example, potassium permanganate crystals. Healing and regeneration following more severe damage take time and will be facilitated if the wound is cleaned and protected. Drying must be avoided as this can result in infection and necrosis. The clipping ('coping') of talons and their routine care are discussed elsewhere.

Drying and cracking of the skin can be a feature of larger birds, especially eagles (Harcourt-Brown, 1996b,c), and can lead to dermatitis or dermal ulceration. Early attention, including the application of skin-softening preparations, will help to forestall this – as will ensuring that feet do not become excessively or frequently wet.

Congenital (developmental) abnormalities sometimes occur (Harcourt-Brown, 1966b), for instance, duplication of digits or syndactyly. These are covered in Chapter 13. Feather conditions are also discussed in that chapter.

A leiomyoma affecting the toe of an eagle was amongst the tumours reviewed by Forbes *et al.* (2000a). Neoplasms and gout are also discussed in Chapter 13.

In conclusion, foot conditions remain an important – and sometimes difficult – part of veterinary care for captive birds of prey. Their prevention and their treatment require a logical and systematic approach and a sound understanding of both the anatomy of the foot and the natural history of the bird.

Neurological (Nervous) Disorders

'There is a disease in the head of some, called Vertego, it is a swimming of the braine.'

Edmund Bert

INTRODUCTION

The nervous system of the Class Aves has long attracted the interest of biologists and physiologists; Severino (1645), in his *Zootomia Democritaea*, depicted the brains of birds, amongst them a hawk. The chapter on anatomy in the present book, appropriately written by an Italian colleague, Paolo Zucca, provides some up-to-date information on this subject, including new theories about the cognitive powers of birds. The history was reviewed in *The Avian Brain* (Pearson, 1972) and that book is still recommended to all who are involved in veterinary work with birds. Most of the earlier research was concerned with gross anatomy but recently there has been more interest in microscopical structure.

Over the past 25 years brain function has attracted considerable attention, particularly that relating to stereotyped behaviour and the relationship of brain growth and differentiation to the activity of young birds. Much of the work has involved the use of experimental birds, particularly pigeons, and a considerable amount of surgery has been carried out to assess the effect of lesions in different areas of the brain – an example was the work on feeding behaviour by Zeigler and Karten (1973).

In this chapter neurological diseases and their investigation are considered. Behavioural ('psychological') disorders, some of which have a neurological aetiology, are discussed in Chapter 13.

Despite this history of research on the avian brain, its pathology has not been studied in detail, even in domestic species. A number of diseases that produce nervous signs are recognised in non-domesticated birds but relatively little is known of the aetiology and pathogenesis of most of them. Only recently has any attempt been made to relate them to modern neurology. For example, 25 years ago Arnall and Keymer (1975) discussed fits, convulsions, 'epilepsy', fainting, vertigo and 'hysteria' in cagebirds. Earlier Hasholt (1960) divided the 'diseases of the brain' in cagebirds into three main categories, these being encephalitis, nutritional and toxic encephalomalacia, and functional encephalopathy but he too confirmed that a definite diagnosis is often not possible. More recent texts provide information about nervous diseases of birds in general but the cause in most cases remains unclear.

In the case of birds of prey, nervous diseases warrant a separate chapter for a number of reasons. First of all, 'fits' and other disorders have, for a long time, been recognised by falconers, especially in the short-winged hawks or accipiters, for example the description above by Bert in the seventeenth century. Two hundred years later Salvin and Brodrick (1855) wrote of 'fits' which they described as 'not necessarily fatal, as the Hawk may live for weeks after experiencing the attack'. Even in the second half of the last century while the majority of authors of falconry texts described nervous diseases of hawks and emphasised their importance, knowledge of the causes remained obscure. Thus, Woodford (1960), himself a veterinarian, stated that 'no one has the slightest idea of the cause of these convulsions or how to treat them'. 'Fitting' and incoordination remain important in captive birds of prey to this day (Cooper, 1978a, 1985b, 1996c). The second reason why special attention is paid in this book to nervous diseases is because they constitute one of the emergencies that warrant prompt attention. The third reason is because they also occur in free-living birds.

CLINICAL FEATURES OF NERVOUS DISEASES

The clinical signs seen vary considerably. They can include general signs, such as convulsions, or local, such as paralysis. In the case of classical 'fits' the bird shows incoordination and inability to use its legs. It has a vacant staring appearance and its head is usually on one side (Plate 20), with mouth often slightly open and respiration accelerated and pronounced. Regurgitation of food sometimes occurs. The bird may recover within 2–3 hours and never have another fit, or, more probably, it will have further attacks within the next few hours or days.

A variety of other clinical signs may be seen in raptors and it is often not clear as to whether these represent different syndromes or other manifestations of one disease. Muscle fasciculation is not uncommon and there may be weakness or paralysis of the limbs. In some cases there is opisthotonos and the bird may call out, as if in pain. The bird may be able to stand and walk but sometimes holds its head at an angle or upside-down.

Peripheral nerve lesions, which usually cause more localised clinical signs, are covered separately later in this chapter. Behavioural changes are discussed in Chapter 13. Syndromes known as 'apoplexy' and 'stroke' may produce clinical signs that are somewhat similar to those in nervous disease but these are usually considered to be cardiovascular in origin and are discussed in Chapter 13.

It will be apparent from the above that a variety of 'neurological' clinical features may be encountered in birds of prey, usually but not exclusively when they are kept in captivity. That some of these clinical signs may be unrelated to the nervous system can complicate examination, diagnosis and prognosis.

NEUROLOGICAL EXAMINATION

General clinical examination of a bird of prey is discussed in Chapter 4. When a nervous disease is suspected, the approach is similar but there are some important differences. The recommended approach is given in Fig. 9.1. Full clinical history and records are essential and here the use of a 'check list' (questionnaire), completed *before* the bird is examined, is very useful (see Appendix II). Important features of history are the age and source of the bird, its previous health, the diet being fed and *detailed* information on the onset, duration and features of the nervous syndrome.

Observation of the bird from a distance or without the bird being aware of the observer is most important since premature handling or disturbance may precipitate a fit or radically influence minor locomotory abnormalities. A 'peephole' in the consulting room door will permit observation of this kind. Even better is a video, usually taken by the owner, showing the clinical signs.

Much depends upon the severity of the clinical picture. A bird with mild nervous signs, such as muscle tremors, can usually be examined on the falconer's fist or on a table. A bird which is having fits poses problems of restraint and it may be wiser to wait for the fits to subside, or to reduce their severity before commencing examination. The water soluble benzodiazepine midazolam has proved useful in raptors and can be given intramuscularly or intravenously. When administered by the former route it appears to be less painful and more effective than diazepam. A comatose bird can be handled with relative ease.

Subdued lighting – for example, by use of a dimmer switch – should always be used when examining a bird with nervous disease and basic aids to handling, such as a towel or falconer's hood, must be at hand.

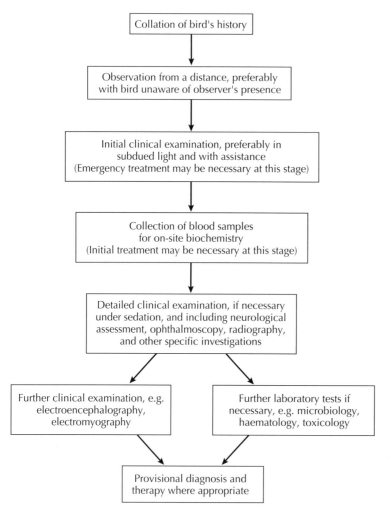

Collation of bird's history

Observation from a distance, preferably
with bird unaware of observer's presence

Initial clinical examination, preferably in
subdued light and with assistance
(Emergency treatment may be necessary at this stage)

Collection of blood samples
for on-site biochemistry
(Initial treatment may be necessary at this stage)

Detailed clinical examination, if necessary
under sedation, and including neurological
assessment, ophthalmoscopy, radiography,
and other specific investigations

Further clinical examination, e.g.
electroencephalography,
electromyography

Further laboratory tests if
necessary, e.g. microbiology,
haematology, toxicology

Provisional diagnosis and
therapy where appropriate

Fig. 9.1 Recommended approach to birds with signs of fits, incoordination and coma.

When the earlier editions of this book appeared there were few sophisticated aids to neurological examination of raptors. Ophthalmoscopy was a key part then and remains so (Korbel, 2000) (see Chapters 4 and 13). Electroencephalography (EEG), electromyography (EMG) and nerve-conduction studies are of value and in specialist avian practices may be used as a routine. Smith (1993b) used EMG and nerve-conduction studies to diagnose brachial plexus avulsion in owls.

Computerised tomography (CT) and magnetic resonance imaging (MRI) are likely to assume increasing importance as such units become more widely available.

Nerve and muscle biopsies are used to aid diagnosis in mammals (Wheeler, 1995) but demand special care in sampling. Such techniques may be applicable to birds of prey, but have been little used and clearly need further evaluation.

Until specific investigative methods are agreed, one must use standard clinical techniques. I have been guided in some of my investigations by methods used in toxicological studies in poultry where, for example, an 'ataxia grading' is utilised to assess the effects of neurotoxicity. Neurological diagnostic procedures employed in domestic mammals can also sometimes be applied (Lawton, 1995; Wheeler, 1995).

General behaviour can be assessed before the patient is restrained. A considerable amount of valuable information can usually be obtained from the owner's descriptions coupled with observations and, if available, video film of the clinical signs. The gait or stance of the bird should be noted as should any tendency to hold its head on one side, or to 'circle'. A word of caution here is that a falconer's bird that is hooded sometimes shows abnormal head movements, particularly if it has some limited vision through the hood. If in doubt, the hood should be removed.

It is important to see the bird in motion and here again the task is easier with a falconer's bird which will step or fly to the fist. If the bird has come from an aviary it can be released in a suitable room, with reduced illumination, and observed. Important points to note are whether (a) the bird walks or flies into objects, (b) is incoordinated when walking or flying, (c) shows inability to use a limb or limbs properly. The reaction of the bird to sound can be assessed in a trained hawk by use of a familiar call or whistle and in an aviary bird by sounding a small bell or tapping two metal objects together – the bird should turn its head and show evidence of having heard.

Assessment of postural reactions is again much easier in a trained hawk. There are a number of investigations that can be carried out but tests I recommend are:

(1) Will the bird step on to a perch, or another gloved hand, if pressed backwards so that its legs touch that object?
(2) If the hand carrying the bird is lowered abruptly, does the bird extend its wings and retain its balance?
(3) If a falconer's bird 'bates' off the fist, can it return to it satisfactorily?

If the patient is not a falconer's bird such tests are not always practicable but it is still often possible to carry out (1) and (2) in a darkened room. Rotating a horizontal bar while the bird is standing on it is another useful technique; normally a bird is able to adjust the position of its feet, and, often with the occasional help of its wings, retain its balance and posture. In many cases of nervous disease it is unable to do so and falls, or flutters, off.

The detailed clinical examination must be systematic. There is merit in doing it in a darkened room. My own approach, with any suspect nervous disease, is to start at the bird's head and progress to the wings, body and legs. When the head is examined it should be checked for evidence of symmetry, for example whether both eyes are equally open. One or both of the nictitating membranes may be conspicuous or perhaps excessively active. The pupillar reflexes should be checked using a pinpoint source of light. The eyes should each be examined, if necessary with the assistance of a colleague who is experienced in avian ophthalmology (see Chapter 13). Nystagmus is rare in birds of prey as the majority cannot move their eyes and instead rotate the head.

The wings, body and legs are gently palpated and sensation is assessed with a sterile 21 gauge needle which is used to prick the skin gently. Areas of sensation can be plotted on a rough drawing. Any hyperaesthesia should be noted. If there is evidence of paralysis or impaired use of a limb this must be examined carefully. In particular, it is important to assess whether the paralysis is flaccid or spastic. The filming of an affected bird will enable a particular neurological or locomotory sign to be viewed on repeated occasions.

I cannot claim that a detailed examination as outlined above will lead to definitive diagnosis and specific therapy. Still the treatment finally chosen for the bird can be empirical and symptomatic, with the 'success' of the case being judged on whether the bird improves – and this may or may not be due to the treatment. There remains a dearth of scientific information on nervous diseases in birds and it is therefore necessary for each case to be investigated methodically and for 'clusters' of cases to be properly analysed. Only in this way will data be accumulated and some light thrown on the perplexing range of 'nervous' conditions seen in raptors.

TERMINOLOGY AND AETIOLOGY

Many lay persons' terms have been used to describe nervous diseases in birds of prey, and some of these date from the Middle Ages. The word 'encephalitis' was used fairly commonly amongst falconers in the middle of the nineteenth century, apparently on the erroneous assumption that intraosseous haemorrhages seen in the skull *post mortem* could be equated with inflammatory lesions in the brain (Plate 21). This is totally incorrect and, with the exception of proven cases of brain infections (for example following otitis media), the term 'encephalitis' should not be used.

The word 'epilepsy' was used 150 years ago by Salvin and Brodrick (1855) and was presumably coined on account of the clinical similarity between fits in hawks and epilepsy in humans. However, nowadays the pathogenesis of epilepsy is better understood – the important feature being overactivity of the motor cortex, which causes marked locomotory signs – and we do not have sufficient evidence to suggest that this is what occurs in birds of prey. However, in view of the clinical features of fits it is probably justifiable to apply the term 'epileptiform', as was used by Woodford (1960). Epileptiform seizures of unknown aetiology were reported in captive African vultures by Mundy and Foggin (1981). They suspected an infectious disease but bacteriological and virological investigations proved negative.

Since the term 'fits' is used commonly by falconers and others to describe any condition where general signs of incoordination or nervous derangement are present, I use the word in that general sense here. I am assuming that 'convulsions' and 'seizures' are synonymous with fits. Nevertheless, I must emphasise that the overt nervous signs seen in clinical cases are often only one manifestation of an underlying disorder and when improved investigative techniques are available, differential diagnoses are easier.

Greenwood (1973) divided nervous diseases of raptors into five groups – nutritional, infectious, poisoning, CNS lesions and peripheral nerve lesions. These have proved to be convenient headings and will be used as a basis here.

TYPES OF NERVOUS DISEASE

Nutritional

A number of nutritional/metabolic disorders can cause fits, incoordination or coma in birds of prey. The main categories are hypoglycaemia, hyperglycaemia, thiamine deficiency, hypocalcaemia and 'hepatopathy' (Cooper, 1996a).

Hypoglycaemia is often a cause of fits. Birds of prey which are *in extremis* may have convulsive seizures before death and these are particularly common in birds that are found *post mortem* to have died of inanition.

Fits are also seen in birds in low condition which are subjected to exercise, stress or exposure to low temperatures. For example, a falconer's bird will sometimes have a fit after a flight or even following several hours on the fist on a cold windy day when it is expending considerable energy in keeping its balance and maintaining its body temperature. Birds that have fasted may already have blood glucose values that are towards the bottom of the normal range although this is not always the case (see Chapter 10).

It is possible that fits in birds which are not in low condition may also be due to hypoglycaemia if their food intake is being reduced. For example, Woodford (1960) mentioned the occurrence of fits at the end of the moult and this may be associated with the reduced or poorer quality food that is usually offered at that time. Forbes (1996b) described hypoglycaemic fits in falcons with 'hepatopathy' and suggested that the latter might be due to an infectious agent.

Investigation of blood glucose values can be hampered by the difficulty of getting samples from small birds, especially if they are showing nervous signs, and the possibility that handling and restraint may influence the results. In this context, however, it is worth noting that Nelson *et al.* (1942) could detect no influence on blood sugar levels when great horned owls were handled and anaesthetised with phenobarbitone.

Theoretically the initial clinical feature of hypoglycaemia is flaccidity – in contrast to epilepsy, where motor activity is predominant – but in practice this stage is quickly superseded by neuronal activity, possibly on account of hypoxia or metabolite accumulation (Palmer, 1976). Specific clinical diagnosis is, therefore, probably not practicable, although premonitory signs of muscle weakness may be suggestive of hypoglycaemia. Probably the bird's history is the most important information.

Glucose can be given to birds by either the oral or parenteral route. If the latter is used, a 10% dextrose solution is injected subcutaneously, intravenously, intraosseously or intraperitoneally. The administration of glucose is often associated with a clinical improvement although fits may recur some hours later.

In other cases of fits a thiamine deficiency may be involved. The effect of such a deficiency in both birds and mammals has been long recognised; chickens, and later pigeons, were used in experimental work on human beriberi – a disease that is characterised by demyelination and other nervous lesions. So called 'Chastek paralysis' in foxes (*Vulpes vulpes*) and mink (*Mustela vison*) fed on raw fish has also been studied in detail and found to be due to the enzyme thiaminase in the fish. Many years ago Wallach (1970) discussed thiamine deficiency in exotic animals and stated that it 'occurs often in . . . carnivorous birds (e.g. eagles, penguins, storks, seagulls) because they consume diets high in fish'. That it can be a problem in (for example) ospreys is now clearly recognised (Redig and Ackermann, 2000).

In non fish-eating birds of prey the situation is less clear. There was a published account of thiamine deficiency in a peregrine in the United States some years ago (Ward, 1971). That bird showed clinical signs of opisthotonos followed by seizures that showed no response to antibiotics, small doses of a vitamin/mineral mixture or sedative drugs; a slow recovery followed the administration of thiamine. The author attributed the thiamine deficiency to the use of day-old cockerel chicks. I have seen similar clinical signs of 'star gazing' and demyelination in a number of cases (Fig. 9.2) and both Heidenreich (1997) and Redig and Ackermann (2000) confirmed it as an entity, especially in large falcons. Interestingly, Heidenreich attributed the condition to enteritis and impaired absorption of B vitamins.

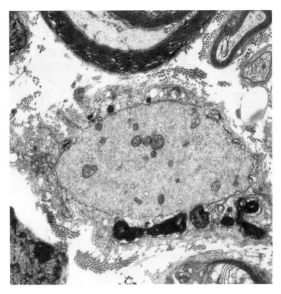

Fig. 9.2 Transmission electronmicroscopy (TEM) of a nerve of a merlin showing demyelination (gaps in the myelin sheath of the lower nerve fibre), probably as a result of thiamine deficiency (TEM ×1000).

Thiamine can be administered to birds orally (see Chapter 10 and Appendix IX) or by injection. Not all cases respond: some remain with residual signs.

Another cause of nervous signs in raptors is hypocalcaemia following nutritional osteodystrophy and hyperparathyroidism, as originally postulated by Wallach and Flieg (1970). Hamerton (1938) reported cases of fits in young buzzards at the London Zoo and described clinical signs 'suggestive of tetany'; in view of their age, these may have been cases of nutritional osteodystrophy but it is noteworthy that Hamerton reported no significant lesions in the parathyroid. Radiography and clinical chemistry play an important part in the confirmation of a diagnosis of osteodystrophy and hypocalcaemia (Cooper, 1975d).

Administration of calcium in cases of fits should be subcutaneous or intravenous. The long-term treatment of hypocalcaemia consists of supplying an adequately balanced diet, but, as is stressed in Chapter 10, the bone changes may be irreversible.

There are other nutritional factors that might cause nervous signs in birds of prey and these include deficiencies of vitamin A and/or E. Certain metabolic disturbances, such as hypoxia, uricaemia and electrolyte imbalance, may produce clinical signs suggestive of neurological disease and thus must be differential diagnoses.

Infectious

A number of infectious diseases can produce central nervous signs. Those listed by Cooper (1996a) were (a) bacteria producing a bacteraemia, septicaemia or toxaemia, (b) bacterial sinusitis causing pressure, (c) Newcastle disease (d) trichomoniasis, and (e) sarcocystosis. To these can be added infections of the brain (encephalitis/meningitis) itself and otitis; (a)–(e) are discussed in more detail elsewhere.

Encephalitis/meningitis can be due to a number of organisms, especially bacteria and viruses, but also protozoa (Raidal & Jaensch, 2000). The brain lesions may be primary or secondary. Although rare, viral infections with zoonotic potential, such as West Nile (Steele *et al.*, 2000) should be considered in differential diagnosis.

Bacterial otitis media is common in raptors; it may occur 'spontaneously' or follow trichomoniasis.

Cawthorne (1993) gave aberrant parasitism as a cause of CNS disorders, citing *Sarcocystis* as an example (Aguilar *et al.*, 1991). Such conditions are likely to be diagnosed *post mortem*, not in the live bird.

Careful clinical examination is necessary to diagnose an infectious cause of nervous disease and must include appropriate laboratory techniques. Therapy of a suspected bacterial infection should comprise intravenous administration of a suitable broad-spectrum antibiotic which is likely to cross the blood–brain barrier and an intramuscular dose of a corticosteroid.

Poisoning

Nervous signs can be a feature of poisoning with a number of agents and this subject is discussed in more detail in Chapter 10. Both captive and free-living birds are susceptible. In the case of chlorinated hydrocarbon poisoning affected birds are weak and incoordinated and may show convulsions

(Plate 20). In addition, as will be mentioned later, occasional episodes of nervous disease may be due to sublethal levels in older birds. Greenwood (1973) made the important diagnostic point that such poisons produce hypersensitivity and a continuous overall tremor as well as fits.

Many other organic poisons can also produce nervous signs, amongst them organophosphorus compounds and other cholinesterase-inhibitors, but there are problems of relating clinical signs to individual poisons. In addition, there may be species differences in susceptibility and the reaction of a raptor to poison may not be the same as a mammal or a galliform bird – on which most toxicological tests are done. Diagnosis and treatment of suspected cases are covered in Chapter 10.

Certain inorganic chemicals can cause similar clinical signs – for example, violent muscular contractions and incoordination with strychnine, and immobility and loss of righting reflex with thallium sulphate (Bean & Hudson, 1976). Falconers' birds dosed with ammonium chloride may show 'fits and spasms' (Naldo & Samour, 2001). Lead poisoning can cause nervous signs and should always be considered: diagnosis and treatment of this are discussed in more detail in Chapter 10. Work by Koeman *et al.* (1971) showed that a feature of methyl mercury poisoning in captive kestrels was demyelination of the medioventral part of the abdominal spinal cord. Affected birds showed clinical signs of paralysis. Similar clinical and pathological features are seen in poultry poisoned with tri-ortho-cresyl phosphate (TOCP). The extensive studies on this subject have provided data on myelin degeneration in birds (Glees, 1961), which could be of great value in work on nervous diseases in raptors.

Toxic algae may possibly play a role in neurological diseases of birds of prey. This has been hypothesised in the USA where avian vacuolar myelinopathy (AVM) has been seen in both coots (*Fulica atra*) and bald eagles (Miller *et al.*, 1998; Pollack, 2000).

Certain soft ticks, *Argas* spp., can produce paralysis in domestic birds in Africa (Walker *et al.*, 1978) and are sometimes found on raptors but whether they ever have the same effect on these hosts is unclear. Marked reactions to *hard* ticks, *Ixodes ricinus*, in birds of prey were reported by Forbes (1995) but were essentially inflammatory and toxaemic.

Neurological reactions to therapeutic agents may be seen from time to time. The compound may be directly toxic to birds or, alternatively, an overdose or impaired metabolism/excretion can result in toxicity. An example of the former is procaine penicillin; an injection of the drug into a bird of prey can result in clinical signs ranging from muscle tremors and ataxia to opisthotonos and collapse (see Chapter 12). Recovery from parenteral anaesthesia can be manifested by stupor and muscle tremors.

Treatment of poisoning is discussed in Chapter 10. A definitive diagnosis is often difficult and specific therapy is rarely practicable. Symptomatic and supportive treatment should be attempted.

Central nervous system (CNS) lesions

Traumatic damage to brain or spinal cord can result in nervous disease. A few road casualty cases exhibit nervous signs but usually these are characterised by 'concussion' – the bird shows reduced response to stimuli, slow pupillar reflexes and depression ranging from unusual tameness to complete unconsciousness. *Post-mortem* examination usually reveals subcutaneous, intraosseous and meningeal congestion and/or haemorrhage. Occasionally the whole head is rotated clinically but, surprisingly, in my experience pathological examination of such cases often reveals no specific lesions.

Leadshot in the brain or spinal cord can be diagnosed by radiography. It can cause nervous signs, including rotation of the head.

Treatment of traumatic injuries is discussed in Chapter 5. In the case of nervous lesions, supportive treatment should also be given as outlined later.

Hyperthermia can also cause clinical signs suggestive of nervous disease (Cooper, 1996a).

Tumours (neoplasms) of the brain are another possible cause of nervous signs but only one such case has been located – in a great horned owl (Halliwell & Graham, 1978b) – and that was diagnosed *post mortem*.

General treatment of central nervous signs

Although I have discussed specific treatment under each of the four headings covered so far, it is frequently difficult to distinguish distinct syndromes, and general therapy is then necessary.

Initial treatment should be to reduce stimuli by placing the bird in a padded box in the dark or by hooding it. Thereafter therapy may be attempted. My own approach is to administer glucose by mouth with calcium boragluconate and thiamine (or B-vitamin complex) by injection. If poisoning is also considered a possibility, I inject atropine (see Chapter 10). Fits may be reduced in severity by the use of benzodiazepines such as diazepam or midozolam. Corticosteroids appear to alleviate certain clinical signs and can be given by intramuscular injection.

Following initial and supportive treatment, attempts at a definitive diagnosis can be made although in some cases therapy will have influenced the results of blood tests and other procedures. A neurological examination should be carried out, as outlined earlier, together with radiography and other investigations.

If a lay person has a bird which has a fit he or she is probably best advised to keep the bird warm, in the dark, if necessary, wrapped in a blanket to reduce self-inflicted damage. Oral glucose or sucrose should be given, together with vitamins (again by mouth) if available. A number of cases have apparently responded to such therapy and it is well worth following if professional advice is not readily available.

Peripheral nerve disease (lesions)

Peripheral nerve damage is a common sequel to traumatic injury and is discussed in that context in Chapter 5. The usual picture is impaired use of a wing or leg but other regions may be involved. A case of right cranial nerve paralysis in a (casualty) red-tailed hawk was described by Chubb (1982): the bird was successfully treated and released after 5 weeks.

Brachial plexus avulsion (damage to the roots of the brachial plexus) can cause paralysis of the affected wing, sometimes together with other paralysis and analgesia. Diagnosis in the live bird is by EMG, in the dead bird by histology. There is no specific treatment. Amputation of the affected wing can be considered (Smith, 1993b).

Other causes of peripheral nerve dysfunction are vertebral column injuries (especially cervical, notarium-synsacrum and caudal to synsacrum), posterior paresis due to pressure (e.g. renal disease, tuberculosis), aspergilloma of the lumbar vertebrae and nutritional deficiencies (riboflavin, vitamin E/ selenium). Differential diagnosis requires careful clinical investigation, including in some cases radiography/ultrasonography, MRI, laparoscopy (aspergillosis), biopsy and blood tests (space-occupying lesions) and response to therapy (deficiencies).

A specific syndrome, probably of nervous origin, is a bilateral paralysis of the legs that is seen in raptors, especially goshawks. The paralysis may be complete or only partial. Usually the digits are tightly clenched and there is considerable tone in the leg muscles. Sensation appears to be present, but impaired. Some cases seem to respond to multiple injections (at 1–2 day intervals) of a B-vitamin complex, suggesting that a B-vitamin deficiency is involved, as has been described in a golden eagle (Stauber, 1973). Some cases treated thus recover fully in 7–10 days. Others, however, show no response and remain paralysed. The digits become abraded, the wing tips damaged and the underparts soiled. There is no response to antibiotics or corticosteroids. Current thinking is that many of these cases are attributable to heavy metal toxicity. *Postmortem* examination of affected goshawks has revealed no specific lesions; inflammatory lesions of the legs, including low-grade lymphocytic infiltration around the sciatic nerves, have been attributed to secondary damage.

Other causes of leg 'paralysis' can be infectious (Harcourt-Brown, 1996b,c) – for example, paramyxovirus (PMV) infection or aspergillosis, especially if the latter involves the abdominal air sacs. There may be radiographic evidence of vertebral lesions (Fig. 9.3a,b). Renal disease may cause an increase in pressure on the sciatic nerves.

Apparent paralysis of the legs may also follow

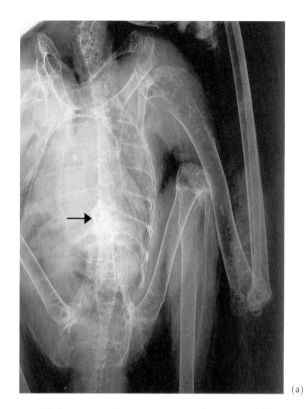

(a)

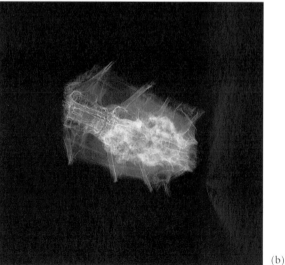

(b)

Fig. 9.3 Radiograph of a common buzzard, which presented with clinical signs of leg weakness. A vertebral lesion is visible (a) (arrow). The affected region removed by dissection and radiographed is shown in (b). This was a proliferative osteo-arthritis.

other diseases. For example, a bird with severe enteritis may 'go off its legs' and lie down; usually it will stand again so long as it receives prompt treatment. 'Cramp' may produce similar clinical signs (see Chapter 13), and was recognised centuries ago (Fig. 9.4). Lesions of tuberculosis or neoplasms, as well as renal distension, may press upon the sciatic nerves and cause paralysis of the legs, as may any intra-abdominal space-occupying lesion – even an egg!

Other possible causes of paralysis may include emboli from an infection or resorbed yolk and from lesions of atheromatosis.

Paralyses of wings and/or legs are also seen from time to time. I have had many such cases, some clinical, others *post mortem*. Sometimes a degree of demyelination is seen on histology/electronmicroscopy but it is not clear whether this is a cause or an effect (see earlier).

Damage to nerves may also follow surgery and this is discussed in part in the context of bumblefoot, in Chapter 8. Intramuscular injections will occasionally cause paralysis of wing or leg but this usually resolves spontaneously over a period of 5–7 days. Trauma to the vagus is more serious and may follow surgery on the crop or thyroid. I have not seen this myself but Voitkevich (1966) described clinical signs of 'paralysis of the crop' in pigeons and fowls. The patient eats well initially but the crop becomes full of food and is not 'put over'; the bird finally dies of inanition. Voitkevich also described impairment of respiratory rhythm following such damage.

Self-mutilation is discussed in Chapter 13. This sometimes occurs following surgery or an injury and it is possible that hyperalgesia, due to nerve damage, is a cause. It can also be a behavioural trait.

Studies on nociceptors in poultry (Gentle & Tiltson, 2000) involved the recording of electrical activity and measuring the response to stimuli. This is but one example of where work in other species, for other reasons, may be applicable to raptors.

POST-MORTEM EXAMINATION

Many birds with nervous disease will die or have to be euthanased and it is important that a *post-mortem* examination and full laboratory investigations are performed. Unfortunately, however, autolytic changes occur quickly in the nervous system and even if material is fixed by immersion immediately after death, the fixative takes some time to penetrate the tissues. It follows that if brain tissue from a bird of prey is sent for examination by post it is often too autolysed for meaningful interpretation – certainly for histological and/or electron-microscopical changes (Fig. 9.5). Under such circumstances it is wiser to arrange to have samples taken by the owner, or another veterinary surgeon, immediately after death. Perfusion of the bird with formol saline is probably the most reliable method of fixation but, as is mentioned in Chapter 4, this will render it useless for microbiological examination. Often, therefore, fixation by immersion has to be used.

Ideally brain material should be taken for histopathology, microbiology and toxicology. My own technique is outlined in Chapter 4. If the skull is split longitudinally, one half of the brain can be fixed immediately for histopathology and pieces of the other portion kept fresh for bacteriological culture, virus isolation and toxicology. If material for toxicological examination is deep-frozen it is

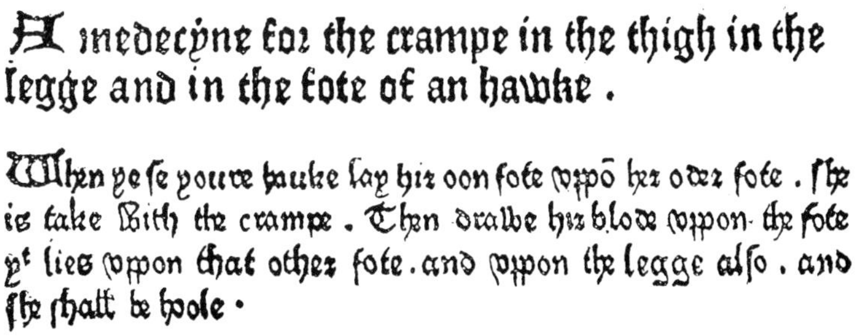
A medecyne for the crampe in the thigh in the legge and in the fote of an hawke.

When ye se youre hawke lay hir oon fote vppō her oder fote. she is take with the crampe. Then drawe hir blode vppon the fote yt lies vppon that other fote. and vppon the legge also. and she shall be hole.

Fig. 9.4 'Cramp' was recognised in falconers' birds centuries ago – here 'crampe in the thigh' from the *Boke of St Albans* (1486).

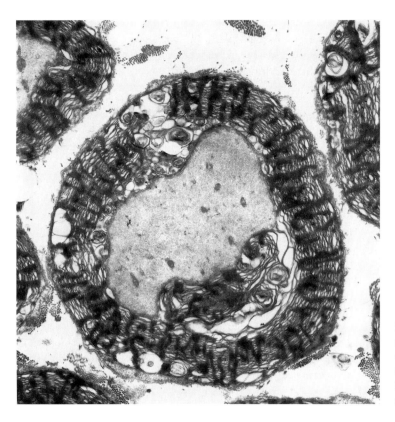

Fig. 9.5 Transmission electronmicroscopy (TEM) of a nerve of a common kestrel, showing changes in the myelin that are not pathological but a result of poor fixation (TEM ×2500).

often possible to use it again later for microbiology.

I have had limited success in dissecting and fixing the spinal cord from raptors without damaging it. I prefer to remove a portion of vertebral column, including the cord, from the cervical and lumbar regions. Following fixation and decalcification, transverse sections can be cut. Peripheral nerves should also be taken, preferably the sciatic or brachial; according to Wallach (1970) the vagus is important in the diagnosis of thiamine deficiency. Wheeler (1995) discussed the sampling of nerves and muscle from domestic mammals for light and electronmicroscopy and the advice given is applicable also to birds.

In addition to the preparation of paraffin sections, nervous tissue should be kept in fixative for fat and myelin stains and, whenever possible, retained for possible electronmicroscopy at a later date.

CONCLUSION

It will be obvious from the foregoing that relatively little is still known about nervous diseases in birds of prey and there is a need for research. Studies using experimental birds are probably justifiable. In the case of naturally occurring disease, if an affected bird has to be killed, every effort should be made to ensure that full pathology, including clinical chemistry, histopathology and electronmicroscopy is performed.

Even though our knowledge of nervous diseases of raptors is so sparse, there can be no doubt that the importance of the brain, especially of regal species, was early recognised and exploited. A seventh century Assyrian text contains the following recipe for use in humans: 'If a man's eyes are sick . . . thou shalt pound the brain of an eagle in harlot's milk and apply'.

Nutritional Diseases, including Poisoning, in Captive Birds

'The wild hawk preserveth herself in all Times and Seasons in a Moderate state by her continual Exercise and Good Feeding.'

Richard Blome

INTRODUCTION

In a paper on the nutrition of raptors at the Oxford Conference, a quarter of a century ago, I drew attention to the paucity of scientific data on the nutritional requirements of these birds. This is still largely the case, as pointed out by Forbes and Flint (2000) in their excellent notes and bibliography, although some advances have been made, especially in our understanding of the deficiency diseases. In this chapter I outline some such developments and at the same time emphasise the fields in which further work is urgently required.

Many of the points made many years ago about the feeding of raptors need to be regularly repeated as both familiar and novel nutritional diseases continue to be recognised (Forbes & Rees Davies, 2000).

Birds of prey are, by definition, essentially carnivorous. In the wild they feed upon animals ranging from grasshoppers, snails and earthworms to small gazelle. In captivity they are usually given meat or dead animals, mainly mammals or birds, although (as will be mentioned later) commercial diets are now also widely used. Aviculturists will offer the smaller species a range of insects, such as locusts, while Leese reported, in 1927, that the Arabs fed camel ticks to their falcons.

A few birds of prey will take food other than flesh – for example, the African harrier hawk will eat oil palm nuts (Brown & Amadon, 1968) – but this is exceptional.

Cannibalism is well recognised amongst the nestlings of free-living birds, particularly the larger species such as eagles, and it can occur in captivity. In very cold climates, such as certain areas of Canada, it may be prudent to separate male and female birds during the winter since, if food becomes frozen, the female may eat the male. A bird that dies in an aviary is very often eaten by one of its cage mates. Eggs are also devoured from time to time and such behaviour may indicate a nutritional deficiency (Porter & Wiemeyer, 1970).

In contrast to the situation for free-living birds, information on the nutrition of captive birds of prey is surprisingly sparse, other than limited studies on certain species, mainly in zoos, and scattered reports of diseases supposedly of nutritional origin. Valuable research on the nutrition of raptors was carried out in the 1970s and 1980s by James Kirkwood, including comparative studies on energy requirements of the kestrel and barn owl in captivity (Kirkwood, 1979), and of the young free-living kestrel (Kirkwood, 1980), and a review of data on various other raptorial species (Kirkwood, 1981). A study on food deprivation that is pertinent to the nursing and treatment of raptors was that by Shapiro and Weathers (1981). Tabaka *et al.* (1996) studied diet, the composition of pellets and energy and nutrient intake in three species of raptor, using captive birds and there have been other, similar, projects elsewhere.

More systematic studies on the nutrition of captive birds would undoubtedly prove of use to the field biologist as well as to the falconer, aviculturist or curator of birds and in this respect it should be noted that in *Eagles, Hawks and Falcons of the World* Brown and Amadon (1968) referred to work with captive species. More recently there have been scientific studies on the effect of different diets in raptors (Lavigne *et al.*, 1994) and on comparative digestive efficiency (Barton & Houston, 1993).

A useful review of raptor feeding and nutrition, including data on pellet (casting) analysis and study of uneaten prey remains was included in the *Raptor Management Techniques Manual* (Pendleton *et al.*, 1987). Studies on the nutrition of raptors have been enhanced by the use of 'stable isotope ratio analysis' (SIRA), whereby one can measure the type of ecosystem and relative trophic level in which raptors are feeding. The analyses can be carried out on feathers – another example of minimally invasive monitoring (Cooper, 1998). Duxbury (1998) discussed the use of SIRA, in combination with more traditional methods, in the context of work on raptors in Alberta, Canada.

The anatomy and physiology of the raptor's gastro-intestinal tract are discussed in Chapter 3 (Figs 3.11 and 3.12). A knowledge of these is essential to a proper understanding of both normal and abnormal function. It also provides information that is relevant to hunting strategies and how best to measure 'body condition' (Barton & Houston, 1996). Students sometimes bemoan the absence of detailed information on the anatomy of the GIT (and other organ systems) in modern books. In fact, dissections of some species were carried out centuries ago, especially by the various anatomy schools. Excellent descriptions and drawings of several European species were provided by the nineteenth century naturalist and taxidermist William MacGillivray (1836) who reminded us of the importance of examining birds internally as well as recording their exterior:

'To those really desirous of information respecting our native species, I would say, Let us betake ourselves to the fields and woods; let us traverse the hills and valleys study our favourites . . . inspect their exterior, look closely to their bills, feathers and feet, and not resting content with this, open them up, examine their internal organs, and record as much of our observations as we may judge useful to ourselves and others.'

Information on the morphology of the digestive tract continues to provide valuable information that can help in the interpretation of clinical signs and pathological lesions. Studies on the anatomy and histology of the digestive tract of the (African) whitebacked vulture preceded research on the possible role of this species in the spread of pathogens (Houston & Cooper, 1975). General data on the anatomy of the digestive tract of birds are given in a number of textbooks – for example, King and McLelland (1975) – and more specific studies on raptors have been carried out by Barton and Houston (1994, 1996), relating morphology to feeding ecology.

Developmental abnormalities of the digestive tract appear to be rare but cystic dilatation of the gizzard has been reported on at least two occasions (Cooper, 1973c).

Many data are available on the nutrition of poultry and some on the requirements of psittacine, columbiform and passeriform birds but there are significant gaps in our knowledge and extrapolation from other species is not always reliable.

DIET

A diet for captive birds of prey should be:

(1) Sufficient in quantity
(2) Sufficient in quality
(3) Free from deleterious effects
(4) Acceptable and digestible
(5) Easily and cheaply obtained.

Quantity

Figures for food consumption for some falconiform species are given in Table 10.1 and examples of reduction in intake in Table 10.2.

Table 10.1 Figures for food consumption for some falconiform species.

Species	Bodyweight (g)	Daily intake (g)	Approximate % of bodyweight
Sharp-shinned hawk	100	25	25.0
Sparrow-hawk	200	53	26.5
Peregrine	683	104	15.0
Red-tailed hawk	1150	127	10.7
Golden eagle	4047	251	6.25
Steller's sea eagle	7030	240	3.5

From Brown and Amadon (1968), with the permission of the publishers.

Table 10.2 Reduction in food intake in warm weather.

Species	From (%)	To (%)
Sharp-shinned hawk	25.0	23.0
Peregrine	15.0	11.5
Red-tailed hawk	10.7	8.6
Golden eagle	6.25	5.26

From Brown and Amadon (1968), with the permission of the publishers.

It will be noted that, the smaller the bird, the greater the percentage of bodyweight that is consumed daily. This reflects the higher metabolic rate of small birds and their high energy requirement. Food consumption increases when temperature drops or when a bird is active as opposed to being sedentary, or when it is laying eggs. Growth and moulting also require increased food intake. Inclement weather can have particularly profound effects on reproductive success of free-living raptors and part of this is the production of smaller and lighter fledglings, probably because they receive less food from their parents (Dawson & Bartolotti, 2000). Parasitic numbers may be affected by abundance and intake of food, in free-living birds as well as captive (Appleby *et al.*, 1999).

Digestive efficiency is an important component of nutrition and will influence the value of a diet. Barton and Houston (1993) studied the digestive efficiency of different raptors and compared values in summer and winter.

In captivity a raptor must receive sufficient food to keep it alive and healthy. In the case of falconers' birds the food intake is deliberately controlled so as to make the hawk 'keen' and thus more easily trained. As will be mentioned later, under 'Inanition', inexperience in this technique can prove disastrous. Overfeeding is more likely in birds maintained in zoological and private collections; it too should be avoided since obesity can also result in disease and death. For example, Fisher (1972) postulated that calorific restriction is an important factor in reducing the incidence and severity of atherosclerotic lesions and Wallach (1970) discussed the role of excessive calorific intake in producing zoo animals which were obese, lazy, infertile and less resistant to high temperatures. He recommended: 'When keeping exotic animals in captivity they should be thought of as animals at rest and fed accordingly'. One way of achieving this with raptors is not to feed the birds on 1, or possibly 2, days a week.

Regular weighing of captive raptors is an important guide to condition but is not easy when the birds are maintained for breeding. Under such circumstances it is probably best to feed an excess of food. Indeed, since precopulatory behaviour may include the offering of food to a mate, even when both have full crops, underfeeding may have deleterious effects on breeding. There is also increasing evidence that some species kill surplus food and then hide (cache) it – the American kestrel, for example (Nunn *et al.*, 1976). When birds are rearing youngsters underfeeding may result in the offspring being killed and eaten, and again supplying food *ad libitum* is probably desirable. One disadvantage of overfeeding is that uneaten food attracts rats and flies and may harbour pathogens; a careful check must therefore be kept upon the food supplied.

It may be advisable to maintain a high plane of nutrition throughout the winter for females intended for breeding. It is also important that the diet is optimum prior to, and during, egg-laying – as Frazer (1977) stated, 'within the egg . . . the development of the young is confined both spatially and by the food available a few months earlier'.

Overfeeding and obesity can result in the deposition of excessive quantities of fat under the skin and within the body cavity as well as fatty change in various organs (Wadsworth *et al.*, 1984) (see Chapter 13). In addition a 'fatty liver–kidney syndrome of merlins' (Plate 22) has been recognised and reported (Cooper & Forbes, 1983; Forbes & Cooper, 1993). The cause is unclear but factors that may contribute include excessive feeding of day-old chicks and inbreeding.

Inanition

This can be defined as 'exhaustion from lack of nutrients' and may be due to an absence of food, an unwillingness or inability to ingest food or an inability to absorb or use nutrients. 'Lowness of condition' was well recognised by early falconers and is, for example, referred to in the *Boke of St Albans* (Fig. 10.1).

Starvation due to unavailability of food kills large numbers of free-living birds, for example young European kestrels (Snow, 1968) where, as was mentioned earlier, the mortality rate is high in the first year of life. Although a small bird, such as a kestrel, may starve to death within 72–96 hours, a large eagle can survive for weeks. If the bird does not have access to water, it may die as a result of dehydration before starvation supervenes. Starvation due to insufficient food should occur only rarely in raptor collections but in falconry, where a hawk is encouraged to fly by reducing its weight, it can be a cause of death. I have examined many cases of inanition *post mortem*; while the majority of these were due to a reduction in food intake and associated factors, this is not always the case. For example, one peregrine died from inanition following damage to the mandible which prevented the bird from feeding; other birds had a localised infection which produced the same effect.

Alternatively, a raptor may receive adequate food in terms of weight but its carbohydrate content may be inadequate. As a result the bird fails to thrive and finally dies of 'calorific exhaustion' (Wallach, 1970). In the case of birds of prey approximately 2000 total calories per g of diet should be provided. An important point here is that the calorific value of whole animal diets may vary. Brisbin (1970) reported that wild-caught mice may show significant deviations in 'caloric' density from those individuals raised in captivity, and referred to work with the rodent *Peromyscus polionotus* which showed that laboratory-raised animals had twice as large fat indices as wild-caught specimens.

In his book *A Hawk for the Bush* Mavrogordato (1960) stated that 'lowness of condition' was the chief cause of disaster to trained sparrow-hawks and gave an excellent description of clinical features. He drew attention to the change from early signs of being ravenously hungry to a terminal stage of

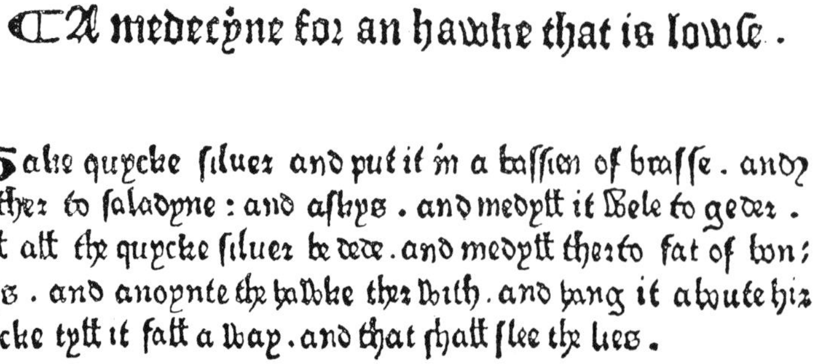
A medecyne for an hawke that is lowe.

Take quycke siluer and put it in a bassyn of brasse. and do ther to saladyne : and asshys . and medylt it wele to geder . tyll all the quycke siluer be dede . and medyll therto fat of swyn; nys . and anoynte the hawke ther with . and hang it aboute hir necke tyll it fall a way . and that shall slee the lyes .

Fig. 10.1 How to treat 'lowness' of condition in a hawk. From the *Boke of St Albans* (1486).

apathy. As he rightly pointed out, the condition should be easily prevented. Birds that are 'low in condition' must be carefully nursed and fed good quality food, without roughage, in small amounts. At the same time they should be kept warm to prevent unnecessary energy expenditure while the administration of oral or parenteral glucose appears to help prevent hypoglycaemia.

Stehle (1965) described a rather similar condition ('Verdauungsinsuffiziens') in Germany but in his cases food was retained in the crop and had to be removed manually before treatment (small meals of warm meat in milk) could be commenced. This condition is now well recognised and termed 'sour crop' in English; it is discussed further in this chapter and Chapter 6.

Diagnosis of inanition is usually based upon history, clinical signs and the bird's low weight. Plasma total protein may be low. Treatment consists of fluids (containing dextrose) and, if the bird is not willing to take food for itself, crop-tubing with readily digestible nutrients. Care must be taken not to overload the bird. Probiotics may also be beneficial.

The *post-mortem* findings in birds that have died of inanition are largely negative. The bird is thin and may be slightly dehydrated. The pectoral muscles in particular are wasted in appearance; they play an important part in metabolism, and at times of reduced food intake are used as a source of amino acids. Internally there are usually no fat reserves and either the gastro-intestinal tract is empty or the crop is full of food. The latter is usually due to the owner's realising, too late, that the bird is in low condition. There may be mild congestion of the lungs and pale internal organs. The liver may appear small and contracted and weigh less than normal – usually calculated on a liver weight:bodyweight basis. The gall bladder is enlarged.

Birds suffering from inanition often ingest vegetation and stones and these are found in both crop and gizzard. However, it should be noted that up to 10% of castings from free-living European kestrels may consist of earth in the winter and early spring (Davis, 1975). In cases where terminal fits have occurred, or the bird has been tethered on a perch and at death perhaps hung from its jesses, agonal intraosseous haemorrhages are visible in the skull. Petechial haemorrhages may be seen occasionally in visceral organs in histological sections but usually there are no significant microscopical lesions.

Green mutes are often a feature of inanition but are also seen under other circumstances. They are generally indicative of a period of low food intake; the green coloration is due to bile. Usually the colour returns to normal once adequate feeding resumes but some birds regularly produce rather greenish faecal material, often intermittently, and this may cause alarm to the owner. No treatment appears necessary but I routinely culture the faeces of such cases bacteriologically and check for parasites.

Although the answer to inanition in practical terms is relatively simple, the whole question of starvation in birds has attracted considerable interest, mainly on account of the unusual features of carbohydrate metabolism in this group of vertebrates. Fisher (1972) reviewed the subject in detail and the reader who is interested in the mechanisms involved is advised to read his chapter; it should be noted that Fisher stated that 'unfortunately, virtually no information relative to tissue metabolic patterns of non-domestic species is available' and this situation is virtually unchanged insofar as birds of prey are concerned.

Captive birds should not suffer from starvation and, so long as they are in the hands of an experienced and conscientious falconer, even those kept for hunting will not do so. Imprinted hawks tend to be flown at a higher weight than non-imprints. This makes inanition/hypoglycaemia less likely but these same imprints sometimes consume food in excess of their requirements and may show 'selective feeding'.

All trained birds must be weighed regularly; only in this way will a drop in condition be quickly diagnosed. The size of the pectoral muscles is an important clue but, as has been emphasised in other species (Owen & Cook, 1977), does not take into account the size of the fat reserves. Another feature that is frequently overlooked is that, while an increase in weight may take several days to achieve, a corresponding drop can occur very rapidly.

Appetite stimulation in raptors was discussed by

Suarez (1993). Analgesics will often help in this respect, as part of stabilisation.

Anorexia can lead to inanition and anorexia can be due to infectious agents, such as *Trichomonas* and *Candida*, or to 'secondary' causes, such as low condition/sour crop and aspergillosis or foreign bodies (ranging from fish hooks to bones of food items). Anorexia may also be a sequel to a number of less severe disorders. Careful investigation of the anorectic bird is, therefore, essential.

According to Redig (1996b), the most life-threatening form of anorexia is that associated with 'sour crop' and low condition/starvation. He attributed most such cases in captive raptors to their being trained for falconry and, in some cases, developing a net catabolic state following a period of being maintained in a state of 'lean body mass' for hunting. Such birds are not usually hypoglycaemic but dehydrated and unable to put over a crop of food. As a result bacterial endotoxins form in the crop and these are absorbed, producing a 'toxic' state. Treatment consists of dilution of crop contents and encouraging digestion or regurgitation. Fluids and supportive care are essential concomitants. If, after 2 hours treatment is clearly not effective, the crop contents need to be removed under anaesthesia. 'Sour crop' is discussed in more detail in Chapter 6, as are some other conditions affecting the digestive tract.

Quality

A diet may be sufficient to assuage hunger but still be unsatisfactory in terms of content. The important constituents of a diet are water, protein, fat, carbohydrate, minerals, vitamins and roughage and insufficient or excess of any of these may result in disease.

Only recently has analysis of diets fed to raptors attracted serious attention. Thus, for example, Clum *et al.* (1997) reported on the nutrient content of five species of domestic animal that are commonly fed to captive birds of prey, and Crissey *et al.* (1999) investigated cholesterol, fat and fatty acids in mice used as a food source.

Water and roughage are related in that both influence consistency. A diet containing low amounts of roughage for over 14–21 days can cause diarrhoea (loose droppings) and birds on such a diet may try to ingest soil or plant material. It is therefore important to ensure adequate feather, fur or artificial roughage such as cotton wool. Impaction of the proventriculus and/or gizzard occasionally occurs, however, and in one case in my experience it was associated with ulceration. Hamerton (1938) reported the death of a falconet due to impaction of a hard ball of mouse fur in the gizzard and consequent obstruction of the intestinal tract. He made the comment: 'these insectivorous falcons seem to be unable to thrive on the ordinary meat diet provided for birds of prey'. Forbes and Rees Davies (2000) discussed 'Obstructions' and listed as examples casting, inadvertent ingestion of indigestible matter, ingestion of oversized food items and decreased gastro-intestinal motility.

Impaction of the crop by casting or by ingested food (especially indigestible or oversized items) is common and was reported as long ago as the fifteenth century (Fig. 10.2). Many cases respond to oral liquid paraffin (mineral oil) or fluids and manual 'milking out' of the crop but occasionally surgical removal of crop contents is necessary. Such conditions are less likely to occur if one ensures that the moisture content of the diet is adequate.

Other physical features of the food may influence the health of the bird. Bones can become lodged in the crop or, rarely, penetrate its wall and cause infection. Such bones can be removed surgically or, in some cases, milked out manually. Many raptors are kept on sand and will, inevitably, ingest some with their food. Not only may this reduce palatability but, according to some authors, it can cause enteritis. For example, Hamerton (1935) described acute gangrenous gastroenteritis in a peregrine and reported: 'the alimentary tract was packed with fine sand, a condition that is frequently found in acute enteritis among small birds of prey'. This has not been my experience; many people maintain raptors on sand without any ill effects and soil is commonly found in the castings of free-living birds (Davis, 1975). Indeed, I sometimes find the presence of small amounts of such material in the alimentary tract a useful landmark in radiography! Nevertheless, if complications due to ingesting sand were diag-

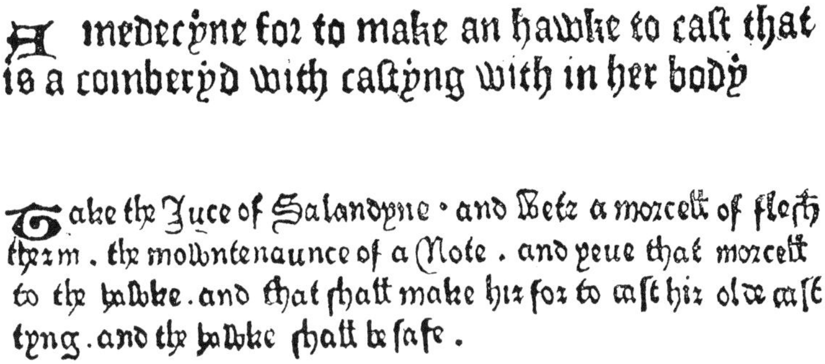

A medecyne for to make an hawke to caſt that is a comberyd with caſtyng with in her body

Fig. 10.2 Fifteenth century guidance on how to make a hawk cast (bring up a pellet). From the *Boke of St Albans* (1486).

Take the Juce of Salandyne · and Betz a morcell of fleſh therm . the mowntenaunce of a Note . and yeue that morcell to the hawke. and that ſhall make hir for to caſt hir olde caſt tyng . and the hawke ſhall be ſafe .

nosed early, I would expect liquid paraffin (mineral oil) to be of use in treatment.

Occasionally a young bird, especially if hand-reared, will swallow air which is then visible and palpable in the crop. The bird may show discomfort, craning its head as if to regurgitate. The condition is recognised by aviculturists in other birds; often it resolves spontaneously but it may be necessary to pass an oesophageal tube through which the air will escape. It is important to distinguish this condition from subcutaneous emphysema, which is discussed in Chapter 5.

When considering consistency it must be remembered that food that has been deep-frozen should be thawed slowly and then, if possible, soaked in water or physiological saline before being used. If this is not done the moisture content may be reduced excessively. This can be a danger if food is partially thawed and then refrozen. Food that contains ice should not be fed.

Water itself must also be discussed. Traditionally falconers rarely gave their birds water on the grounds that they were not often seen to drink. But raptors need fluid (40–60 ml/kg bodyweight) and it is now generally accepted that water should be available for captive birds even if they take very little of it. Birds that are unwell, egg-laying or rearing young will often take small amounts of water to supplement that obtained from their food. Some sick birds will refuse to feed until they have taken water and a bird that is not eating will rapidly become dehydrated as well as lose condition. Renal disease, including uricaemia and visceral gout, can be the sequel (see Chapter 13).

Water containers are, therefore, an integral part of managing captive raptors. They must be properly maintained and in temperate climates it must be remembered that they may freeze on particularly cold days. Hygiene is of the utmost importance as bacteria (especially *Pseudomonas*) and other organisms, including some metazoan and protozoan parasites, will survive and in some cases multiply in containers and in hosepipes. Water baths should have their water changed every 24 hours and the use of *hot* (boiled) water, which is then allowed to cool, will help to reduce numbers of organisms. Diluted disinfectants are used by some people to discourage multiplication of pathogens. Slight acidification of the water can reduce bacterial and algal growth and may be helpful in the treatment of candidiasis.

Care must be taken in the choice of water container. Water baths that contain galvanised material may be a source of zinc poisoning (see later). The addition of acid, referred to earlier, may exacerbate the risk. It may be wise to use plastic containers.

Water testing can be a useful important addition to the diagnostic and health monitoring investigations carried out on both captive and free-living birds. The tests should include bacteriology, chemical assays and routine measurements of pH and hardness. Much has been published on water quality: a useful general reference, used internationally was produced by WHO (1984).

A subject which should be mentioned is that of 'rangle'. That captive hawks will swallow small stones was known to the earliest falconers; in 1615 Latham described the way his peregrine would later regurgitate these stones and, if they were placed near the block, swallow them again. Falconers have traditionally believed that 'rangle' stirs up mucus and fat in the stomach and that this has a beneficial effect, as evidenced in Latham's advice:

'Wash'd meat and stones maketh a hawk to flie, but great casting and long fasting maketh her to die.'

An interesting discussion on the history and possible role of rangle was provided by Fox (1976) who concluded that captive birds of prey benefit from having 'appropriate stones available to them at all times'. He went on to mention captive hawks dying following the use of diets with a high fat content but did not elucidate: stones are occasionally found in the gizzard of birds at *post-mortem* examination or may be detected radiographically.

The protein content of a diet is important and in this respect one can to a certain extent extrapolate from the situation in poultry where the protein percentage used for young chicks is usually 18–20% and this is reduced to 12–14% for growers; layers and breeders require higher levels, usually 14–18%, but adult non-breeding birds will thrive on less than 10%. Comparable figures apply to birds of prey: a figure of 15–20% is desirable, with young birds receiving higher levels than non-breeding adults. As Bird and Ho (1976) pointed out, rodents, chickens and day-old chicks show comparable levels of protein. It is not just protein levels that are of concern, however; the amino acids present are also important and here again few scientific data are available. In poultry the amino acid requirements can differ between strains of fowl, and from this one would assume that there are likely to be variations between species of raptor. In the absence of reliable data one should rely on 'natural' foods rather than attempt to formulate an artificial diet.

Excess protein must also be avoided. It has been postulated that it may produce visceral and arthritic gout (Wallach, 1970).

Even less is known of the importance of dietary fat to raptors. Again, Bird and Ho (1976) found little difference in levels in the species they analysed and since raptors appear to thrive on such diets it may be reasonable to assume that a crude fat % (of dry matter) of 20–25% is acceptable. However, I would refer the reader to my comments earlier, under 'Quantity', concerning the difference in fat content between free-living and laboratory-reared rodents.

A similar situation applied to carbohydrates: figures by Bird and Ho (1976) for gross energy, which reflect other constituents as well as carbohydrates, ranged from 5.78–6.02 kcal per g of dry matter and conformed closely with those of Duke *et al.* (1973) for mice and young turkeys.

Of the minerals, only calcium and phosphorus have been investigated in any detail in birds of prey, largely on account of the prevalence of osteodystrophy (metabolic bone disease (MBD) or nutritional secondary hyperparathyroidism). Osteodystrophy is usually attributable to a calcium/phosphorus imbalance, and is discussed in detail later in this chapter. A useful review of MBD, in different species, was written by Fowler (1986).

Wallach and Flieg (1970) recommended a calcium level of 2% of the diet for raptors, and Bird and Ho (1976) suggested that day-old chicks which contain less than this on a dry matter basis should be rolled in bonemeal to increase their calcium content. In Bird and Ho's study rats and mice contained 2.06% and 2.38% calcium, respectively. However, the commercial diet mentioned earlier is described as having a minimum of only 0.4% calcium and one wonders if this is adequate for breeding birds. Other minerals may influence calcium metabolism, especially phosphorus and manganese, and, as Wallach and Flieg (1970) pointed out, exceptionally high levels of these should be avoided.

Bird and Ho (1976) also investigated levels of zinc, copper, manganese and iron and, extrapolating from poultry, suggested that rodents and poultry used to feed raptors were adequate in terms of zinc and iron, possibly marginal for copper and very likely deficient in manganese. In view of the known effect of manganese deficiency in causing infertility of poultry, they suggested that supplementation of these diets with the mineral may be necessary. In my view, however, there is as yet no evidence of such an effect in birds of prey and one should be wary of interference with the diet until more information is available. Care *must* be taken with some elements: zinc poisoning can easily result from excess intake by birds.

Vitamins follow the same pattern as minerals – there is only limited information on their importance in birds of prey. Certain deficiencies have been reported in raptors and these will be discussed later. Bird and Ho (1976) were sceptical of the claim that day-old chicks may be deficient in thiamine – in their study comparable figures were obtained for rats and for one strain of chicks. They drew attention, however, to the marked variation in values between strains of day-old chicks and this is an important point to remember whenever the nutritional value of chicks is being discussed. One must also bear in mind that even if the thiamine in the diet is adequate, it may not be available if there is also thiaminase present – for example, in chicks or fish. Redig and Ackermann (2000) recommended supplementing frozen fish with thiamine (1–3 mg/kg) when these are fed to bald eagles or ospreys.

Biotin deficiency may be involved in conditions in which the beak (and sometimes talons) are of poor consistency and tend to break or crumble easily. This and other deficiencies may contribute to abnormal plumage, including colour changes (see Chapter 13).

Although the indications are that the mineral and vitamin contents of diets fed to raptors are adequate, one must bear in mind that this may not apply when birds are breeding, unwell, or perhaps, when wounds are healing. It must also be remembered that the young growing bird needs a diet of high quality and will fail to thrive on one that appears to be satisfactory for an adult. Another important point is that work on the fowl has shown that abnormal embryonic development, including peaks of mortality, can be due to nutritional deficiencies in the diet of the hen (Couch & Ferguson, 1975). Such deficiencies can include riboflavin (embryonic abnormalities from 9–14 days incubation), biotin (3 and 18–21 days), phosphorus (12–14 days), vitamin B12 (16–18 days), manganese (20–21 days) and vitamin E (2–4 days). Turkey embryos from eggs laid by hens deficient in pantothenic acid do not die in the egg but are unable to pip the shell, and show morphological abnormalities. It is reasonable to assume that vitamin deficiencies in raptors could have comparable results – but hard data are difficult to find and controlled research is needed.

As was mentioned earlier, metabolic bone disease (MBD) associated with a relative deficiency of calcium can be a problem in captive birds of prey. There is confusion about the nomenclature used for this condition; some authors still speak of 'rickets' and 'osteomalacia' but these terms are best reserved for a specific vitamin D deficiency. The word osteodystrophy is generally used throughout this book, or nutritional secondary hyperparathyroidism and/or hypocalcaemia, when non-skeletal effects are being discussed.

Osteodystrophy was probably not so rare in falconers' birds as Keymer (1972) suggested. It is particularly prevalent in young birds that are hand-reared prior to training. It may even occur in captive-bred birds on an adequate diet if they are offered only muscle and viscera by their parents instead of bone (Cooper, 1975d). Such 'selective feeding' can contribute to other nutritional disorders also. Small species of raptor, such as little owls and falconets, may develop osteodystrophy if fed on a diet of insects, such as crickets, supplemented only with meat; some bird keepers believe, erroneously, that the exoskeleton of such insects contains calcium. Forbes and Rees Davies (2000) warned that young secretary birds fed on standard raptor diets may suffer a $Ca:PO_3$ imbalance because their principal food in the wild is snakes, which are high in calcium phosphate.

The cause of osteodystrophy is usually an all-meat diet (or sometimes, overfeeding so that meat alone is selected by parents for young birds). Meat supplies plenty of protein but offers an inverted calcium/phosphorus ratio – often 1:15–1:40. The optimum ratio is 1.5:1.0 (Wallach & Flieg, 1969) and hence, on the meat diet, a disparity in levels of available calcium and phosphorus results. Serum calcium levels are initially maintained by resorption of calcium (demineralisation) from the bones; as a result, there is a breakdown of osseous structure: spontaneous fractures, 'folding' of long bones and locomotor signs result (Fig. 10.3). Wallach and Flieg (1970) discussed the early signs of the disease and described such clinical signs as drowsiness, poor growth, feather pecking and diarrhoea although it is not my experience that these are generally seen in raptors.

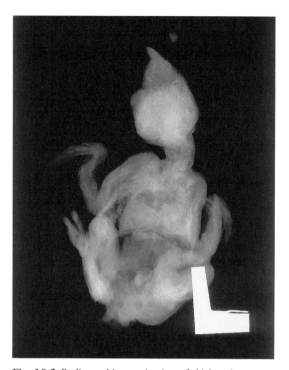

Fig. 10.3 Radiographic examination of chicks prior to necropsy can prove useful. This young barn owl shows metabolic bone disease with folding fractures of long bones. Locomotion was severely impaired.

Both prevention and treatment are based primarily on increasing the dietary calcium intake; calcium lactate may be used, or bonemeal, or a 'natural diet' of adult mice or birds. Vitamin D should not be administered as such since it may cause further reduction of bone calcium.

In severe cases of osteodystrophy, where bone changes are irreversible, euthanasia will be the most humane option. However, Forbes and Flint (2000) emphasised the role of vitamin D3 in *preventing* metabolic bone disease and pointed out that exposure of raptors to unfiltered sunlight will result in D3 production in the preen oil, some of which is ingested by the bird during feather maintenance.

Older birds of prey on an apparently adequate diet may show decalcification of the bones and the clinical signs seen are similar to those in osteodystrophy. This possibly has a different aetiology. For example, Hamerton (1938) described 'spontaneous fractures

due to senile rarefaction of the bones' in a Javan fish owl.

The production of soft-shelled eggs by female birds is another problem that can be associated with an inadequately balanced diet. Work with poultry (Antillon *et al.*, 1977) showed that the recommended levels of calcium and vitamin D3 (3.6% and 1180 ICU/kg respectively) resulted in high egg production and good eggshell strength. A decrease from 0.55 to 0.26% in dietary phosphorus gave higher egg production and increased eggshell strength, but reductions in calcium and vitamin D3 had the opposite effect. It is probable that a similar situation applies in birds of prey and therefore every effort should be made to ensure that breeding birds receive adequate calcium and vitamin D in their diet. Commercial strains of poultry show differences in eggshell strength and it is possible that there are similar variations within raptorial species.

Other causes of soft or thin eggshells in birds of prey include old age, systemic and local infectious diseases and certain forms of poisoning. Disorders of the oviduct, which may be infectious, developmental or metabolic in origin, are a particularly common aetiology.

Calcium metabolism in birds of prey needs more investigation. Cummings *et al.* (1976) showed that falconiform birds digest the bones of their prey more thoroughly than do strigiforms because of greater gastric acidity and it is therefore possible that an owl is more likely to suffer a calcium deficiency on a low-bone diet.

There is interest in calcium metabolism in free-living birds of prey and this is a field where captive specimens could play a useful part in research. Mundy and Ledger (1976) first reported Cape vulture chicks with broken or deformed limbs (unfortunately termed 'rickets'), apparently on account of insufficient calcium in the diet; they postulated that griffon vultures depend upon carnivorous mammals for a supply of suitable pieces of bone which they feed to their chicks. This was a novel theory since previous authors (Houston, 1972) had questioned how vulture chicks, which appear only to eat meat, obtain calcium. Further work on (free-living) Cape vultures was carried out by Evans and Piper (1981) who described the bone abnormalities seen in those birds as 'juvenile osteoporosis' or 'nutritional osteodystrophy' and attributed the condition to a calcium/phosphorus imbalance following a lack of calcium intake. Vultures tend to have a calcium-deficient diet because they usually ingest meat and viscera that have a high phosphorus/calcium ratio (Houston, 1978). Mundy and Ledger (1976) and Richardson *et al.* (1986) showed that African vultures depend upon the presence of large predators to provide them with bone fragments that can correct this deficiency. Elsewhere in the world, where large carnivores are absent, alternative strategies are needed. Thus Bertram and Margalida (1997) reported griffon vultures in Spain making use of bone splinters obtained from bearded vulture ossuaries, where large bones are deliberately dropped on to rock slabs.

Calcium deficiencies can also arise when free-living birds of prey select meat (muscle) rather than whole carcasses, for instance during myxomatosis outbreaks in Europe when rabbit carcasses are available in abundance and there is little need to take bones. This is a reminder that both in the wild and in captivity 'selective feeding' can prove deleterious in terms of health.

It is important to distinguish nutritional osteodystrophy from rickets (vitamin D3 deficiency) since the treatment of the two conditions is very different. Clinically rickets produces similar lesions to nutritional osteodystrophy but radiographically there is an important distinguishing feature in that in rickets the epiphyseal plates are widened and the articular surfaces of long bones are enlarged (Wallach, 1970). Unfortunately, as with other vitamins, it is possible that there may be a combination of deficiencies and imbalances in which case definitive diagnosis is not always possible. In such instances one often resorts to supplementation with both multivitamins and minerals, sometimes with surprisingly good clinical results. It must be emphasised that raptors need vitamin D3: some supplements may contain vitamin D2, which cannot be utilised.

Various vitamin deficiencies have been reported in birds of prey but only rarely has a full diagnosis been possible. Ward (1971) described a thiamine deficiency in a peregrine which showed nervous signs

(see Chapter 9). Wallach (1970) stated that thiamine deficiency was common in carnivorous birds fed diets high in fish on account of the high thiaminase content of the latter. He also drew attention to the paper by Friend and Trainer (1969) which indicated that thiamine-deficient birds frequently die of aspergillosis. Stauber (1973) described a syndrome in an immature golden eagle which showed leg paralysis and he postulated that this was a riboflavin deficiency; a rapid clinical response followed the oral administration of a B-vitamin complex. A similar response to B vitamins has been seen in birds showing leg paralysis in Britain, especially goshawks, and I discuss this syndrome in Chapter 9.

The possible role of vitamin D in the maintenance of eggshell strength was mentioned earlier. While it is wise to ensure that a diet is not likely to be deficient in this vitamin, it must also be remembered that excess D3 may prove toxic. Some caution must, therefore, be observed. The true role of sunlight in the metabolism of vitamin D in raptors is unknown.

I have often noticed small subcutaneous haemorrhages in birds that are in poor condition, and interestingly, this has usually been by the use of a magnifying lens during my clinical examination: they are easily missed with the naked eye. These haemorrhages usually overly joints and I tend to attribute them to physical damage but a vitamin K deficiency should perhaps be considered. Unexplained internal haemorrhage in birds at *post-mortem* examination might also be due to a deficiency of this vitamin (although anti-coagulant rodenticides and trauma remain the most common causes).

There seems little doubt that vitamin A deficiency plays a part in raptor disease although sound data are again difficult to obtain. I have seen birds with clinical signs of conjunctivitis, swollen eyelids, poor scaling and stomatitis, which I consider suggestive of a vitamin A deficiency, possibly combined with other deficiencies. Such birds have usually responded to nursing and dietary supplements. Graham (1970) described similar lesions and also attributed 'corns' on the feet, anorexia and mouth lesions in hawks on an all-meat diet to a vitamin A deficiency. Ocular lesions in hand-reared birds may also be associated with such a deficiency.

Some other diseases show a clinical response to vitamin therapy and it is probable that a deficiency may be involved in the condition, possibly by retarding healing. For example, I treated a goshawk which showed loss of weight, a change of voice and a degree of dyspnoea with intramuscular vitamin A and there appeared to be a rapid and spectacular response. Other respiratory conditions have also appeared to respond to multivitamins by mouth or injection.

The possible role of vitamin A deficiency in foot conditions is discussed in Chapter 8.

Pansteatitis was reported by Wong *et al.* (1999) in a free-living red-tailed hawk. The bird died and the diagnosis was made *post mortem*. The authors suggested that the changes might be due to a vitamin E deficiency, as in mammals and fish-eating birds. Forbes and Flint (2000) pointed out that vitamin E deficiency may result from excessive storage of food and associated rancidity. Dierenfeld *et al.* (1989) reported significant improvement in libido, hatchability of eggs and activity of chicks when falcons were fed quail which had been supplemented with vitamin E.

Perosis, similar to 'slipped tendon' in poultry, was first reported in peregrine falcons by Sykes *et al.* (1982) who suspected that marginal manganese levels in the whole pigeon diet might be responsible. I have seen similar cases in peregrines and eagle owls in Britain: again the cause has been unclear. In other birds, e.g. ratites and cranes, excessive growth rate has been implicated. More research is clearly needed.

Caution must always be taken in the use of vitamins. There is a tendency amongst some falconers and aviculturists to assume that, because small quantities of vitamins can be beneficial, large amounts must be even more so. As a result some feed enormous quantities of vitamin supplement to their birds. I have investigated non-specific diseases in such birds with vague clinical signs of lethargy or poor condition, and believe that in some cases a nutritional disorder is resulting from *overuse* of vitamins.

An exception may be in the newly hatched chick.

Broiler chick survival and weight gain are enhanced by the oral administration of multivitamins and it is possible that a similar situation applies to raptors.

An important point in any consideration of the quality of a diet is that gastric digestion appears to be more efficient in falconiforms than strigiforms. Duke *et al.* (1975), using captive raptors of seven species, showed that falconiform birds were able to digest a greater proportion of their diet than owls and as a result a smaller amount of the food consumed reappeared in their pellets.

Analysis of diets fed to captive raptors is recommended. Often this can be performed by university or private laboratories; at least one company (in Canada) offers such analysis to raptor biologists on a commercial basis.

Deleterious effects

The main deleterious effects of diet are (a) infectious and parasitic diseases, (b) poisoning. Diseases due to deficiencies or antagonists in the diet were discussed earlier.

Infectious and parasitic diseases derived from the food

These may be attributable to either infected or contaminated food and can present a hazard to free-living and captive raptors alike.

Whilst the feeding of 'natural' food, such as dead birds, to captive raptors will probably prevent the development of deficiencies, it can also be dangerous. A number of infectious diseases may be transmitted thus, amongst them such potentially dangerous conditions as Newcastle disease and tuberculosis, and these and other examples are discussed in Chapter 6. Other organisms may be contracted from food, even if not of 'natural' origin and precautions need to be taken, in the case of large establishments, to have proper quality control. This should include regular checks for bacteria, such as *Salmonella* spp. using appropriate media (June *et al.*, 1995).

Certain parasites may be contracted from food, especially if it has become contaminated with faeces but also if the prey item is itself infected – for example, with *Syngamus trachea* or *Trichomonas gallinae* (see Chapter 7). Botfly (*Gasterophilus pecorum*) larvae can be acquired by African vultures if they feed on infected zebra (*Equus burchelli*) (Houston & Cooper, 1975). Keymer (1972) suggested that *Capillaria* worms might be transmitted from prey to predator, citing as his example ptarmigan (*Lagopus mutus*) and gyrfalcons in Iceland. Certain ectoparasites can also be contracted in this way, especially fleas. It is not unusual to find avian lice and fleas in the faeces of raptors fed on wild birds; these parasites are ingested and then pass through the intestinal tract and can provide information on the food items taken.

Poisoning

Food can also be the source of poisons and the broad subject of poisoning is therefore included in this chapter even though some chemicals may be acquired through routes other than the alimentary tract.

Poisoning of free-living birds of prey is covered in Chapter 11, contributed by David Peakall, and provides information on the different groups of chemical involved. The emphasis in this chapter is on captive birds, which can also be affected by poisons in the environment. Thus, in and following the heyday of chlorinated hydrocarbon use, Woodford (1960) and Jefferies and Prestt (1966) recorded deaths in captive birds due to their being fed on woodpigeons which had ingested seed corn dressed with dieldrin and more recently Lumeij *et al.* (1993) reviewed cases diagnosed *post mortem* in the Netherlands.

The susceptibility of birds of prey to poisoning by chlorinated hydrocarbon insecticides was recognised following extensive work on free-living birds in Europe, North America and elsewhere (see Chapters 1 and 11). The main hazard to captive birds is from contaminated food or quarry and experimental work with raptors has confirmed this threat (Porter & Wiemeyer, 1972). Affected birds are usually incoordinated and weak and refuse to feed. Fortunately, most bird keepers are aware of such dangers and acute poisoning is now very much less common, although, as Wheeldon *et al.* (1975)

pointed out, it may still occur and diagnosis can prove difficult. Those who keep the smaller species and feed them on insects should be wary of insecticides. Food items should be obtained from a reputable source.

In addition, birds in captivity may suffer from sublethal effects. Falconers sometimes report transient fits or muscle tremors in older birds, which resolve spontaneously with supportive treatment. It is possible that these clinical signs are associated with pesticide levels since they often occur following a drop in condition (such as reduction in weight prior to flying) which is not sufficiently critical for hypoglycaemia to be a likely cause. A possible effect of pesticides on breeding is mentioned later.

Chlorinated hydrocarbon insecticides may accumulate in captive raptors: such chemical burdens are probably acquired from the diet but this is often difficult to prove. Birds that die unexpectedly and which show no *post-mortem* evidence of disease should be analysed. Clinical diagnosis may be facilitated by the use of blood tests (Henny & Meeker, 1981).

Owls from the Zoological Society of London succumbed some years ago to dieldrin poisoning as a result of being fed laboratory rodents which had been housed on sawdust impregnated with the insecticide (Jones, 1977a). Affected birds either died unexpectedly or were found *in extremis*, often with torticollis or in convulsions. Gross *post-mortem* findings were generally absent although some showed incidental lesions, such as interstitial nephritis, or changes secondary to nervous signs. A falconer who fed his hawks on rodents from the same source also had a number of unexplained deaths and the same negative findings were noted at *post-mortem* examination. In his case it was not possible to analyse the tissues of the dead birds but it is reasonable to assume that dieldrin poisoning was again involved. These incidents made many falconers and aviculturists aware of the continued danger of pesticides, even from apparently healthy laboratory mice, and it was postulated at the time that some of the failures to breed birds of prey, and behavioural changes noted in them, might be attributable to non-lethal doses of such chemicals.

Even commercial diets may pose a threat of pesticides. Kisling (1974) gave figures for chlorinated hydrocarbon levels in a variety of commercial zoo diets. The latter were not high (maximum 0.36 ppm) but they emphasise the point that a 'synthetic' product is not necessarily free of those contaminants that one associates with a 'natural' diet. Quality control is always needed and this should include toxicological assays as well as analysis of nutrients and health monitoring.

Unfortunately, financial considerations often preclude the analysis of tissues from captive birds and, as a result, diagnoses of poisoning may be missed.

A definitive diagnosis of chlorinated hydrocarbon poisoning in birds of prey can usually only be made on the basis of toxicological examination. However, the combination of history and clinical signs may be suggestive of poisoning. Specific *post-mortem* lesions are rarely seen, although Bell and Murton (1977) reported internal haemorrhage as a common feature of organochlorine poisoning.

A possible source of poisoning in captive birds of prey is the use of insecticidal preparations, and great care should be taken in their use. My first example – from which I learned a great deal – was when a lanner falcon died of lindane poisoning following the administration of an allegedly 'non-toxic' poultry aerosol. In this case the product contained lindane (a form of benzene hexachloride) in addition to its pyrethrum base. It is most important that one checks the constituents of any insecticide intended for use on birds and that the manufacturers' instructions are followed exactly. If in any doubt the compound should not be used and, instead, a safer method of control followed. Tight regulations in some parts of the world (e.g. the European Union) mean that preparations are properly labelled but this is not necessarily the case elsewhere.

It is not only the chlorinated hydrocarbon insecticides that are a hazard to captive birds of prey. A possible danger is alphachloralose used as a stupefying bait for pigeons and other species. In raptors the chemical can produce incoordination and lethargy which will usually wear off, without specific treatment, in 24–36 hours. Death has been reported in free-living eagles, buzzards and hen harriers (van Nie, 1975).

Organophosphorus (OP) compounds and carbamates may also cause disease or deaths. The effect of these is due to cholinesterase inhibition and again a possible source is insecticidal preparations (Porter, 1993). Affected birds show muscle tremors, limb contractions and/or paralysis and diarrhoea. There is very little information on the therapy of such cases in captivity but atropine sulphate can be used (Redig & Ackermann, 2000), coupled with a benzodiazepine such as diazepam or midazolam, to control muscle contractions. If there is no response within 6 hours, the prognosis is poor. Shimmel & Snell (1999) used a variety of agents when treating a bald eagle with presumed OP toxicity. Shlosberg (1976) successfully treated wild raptors that had ingested voles (*Microtus* sp.) containing the insecticide monocrotophos. He used pralidoxime iodide intramuscularly, and drew attention to the apparent varying response in different avian species; this should be borne in mind when treating captive birds.

Contamination with oil is also discussed in Chapter 13. The subject is a complex one. Oiling produces both external and internal damage (Croxall, 1979; Robinson, 2000). The former results in heat loss and chilling, or drowning if the bird is in the water. Internally, oil can produce enteritis and damage to kidneys, liver and lung. It is vital, therefore, to ensure that a bird which has oil on its plumage does not try to preen and hence ingest it. The bird should be wrapped up to prevent such an occurrence and this will also keep it warm; nursing is most important.

The effect of ingested oil on American kestrels was studied experimentally by Pattee and Franson (1982) who concluded that crude oil from a spill posed little hazard to this and other falconiform species.

Those who feed day-old chicks or rodents to their birds should check how they have been killed. I have examined histologically tissues from birds of prey which died in unusual circumstances after being fed chicks killed with excess amounts of carbon tetrachloride; the livers showed severe fatty change. This suggests that carbon tetrachloride may act as a poison to raptors and care should be taken when it is used. Other chemicals used to kill chicks have not, apparently, been associated with toxicity in birds of prey but the use of ether or chloroform may result in the chicks being refused as food, probably on account of their taste. Such agents are also likely to be toxic in large amounts. It is therefore best, whenever possible, to use (humanely) carbon dioxide to euthanase chicks and rodents, or to kill them manually.

Barbiturate poisoning can occur, even in the wild, if disposal of carcasses is inadequate. Langelier (1993) described such an incident.

Although not true 'poisons', antibacterial and antiprotozoal drugs may be present in the food offered to raptors. Excessive quantities could prove toxic and, in addition, ingestion of small amounts of such drugs may encourage drug resistance.

A number of inorganic chemicals are known to pose a hazard to free-living birds of prey, amongst them mercury compounds (Fimreite *et al.*, 1970) and thallium (Clausen & Karlog, 1977). Such poisons should be suspected whenever one is dealing with sick birds only recently taken from the wild – casualties, for example. Koeman *et al.* (1971) used five captive kestrels to investigate the toxicity of methylmercurydicyandiamide. The chemical was fed to the birds in their diet of laboratory mice. The clinical signs seen in the kestrels consisted of paralysis, and *post-mortem* examination revealed heart lesions, demyelination of the spinal cord and mild peritonitis. Subsequent work by Spalding *et al.* (2000a,b) on captive egrets (*Ardea albus*) provided more information as how methylmercury exerts its effects.

In the case of thallium, experimental work carried out using captive eagles suggested that the acute oral LD50 lies between 60 and 120 mg/kg/day. Clinical signs associated with ingestion included incoordination, loss of appetite, distress calls and brachypnoea (Bean & Hudson, 1976).

Selenium is well recognised as a cause of both lethal and sublethal poisoning in a wide range of vertebrates. It is often associated with loss of body mass ('wasting') as well as more subtle effects on immune response. Yamamoto and Santolo (2000) studied its effects on body condition in American kestrels.

Thirty years ago lead poisoning did not appear to be an important problem in raptors and it was assumed by most veterinarians and raptor biologists that this was because ingested lead shot (the usual source of toxicity in other birds) is regurgitated in the pellet or passed rapidly through the intestine. However, the possibility that this might not be so clear-cut followed the report by Locke *et al.* (1969), who reported the death of a captive Andean condor due to aspergillosis and lead poisoning. The bird had been fed on shot animals. There were clinical signs of unthriftiness, and lead poisoning was originally suspected on finding characteristic acid-fast intranuclear inclusions in kidney tubular cells. Subsequently Benson *et al.* (1974) reported fatal lead poisoning in a captive prairie falcon, which had been fed largely on duck heads containing lead shot. The bird showed clinical signs of visual disturbance and, occasionally, ataxia. Gross *post-mortem* findings included an accumulation of serosanguineous fluid in the pericardial sac and a green discoloration of the intestinal tract. They suggested that the long-term feeding of material containing lead shot might cause chronic or even acute poisoning.

Lead poisoning is now recognised as a significant cause of illness and death in captive birds of prey in both North America and Britain (Redig *et al.*, 1980b; Beynon *et al.*, 1996) and has been studied experimentally by a number of researchers including Meister (1981), Pattee *et al.* (1981) and Reiser and Temple (1981). It is increasingly being recognised as a cause of death in bald eagles and other species in the wild (Hoffman *et al.*, 1981). Saito *et al.* (2000) reported deaths in two species of eagle through ingestion of carcasses of deer and pointed out that raptors may select the area of the body where bullets entered, as this is easier to consume.

Lead poisoning is usually acquired by raptors as a result of ingesting birds or mammals that contain lead shot. Affected raptors are lethargic and anorectic and may show paralysis of the upper gastrointestinal tract, ataxia, diarrhoea and paralysis. Haematological examination may reveal anaemia and abnormalities of erythrocytes. Lead values (on blood of live birds, kidney of dead birds) are elevated. Particles of lead shot may be seen in the stomach on radiography: these can sometimes be removed using an endoscope or by gastric lavage, or be allowed to pass through the tract. Treatment of plumbism (lead poisoning) is with sodium calcium EDTA – see Appendix IX.

Shot carcasses should be used with great caution: Forbes and Rees Davies (2000) went so far as to say that 'shotgun-killed quarry should never be fed' and even cautioned against rifle-shot food, on the grounds that fragmented bullets might be present.

Zinc poisoning has been increasingly recognised in birds in recent years – particularly parrots but sometimes in captive birds of prey. The cause in the latter may be galvanised metal (used for a water bath or washed out from a fence) or zinc-containing paint or wood preservative. The clinical signs of zinc toxicity can be very varied – anorexia, lethargy, skin pruritus and lesions or neurological signs. A diagnosis is usually made on the basis of history and/or circumstantial evidence and blood tests.

It has long been assumed and generally agreed that lead shot embedded in the tissues of a bird is unlikely to be toxic to that individual. Surgery to remove such shot is not therefore usually advocated unless the particle is mechanically interfering with function. Sometimes the shot serves as useful identification on radiography.

Lead and steel shot can be readily distinguished using a magnet (Miller *et al.*, 2000).

Other poisons which may prove lethal to raptors and which should be borne in mind in diagnosis include strychnine (Redig & Arendt, 1982) and anti-coagulant rodenticides (Mendenhall & Pank, 1980; Townsend *et al.*, 1981); these may be acquired as a result of feeding on other species which have been accidentally or intentionally poisoned. Anticoagulant poisons are commonly associated with haemorrhage – seen usually *post mortem*. In the Middle East ammonium chloride (known in Arabic as 'schnather') is used by many falconers as a means of improving the hunting ability of trained hawks: Samour *et al.* (1995) pointed out that this practice can lead to death due to toxicity, and it was a major cause of mortality in sakers during a hunting trip in Pakistan (Naldo & Samour, 2001).

Carbon monoxide gas can prove hazardous to captive birds of prey. A bird kept temporarily in a garage may be poisoned if the ventilation is poor, and MacPhail (1964) described a probable case of carbon monoxide poisoning in a goshawk which was

'manned' (accustomed to humans and disturbance) by being carried on a perch in a car. The bird was lethargic and breathless and finally became unconscious and died. The cause of death was not confirmed *post mortem* but was almost certainly due to car fumes. Any clinical or *post-mortem* case in which the tissues appear exceptionally bright pink should be considered a possible carbon monoxide poisoning case.

Toxins from bacteria may cause disease or death in birds of prey. These are discussed in Chapter 6. A toxaemic state may also arise if a bird becomes constipated or suffers an impaction of the crop, intestine or cloaca: the affected bird is depressed and, in the case of intestinal or cloacal involvement, shows abdominal distension and discomfort.

There is a report of toxaemia in two young peregrines which was traced to 'toxic' (presumably rancid) halibut liver oil (Woodford & Glasier, 1955). Care should be taken to ensure that any fish oils used are fresh and uncontaminated.

Snakebite has rarely been reported in birds of prey although it is a cause of death in domestic birds, especially those that are free-ranging. It is not easy to diagnose, clinically or *post mortem*: three raptors examined by Heckel *et al.* (1994) showed haemorrhage and gangrenous necrosis that was attributed, partly on circumstantial evidence, to the bite of venomous snakes.

Tick toxicity is discussed elsewhere.

Examples of environmental pollution, although not strictly poisons, are anthracosis and silicosis. *Post-mortem* and histopathological examination of birds that have spent much of their lives in a city will often reveal black debris (anthracosis) – sometimes siliceous material (silicosis) – in the lungs and air sacs. This is normal and does not appear to be associated with disease.

Anthracosis was common in Arab falcons in the past but nowadays silicosis due to fine sand is the more likely cause of pigment in the lung. Talc particles are also sometimes seen – presumably these originate from surgical gloves.

Air pollution may or may not play a significant role in the health of birds of prey: few reliable data are available. However, concern over the effects of air pollution on humans – over one billion people are regularly exposed to levels exceeding WHO Guidelines (WHO, 2000a) – suggest that it needs to be looked at afresh in animals, including birds. It is possible, for example, that pollutants from burning wood, coal, dung and crop residues, could have an adverse effect – possibly in combination with other factors – on both free-living and captive raptors.

Vegetation fires can also prove toxic because of emissions (WHO, 2000b). The role of hyperthermia, which may be combined with exposure to toxic substances, is discussed in Chapter 5.

Fumes from household appliances can be toxic or irritant to captive birds. For example, plastic light fittings sometimes burn and may cause death or respiratory distress in small cage birds. More common in such birds is polytetrafluoroethylene (PTFE) poisoning as a result of exposure to fumes from overheated cooking utensils. I have not confirmed cases in raptors but have seen gross and histological changes in lungs that appear typical of the condition.

Although there are specific antidotes for a few poisons, some of which have been mentioned, usually it is necessary to apply general treatment. Rees Davies (2000b) provided a useful review of acute toxicities in birds and emphasised, in addition to combinations of therapy, the importance of a controlled environment, with the patient in the dark. Nursing is always of importance and a free respiratory passage must be maintained. If there is severe respiratory distress oxygen should be given. Nervous signs can be controlled with phenobarbitone, diazepam or midazolam. If the poison has been ingested the crop or stomach should be washed out with saline. A useful emetic is a strong salt solution while liquid paraffin (mineral oil) or glycerine can be used as a purgative (see Appendix IX). A general safe antidote recommended some years ago consists of a combination of activated charcoal, kaolin, light magnesium oxide and tannic acid (Cooper, 1971, 1975a) and although doubt has been expressed in both medical and veterinary circles over such 'universal antidotes', it is worth a try. It is of interest to note in this context that Redig and Ackermann (2000) recommended similar supportive care for birds of prey when a toxin is sus-

pected but the precise identity of the poison has not been ascertained. Activated charcoal by mouth will reduce absorption, diazepam will help to control seizures and fluids will give systemic circulatory support.

Case studies on two eagles, one with lead poisoning and the other with cholinesterase-inhibitor poisoning, were detailed by Shimmel and Snell (1999), and their paper provides practical guidance on how to deal with similar cases.

Care must be taken on radiography to distinguish shot in the gastro-intestinal tract from any lodged in the muscle. A useful way of detecting tiny particles of lead in stomach contents *post mortem* is to radiograph the latter in a Petri dish.

There are many other substances that may cause poisoning in birds of prey but on which little scientific information appears to be available. Examples are disinfectants, such as phenols, formaldehyde and many herbicidal and fungicidal compounds. It is important that instances of poisoning are recorded, even individual cases, since these may be relevant to conservation and management programmes – for instance, the report of ethylene glycol toxicosis in a released California condor (Murnane *et al.*, 1995). Poisoning, often carried out maliciously, continues to threaten introduction and reintroduction programmes: for instance, a recent report of mevinphos poisoning in red kites (Anon, 2000b), a species that has been the subject of a lengthy and expensive translocation and release programme in the UK.

Useful primary sources of reference on poisoning in birds are the chapter by Peckham in *Diseases of Poultry* (1972) and the section on poisons in Arnall and Keymer's *Bird Diseases* (1975): these and similar texts are always worth consulting initially if poisoning is suspected. Many chemicals have been incriminated in cases of poisoning in domestic and wild non-raptorial birds and the absence of any reports of them in captive birds of prey is no reason to believe that they do not, or will not, occur.

Acceptability and digestibility

If a diet is to achieve maximum results it must be acceptable to the bird and satisfactorily digested by it. The digestibility is related to both the diet itself and the species of bird and will not be discussed here; the reader is referred to standard publications on the subject, especially those dealing specifically with raptors such as the papers by Duke *et al.* (1973, 1975) alluded to earlier.

I assume here that the term 'acceptable' includes 'palatable'. Some items are totally unacceptable to birds; a bizarre example was the piece of sliced orange offered by airline staff to a black sparrow-hawk that I transported by air from Nairobi to London! Even carnivorous diets may, however, prove unacceptable for a variety of reasons. The raptor might not recognise it as food; for example, a newly captured buzzard may ignore a white mouse unless the latter is first opened to expose blood, muscles and viscera. A small bird, such as a merlin, may recognise that a dead hamster is edible but be unable to pierce the rodent's skin with its beak. Some species, which in the wild take only birds, may at first refuse to eat laboratory rodents but this atti-tude usually changes after a few days, particularly if efforts are made to introduce the new diet gradu-ally. Often it is an individual bird that shows marked distaste for a certain item and such fastidiousness must be borne in mind by the veterinary surgeon who hospitalises a sick bird and, perhaps, offers it a different diet. Birds in aviaries will also become accustomed to certain foods and take some time to accept something unusual. A sudden change from chicks to mice, or even the inclusion of black chicks as well as the usual yellow ones, may result in uneaten food being left at the end of the day. If birds are rearing youngsters the result can be hungry nestlings or even cannibalism.

Although live food is used for captive birds of prey in certain parts of the world its use is, in general, undesirable and in some countries may even lay one open to prosecution for example, in Britain under the Protection of Animals Acts (see Appendix XI).

The parts of a dead animal eaten also vary between species and individuals. Much depends on size. A buzzard will swallow a mouse whole while a kestrel tears portions off it and may discard the intestines and stomach. Many species of falcon avoid eating heads of chickens and internal organs of quail and rodents. Some raptors carefully pluck a bird before eating it, possibly in order to minimise intake of roughage. All these variables have to be consid-ered when investigating a disease problem that may be associated with nutrition.

Under the heading 'acceptability' I shall discuss the main diets available for feeding to the larger birds of prey. I shall not refer to the use of maggots, mealworms and other invertebrates, nor the provi-sion of lower vertebrates such as fish, amphibians and reptiles, other than to make the general point that *any* diet must be clean and from a reliable source. Food must be hygienically stored and pests of all types (vertebrate and invertebrate) denied access. When using rodents or chicks it is wise to deprive them of food for 2–3 hours prior to death; this will result in empty stomachs and the birds are less likely to leave the viscera uneaten.

There are three main groups of diet available for the feeding of captive birds of prey. These are (a) butcher's meat – with or without supplementation, (b) commercially prepared diets, (c) 'Natural' diets of either wild or laboratory-bred mammals or birds, commercially produced poultry or (for species such as the osprey or African fish eagle) fresh or frozen fish.

Butcher's meat

Butcher's meat *per se* cannot be recommended as a standard diet even though some birds appear to thrive on it. It must be supplemented – certainly with calcium and probably with other minerals.

Commercially prepared diets

In view of our lack of detailed knowledge of the nutrient requirements of raptors I am a little scepti-cal of commercial diets, certainly if used on their own, although I recognise that these are being used successfully in both Europe and North America (Redig & Ackermann 2000).

'Natural' diets

Wild birds and mammals are a convenient source of food – they can be shot, trapped or picked off the road – but are an unknown entity and may harbour pathogens or poisons. They might even have been killed by a vehicle because they were already debilitated by infectious or non-infectious disease. If they are to be used, they should be cut open and any showing pathological lesions, such as white foci in the liver, discarded.

Whenever possible I recommend a 'natural' diet of laboratory-bred rodents which can either be obtained from a medical or veterinary institution or be bred specifically for the purpose. Studies on mice by Crissey *et al.* (1999) showed that high lipid values in some mice might be disadvantageous but in general terms captive-bred rodents represent a satisfactory diet for most carnivorous species. Mice and rats, like any other species, can be a source of infection to both birds and humans and one must ensure that any used are from a clean source. They should not be purchased from a petshop or private individual but from a recognised laboratory. There is merit in carrying out health checks on *all* species that are used as food for raptors (Blundell, 1990).

Commercially produced poultry, especially day-old (usually cockerel) chicks, were discussed in some detail earlier in this chapter. They are certainly very convenient in terms of storage and allocation of individual rations. However, I have many misgivings about them, primarily because with food of avian origin there is always an added danger of infection with pathogens that might affect other birds: Kirkwood *et al.* (1994) stressed this when they investigated the source of *Salmonella enteritidis* that was cultured from owls (all asymptomatic) that had been fed on day-old chicks.

There may also be some doubt about the nutritive value of chicks, especially in view of the variation between strains and, probably, batches. Their use may contribute to hepatic lipidosis (Plate 22). However, many establishments have used day-old chicks successfully, sometimes with a vitamin/mineral supplement, and reported excellent captive breeding results. Doubts over their nutritive value could be reduced if they were reared for a few weeks before being killed but this is both time-consuming and expensive. There are also, it appears, differences relating to the species of raptor being kept: common kestrels seem to thrive on day-old chicks alone whereas merlins do not. As a general rule, a total diet of day-old chicks is probably not advisable.

Quail (*Coturnix coturnix*) too can be a source of infection – as was postulated in e-mail communications when the Peregrine Fund World Center (Idaho, USA) lost Aplomado falcons to a herpes virus in 1996 – but this may be less likely if they come from a clean source and have been bred under laboratory conditions.

Pigeons are known to be a potential source of many raptor pathogens – *Trichomonas* and herpesvirus being the most significant – and I do not recommend them. If they *must* be fed, they should first be frozen and the viscera should at least be inspected, preferably discarded.

The nutrient value of five species – quail, chickens, rats, mice and guinea pigs – were studied by Clum *et al.* (1997) who showed that there was little significant difference other than in lipid and vitamins A and E: the choice may, therefore, depend more on safety than on composition.

Fish are a useful and very acceptable item for piscivorous species. They need to be supplemented with thiamine, as already discussed. They too can harbour organisms that may be pathogenic to raptors. Blundell (1990) carried out health monitoring of lizards intended as food for captive Mauritius kestrels and as a result advised that these reptiles should not be used at Jersey Zoo.

The foregoing points apply primarily to the feeding of captive birds: in theory humans have little say in how free-living raptors obtain their food. In fact, there is some overlap, especially when either (a) captive birds are being 'hacked' back to the wild, or (b) free-living birds are being provided with supplementary feeding – the so-called 'vulture restaurants' established in the European Alps being an example, or depend upon livestock carcass disposal sites for food (Larraz, 1999). In such cases many of the precautions above are important, especially since pathogens (including prions) and poisons may be introduced.

The digestibility of diets cannot be discussed in detail here. It relates to a wide range of factors including the anatomy and physiology of different species (see the work of Barton and Houston (1996) on organ weights of raptors) and the type and consistency of the food. Research in this field is yielding some interesting results: for example, Akaki and

Duke (1998) investigated ingested chitin and suggested that the lower GI tract contributes to total chitin digestion in American kestrels.

Purchase

It is important that food is readily obtainable, even if the weather is bad or transport is not available. Cost is also a factor but should not compromise quality or quantity.

Conclusions

The answer to the feeding of captive birds of prey is variety. This should help to eliminate the possibility of dietary deficiencies and may reduce the danger of poisoning from a single source. It will also facilitate a change of diet, if one item becomes unavailable. Much, however, depends upon the size and financial status of one's enterprise, the birds being maintained, and the sources of food available. It is important that records are kept of the food items that are used and the results obtained. Increasingly, zoos maintain written/computerised descriptions of feeding regimes and make these available to other interested parties. They have proved particularly useful when dealing with new, sometimes rare, species and have brought consistency and quality assurance to the whole question of what to feed to captive birds of prey: a good example is the diet used for the first Mauritius kestrels to be maintained outside the island of Mauritius, catalogued by Courts (1995).

Poisoning in Wild (Free-living) Raptors

CONTRIBUTED BY THE LATE D. B. PEAKALL

INTRODUCTION

In this chapter the programmes that have been set up to record kills of raptors (and other species) are considered first. Then the main classes of chemicals involved – the organochlorines, acetylcholinesterase inhibitors (organophosphorus and carbamate pesticides), rodenticides and heavy metals – are considered in turn. This is followed by discussion of the vulnerability of specific species and the possible impact on populations.

WILDLIFE INCIDENT PROGRAMMES

Most of the poisoning of raptors is caused by pesticides. A number of countries have national schemes to report incidents where poisoning is suspected. In the UK the Wildlife Incident Investigation Scheme is run by the UK's Ministry of Agriculture, Fisheries and Food (now DEFRA). In the USA the Biological Resources Division at the National Wildlife Health Center at Patuxent is the main agency and in Canada the Canadian Wildlife Service and Canadian Co-operative Health Centers.

In the UK incidents shown to involve pesticides are divided into four categories:

(1)   Approved use. Incidents occurring when the product was used according to the specified regulations.
(2)   Misuse. Careless, accidental, or wilful failure to adhere to the correct procedures for the use of the product.
(3)   Abuse. When pesticides were used for the deliberate, illegal poisoning of wildlife.
(4)   Unspecified use. Those cases where the incident could not be assigned to any of the above.

In the UK during the period 1993 to 1997 the percentages of all poisoning incidents of vertebrates for the above categories have ranged as follows: approved use 1–7%, misuse 10–12%, abuse 55–74% and unspecified 12–22%. Mineau *et al.* (1999), reviewing the literature, found that the ratio of approved use to abuse cases was similar in the UK, France and The Netherlands, but in North America many more incidents following approved usage occurred, with a ratio of approximately 1:1 in the USA, and in Canada approved usage outnumbered abuse cases by 2:1.

The fraction of cases that are reported is unknown and probably highly variable. Fletcher (personal communication) has suggested for red kites that, based on calculations on the numbers of birds released and fledged and known survival rates, that one in four birds that die are ever found. One would suspect that the proportion found is higher in the UK with its large numbers of naturalists and high population density than in the wide open spaces of Canada. Then, particularly in the case of misuse or abuse, there is considerable likelihood that the incident will be covered up.

CHEMICALS OF CONCERN

Organochlorines

In the developed world the use of this class of compounds has been greatly restricted, starting in the early 1970s. The change that this has made has been clearly demonstrated by the titles of two major symposia on the peregrine falcon in 1965 (Hickey, 1969) and 1985 (Cade *et al.*, 1988). The first was entitled *Peregrine Falcon Populations: Their Biology and Decline* and the second *Peregrine Falcon Populations: Their Management and Recovery*. In the United States the species which was extirpated in the eastern part of the country has now been removed from the endangered species list. In the UK the population was reduced to 40% of pre-war numbers by the mid 1960s but by 1991 the population was larger than the population in the 1930s (Ratcliffe, 1993). A new survey of the population of the peregrine in the UK is to be carried out by the British Trust for Ornithology (BTO) in 2001.

Another species that has been studied in detail is the European sparrow-hawk. The decline and recovery of this species in the UK have been detailed by Newton (1986). The effect of the cyclodiene insecticides on this species has been recently reappraised (Walker & Newton, 1999). In the period 1963–1975 the distribution of the dieldrin residue levels in the livers of sparrow-hawks was biphasic with peaks at 20 and 1 ppm (wet weight). In 1976–1982 the pattern was still biphasic with peaks at 0.75 ppm and 4.8 ppm, the latter peak being considered to represent birds dying from chronic neurotoxic effects. In recent years (1983–1986) there is only a single peak at 0.75 ppm. The impact of the effect of these residues on the population dynamics of the species was considered by Sibly *et al.* (2000). A number of scenarios are proposed.

Newton *et al.* (1993) calculated the levels in the livers of sparrow-hawks and European kestrel of dieldrin, dichlorodiphenyldichloroethane (DDE), polychlorinated biphenyls (PCBs) and mercury for five time periods. These are given in Table 11.1.

There has been a marked decrease of the levels of both dieldrin and DDE especially in the last two time periods; however, PCBs show no definite trend in either species.

Liver levels of more than 10 ppm dieldrin or 100 ppm DDE have been considered to be associated with lethality (Cooke *et al.*, 1982) but the latter figure has been criticised as too low by Blus (1996). The values used by UK Wildlife Incident Investigation Scheme are 10 ppm dieldrin and 150 ppm DDE.

The causes of death of bald eagles found dead in the United States were determined from 1964 to 1983. The percentage of eagles dying from dieldrin poisoning decreased markedly over this period from over 10% for the period 1966–1972 to 1.7% by 1978–1983 (reviewed in Peakall, 1996).

That poisoning by organochlorine pesticides is not a thing of the past, even in the developed world, is shown by the poisoning of 425 birds in New Jersey over the period 1996–1997 (Stansley & Roscoe, 1999). Most of the birds affected were passerines but four species of raptor were involved, including nine Cooper's hawks. The brain levels of heptachlor epoxide were in the range 2.5–5 ppm, oxychlordane 1.5–5.5 ppm and trans-nonachlor 1.4–4.6 ppm. All birds were considered to have died from chlordane poisoning; there was no sign of acetylcholine esterase (AChE) depression.

Serious, but non-lethal, effects have been found at much lower levels. Indeed, from a population viewpoint, decreased reproduction can be more serious than outright mortality. Newton (1986), examining the large database for sparrow-hawks, concluded that levels in the liver above 1 ppm were associated with population declines. Levels of DDE (dichlorodiphenyldichloroethane) in eggs associated with population declines in the peregrine have been estimated at 15–20 ppm (Peakall & Kiff, 1988)

For the developing world there are many fewer data. Mendelsohn *et al.* (1988), reviewing the limited data for southern Africa, found that 83% of the eggs analysed had DDE levels greater than 5 ppm, a level that has been associated with lowered productivity (Newton, 1979). Seven of the 27 sam-

Table 11.1 Residue levels (in ppm, wet weight for the organochlorines, dry weight for mercury) in the livers of kestrels and sparrow-hawks in the UK over five time periods. Figures are geometric mean (sample size) and range.

Species	Period	Dieldrin	DDE	PCB	Mercury
Sparrow-hawk	1963–1970	0.57 (104)	4.84 (104)	1.99 (60)	4.60 (3)
		0.09–3.72	0.90–26.08	0.23–17.48	2.55–8.28
	1971–1975	0.63 (107)	4.11 (107)	2.07 (107)	5.64 (67)
		0.08–5.18	0.60–27.92	0.22–19.97	3.28–9.72
	1976–1980	0.51 (198)	5.08 (204)	2.75 (204)	3.52 (123)
		0.12–2.28	0.97–26.66	0.50–15.19	1.50–8.29
	1981–1985	0.44 (288)	2.85 (296)	1.80 (296)	2.26 (294)
		0.10–1.96	0.54–14.92	0.23–14.09	0.65–7.87
	1986–1990	0.28 (290)	1.77 (290)	2.72 (290)	0.98 (290)
		0.05–1.44	0.31–10.25	0.37–19.96	0.15–6.28
Kestrel	1963–1970	0.97 (249)	1.77 (249)	1.27 (108)	5.77 (11)
		0.20–4.61	0.30–10.46	0.17–9.62	2.98–11.17
	1971–1975	1.44 (195)	1.66 (194)	0.98 (194)	3.90 (168)
		0.20–10.41	0.25–11.00	0.09–10.77	1.77–8.62
	1976–1980	0.58 (168)	1.59 (175)	1.17 (175)	1.27 (115)
		0.15–2.26	0.18–14.09	0.15–9.33	0.43–3.74
	1981–1985	0.46 (266)	0.67 (282)	1.04 (282)	0.77 (276)
		0.15–1.42	0.07–6.75	0.17–6.31	0.19–3.11
	1986–1990	0.25 (174)	0.37 (174)	1.93 (174)	0.22 (174)
		0.05–1.24	0.04–3.08	0.32–11.47	0.02–2.21

DDE = dichlorodiphenyldichloroethane; PCB = polychlorinated biphenyl.

ples analysed for dieldrin had levels above 1 ppm. The authors concluded that 'organochlorine residues in southern Africa are high enough to have a significant impact on the dynamics of some raptor populations'. Douthwaite (1992) examined the effect of DDT (dichlorodiphenyltrichloroethane) on the fish eagle population of Lake Kariba in Zimbabwe. Eggshell thinning of greater than 20%, high enough to have an effect on reproduction, was found in one part of the lake. However, Douthwaite concluded 'DDT contamination is reducing hatching success on Lake Kariba but does not appear to be limiting population size'. In South Africa significant eggshell thinning was recorded for this species (Davies & Randall, 1989). In the period 1971–1980 the decrease averaged 12% but had recovered to only 8% thinning by 1981–1986. The degree of thinning recorded was not large enough to produce population effects although some loss of eggs would

be expected. In India reproductive problems have been found for the grey-headed fishing eagle in the Corbett National Park (Naoroji, 1997). Organochlorines were considered to be the cause but no details are given in the note.

Organophosphorus (OP) and carbamate pesticides

During the period 1985–1995 the minimum number of raptors killed by pesticides in the UK was 136, based on the records of the Central Science Laboratory cited in Mineau *et al.* (1999). By far the commonest species affected was the common buzzard with 71 records, but the most serious from a population point of view were the deaths of 29 red kites. The population of this species in the UK in 1995 was only 144 pairs (Ogilvie, 1998). In North America the commonest species poisoned was the bald eagle with 243 out of 736 in the USA and 64 out of 126 in Canada. In the USA the next highest figures were for the golden eagle (144 birds) and red-tailed hawk (133) whereas in Canada, where the reporting period was only 1990–1995, they were the hen harrier (30) and the red-tailed hawk (24). The USA data come from the US Fish and Wildlife Service, the Environmental Protection Agency and the Biological Resources Division of the US Geological Survey, and the Canadian data from the Canadian Wildlife Service and Canadian Co-operative Wildlife Health Centers. Again, these data were compiled by Mineau *et al.* (1999). By far the commonest pesticide involved in the deaths of raptors in the USA was carbofuran (406 out of 734); in Canada the pesticides causing the most problems were phorate (34 out of 122) and carbofuran (28 cases). In the UK the leading pesticides were mevinphos (56 out of 136) followed by fenthion (36), and carbofuran was in third place with 20 cases.

The hazards to raptors from pest control programmes in Sahelian Africa have been recently reviewed by Keith and Bruggers (1998). They concluded that the use of pesticides (malathion, fenitrothion and chlorpyrifos) to control locusts, grasshoppers, birds and rodents in the Sahel have caused only minimal raptor losses. In contrast, the use of fenthion to control red-billed quelea (*Quelea quelea*) has led to considerable mortality of raptors. Many dead or dying hawks and owls were reported after a spray operation in Kenya in 1984 (Thomsett, 1987, cited in Bruggers *et al.* 1989). Detailed studies were made by Bruggers *et al.* (1989) following spraying of quelea colonies with the organophosphate, fenthion. These workers trapped a number of raptors and fitted them with radio transmitters. Of the 24 raptors only two were found moribund despite the fact that large numbers of quelea were killed and that the area in which quelea were found dead or dying was 35 km². However, 16 of 23 raptors examined had depressed levels of blood AChE. In a programme to control red-winged blackbirds (*Agelaius phoeniceus*), using parathion, in the United States, 14 Mississippi kites were killed, a considerable mortality for a scarce species (Franson, 1994).

Massive kills of Swainson's hawk have been reported from the pampas of Argentina following the use of monocrotophos (MCP) to control grasshoppers (Goldstein *et al.*, 1999a). Nineteen incidents were investigated during the austral summer of 1995–1996: a total of 5095 dead hawks was reported. Forensic analysis at six sites which accounted for over 4000 of the mortalities showed that brain AChE was lethally inhibited (>95%) and MCP residues were found in the contents of the gastro-intestinal tract. No other residues were detected.

Subsequently meetings were held between Argentine, USA and Canadian government agencies (Swainson's hawk breeds in the latter two countries), non-governmental agencies and representatives of the agrochemical industry. An exclusion zone covering the main wintering areas was set up and the use of MCP was banned from this area. Less toxic chemicals – dimethoate, chlorpyrifos and cypermethrin – were recommended. This exclusion zone was monitored in 1996–1997 and no mortality incidents were recorded (Goldstein *et al.*, 1999b). It would be valuable to examine whether problems with MCP are occurring in other countries.

Rodenticides

Mass mortality of raptors was reported in Switzerland when bromadiolone was used to control ground voles, with the deaths of 185 common buzzards and 25 red kites (Beguin, 1983). On a Malayan oil palm plantation the heavy use of brodifacoum extirpated the population of barn owls that fed almost exclusively on rats (Duckett, 1984, cited in Newton and Wyllie, 1992). In North America radio-tagged screech owls were used in a study to evaluate the effects of brodifacoum used to control voles in orchards (Hegdal & Colvin, 1988). The mortality recorded was 58% when 20% of the home range was treated and 17% when 10% was treated. At least half of the deaths were caused by the rodenticide. A long-running survey into the causes of mortality of barn owls has been carried out in the UK. During the period 1963–1996 more than 1100 carcasses of barn owls were received by the Institute of Terrestrial Ecology (ITE) (Newton *et al.*, 1997).

Of these, 53.7% were diagnosed as road traffic deaths, 25.8% as starved and only 6.1% as poisoned. The pattern of poisoning has altered over the period, with aldrin–dieldrin predominating in the 1960s and 1970s. These compounds remained in common use until 1976; complete banning of organochlorines did not take place in the UK until 1986. The proportion of barn owls containing rodenticide residues has risen markedly from 1% in 1983–84 to 32% in 1993–94. However, only eight birds were diagnosed as having died of rodenticide poisoning. Although the percentage dying from rodenticides is small, the authors caution against complacency as the proportion exposed is increasing and the sampling is likely to be biased against rodenticide victims, and the levels of rodenticide needed to affect free-living birds may be lower than the levels determined from experimental studies.

The possibility that programmes to control rats in seabird colonies cause poisoning of scavenging birds has been examined by Howald *et al.* (1999). They made studies on an island in the Queen Charlotte archipelago in British Columbia by putting out radio-tagged rats during the baiting programme. Ravens were found poisoned; bald eagles were trapped and their blood sampled for brodifacoum. Some 15% of the sampled population of eagles showed detectable residues but no adversely affected birds were found.

Heavy metals

Lead

Although the largest – but now declining – source of lead in the environment is leaded petrol, it is ingestion of lead shot which appears to be by far the most serious source of lead poisoning in raptors. The poisoning of waterfowl by lead shot has been known for over a century (Grinell, 1894) but action has only been taken during the last decade with a total ban in the USA from the 1991–92 hunting season onwards and restrictions have been made in a few other countries. Raptors that scavenge on crippled or unretrieved birds can suffer from lead poisoning (see also Chapter 10).

Franson (1996) summarised the tissue levels of lead associated with effects in the Falconiformes. For blood he considered that 0.2–1.5 ppm (wet weight) is associated with sub-clinical effects, >1 ppm with toxic effects and >5 ppm with mortality. For liver the levels are 2–4, >3 and >5 ppm, respectively, and for the kidney 2–5, >3 and >5 ppm.

In the United States mortality of seven species of raptors was reported (Locke & Friend, 1992), including approximately 200 cases of lead poisoning of the bald eagle. The widespread mortality of the national bird was one of the reasons for the ban on the use of lead shot in wildfowl hunting that was introduced nation-wide in 1991.

In France 222 liver samples of 17 species of raptors sent to Centres de Sauvegarde de la Faune Sauvage between 1989 and 1991 were analysed for lead (Pain & Amiard-Triquet, 1993). These workers considered that levels of lead (Pb) over 5 ppm (dry weight) to be elevated and those over 20 ppm to indicate probable mortality from lead poisoning. Elevated lead levels were found in five common buzzards, two sparrow-hawks and one goshawk. One sparrow-hawk and the goshawk had levels above 20 ppm although three of the buzzards were only just below this figure. In a study on marsh harriers in southern France (Pain *et al.*, 1993) it was found that of the 94 birds captured (baited clap traps or in mist nets at night roosts), 29 had elevated levels of Pb in their blood (>30 µg/dl) and 13 had concentrations indicative of clinical poisoning (>60 µg/dl). Lead shot pellets were found in regurgitated pellets, demonstrating that eating crippled or unretrieved waterfowl was a source of lead.

In the UK a study of the levels of lead in the livers of 424 individuals sent for analysis at the Institute of Terrestrial Ecology over the period from the early 1980s to the early 1990s showed lead levels high enough to cause mortality in only two cases – a peregrine and a common buzzard (Pain *et al.*, 1995).

A detailed risk assessment of lead shot exposed to avian species other than waterbirds was recently published (Kendall *et al.*, 1996). The most detailed assessment was made for the mourning dove but the data on raptors were also considered. The panel concluded that this risk assessment did 'not clearly define a significant risk of lead shot exposure to upland game birds, but this issue merits continued scrutiny to protect our upland game birds and raptor resources'. The progress that has been made towards banning lead shot was reviewed by Scheuhammer and Norris (1996).

Mercury

Although mercury compounds were earlier used as fungicides to protect seed, the main interest in mercury contamination of wildlife has been in the aquatic environment. The paper and pulp industry at one time used considerable quantities of mercury as fungicides, and increased mercury levels have been found due to acidification and flooding of areas associated with hydroelectric projects. Thus, among birds, the attention has focused on fish-eating species such as the osprey, white-tailed sea eagle and bald eagle. An exception to this was the study by Newton and Haas (1988) on the merlin. These workers found an inverse relationship between mercury level and brood size although they noted that some clutches with high levels managed to produce three or four young. One strange finding was that in the islands of Orkney and Shetland where the levels of mercury were high, there was no relationship between mercury level and brood-size. It is possible that on mainland Britain the proportion of organomercury was higher but since only total mercury was measured, it is impossible to test this hypothesis. In a subsequent study on the merlin (Newton *et al.*, 1999a) it was found that, although the levels of mercury in eggs decreased from 1978 to 1985, the levels subsequently increased in the late 1980s although there was some decrease again in the 1990s.

The mercury levels of ospreys have been studied in both North America and Europe. In the Great Lakes all of the samples collected over the period 1971 to 1992 were well below the threshold value of 0.5 ppm (Environment Canada Fact Sheet, undated).

Nygård and Skaare (1998) found that mercury levels in the eggs of white-tailed sea eagles collected in Norway between 1974 and 1994 were well below critical levels. Bowerman *et al.* (1994) reported no significant relationships between adult or nestling feather concentrations and any parameters of nesting success of bald eagles in the Great Lakes

region. The means of levels in feathers for various regions along the shores of the Great Lakes were 13–21 mg/kg whilst inland areas had lower values. The maximum figure recorded was 66 mg/kg. These workers concluded that mercury was not affecting bald eagle reproduction in the region. On the Pacific coast of Canada Elliott *et al.* (1996) found that, although the levels of mercury in eggs of birds near pulp mills were higher than reference sites, the levels were below critical levels.

Heinz (1996) gave 20–60 ppm (wet weight) in the liver as the level causing mortality in birds. As with the organochlorines, adverse effects are found at lower levels. In their review of the literature, Zillioux *et al.* (1993) came up with a threshold for major adverse effects in waterbirds of 5 ppm (wet weight) in the liver and between 1 and 3.5 ppm in eggs. Thus, the liver levels reported in Table 11.1 are well below the threshold level as they are given in dry weight and thus need to be divided by 5 to express the values on a wet weight basis.

VARIATION IN SPECIES SENSITIVITY

With the organochlorines the most vulnerable species were the bird-eaters, such as the peregrine and sparrow-hawk, and fish-eaters, such as the osprey, due to accumulation of residues up the food chain. Species such as the buzzard, which feeds on small mammals, and carrion or the hobby, whose diet includes a substantial amount of invertebrates were less affected (Newton, 1979).

With organophosphorus compounds and lead it is scavengers that are at the greatest risk. With OPs in North America three species (bald eagle, golden eagle and red-tailed hawk) accounted for 70% of all kills recorded. In the UK the buzzard represented over half of the cases. The massive kills of Swainson's hawk (closely related to the red-tailed hawk and buzzard) are considered in the next section. Lead poisoning is most prevalent among species that scavenge on dead or injured waterfowl. Thus, species such as the marsh harrier in Europe and the bald eagle in North America are at greatest risk. A recent preliminary report that two of the four

Steller's sea eagles (Kim *et al.*, 1999) found dead in Japan died from lead poisoning is disturbing in view of the rarity of this species.

With rodenticides it is those species that prey on or scavenge rats that are at risk. Detailed studies on one candidate species – the barn owl – in the UK does not indicate a serious problem. The possibility that the red kite is seriously affected is considered in the next section.

EFFECTS AT THE POPULATION LEVEL

Ecotoxicologists are mainly interested in effects at the population level. That chemicals can affect populations of raptors was all too clearly demonstrated by the crash of the peregrine population throughout much of the Holarctic (see Chapter 1). As Cade (1968) put it, 'down through the centuries, not all the falcon trappers, egg collectors, war ministries concerned for their messenger pigeons or misguided gunmen have been able to effect a significant reduction in the numbers of breeding falcons. But the simple laboratory trick of adding a few chlorine molecules to a hydrocarbon and the massive application of this unnatural class of chemical to the environment can do what none of these other grosser, seemingly more harmful agents could do.' The main mechanism of the decline is considered to be due to DDE-induced eggshell thinning. The history of the investigation into the chemical causes of the decline was reviewed by Peakall (1993).

Eggshell thinning may still be causing an influence on the population of burrowing owls in California (Gervais *et al.*, 2000). Eggshell thinning was found to be negatively correlated with DDE residue levels and, on average, the eggshells were 22% thinner in 1996 compared with those from the pre-DDT era. Decreases of eggshell thickness of 18–20% have been associated with population decreases (Hickey & Anderson, 1968; Peakall & Kiff, 1988).

Two cases in which poisoning may have effects at the population level at the present time are the red kite in the UK and Swainson's hawk in the Americas. The effect of lead on the Californian

Condor in the 1980s was considered to have a serious impact.

Over the period 1971–1993, 44 red kites were confirmed as having been poisoned in the UK (Evans *et al.*, 1997). A number of different chemicals was involved although the organophosphorus and carbamate ones are the most important (Mineau *et al.*, 1999). Recently there have been concerns about rodenticides and red kites (Mark Fletcher, personal communication). The kite is a generalist scavenger and its diet dominated by carrion sets it apart from all other British birds of prey. Rats form an important part of the diet throughout the year in England (in contrast to the populations in Wales and Scotland) and kites are found feeding close to human habitation. There were two confirmed and one suspected case of rodenticide poisoning in England in 1998. While these numbers are small, calculations suggest that only one in four birds that die are ever found. In one case – a juvenile poisoned in the Midlands – it was one of seven found dead within a 2-week period, but other carcasses were too decomposed for analysis (Mark Fletcher, personal communication).

The re-introduction programme into England and Scotland has been going well. In England, the number of breeding pairs has increased from two in 1991 to 37 in 1996 and in Scotland from one in 1992 to 16 in 1996 (Evans *et al.*, 1997). However, any calculation of the dynamics of the population must take into account that 186 kites from Sweden and Spain have been released.

Serious concerns have been raised about the impact of large-scale kills of Swainson's hawks in Argentina. Goldstein *et al.* (1996b), studying this problem, considered that it was 'likely that pesticide-related mortality may well exceed 5% of the world's population' and concluded that 'continued large-scale mortality from OP pesticide applications in Argentina wintering areas may threaten the future status of this species'.

Lead poisoning of Californian condors was a major factor in the decision to take the remaining wild birds into captivity in 1987. Between 1980 and 1986 36% of the remaining wild condors had elevated blood levels and three of the five necropsied were considered to have died from lead poisoning

(Wiemeyer *et al.*, 1988). Re-introduction started in 1992 (Snyder & Snyder, 2000) – by which time a ban on lead shot for waterfowl hunting was in place, but even in 1999–2000 there continued to be major morbidity and mortality from lead (P. T. Redig, pers. comm.). This illustrates the difficulty in preventing poisoning incidents unless the provenance and means of dissemination of the toxic substance are known. Kramer and Redig (1997) discussed this in detail in a paper that assessed differences in the prevalence of lead poisoning in bald and golden eagles over a sixteen-year period. They suggested that existing theories regarding the source of lead for eagles should be reviewed and advocated study on the mechanisms by which such poisoning occurs. Similar reappraisal is needed in other parts of the world for various species of raptor.

CONCLUSIONS

In general, the situation as regards the poisoning of birds of prey has improved over the last few decades. Most populations of raptors are now stable or increasing. In the UK the greatest threat to avian populations is the impact of intensive agriculture on farmland birds (Peakall & Carter, 1997).

ACKNOWLEDGEMENTS

The author is grateful to Mark Fletcher for supplying unpublished information on the red kite and to Richard Sibly for data on sparrow-hawk populations. Charles Henny and Jim Keith supplied valuable references.

Anaesthesia and Surgery

'*Dr Snow gave that blessed Chloroform and the effect was soothing, quieting and delightful beyond measure.*'

Queen Victoria (describing her labour)

ANAESTHESIA

The term 'anaesthesia' is used in this chapter in a broad sense, to cover various forms of chemical immobilisation as well as true general anaesthesia and analgesia.

Competent handling or restraint can sometimes replace the need for anaesthesia. Some such techniques are discussed and depicted in Chapter 4. However, painful procedures should not be inflicted upon a raptor without adequate anaesthesia or analgesia.

Enormous advances have been made in the anaesthesia of birds, including raptors, over the past 20 years and it is now difficult to believe that, even in the early 1960s, general anaesthesia was thought by many falconers to be synonymous with a death sentence for their bird. The turning point was in the late 1960s and early 1970s when new anaesthetic agents appeared for use in mammals and many of these proved to have a place in avian work. Lawton (1996) referred to Paddleford when he wrote: 'Raptors have previously been considered difficult patients to anaesthetise and poor anaesthetic risks', but in fact anaesthesia of these birds was already being carried out successfully and relatively safely even before the advent of 'newer, safer anaesthetics', such as isoflurane.

A whole range of agents, both inhalation and injectable, is now available for use in birds of prey and although a few – notably isoflurane – are often considered to be ideal or the 'gold standard', it remains important for the clinician to be aware of the others, which may need to be used in field work or in poorer countries where the preferred agents are unavailable. Therefore, as well as for historical reasons, some knowledge of the evolution of avian anaesthesia is desirable.

Early research was carried out on the physiological effect of anaesthetic agents in raptors by Bonath (1972a,b), who used buzzards, amongst other birds, in his research on the effect of inhalation anaesthetics on various parameters. Since then there have been studies on many aspects, some of which will be mentioned later.

The veterinary surgeon who deals with birds should be aware of the particular features of this class of animals. Many species have a high metabolic rate; as such they usually absorb, metabolise and excrete drugs rapidly. They can be particularly sensitive to anaesthetic agents. Inhalation anaesthesia can be complicated by the presence of air sacs which permit gaseous exchange during both inspiration and expiration (Fig. 3.13). Assessment of depth of anaesthesia may prove difficult because the abolition of reflexes does not always follow a set pattern.

Local analgesia

Local analgesia can also pose problems in birds. Evidence of sensitivity to the effects of the procaine group was published four decades ago (Friedburg, 1962) but it was subsequently suggested that the LD50 of procaine in birds is comparable to that in mammals and that the reason for toxicity in the past was overdosing. The safe use of small volumes of 2% lignocaine in larger birds, including raptors, helps to substantiate this view but it is obvious that more work is needed. I have not personally encountered toxicity to local analgesics in birds of prey. However, I have seen and treated hawks which have reacted adversely to procaine penicillin. These birds (which were not injected by myself!) developed almost immediate clinical signs of incoordination, ataxia and muscle rigidity, including a degree of opisthotonos. In each case a small dose of corticosteroid was administered and there was recovery within 15 minutes.

I am therefore generally wary of the procaine group in birds of prey. I would suggest that caution continues to be exercised in the use of local analgesics; one approach that appears safe is to use them diluted 1:5 in saline. Other colleagues remain unconvinced: Rees Davies (2000b) reported 'birds with non-specific systemic signs even after application of wound powder containing benzocaine'.

Local analgesics have long been used for ocular work; for example, Martin *et al.* (1975) used 4% benoxinate hydrochloride to anaesthetise the cornea of tawny owls.

Sedation

Few sedative or ataractic (tranquilliser) drugs are of great practical value in birds of prey, although diazepam and midazolam are useful. Low doses of some of the parenteral anaesthetics will produce a hypnotic state and it is to this that I refer when I use the term 'sedation' in this book. However, such sedation is usually of limited use as the bird is generally unsteady on its feet and can be roused.

Until very recently there was no proven systemic analgesic for the relief of pain in raptors. In my early studies small quantities of sodium salicylate appeared harmless when given orally and may have reduced pain or discomfort but was never properly evaluated. More recently it was listed by Dorrestein (2000) as a possible analgesic agent for birds *per os*. Now new agents are available that are proving efficacious as analgesics in certain birds (Clyde & Paul-Murphy, 2000; Paul-Murphy & Ludders, 2001): examples are given in Appendix IX. However, caution should be exercised in extrapolating from work on one group of birds (psittacines) and assuming that the findings are applicable to raptors. Buprenorphine, which has played such a large part in analgesia of small mammals, does not appear to be effective in birds of prey, although Lawton (1996) listed it, together with carprofen (see Appendix IX). Valuable work has been carried out on the domestic fowl that demonstrated the value of carprofen in lameness (McGeown *et al.*, 1999) and similar controlled studies would be helpful in raptors. Gentle (1992) reviewed the question of pain in birds and that paper provides useful background to the subject.

Systemic analgesia

Analgesia for raptors can be provided directly by the use of systemic analgesic agents (Appendix IX) and by administering nitrous oxide with inhalation anaesthetic agents as well as by the careful use of local analgesics, such as diluted lignocaine, which has already been covered. Interestingly, with the advent of isoflurane, a remarkably safe and easily administered agent that has a better muscle relaxant effect than halothane, many veterinarians seem to have forgotten the value of nitrous oxide. As an adjunct to other agents, nitrous oxide provides analgesia, enhances muscle relaxation and (important from the point of view of both cost and safety) reduces the amount of inhalation anaesthetic agent that needs to be used. It remains a key component of avian anaesthesia in countries and situations where halothane has still to be used – and in my view should be reinstated elsewhere!

Prevention or control of pain is important on welfare (and often legal) grounds but also because

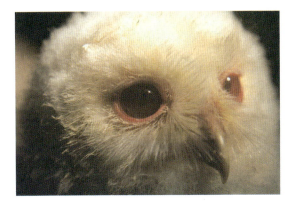

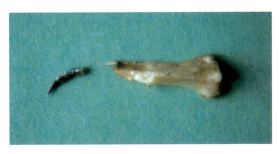

Plate 1 An albino Eurasian tawny owl – details of head and eyes. (Courtesy of Paolo Zucca.)

Plate 2 Alula of peregrine, showing claw. (Courtesy of Paolo Zucca.)

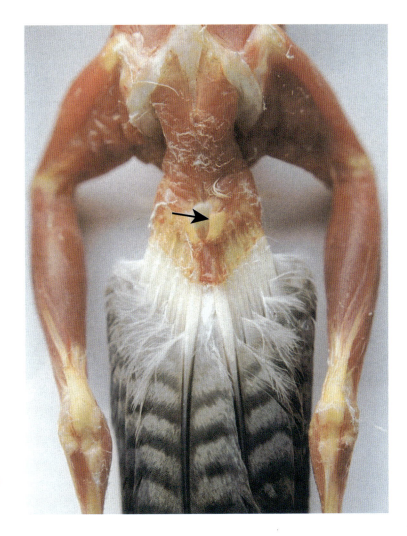

Plate 3 *(Right.)* Peregrine – anatomical preparation, showing tail with uropygial gland (arrow). (Courtesy of Paolo Zucca.)

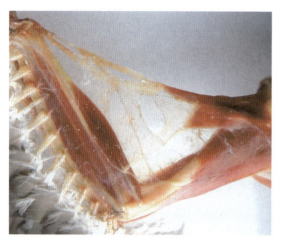

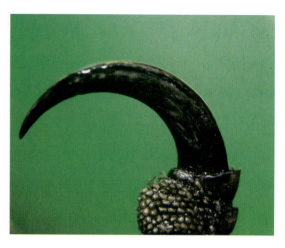

Plate 4 Peregrine – anatomical preparation of left wing of peregrine, showing propatagium. (Courtesy of Paolo Zucca.)

Plate 5 Details of the talon and distal end of terminal phalanx of an osprey. (Courtesy of Paolo Zucca.)

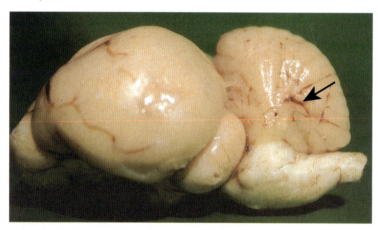

Plate 6 *(Left.)* Lateral view of the brain of a griffon vulture (note the well-developed cerebellum, arrowed). (Courtesy of Paolo Zucca.)

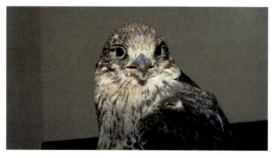

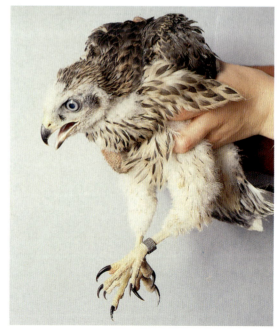

Plate 7 A sick lanner falcon, with oval eyes and soiled plumage. Such a case needs full clinical examination with supporting tests. (Courtesy of Margaret E. Cooper.)

Plate 8 *(Right.)* Handling a young Northern goshawk by restraining the wings: care must be taken to avoid the talons.

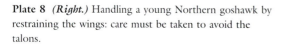

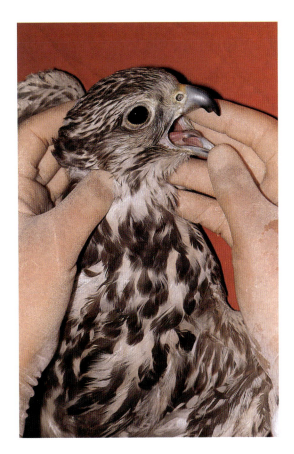

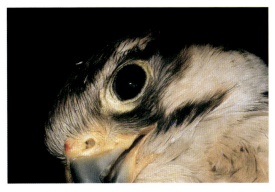

Plate 10 Normal eye and slightly damaged cere of a lagger falcon. The eye is apparently normal: however, the other eye, hidden from view, was partly closed on account of sinusitis.

Plate 9 *(Left.)* Clinical examination of a lightly anaesthetised saker.

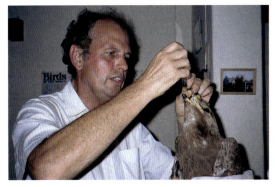

Plate 12 Tube-feeding a tawny eagle: a competent assistant is needed for such tasks, and knowledge of normal anatomy is essential. (Courtesy of Margaret E. Cooper.)

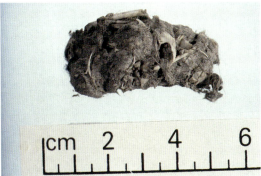

Plate 11 Casting (pellet) of an owl prior to dissection and laboratory investigation: note the bones and hair.

Plate 13 *(Right.)* First aid treatment of an injured harpy eagle in the field (Guyana, Central America). Field equipment is essential in such cases. (Courtesy of Margaret E. Cooper.)

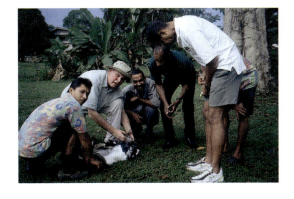

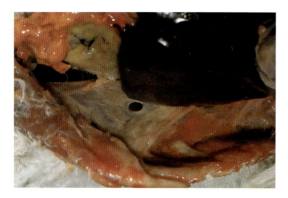

Plate 14 Air sacculitis in a hawk eagle: the grossly thickened (yellow) air sacs are apparent.

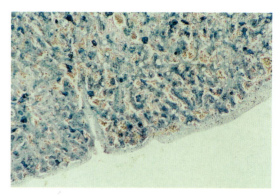

Plate 15 Iron pigment in the liver, appearing blue with Perls' stain: iron deposits can interfere with hepatic function.

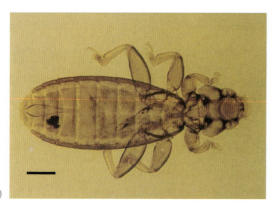

(a)

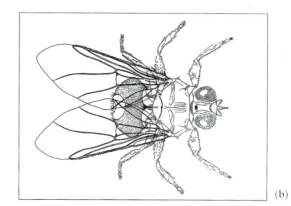

(b)

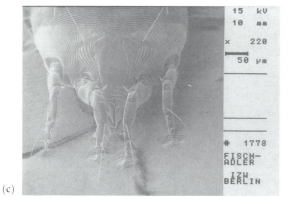

(c)

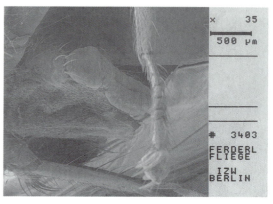

(d)

Plate 16 (a) *Laemobothrion tinnunculi* from a peregrine falcon, bar scale 1 mm; (b) hippoboscid fly, *Ornithomyia* sp. (courtesy of Oliver Krone); (c) feather mite, *Bonnetella* *(Bucholzia) fusca*, from an osprey; (d) hippoboscid fly as vector for *Degeeriella* sp. (courtesy of M. Rudolph).

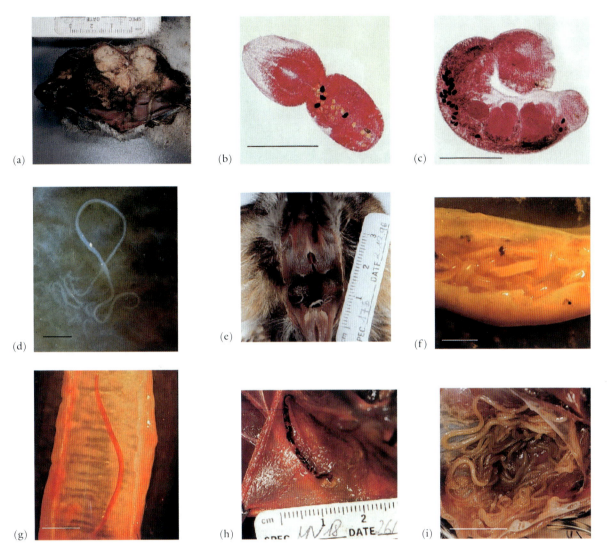

Plate 17 (a) Caseous abscess in the lateral pharynx of a 30-day old Northern goshawk (*Accipiter gentilis*); (b) *Neodiplostomum attenuatum* (stained); (c) *Strigea falconispalumbi* (stained, bar scale 1 mm); (d) *Eucoleus dispar* embedded in the mucous membrane of the oesophagus (bar scale 2 mm); (e) *Synhimantus laticeps* in the prepharynx of a long-eared owl (*Asio otus*); (f) small intestine of a Eurasian buzzard (*Buteo buteo*) partially blocked by *Porrocaecum* sp. (bar scale 3 mm);

(g) *Hovorkonema variegatum* in the trachea of a sparrow-hawk (*Accipiter nisus*) (bar scale 0.5 cm); (h) *H. variegatum* in the cranial thoracic air sac of a white-tailed sea eagle (*Haliaeetus albicilla*) causing air sac wall thickening; (i) *Serratospiculum tenda* between the two layers of the caudal thoracic air sac of a peregrine falcon (*Falco peregrinus*) (bar scale 1 cm). (Courtesy of Oliver Krone.)

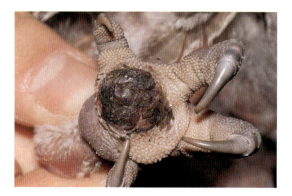

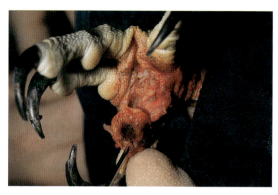

Plate 18 Type 2 bumblefoot in a young tawny owl: the sole of the foot bears a large scab and there is inflamed and infected tissue beneath. (Courtesy of Margaret E. Cooper.)

Plate 19 Surgical excision of infected and damaged material from a case of bumblefoot.

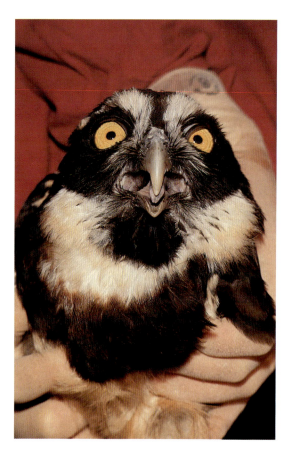

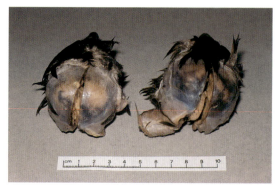

Plate 21 The skulls of two Northern goshawks that died following convulsions. The dark areas are 'intraosseous haemorrhages', which are agonal and often associated with an abnormal posture at the time of death.

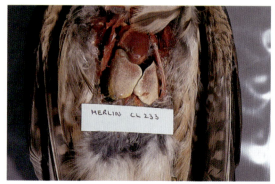

Plate 20 A spectacled owl, having 'fits', as a result of dieldrin poisoning.

Plate 22 A pale, markedly fatty liver in a merlin: the kidney was similarly affected.

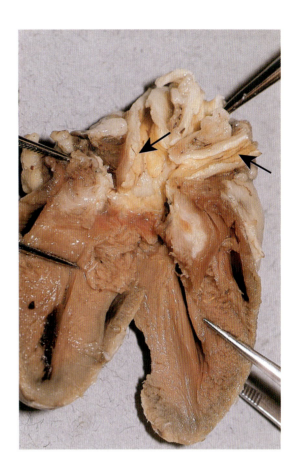

Plate 23 *(Right.)* The heart of an eagle, showing raised, yellow, atheromatous plaques in the aorta (arrows).

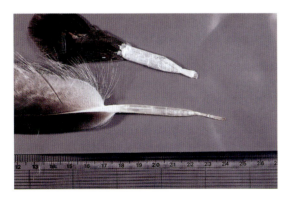

Plate 24 Two feathers of an eagle showing 'pinching off' at the bases.

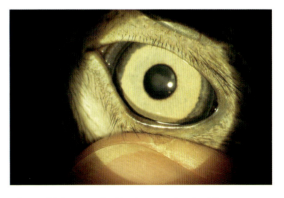

Plate 25 The eye of a Northern goshawk with a cataract. The affected lens was successfully removed.

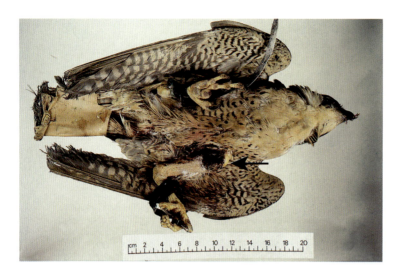

Plate 26 *(Left.)* A Barbary falcon with a chronic lesion of the medial aspect of the thigh (arrow) that proved to be a carcinoma.

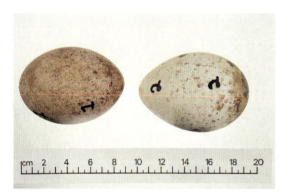

Plate 27 Eggs of a black vulture, submitted for pathological examination. A description of the external appearance of eggs is essential and they should be weighed and measured before being opened.

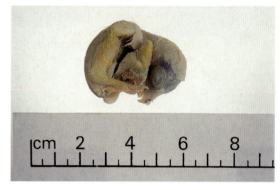

Plate 28 Embryo of the Mauritius kestrel, which failed to hatch and was found to be 'dead-in-shell'. The embryo has been swabbed for bacteriological examination and is now to be examined for morphological abnormalities.

painful lesions can have adverse effects on a bird's physiology and behaviour, retarding healing and regeneration. It was encouraging to note that the Morris Animal Foundation in the USA has funded a study on pain relief for uncomplicated fracture repair in wild (free-living) raptors (Anon, 1995).

Assessment of pain

Assessment of pain is not easy in birds (Gentle, 1992; Flecknell & Waterman-Pearson, 2000). These animals often hide clinical signs, as a defence mechanism, and when handled may appear not to respond to 'painful' stimuli. Frequently the assessment is subjective, with the bird given the benefit of the doubt – probably the better option. Some valuable work was carried out by Vestergaard and Sanotra (1999) on broiler chickens, relating the severity of lameness and the presence of tibial dyschondroplasia to behavioural changes. The study confirmed the value of using behaviour as one indicator of pain and such an approach has already proved useful under certain circumstances in raptors (see Chapter 13). In the study on pain relief referred to above (Anon, 1995), behavioural changes are assessed in conjunction with physiological and metabolic studies. Another valuable way of determining whether a bird is in pain is to administer analgesics and to see if clinical signs that were present are then abolished or reduced in severity, as has been done experimentally with lame chickens (McGeown *et al.*, 1999).

It is not only specific analgesics that can contribute to reducing pain in raptors. Other agents, such as sedatives and non-steroidal anti-inflammatory drugs may have a direct or indirect effect. Management and nursing can also play an important part in pain relief – for example, providing a bird with a damaged foot with chopped food so that it does not have to tear it up (see Chapter 8). Likewise, supporting injuries with a light dressing or sedating a bird for routine examination can minimise pain, as can providing padded perches for bumblefoot cases.

I have never used a muscle relaxant in a bird and have been unable to trace any reference to the subject.

General anaesthesia

General anaesthetic agents for birds of prey can be divided into those that are given (a) by inhalation and, (b) parenterally.

Inhalation anaesthetic agents

Inhalation agents may be administered by facemask, by intubation, by infusion into an airsac ('airsac intubation') or by using an anaesthetic chamber.

A transparent facemask can be placed over the head of a bird to induce anaesthesia. Anaesthesia cannot be induced using an endotracheal tube except in birds that have, for example, been concussed or are comatose following poisoning or electrocution and thus permit intubation.

Anaesthetic chambers are ideal for the induction of anaesthesia in stressed birds (especially casualties) that respond badly to being 'masked down'. This is also a good technique if one has to use agents that take longer than isoflurane to produce a state of anaesthesia or a series of birds has to be anaesthetised.

Anaesthesia can be maintained by facemask or by endotracheal tube. Where purpose-made tubes are not available – a common scenario in less wealthy countries – it may be necessary to fashion something suitable. The tube part of 'butterfly' needles can be used for this purpose, or disposable intravenous drip tubing. The glottis is readily visible at the back of the tongue. Local analgesia of the area is not necessary and the tube will slide down with ease to the bifurcation; it should then be withdrawn slightly to ensure that it does not accidentally enter one bronchus only and occlude the other. It is not necessary to use a cuff but careful positioning of the head and neck is important to prevent kinking or obstruction of the tube. Green (1979) suggested that inflowing gases should always be warmed and moisturised to help prevent loss of bodyheat. He also recommended a gas flow of approximately three times the respiratory minute volume of the patient – a 300 g bird has a minute volume of approximately 250 ml.

Air sac intubation can be very useful when, for example, there is airway obstruction or a need to perform surgery on the mouth. The technique is well described, with references, by Lawton (1996). At least one company now manufactures an 'avian air sac ventilation catheter'.

An anaesthetic chamber can be particularly useful under field or laboratory conditions when a series of birds has to be anaesthetised in quick succession. The chamber is attached to an anaesthetic machine and the agents pumped through. A design of an anaesthetic chamber suitable for birds as well as for mammals and reptiles was described by Applebee and Cooper (1989). The sides of the chamber are best covered so as not to disturb the bird unnecessarily. The patient should be removed when it is recumbent, with eyes closed and breathing regularly; anaesthesia can then be maintained by facemask or tube.

Intermittent positive pressure ventilation (IPPV) can be advantageous. Lawton (2000) emphasised that IPPV allows better control of respiration and oxygenation and can prevent hypercapnoea. Small animal ventilators are now available commercially and can be used for birds of prey. Intubation is essential and monitoring of airway pressure important to avoid overinflation.

Fitzgerald and Blais (1993) provided a useful review of the history of anaesthesia of birds of prey. Brief mention will be made here of inhalation agents that are now rarely used, except in emergencies, and sometimes in the field or overseas, but which served raptor medicine well only a quarter of a century ago.

A valuable table, comparing three inhalation agents was provided by Lawton (1996) and is worth ready reference.

Methoxyflurane was a safe but relatively non-potent agent. For many years it proved of great value in wild bird casualties, which are often a poor anaesthetic risk. Analgesia was good. Both induction and recovery tended to be slower than with halothane.

Ether was a very reliable anaesthetic agent which was long used by many veterinary surgeons. Its main disadvantage was its inflammability which rendered it unsuitable for use when thermocautery is involved and potentially dangerous at other times.

Halothane was for many years the inhalation anaesthetic of choice for surgical procedures in mammals and birds. It was, however, potent and had

to be used with care. It caused a marked reduction in blood pressure in birds, together with a drop in respiration rate and body temperature. Bilo and colleagues (1972) made a special study of halothane anaesthesia in birds and their paper (in German) was an important contribution to the literature. It illustrated techniques of induction and discussed both reflexes and the use of the electrocardiogram (ECG) in monitoring anaesthesia.

Isoflurane has largely superseded all the above in the richer parts of the world. Its use in raptors was discussed in detail by Fitzgerald and Blais (1993). Isoflurane is considered by most people to be the anaesthetic agent of choice at the present time – although this opinion could change as new drugs appear and there is always the important point, repeated frequently in this book, that in many parts of the world isoflurane is not available (or too expensive to use) and recourse to older, less reliable, agents is essential. The claim that the safety of isoflurane alone 'makes other agents obsolete' (see, for example, Lawton, 1996 and Rosskopf *et al.*, 1992) may be correct from a Western European/North American point of view but reveals no understanding of the needs of the wider world outside – nor, indeed, of the special problems presented by work on birds in the field. In this book, therefore, a broader perspective is adopted.

The use of isoflurane in raptors is characterised by rapid induction (associated with its low solubility) and a wide safety margin. In addition, excretion is virtually independent of liver and kidney, muscle relaxation is good and there is little respiratory depression. However, it can cause myocardial depression and arrhythmias have been reported in bald eagles anaesthetised with isoflurane (Aguilar *et al.*, 1995). A small number of birds react adversely to isoflurane: Tom Bailey (pers. comm.) reports that fewer than 0.5% of the falcons he and his colleagues see come into this category. Such birds become apnoeic under isoflurane and are therefore given instead ketamine and xylazine.

Dresser *et al.* (1999) studied the effects of repeat blood sampling and isoflurane anaesthesia on haematological and biochemical values of American kestrels. They concluded that the combined effect of isoflurane and repeat blood sampling causes more dramatic changes than bleeding alone. However, this may not apply to other species and it can be argued that the routine use of isoflurane carries many other advantages such as the possibility of performing a full clinical examination.

Sevoflurane and desflurane are not in general use in avian work but preliminary studies and reports – for example, on sevoflurane in raptors (Hawkins *et al.*, 2000; M. P. C. Lawton pers. comm.) and in psittacines (Quandt & Greenacre, 1999) – suggest that they may prove useful.

The use of nitrous oxide was discussed earlier – a valuable adjunct to all inhalation anaesthetic agents. It may, however, prolong recovery time when used with isoflurane.

Parenteral anaesthetic agents

Parenteral anaesthetic agents for raptors are usually given by the intravenous or intramuscular route. Intraperitoneal administration, once favoured in some circles, can be hazardous because of the damage of hitting internal organs, such as the liver.

For intravenous injection the basilic vein is usually used and the technique for locating this was described earlier in Chapter 4; it has the disadvantage that the bird must be cast on its back. Other veins are also available and Tom Bailey (pers. comm.) particularly favours the saphenous vein in small to medium-sized birds because these then do not have to be cast on their backs.

For intramuscular administration either the thigh or pectoral muscles can be used. Clumsy injections into the pectorals may impair flight; I have seen (on histological examination) severe damage to these muscles, confirmed in studies on starlings (Cooper, 1983). The leg muscles can be used in preference and the presence in birds of a renal portal system does not appear adversely to influence the results.

The duration of action of the injectable agents increases with body size: thus, a large bird, such as an eagle, will take significantly longer to absorb, metabolise and eliminate a drug than a small sparrow-hawk or kestrel. It is for this reason that allometric scaling is advisable (see Chapter 4).

Barbiturates were never widely used in birds of prey in view of their respiratory depressant effect and their poor analgesia. However, they filled a niche in the early days. Thus, Nelson *et al.* (1942) described pancreatectomy in the great horned owl using sodium phenobarbital and did not report any adverse effects; they noted that owls needed a smaller dose than ducks of comparable weight. In the 1960s I had to use pentobarbitone sodium, diluted, by the intravenous route when inhalation agents were unavailable – mainly in the field and in Africa. Sawby and Gessaman (1974) employed pentobarbitone when implanting electrodes in American kestrels and reported that 'a few kestrels died'. Methohexitone is an ultra short-acting barbiturate. Its successful use in the domestic fowl was reported 30 years ago (Scott & Stewart, 1972): I have used it, by the intravenous route, in a number of species of bird (Cooper, 1984a). The administration of this and other agents by the intravenous route is facilitated if a butterfly attachment is strapped into position with tape: incremental doses can be given as and when required.

Metomidate was introduced into bird of prey work in the early 1970s (Cooper, 1970b) – when it was called 'methoxymol' – and for some time it proved to be useful in a wide variety of species. The drug appeared to be very safe and in Kenya was used at monthly intervals (with occasional exceptions) for 36 months in two African harrier-hawks; never were ill-effects observed and regular clinical, haematological and parasitological examinations showed no associated abnormalities. It was also the anaesthetic agent that I used for my early work on laparotomy and surgical sexing (Cooper, 1974a). However, Cadle and Martin (1976) reported four fatalities with metomidate in tawny owls. None of these occurred on the first occasion and they suggested that in two cases an antigen–antibody reaction might have occurred. The two deaths were considered a mystery and, unfortunately, neither *postmortem* examination nor histology was performed. Electrocardiography was carried out during anaesthesia and episodes of asystole and bradycardia were noted. I cannot account for the fatalities experienced by these authors. My own good opinion of metomidate at that time was substantiated by Ryder-Davies (1973) who described it as a 'very useful drug and a safe one'.

The dissociative anaesthetic ketamine hydrochloride soon replaced the earlier agents, such as metomidate, as the parenteral agent of choice. Its use in birds of prey was probably first reported by Borzio (1973). Ketamine can be used alone, in combination with other injectable agents or prior to administering inhalation agents. It is administered intramuscularly or by the intravenous route. Redig (1977) reported on ketamine mixtures and stated that he had found ketamine–xylazine preferable to ketamine–diazepam, by the intravenous route. Samour *et al.* (1984) compared ketamine, xylazine and alphaxalone–alphadolone in over a thousand birds, some of them raptors. They reported satisfactory results with ketamine in most species but vultures showed marked salivation, excitation and convulsions and it did not prove possible to achieve adequate surgical anaesthesia. This, however, was not my experience when I used ketamine in black vultures on Mallorca in 1983. Lumeij (1993), however, reported effects on adrenal function and cardiac conduction in pigeons and goshawks and concluded that at 50 mg/kg ketamine and 4 mg/kg xylazine intramuscularly the combination could be life-threatening for the former. In contrast, Raffe *et al.* (1993) described the combination as 'well tolerated' at 15 mg/kg and 3 mg/kg in greathorned owls.

In his paper Borzio (1973) pointed out that ketamine is eliminated by the kidney; he recommended fluid therapy in debilitated birds or when the recovery period is prolonged. The possible effects of ketamine on the avian adrenal are mentioned in Chapter 13.

Other dissociative agents can also be used. Zenker and Janovsky (1998), for example, described immobilisation of the common buzzard with oral tiletamine zolazepam. Use of a steroid anaesthetic agent was first reported in birds of prey in 1973 (Cooper & Frank, 1973). The drug consists of alphaxalone and alphadolone acetate in polyoxyethylated castor oil and was originally designated 'CT 1341'. In my initial work, in Kenya, at a time when only barbiturates and metomidate were regularly used as parenteral agents in birds of prey, 'CT 1341' proved useful and relatively safe in both chickens and birds of prey. Subsequently it established itself, by the intravenous route, as an agent for ultra-short anaesthesia of raptors. Within a few seconds the bird was anaesthetised and the duration of anaesthesia was usually 5–10 minutes. Incremental doses by either the intravenous or intramuscular route were used to prolong anaesthesia. Alternatively it could be used to induce anaesthesia which was then maintained with an inhalation agent. Very few fatalities were reported but Patrick Redig and I encountered adverse reactions to the drug in red-tailed hawks (one of which died) and we later recommended care in its use in this species (Cooper & Redig, 1975). Abnormal cardiac rhythms were observed in six out of seven birds anaesthetised by Frank and Cooper (1974b). Subsequently Cribb and Haigh (1977) carried out electrocardiographic monitoring of birds, including a red-tailed hawk, under alphaxalone–alphadolone anaesthesia and reported a high incidence of sinus arrest and tachycardia. As a result, they also urged caution in its use and it is now not regularly employed for raptors.

Propofol has been used in birds, including raptors, and a study on its safety and efficacy in pigeons was carried out by Fitzgerald and Cooper (1990). Hawkins *et al.* (2000) recently re-evaluated it as an agent in birds of prey and concluded that, while infusion allowed for a light plane of anaesthesia, cardiopulmonary monitoring and ventilatory support are advisable.

Dosages of injectable anaesthetic agents are usually cited in 'mg/kg bodyweight' but, as mentioned earlier (and in Chapter 4), allometric scaling would probably provide more reliable and consistent figures. The question of scaling and its relevance to veterinary anaesthesia was recently reviewed by Morris (2000).

The pre- and post-operative care of raptors plays an important role in ensuring successful anaesthesia. Pre-operatively the bird should be observed carefully for 48 hours and monitored clinically and haematologically. The bird should generally not be fed in the period preceding anaesthesia but starvation of small birds for longer than 18 hours can prove dangerous. My own approach is therefore to feed birds 6–12 hours beforehand but I ensure that this does not include roughage since this can result in regurgitation or increased intra-abdominal pressure. I also check carefully that no food remains in the crop. Atropine given by injection 15 minutes before induction will help to reduce salivation: this was particularly advisable when metomidate was being used. Tom Bailey (pers. comm.) reports the reflux of 'stomach' juices during anaesthesia of falconers' hawks, probably because these birds have not been starved for long enough, and stresses the importance of removing this fluid.

Induction of anaesthesia in birds is usually not accompanied by marked excitation since even by the intramuscular route induction time is short. During induction with an injectable agent the bird may shake its head, fluff out its feathers and extend its limbs. Induction by inhalation may again be accompanied by head shaking and occasionally wing flapping. Once a bird starts to become unsteady on its feet it is often wise to restrain it for further induction.

During anaesthesia the bird must be maintained at a constant temperature, preferably 32–35°C. An operating light will provide overhead warmth but it is also advisable to lay the bird on a heating pad or to wrap it in well insulated material.

Monitoring during general anaesthesia

Assessment of depth of anaesthesia depends in part upon the use of monitoring equipment, which is discussed later, but also upon careful observation of the bird. Under field conditions in poorer parts of the world the latter may be all-important. I rely on respiratory rate, the response to pressure (squeezing of the foot) and to pain during surgery. In addition, muscle tone (extending a wing or opening the mouth), heart rate and colour of mucous membranes can be used. In some species other indicators may be useful; a rather unusual example to which I have referred elsewhere (Cooper, 1974a) is the change of face colour in the African harrier hawk from red to yellow as anaesthesia lightens!

During surgery observation of the bird may be difficult on account of operating cloths but the use of transparent drapes is increasingly common and overcomes this problem. The head in particular should be exposed. Movement of the base of the tail will correspond with respiration and it is important

that this too is visible. Attention must be paid to the respiratory tract to ensure that pellet material, undigested food or mucus is not occluding the glottis or oropharynx. If a bird has obstructed nares it must either have its beak held open or be intubated. The use of an endotracheal tube is always useful, even if no inhalation anaesthetic agent is being used, as it helps to ensure a clear airway and reduces the risk of ingesta being inhaled. In the case of vultures the positioning of the head is important since asphyxia can occur if the neck becomes twisted (Cooper, 1973a).

The monitoring of avian patients is vital (Lawton, 2000) and in modern small animal (dog and cat) veterinary practice the minimal equipment assumed necessary for monitoring anaesthesia is an oesophageal stethoscope and a pulse oximeter. Other monitors that are available include display electrocardiography (ECG) equipment, non-invasive blood pressure monitors, temperature and respiratory monitors. Some modern units permit the monitoring of heart/pulse rates of up to several hundred and respiratory rates of up to 90 per minute. With the possible exception of pulse oximeters, these monitors can all be used for raptors – certainly captive birds and in cases where the equipment is portable, runs on batteries and can be taken into the field, for free-living birds. However, all this sophisticated equipment cannot substitute for a clinician or nurse who is monitoring the patient – mucous membranes, respiration rate and quality, heart rate and quality, response to stimuli – throughout the operation. A competent assistant should do the monitoring: it is not satisfactory for one person to attempt to be anaesthetist and surgeon.

Anaesthetic emergencies

Anaesthetic emergencies can occur. Apnoea is the most common. It is often seen following the use of alphaxalone–alphadolone by the intravenous route but usually respiration recommences within a minute. Birds that react adversely to isoflurane will also develop apnoea that may not be transient. In such cases, or if a bird suddenly stops breathing during surgery, the tongue very soon appears cyanosed. The first step is to ensure that the mouth and glottis are clear of mucus or other material and to place the bird on its breast, when respiration will often resume spontaneously – respiratory embarrassment is more of a problem when a bird is on its back. If breathing does not start, oxygen should be given and artificial respiration (squeezing of the rib cage) carried out every 20–30 seconds. If oxygen is not available, a piece of tubing can be placed in the trachea (an endotracheal tube can be used) and a 20 ml syringe used to pump air backwards and forwards over the lungs. In cases when an inhalation agent is being used and apnoea occurs it is possible that a reservoir of anaesthetic remains in an air sac – an early example of mine was an osprey that took several hours to recover from ether – and in such cases it might be useful to insert a needle into an abdominal air sac and draw off some anaesthetic.

Exaggerated breathing movement may indicate airway obstruction: the bird's mouth must be opened to ensure that the glottis is patent. As Green (1979) pointed out, this can be mistaken for a lightening of anaesthesia – with possible fatal results.

Cardiac arrest may occur. Occasionally it lasts only a few seconds and the heartbeat recommences but it usually persists and, in my experience, shows no response to external massage. I have injected adrenaline into the heart in such cases but with no success. Cardiac arrhythmias are not at all uncommon during anaesthesia: I am uncertain of their significance.

Overdosage of an anaesthetic agent can occur and may result in respiratory depression and failure to respond to stimuli. The former can be treated as outlined earlier for apnoea. Respiratory stimulants such as doxopram (given intravenously or on to a mucosal surface) are valuable.

These and other possible emergencies justify the use of a 'crash kit' and a written, readily visible, avian resuscitation protocol. Those recommended by Tom Bailey (pers. comm.) are reproduced, with his permission, as part of Appendix IX.

Post-operative care

Immediately following anaesthesia a raptor should be wrapped firmly in a towel or similar material and kept warm, if possible on a heating pad or in an insulated container. The optimum temperatures are 32–35°C. Administration of oxygen will help to hasten recovery from an inhalation agent. Failure to restrain the bird adequately can result in postoperative trauma if there is wing flapping and other uncontrolled activity. Physical restraint by wrapping the bird will help to prevent this and will also enable the bird to be fed by hand or given fluids. Alternatively a small raptor, such as a merlin, can be placed in a cloth bag which is suspended so that the bird inside cannot strike anything. This method may sound crude but is usually very successful, especially under field conditions. Once a bird is able to stand, it can be returned to its enclosure but is usually best kept warm in a recovery box for at least a further 6–12 hours.

Drugs used for baiting

Occasionally it may be necessary to capture freeliving raptors or to recapture an escaped captive bird. Although mechanical methods of capture are probably preferable, drugs can be employed in a bait (Zenker & Janovsky, 1998; Belant & Seamans, 1999). Ebedes (1973) used phencyclidine to capture free-living vultures, and Zenker *et al.* (2000) tiletamine–zolazepam for Eurasian buzzards. In their section on 'sedating lost birds', Forbes and Harcourt-Brown (1996) referred only to baiting with oral diazepam and oral ketamine. In addition to the agents mentioned above, I have found oral phenobarbitone or pentobarbitone valuable but somewhat variable in effect. Phenobarbitone is given in tablet form and hidden in the food. Pentobarbitone is best injected intraperitoneally into a mouse or chick and then the dead animal offered to the escaped bird. In many countries a licence is needed to bait birds, even escaped ones (see Appendix XI), and great care has to be taken to avoid non-target species.

Euthanasia

Euthanasia must be mentioned. If it is necessary to kill a raptor on humanitarian or other grounds, this must be done with the minimum of discomfort or pain to the bird. Physical methods, such as shooting or a blow to the head, are often the most humane and rapid but are frequently repugnant to laypersons. If a chemical method is to be employed then an overdose of an anaesthetic agent is permissible. Carpenter *et al.* (2001) collated data on a number of suitable substances. Pentobarbitone or ketamine can be injected by any route, but if alphaxalone–alphadolone, propofol, thiopentone or methohexitone has to be used, the recommended method is intravenous. Under field conditions, where these agents may be in short supply, it may be necessary to complete the task with intravenous magnesium sulphate. Inhalation agents employed for euthanasia can be pumped into an anaesthetic chamber (Applebee & Cooper, 1989) or given by mask. Only in a real emergency should an old-fashioned 'ether jar' be used. Under no circumstances should a bird be disposed of until it has undergone *rigor mortis*, and care must be taken over disposal of the body if injectable agents have been used. In any case, the carcass should, whenever possible, be submitted for *post-mortem* examination.

When submitting a raptor that has been euthanased for necropsy a note should be made of the method used. If this is not done, problems can result and the pathologist may have difficulty in interpreting the sequence of events. Pentobarbitone given intraperitoneally shows as crystalline deposits on the serosal surface of organs: this can be mistaken for visceral gout. Likewise, physical methods of euthanasia will usually produce signs of haemorrhage and trauma (see Appendix VI).

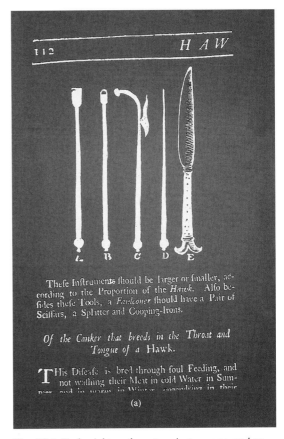

Fig. 12.1 Early eighteenth century instruments used to treat hawks. From *The Gentleman's Recreation* (1686).

SURGERY

> *'In a good surgeon, a hawk's eye: a lion's heart: and a lady's hand.'*
> Leonard Wright

Introduction

Surgical techniques in birds of prey are not new, and instruments for this purpose were in use at least three centuries ago (Fig. 12.1). There have been great advances in surgery over the past two decades. Essentially, however, the techniques do not differ greatly from those used in other birds. Most of the more important surgical procedures in raptors are discussed elsewhere in this book – for example, repair of skin wounds and fractures (Chapter 5) and surgical treatment of bumblefoot (Chapter 8). Others will be described briefly in this section together with mention of general considerations when performing surgery on raptors.

Useful references to surgical techniques in birds of prey include the chapters on the limbs by Nigel Harcourt-Brown (1996b,c) and Greg Simpson (1996) in the BSAVA *Manual of Raptors, Pigeons and Waterfowl*. These are referred to in more detail in Chapter 5 where emphasis is laid upon the importance of having a sound knowledge of anatomy, especially of the limbs, before attempting surgery (Figs 12.2, 12.3 and 12.4).

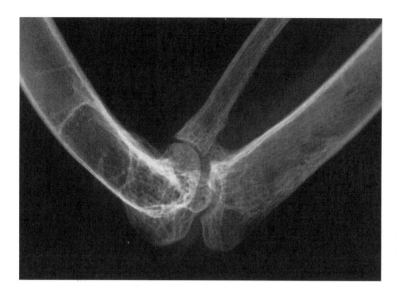

Fig. 12.2 Radiograph of a lanner showing details of the humerus – radioulnar joint. Knowledge of such anatomy is important in surgery. (Courtesy of Paolo Zucca.)

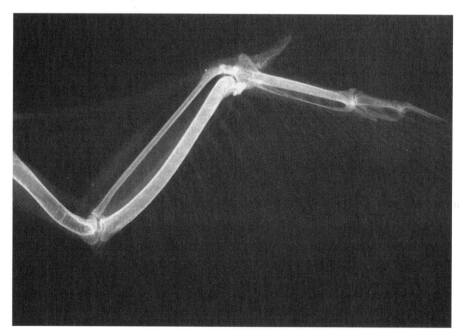

Fig. 12.3 Radiograph of a peregrine showing (normal) osseous structures and feather shafts. The humerus is clearly a pneumatised bone. (Courtesy of Paolo Zucca.)

Pre-operative preparation

Although asepsis is important in surgery, post-operative infections occur relatively rarely in birds compared with mammals. Skin preparation should be thorough but over-enthusiastic plucking of feathers or use of disinfectants must be avoided as these can result in considerable loss of bodyheat and the possibility of shock.

The positioning of a bird for surgery has been

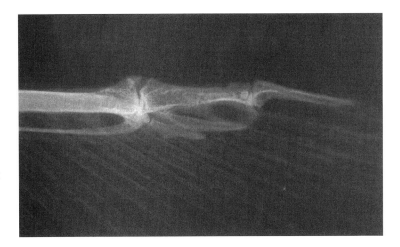

Fig. 12.4 Radiograph of the phalanx of a peregrine, taken with high sensitivity equipment. The 'new' sesamoids are visible (see Chapter 3). (Courtesy of Paolo Zucca.)

mentioned previously and Green (1979) discussed this in some detail. He stressed that birds should not be kept on their backs for long periods since hypotension can develop due to reduced venous return. Nor should limbs be overextended too forcibly. As a general rule, all movements during surgery should be made slowly and gently.

In the smaller birds of prey blood loss can be a problem. If considerable bleeding is expected the bird should be given fluids prior to and during surgery. Every effort must, however, be made to control haemorrhage using artery forceps or thermocautery. Diode laser equipment is likely to become more readily available in future and will make many procedures virtually bloodless.

Surgical procedures

Some procedures can hardly be described as 'surgical' but should be mentioned. In this chapter most are managemental and present no problems to the experienced falconer or aviculturist but occasionally a veterinary surgeon will be asked for advice, especially over difficult cases. The regular clipping ('coping') of talons and beak is an example – probably best carried out using sharp (veterinary) nail clippers or even a pair of garden secateurs. A strong light can help to localise the blood vessels – which should not be cut! Precautions when coping talons

were discussed by Redig and Ackermann (2000). Coping is an art and must be carried out with sensitivity and an understanding of the anatomy of the areas concerned. In the case of the beak, manicuring can be performed with a scalpel blade or sharp knife and a nail file or piece of sandpaper. Pumice stone is very useful for manicuring the beak and talons. If there is extensive damage to the beak, it is often helpful to anaesthetise the bird lightly during the procedure.

Falconers' birds that are kept on stone blocks will tend to keep their own talons and beak short but they too may need to be coped, in which case particular care must be taken to ensure that the end result is good and the bird is able to hunt satisfactorily. Such precision is not so essential for birds that are to live in an aviary, where dead food is provided.

Falconers have a long tradition of experience in the care, and to a certain extent repair, of their birds' feathers and some of the techniques used, applicable to casualty raptors intended for release, as well as for falconers' birds, are discussed in Chapter 13.

Most falconers' birds are now telemetered and the use of a short-acting anaesthetic can make the attachment of the transmitter to a leg or tail much easier and permit health checks at the same time.

Deflighting of captive raptors may be requested, especially involving large species such as vultures and eagles in safari parks. The simplest method is to clip the primaries (or even alternate primaries in some species) on one wing; the outer primary should be left intact on aesthetic grounds and since it helps protect the other feathers. This technique is often moderately successful, and is of course painless, but does not always have the desired effect and flight will be possible again once the bird has moulted. Surgical pinioning (amputation of a wing at the carpus) is an irreversible alternative and should only be performed, under general anaesthesia, after careful consideration of the ethical and welfare implications. Other techniques for restricting or preventing flight are used in waterfowl (Humphreys, 1985), amongst them a patagiectomy whereby a portion of the patagial membrane, on the leading edge of the wing, is removed surgically so that the bird is unable to extend the treated wing (Robinson, 1975). This and other procedures may be of value in raptors but I have no experience of them.

In recent years there has been great concern over the theft of captive birds of prey and owners may seek advice over methods of marking raptors (see Appendix XI). The use of passive integrated transponders (microchips) is becoming standard not only for these birds but also for those destined for release with possible recapture (Lierz & Launay, 2000; MEFRG, undated). Guidelines on recommended sites for implantation of microchips have been produced by several organisations and have been summarised (Anon, 1999). Studies on the effect of transponders on the tissues of dogs (Jansen *et al.*, 1999) are probably relevant to birds – the thin fibrous capsule and absence of any inflammation, for example. Other methods of identification can be cheaper and some of these fall broadly under the heading of 'surgical techniques' – hence their inclusion in this chapter.

Individual identification of raptors was discussed in general terms by Forbes and Harcourt-Brown (1996). Heidenreich's chapter (1997) on 'Marking and identification' is more substantial and includes egg marking and colour marking of chicks. Tattooing of birds is carried out as in mammals, using the skin of the feet or wing. Other methods of recognising individuals include close-up photographs of

the soles of the feet – these are usually different in each individual, especially if it has had foot lesions (see Chapter 3) – or of the scalation of legs. Radiography, which may reveal the presence of lead shot, healed fractures or skeletal abnormalities (Cooper, 1976b) is an additional aid to identifying individual birds. In legal cases such data can be very valuable.

Free-living birds can be marked for recognition in various ways, including the use of rings (bands) and feather bleaching (Frey & Zink, 2000), as well as employing some of the techniques above. Individual plumage patterns and markings may also be used.

Minor surgery may be required for the removal of unsightly or pathological lesions, such as papillomata, or for the taking of biopsies for histological diagnosis. Cautery is very useful in such work, as is cryosurgery, but both techniques cause tissue damage that can hamper histological interpretation.

Regardless of the legal situation, it is important on welfare grounds that a raptor is anaesthetised for a surgical procedure, even if the latter is only brief. As long ago as 1655 Markham writing about the surgical suturing ('seeling') of hawks' eyelids recognised that birds of prey can feel discomfort when he stated:

'But this manner of seeling of Hawkes, is both troublesome, painfull and dangerous to the Hawke.'

It may be necessary to operate on the crop of a raptor in order to remove impacted material or to clean and suture traumatic injuries such as perforations. The procedure is similar to that in the fowl. A stab incision is recommended and the crop and skin should be sutured separately. Crop surgery may also be necessary to repair a fistula – usually brought about by a puncture wound, sometimes as a result of severe trichomoniasis (see Chapter 7).

Occasionally clinicians receive requests for a raptor to be 'devoiced' because it makes too much noise. The usual cause is a bird taken too early from the nest – a so-called 'screamer'. I have always refused to perform this operation, on ethical grounds, but I know that it has been carried out, with varying success, in Britain and the United States. The technique first described for the fowl by Durant (1953) appears to be applicable.

A laparotomy may be necessary for the purpose of diagnosis or treatment (Krautwald & Trinkhaus, 2000). It can be carried out safely so long as the operator is aware of the anatomy of the bird, and is careful to avoid delicate internal organs. When I first carried out laparotomies in the 1970s I used a midline incision, with the bird on its back; careful dissection was often necessary to avoid damaging the underlying gastro-intestinal organs, especially if there was much fat present. Alternatively the lateral approach can be used, as described for endoscopic sexing of birds of prey (Cooper, 1974a).

Endoscopy (laparoscopy) was originally used widely as a method of 'surgical sexing' but has been largely superseded by other, less traumatic, methods (see Chapter 13). It is still an important method of sexing in the field and used in research work to investigate gonad activity. I used an auroscope (otoscope) for laparoscopy in Kenya in the early 1970s (Cooper, 1974a) but this was hardly revolutionary as I was merely repeating, in a slightly more sophisticated fashion, the technique used by some field ornithologists since the 1940s. Now rigid and flexible high quality endoscopes are used routinely in birds of prey in order to investigate normal and abnormal organs and to take samples from lesions for histology and for microbiology. Endoscopic techniques in birds were outlined by Brearley *et al.* (1991) and more recently described in detail by a number of authors, including Heidenreich (1997).

A muscle biopsy can be of value in studies on pesticides, for the investigation of muscular disorders and to collect tissue samples for molecular studies. A technique used successfully in East African species was described some years ago by Frank and Cooper (1974a). The biopsy was taken as a wedge lateral to the keel and in a bird of 500–1000 g bodyweight could measure 2 cm long × 4 mm wide × 3–4 mm deep. The wound was treated topically and the skin sutured with catgut. The technique described takes under 5 minutes and is easily performed under light anaesthesia. Infection of the wound is rare and haemorrhage is not a problem so long as the incision is made in the position described and not more caudal or lateral.

Cauterisation was widely used to treat hawks in the Middle Ages (Cooper, 1979a) and continues to be employed in Arabia and elsewhere but has no role in modern practice other than thermo-electro-cautery, under anaesthesia, for surgical incision, excision and ablation. Neither thermocautery nor cryosurgery (also widely used in birds of prey) is recommended when a biopsy is to be taken and examined, as both techniques cause tissue damage that can hamper interpretation of changes.

A wide variety of modern surgical procedures can now be carried out in birds of prey. Orthopaedic techniques are discussed under Chapter 5. Ophthalmological operations have become increasingly frequent – for example, enucleation (Greenwood & Barnett, 1981) and lens extraction by ultrasonic pharmacoemulsification (Kern *et al.*, 1984). Ocular diseases are covered in Chapter 13.

Experimental surgery is sometimes needed as part of a research project. This is not a new development. The preparation of a gastric fistula was reported over 70 years ago (Reed & Reed, 1928) and pancreatectomies in birds of prey as long ago as the 1890s (referred to by Nelson *et al.* (1942)).

Nelson and colleagues (1942) performed pancreatectomies on great horned owls under phenobarbitone anaesthetic and stated: 'little difficulty was experienced in removing the gland which is quite discrete and located in the loop of the duodenum'.

The Russian biologist Voitkevich carried out thyroidectomies in a wide range of birds, amongst them short-eared owls and kestrels, as part of his investigations into feather development. The surgical techniques used were described in Voitkevich's book *The Feathers and Plumage of Birds* (1966) and will only be summarised here. Feathers were plucked from the ventral aspect of the neck and a midline incision made. The crop (when present) was displaced and the interclavicular air sac either incised or pushed aside. The thyroid was removed by blunt dissection, care being taken to minimise haemorrhage and to avoid touching the vagus nerve. Voitkevich made the point that owls, in common with certain other species, have a very tough thyroid capsule. Ligation of blood vessels was not considered essential, speed of operation being more important. Sutures were placed only in the skin. Voitkevich referred to surgical procedures used by other authors and stressed the importance of ensuring that all thyroid tissue has been removed; if any remains, it may regenerate.

Surgical techniques for the implantation of telemetry equipment and indwelling cannulae may also be required for research purposes. Sawby and Gessaman (1974) were possibly the first to describe the surgical implantation of electrodes for electro-cardiography in American kestrels; their approach was midline, just caudal (posterior) to the sternum, and the electrodes inserted inside the body cavity, dorsal to the sternum. The lead wires were then threaded under the skin to exit points on the flank and back. Rushton and Osgood (1993) used an automated system – on non-releasable 'casualties' – that involved implantation intraperitoneally of a radio transmitter. More recently, Walzer *et al.* (2000) described the intra-abdominal implantation of a multi-sensor telemetry system in a free-living Eurasian griffon: this permitted long-term record-ing of heart rate, body and ambient temperature, altitude and location remote sensing. These and other experimental techniques are likely to provide useful physiological data that might also contribute to improved health monitoring.

Small satellite telemeters are likely to become increasingly used in studies on raptors and their low weight (30 g for birds of 900–1000 g) may mean less chance of their having an adverse effect on a bird's performance or survival (Britten *et al.*, 1999).

Post-surgical care

Care following surgery has been covered in the section on 'General anaesthesia', under 'Post-operative care'.

The use of post-operative analgesia is an impor-tant welfare consideration and analgesia was dis-cussed earlier in this chapter.

Post-surgical complications also occur in birds of prey. They include cardiovascular and neurogenic disturbances (e.g. 'shock'), thromboembolism and infection.

CONCLUSIONS

Although surgery has been performed on birds of prey for centuries, advances in recent years have been remarkable. While some techniques can readily and confidently be undertaken by the general practi-tioner, other more sophisticated procedures may need the expertise and experience of a specialist in veterinary surgery. In the interests of the bird – and to reduce the (increasing) risks of litigation or accusa-tions of malpractice – referral is always a wise option.

'. . . the best surgeon, like the best general, is he who makes the fewest mistakes.'
Sir Astley Paston Cooper

Miscellaneous and Emerging Diseases

'Emergence is none other than the dark side of co-evolution, a typical inexorable, biological phenomenon.'

Joshua Lederberg

This chapter covers diseases that are not discussed fully in other chapters, together with some that are 'emerging' in the sense that it is only in recent years that they have come into prominence. The latter comprise some conditions that have probably just escaped notice in the past, plus others which have clearly increased in prevalence or importance – perhaps on account of new systems of management (captive birds) or environmental changes (free-living birds).

AGE-RELATED DISORDERS

Birds of prey maintained in captivity may live to a considerable age. Heidenreich (1997) published a useful table of 'maximum recorded life spans' of selected raptor species and this ranged from 12 years for the merlin (egg-laying until 10 years of age) to 95 years for a white-tailed sea eagle (egg-laying until 42 years). Birds kept for falconry usually live less long than those in zoos, although some trained birds reach 20 years or more. It is interesting to contrast this with the comments in *Falconry in the British Isles* (Salvin & Brodrick, 1855) where the authors stated that they had 'met with several trained peregrines which reached the ages of five, seven, eight and ten years'. Some of the conditions discussed in this chapter are likely to be associated with increased longevity.

Ageing an old bird is not easy and some reliable clinical and pathological guidelines would be useful. The work of Wyllie (undated), using talon anatomy in order to age owls, may be applicable to other species.

Old age itself can produce clinical signs of lethargy, stiffness of movement (particularly if the weather is cold or wet) and a tendency to 'doze' with the eyes closed. Recovery time from anaesthesia may be extended. Cataracts (see under 'Ocular conditions') and other degenerative conditions are also a feature. Neoplasia may be seen (Forbes *et al.*, 2000a). A raptor that has died of natural causes at an advanced age usually shows no specific lesions. The plumage may be frayed and lustreless and the feet often show calluses. Internally there are often extensive fat deposits within the body cavity itself and on the heart. Atheromatosis may be present (Plate 23). On histological examination there may be evidence of interstitial nephritis and infiltration of the liver by excess numbers of chronic inflammatory cells. If an old bird deteriorates too drastically in physical condition a decision may have to be taken to kill it humanely.

Obesity – an excess of body fat – is common in elderly (and sometimes non-elderly) birds in zoological collections. It is rarely seen in falconers' birds that are being flown and is not a feature of truly free-living raptors (as opposed to those that are free-ranging but receiving supplementary feeding). Obesity is often defined in terms of weight increase: a bird is 'obese' when weight exceeds optimum by 15% or more. An obese bird can appear on observation to be in good condition but palpation may reveal a 'plumpness' of pectoral muscles and fat deposits under the jaw and in interclavicular and pectoral areas. Grossly overweight raptors may appear to have bands of alopecia because of separation of feather tracts.

The 'scoring' of body fat has for long been a popular way of assessing the condition of wild birds (Brown, 1996) but there are many variables in obtaining such data in the field and doubts as to the relevance of a fat score to a bird's status. Nevertheless, those working with live or (especially) dead raptors should be aware of the possible importance of at least attempting to quantify fat and of recording such data.

Obesity can lead, or contribute, to a whole range of health problems. Chief amongst these are hepatic lipidosis, atheromatosis (see under 'Cardiovascular conditions'), reproductive disturbances and bumblefoot (see Chapter 8).

The cause of obesity is usually excessive food intake (especially high fat/energy diets), coupled with a failure to utilise the food by (for example) exercise or thermoregulation. Endocrinological disturbances, such as thyroid dysfunction, might play a part and some captive-bred birds may begin to show a genetic predisposition to fat deposition as is the case with domestic fowls (Leclerq & Whitehead, 1988).

Hepatic lipidosis (excessive fat deposition in the liver) (Plate 22) may be suspected on the basis of radiography or ultrasonography but for confirmation requires biopsy. Some fat storage in the liver can be 'normal' in birds of prey but large quantities of intracellular lipid with nuclear changes in hepatocytes, or (sometimes) accompanied by inflammation, are pathological (Wadsworth *et al.*, 1984). A system of scoring hepatic lipid has been put forward for reptiles (Divers & Cooper, 2000) and may be applicable in part to birds.

Treatment of obesity and its sequelae necessitates a gradual reduction in weight, brought about by dietary changes and exercise. Regular weighing is vital and care must be taken to avoid sudden demands on energy since the bird may not be able to meet these.

FEATHER CONDITIONS

Feathers are a unique feature of the class Aves and proper maintenance of plumage is generally vital to the health and welfare of raptorial birds. Normal preening behaviour is important in the maintenance of plumage. Preening is a combination of physical and chemical attention to feathers. A bird with impaired use of its head or a damaged beak, or even poorly coped talons (see Chapter 8) may be unable to maintain its feathers properly. Chemical care depends upon the production and application of preen oil – a reason why inspection of the uropygial gland is a vital part of clinical examination (discussed in more detail later in this section) and why preen gland abnormalities should be investigated and reported (Cooper, 1996b).

Abnormal changes in colour of plumage may or may not be significant. Many raptors have different colour forms and plumage changes occur with age and wear. Nutritional deficiencies may be responsible for some abnormal coloration, as might infective agents. Albinism sometimes occurs (Plate 1) and is generally of little importance in terms of health. However, I take note when more than one case is seen – for example, when Roger Clarke (pers. comm.) reported partially white young marsh harriers in some locations – because colour change can be a sign of disease, including (in psittacines) certain viral infections. Some colour changes are artificial: for example, rufous coloration on the feathers of bearded vultures was shown to be due to deposits of iron oxide (Brown & Bruton, 1991). It was suggested that the iron oxide, which is spread by preening, assists with camouflage, reduces wear and 'probably helps control ectoparasites'.

Dark (melanic) keratin has mechanical properties that makes it more resistant to damage than is pale (nonmelanic) keratin and this can be reflected in feather wear and damage (Bonser, 1996).

Supernumerary primary feathers and retrices are not common but occur occasionally and are probably a selective disadvantage: Clark *et al.* (1988) reported 17 instances in 11 000 migrating raptors in Israel and the USA.

Feather abnormalities can be particularly significant in free-living birds where any impairment of flight might prove fatal. In captivity plumage disorders are a particular cause of concern to the falconer whose bird's performance may depend on the state of its plumage. Such conditions are of less importance in aviary birds, but traumatic injuries, such as damaged wing and tail feathers, are usually much more common in the latter. In addition, breeding birds may damage one another's plumage during courtship.

In addition to sometimes being pecked by their companions, raptors may pluck themselves, possibly on account of 'boredom' or lack of stimulation. Chitty (2000b) described one such case, in a 'perlin' (peregrine × merlin) that also had a split keel.

Experienced and conscientious falconers are usually knowledgeable about the care of a bird's plumage. Bent feathers are straightened by immersion in warm water. Broken feathers are mended by 'imping' on a new piece of feather and this technique has been described by many authors throughout the years, for example Blaine (1936), Cooper (1968a) and Woodford (1960). The word 'imp' is one of many falconry terms used by Shakespeare, for example in Richard II:

'If, then, we shall shake off our slavish yoke
Imp out our drooping country's broken
wing . . .'

The technique can also be used to advantage by those who wish to return a casualty or captive-bred bird to the wild and who are reluctant to wait until the next moult before being able to give the bird exercise. Imping of feathers is facilitated by the use of light anaesthesia. Falconry books provide advice on imping and the technique is illustrated in more technical texts by Heidenreich (1997) and Redig and Ackermann (2000). A detailed account of the imping of a casualty black vulture, using the feathers of a turkey vulture, was given by Lahr and Lorah (2000): the bird was successfully returned to the wild.

Injury to a wing can result in the production of feathers of poor quality which may be misshapen; this is a common sequel to a number of conditions, including 'wing tip oedema' (WTO) (discussed later in this chapter) and bursitis of the carpus ('blain'), which is discussed in Chapter 5. Skin granulomas can have the same effect. There is no remedy other than to wait until the next moult during which time the tissues will, hopefully, have healed. Sometimes one feather is damaged, for example by striking a projecting object in the mews, and as a result it protrudes at an angle. It can be attached to the adjacent feathers with a stitch but the latter must be removed in time for the moult. Alternatively there may be follicular damage, which may necessitate surgical removal or ablation.

The plumage of a raptor, captive or free-living, may be damaged by oil (see also Chapter 10). In the past, it has been assumed that this does not occur on a large scale but Clark and Gorney (1987) reported oil-based asphalt on 55 birds of nine species out of 1052 captured on migration in Israel. They argued that more than 100 000 raptors may be contaminated with oil every year in the Red Sea area.

The standard treatment for oiled raptors has usually been application of a warm solution of washing-up liquid, repeated if necessary, and followed by rinsing and drying (Croxall, 1979; Robinson, 2000). Industrial products may be more suitable for heavily oiled cases. It is imperative that oil victims are kept warm and not permitted to ingest the oil – for example, by the use of a collar to prevent preening.

Wilson (1976) reported the oiling of a trained hawk by fulmar oil, and Clarke (1977) suggested that oiling by fulmars (*Fulmarus glacialis*) might even be a significant cause of mortality in free-living peregrines. Further evidence as to the effect of fulmar oil on peregrines was presented by Mearns (1983) while Miller-Mundy (1984) described the clinical treatment of a golden eagle (which had been found heavily oiled) using eucalyptus oil and dish-washing soap. However, fulmar oil is very viscous and not always easy to remove, even using warm water under high pressure. An alternative strategy is to use butter, which must be worked into the plumage and then removed – hopefully with some of the fulmar oil.

Biting lice and mites (see Chapter 7) can cause mechanical damage to feathers giving a typically moth-eaten appearance (Fig. 13.1); the eggs or 'nits' of lice may also be seen on the feather barbs. The condition is easily diagnosed and treated. Care must be taken not to incriminate these or other parasites when *dropped* feathers are found to be infested. The culprits in such cases are almost invariably non-pathogenic and may even include clothes moths (*Tinea* spp.).

Inflammation of the base of the feather, folliculitis, is often seen, and can be either primary or secondary to trauma. The characteristic feature on histological or electronmicroscopical examination is an infiltration of inflammatory cells (Fig. 13.2).

Less straightforward are non-specific conditions

of the feather that result in poor feather growth and, often, breakage. They can impair flight and/or appear unsightly. The best known are the bands of weakness termed 'hunger traces', 'fret marks' or 'fault bars'. These defects in the feather are particularly common in young birds reared in captivity and are also seen in free-living birds of prey. My own scanning electronmicroscopy studies (Cooper *et al.*, 1989) confirmed that the lesions are characterised by poorly formed or missing areas of barb (Fig. 13.3). The conventional wisdom is that these lesions are 'stress marks' associated with an interruption in the normal flow of nutrients to a feather (or feathers) during growth. There is ample evidence that they can follow periods of reduced food intake and/or other stressors including (in captivity) a change of environment or (in the wild) a period of inclement weather. Whether, however, these other factors are *per se* a cause, or perhaps result in reduced intake or absorption of nutrients that then affects

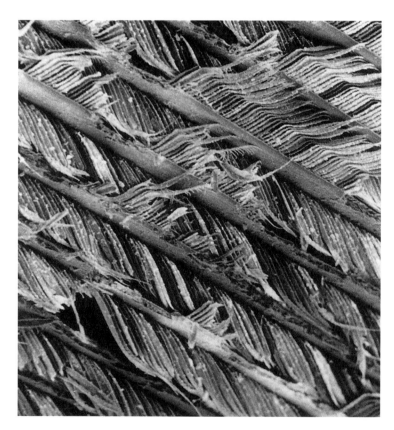

Fig. 13.1 Damage to feathers caused by mites. The barbules have a ragged appearance (SEM × 60).

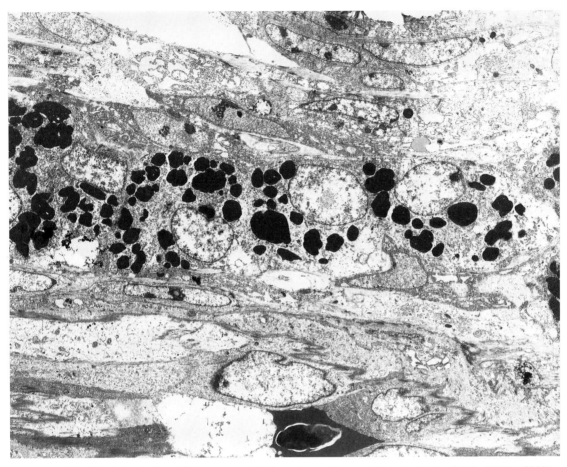

Fig. 13.2 Folliculitis. A band of acute inflammatory cells (granulocytes) is seen within the feather follicle (TEM × 5100).

the growing feather, is not clear. Nor, indeed, is the underlying pathogenesis of poor keratin production, although work on galliform and psittacine species would suggest an effect on follicular epithelial turnover. Malley and Whitbread (1996) gave injury, illness and administration of corticosteroids as alternative causes of 'fret marks' but provided no supporting evidence. The area is ripe for research.

Various other defects occur in raptors and SEM will demonstrate abnormalities that can relate specifically to the barbs and barbules (Fig. 13.4) or to differentiation of keratinous structures (Fig. 13.5a,b).

We still do not know for certain the aetiology of the condition that I christened 'pinching off', where the young vascularised feathers fall out prematurely and on examination are found to have a marked con-

striction at the base of the shaft (Plate 24). Heidenreich (1997) attributed it to quill mites (*Harpyrhynchus* spp.). Viruses might be involved – as in psittacine birds – but no such evidence appears yet to have been published.

There is no treatment for these syndromes other than to wait for new feathers to grow; removal of affected tail feathers will initiate rapid replacement but primaries will usually not develop until the next moult.

A number of other conditions may also be encountered, the aetiology of which remains obscure. More detailed study is needed – as has been carried out in recent years on psittacine birds. Some of these conditions involve the whole feather, others only the shaft or barbs. Individual birds or whole

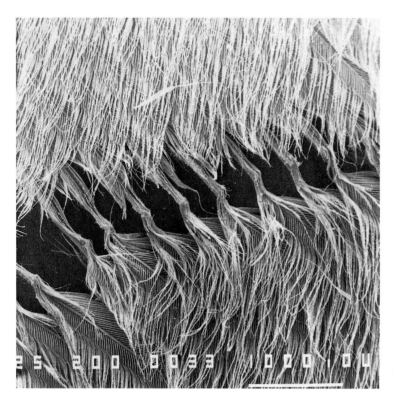

Fig. 13.3 Scanning electronmi-croscopy (SEM) of feather of a common kestrel, showing a well defined band of poor keratinisation, characteristic of a 'fret mark' ('hunger trace'). (SEM ×200)

collections may be involved – suggesting either an infectious aetiology or an underlying management or nutritional problem. I investigated a 'bald thigh syndrome' at one establishment where several birds had lost feathers from the medial surface of the legs. No parasites were seen in scrapings or skin sections and there was no improvement following a dietary change from day-old chicks. The condition eventually resolved spontaneously and no diagnosis was ever made. Other conditions reported by falconers and breeders include a dulling of the plumage with loss of portions of keratin – mainly in juvenile falcons – and this has the appearance of being an infectious and contagious condition.

A feather folliculoma in a barn owl was described by Frasca *et al.* (1999) who claimed: 'This neoplasm has not previously been reported in owls'. In fact their histological description fitted that of hypopteronosis cystica (a 'feather cyst') which I have seen in individual owls and believe to be a developmental/genetic abnormality, as it is in cage birds.

An aspect of the normal flora that has attracted

relatively little attention is that concerning the feathers. Pérez *et al.* (1994) carried out a bacteriological study of the feathers and lice of the common buzzard and suggested that the finding of, e.g. *Staphylococcus hominis* added weight to the theory that humans could contaminate raptors – originally postulated by Cooper and Needham (1976). Chitty (2000b) described a bacterial folliculitis in a merlin × peregrine hybrid and I have diagnosed similar cases, sometimes associated with staphylococci.

It seems very likely that viral infections may affect the plumage, as is the case in psittacine birds, and polyoma has recently been reported in raptors (see Chapter 6).

The plumage can influence or be involved in a whole range of diseases, from ectoparasites to electrocution, and in many respects serves as an indicator of health. Even poisons may be affected by the moult: Spalding *et al.* (2000a) showed that young egrets were initially protected from the adverse effects of methyl mercury because the chemical was deposited in the feathers.

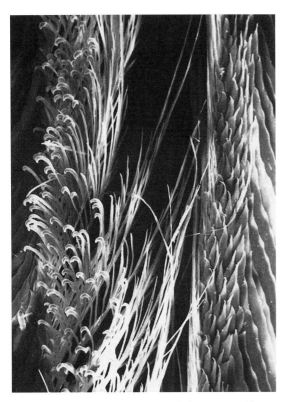

Fig. 13.4 An abnormality of the barbules, on one side only, in a golden eagle. The cause of this condition is unknown (SEM × 150).

Some early cases of feather abnormality appeared to respond to dietary additions of hydrolysed feather meal – a protein supplement used in poultry (Daghir, 1975). A number of agents have been recommended (and used) to treat areas of feather loss in psittacine birds and some of these should perhaps be tried in raptors. Products are available on the market which, it is claimed, will improve the skin and plumage of birds and these usually contain vitamins, minerals (especially zinc) and polyunsaturated fatty acids. An important point to remember in the investigation and treatment of any feather condition is that one is examining lesions which reflect an abnormal situation many weeks or months previously, when the feather was growing. The feather itself is a dead keratinous structure.

Investigation of feather conditions necessitates a full clinical examination as well as specific investigation of feathers and preen (uropygial) gland. A healthy gland is usually firm to the touch and not painful. If it is functioning properly the small feathers around the external orifice appear slightly oily or liquid oil can be extruded by squeezing. A nonfunctional uropygial gland can affect the appearance and health of the plumage but may also have an adverse effect on vitamin D3 intake (Forbes & Flint, 2000).

Assessment of the moult is an important part of clinical examination of birds with feather problems. Although some species, such as African vultures, shed feathers continuously, and a few, such as the steppe eagle, exhibit a bizarre ('chaotic') pattern (Herremans, 2000), the normal moult in birds of prey is annual and lasts between 5 and 7 months. In the Northern Hemisphere it commences in the late spring or summer and the feathers are generally dropped in sequence. As can be imagined, the moult can pose particular problems for the practising falconer if it is delayed or prolonged as birds should not be flown until their plumage is complete.

Factors affecting normal moulting patterns include photoperiod, temperature, nutrition, stressors (Spearman & Hardy, 1985), egg-laying, disease and administration of medicinal agents.

Feather development and plumage type are closely linked to thyroid activity (Parkes & Selye, 1937) and moult can be induced in most species by the use of oral thyroxine. Voitkevich (1966) pioneered early studies on the moult; he discussed the use of thyroxine and referred to experimental work with pigeons which showed that a large single dose had less deleterious effects than several small doses, which tended to cause weight loss. I have never encountered any obvious side effects associated with the use of small (daily) quantities of thyroxine but, until controlled trials have been carried out, I would urge caution in its use. The treatment should certainly be stopped if there is any evidence of excessive feather loss, marked drop in weight, palpitation of the heart or hyperaesthesia (Arnall & Keymer, 1975). Redig and Ackermann (2000) reported the use of 15 g/kg per day for 3–5 days of 'unadulterated thyroid gland of bovine, porcine or ovine origin'.

Other drugs have been recommended by a

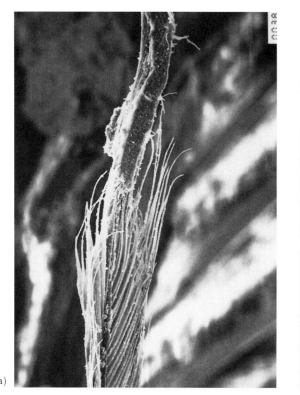

(a)

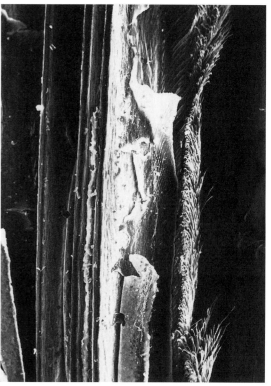

(b)

Fig. 13.5 Two examples of abnormalities of keratinisation: (a) (SEM × 300); (b) (SEM × 50). The cause is unknown.

number of authors, amongst them Beebe (1976), who advocated the use of progesterone; I have no personal experience of such.

Although an irregular or slow moult can pose problems to a falconer, the use of drugs to 'hasten the moult' should be undertaken with caution. Use might instead be made of changing the lighting pattern as suggested by Lawson and Kittle (1970); controlled studies are needed on this subject. Progression of a moult may be retarded when the bird is treated, especially, with corticosteroids, and it may be necessary to bear this in mind with falconers' birds in the summer and autumn. Woodford (1960) reported that hawks moulted faster if kept warm and this appears to be correct. I have encountered a premature moult (early spring) in birds that have been kept indoors, in the warm, during the winter.

It will be apparent that the whole question of feather development is a complex one. There have been no detailed investigations reported into condi-

tions affecting the plumage of raptors and yet such a study, which would be 'minimally invasive', since much of it would involve the collection of dropped feathers, could yield much valuable information. Voitkevich's monograph *The Feathers and Plumage of Birds* (1966) gave an excellent introduction to the subject of feather growth and development, and referred to work, including experimental studies, in raptors: there is a need for this to be followed up.

SKIN DISEASES

These are covered under various headings elsewhere in the book. A useful resumé of diseases of the integument of raptors was provided by Malley and Whitbread (1996) while skin diseases of birds in general were discussed in André (1999). Neoplasms of the integument were amongst those reviewed by Forbes *et al.* (2000a).

WING TIP OEDEMA (WTO)

This syndrome has been recognised for about 15 years. A useful key reference is Simpson (1996). WTO is characterised by the sudden onset of pitting oedema of one or both carpi – vesicular protrusions can be seen and these contain a clear exudate that surrounds the follicles of the primary feathers. The swelling subsides but in some cases the wing tip becomes dark and ischaemic: it will then be sloughed, 4–8 weeks after the first appearance of clinical signs. The cause of WTO is uncertain but its appearance (in Britain, at any rate) in the colder months of autumn and winter has led to the hypothesis that it is associated with frost and/or damp conditions (see Chapter 5). Both the gross features and histological findings (oedema, acute inflammatory reaction, sometimes a granulocytic vasculitis) suggest that the pathogenesis is a peripheral vasoconstriction and a vascular necrosis.

Treatment of WTO consists of applying warmth and encouraging blood circulation using massage and gentle exercise. Corticosteroids may help to reduce swelling and antibiotics will discourage infection. Simpson (1996) advocated vascular stimulants such as isoxoprine and propentofylline.

Prevention is based upon avoiding exposure to damp and cold: a useful rule for falconers is not to let their birds bathe after midday in the autumn and winter because they might not dry out before dark.

MUSCULO-SKELETAL CONDITIONS

Many of the conditions affecting the musculature and skeleton have been described elsewhere in this book (see, in particular, Chapters 5 and 10). However, others are recognised. Care must always be taken not to confuse normal, if unusual, anatomical features with musculo-skeletal disease – for example, the 'double-jointedness' (pronounced antero-posterior rotation) of the intertarsal joint of the African harrier-hawk (Cooper, 1980b). A knowledge of normality is always important in diagnosis.

Both acute and chronic inflammatory lesions of the muscles may follow irritant injections and bacterial infections. Traumatic injuries to the muscles can cause myofibrillar degeneration and chronic inflammatory cell infiltration. I studied this in pigeons and starlings and the findings appear to be applicable to raptors (see Chapter 4).

Inflammatory and neoplastic lesions involving bones and muscles can influence locomotion. Careful investigation of birds with unusual gait, flight or behaviour (e.g. only localised preening) is essential.

Clinical signs that probably relate to the musculo-skeletal system are not uncommon in birds of prey. For example there is a syndrome resembling rheumatism which is seen particularly in older birds. This condition appears to bear no relationship to hypocalcaemia or other nutritional diseases. One or both legs are stiff and may be unwilling to bear weight. There is no palpable swelling and usually no lesions on radiography. The condition may resolve spontaneously, often to recur later. Some birds thus affected also show intermittent signs of collapse, resembling a 'stroke', suggesting that this could be a disease of old age and possibly associated with the cardiovascular system.

'Cramp' is a disease of young birds that has been recognised by falconers for a long time. Cox and Lascelles in *Coursing and Falconry* (1892), stated that:

> 'Hawks that are taken too young from the nest or that have been much exposed to cold when taken are sometimes seized with *cramp* in the legs; this will completely paralyse the limbs and render the bird useless.'

Unfortunately the term 'cramp' probably refers to a number of different disorders, all of which are manifested by stiffness or paralysis of limbs. Hypocalcaemia is probably the most common cause. Salvin and Brodrick in 1855 described cramp as 'the most fatal of all the diseases to which Hawks are subject' and referred to it as 'Tetanus' in parentheses. Blaine (1936) stated that:

> 'Cramp frequently attacks young peregrines taken from the nest at too early a stage. The attack may be so violent as to break the leg bones.'

These and other examples would add weight to a diagnosis of hypocalcaemia. The term cramp is still sometimes used by some falconers but in many of these cases the cause is probably not hypocalcaemia.

Woodford (1960) grouped cramp and paralysis together and, amongst other things, postulated that fowl paralysis (Marek's disease) or a neuritis might be involved in their aetiology. He suggested that the disease might be prevented by keeping young birds warm and dry and feeding a diet of birds and mammals. Hurrell (1967) used the word cramp when he reported a juvenile sparrow-hawk 'with tightly clenched feet and flexed legs, unable to stand or feed, and supporting herself on outstretched wings'. The bird recovered following the administration of calcium, vitamin D, prednisolone and chlordiazepoxide but, as with so many cases, one does not know which, if any, of these drugs played a part in recovery.

My own view is that the term 'cramp' should be avoided. It probably covers many syndromes and it is far preferable to describe the bird's clinical signs and, using appropriate tests, to try to relate them to a particular organ system or systems.

Articular gout is seen in captive birds of prey, especially affecting the feet. Siller (1981) discussed its pathology and emphasised the importance of differentiating it, in terms of pathogenesis as well as location, from visceral gout (which he preferred to call 'visceral urate deposition'). The latter is discussed in more detail later in this chapter.

Tendon damage is mentioned in Chapter 8 as a possible sequel to bumblefoot and in Chapter 5 in terms of treatment. Halliwell (1967) discussed this in some detail and illustrated his paper with drawings of the foot. He emphasised how easily the flexor tendons of the digits can be stretched or torn.

Damage to the keel occurs frequently, especially if a bird is recumbent. Distortion of the keel is also sometimes seen, clinically or *post mortem*, in raptors with no such history – possibly genetic, congenital, or due to earlier skeletal disease.

Studies on musculo-skeletal disorders in birds of prey have been greatly facilitated by the use of improved diagnostic aids such as electromyography (EMG) and by a better understanding of the significance of blood biochemical (enzyme) values.

Electron-microscopical examination of biopsies and *post-mortem* material can also yield information, but sometimes the significance is not clear (Fig. 13.6).

OCULAR CONDITIONS

The eyes of birds of prey play an extremely important part in the detection and capture of their quarry. In captivity the situation may be different but impaired vision can still have a significant effect on the health and welfare of the bird. Ocular defects are an important consideration in the return of casualty birds to the wild.

In recent years there has been considerable interest in the vision of raptors, both in captivity and in the wild (Murphy *et al.*, 1982) and a number of veterinarians have contributed substantially to our understanding of ocular diseases.

In 1981 Greenwood and Barnett drew attention to the largely overlooked book *The Fundus Oculi of Birds* by Casey Wood (1917) and discussed the functional anatomy and clinical examination of the eyes of raptors. They described a number of conditions encountered in these species, many of them assumed to be traumatic in origin. Greenwood and Barnett's own observations bore out Wood's comment that many otherwise normal owls are affected with chorioretinitis: the cause is unknown but nutritional deficiencies and toxoplasmosis are possibly involved. Studies on the retinal structure of owls, using electroretinography, were carried out by Ault (1984).

It is of note that Wood had a particular interest in studying the vision of raptors as he believed that this could provide information of relevance to work with humans. As Paolo Zucca emphasises in Chapter 3, comparative studies using birds of prey can be important but are often overlooked.

The overall conclusion from studies such as those by Murphy (1993) is that the majority of eye lesions in raptors are traumatic in origin. However, there may be bias in the figures as many of the cases recorded were in raptor centres and involved birds injured by traffic or firearms.

While trauma is probably the most important

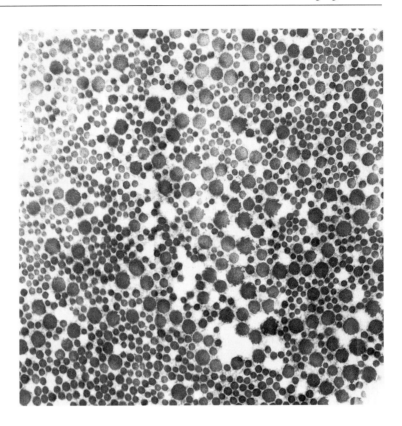

Fig. 13.6 Very little is known about connective tissue disorders in birds. This abnormal collagen was an incidental finding in a Barbary falcon (TEM × 45 000).

cause of ocular disease in raptors, a number of conditions due to other factors, or sometimes multifactorial, have been reported in both captive and free-living birds. A selection is described below.

Useful reviews were those of Murphy (1993), Williams (1994) and Boydell and Forbes (1996). Korbel (2000) discussed disorders of the posterior eye segment. Papers on specific cases include reports of bilateral keratopathy in a barred owl (Murphy *et al.*, 1981), retinal dysplasia in a prairie falcon (Dukes & Fox, 1983), Horner's syndrome in an African eagle owl (Williams & Cooper, 1994), endophthalmitis, glaucoma and scleral osside osteomyelitis in a great horned owl (MacLaren *et al.*, 1995) and the implantation of an intraocular silicone prosthesis, also in a great horned owl (Graham *et al.*, 1999).

Other than the work so long ago by Casey Wood, information on ocular disease in free-living raptors remains surprisingly patchy. The only epizootic involving the eyes of birds of prey that appears

to have been reported was by Raidal and Jaensch (2000) who described a seasonal condition in Nankeen kestrels characterised by central nervous system disease (see Chapter 9) and blindness. Inclusions in leucocytes resembled a *Leucytozoon* species.

Ophthalmological evaluation of raptors is now a specialised task and difficult cases should be referred to a colleague with the appropriate knowledge and experience. However, a basic examination is still an essential part of clinical practice. Thus Davidson (1997) included ophthalmoscopy in a list of general procedures conducted at admission. As elsewhere, a knowledge of the normal appearance of different structures is vital. Redig and Ackermann (2000) provided a useful table of 'parameters for physical examination' and listed such normal ocular features as a white non-inflamed conjunctiva, lacrimal ducts that are symmetrical, a cornea that is not oedematous and does not retain fluoreoscein dye, an iris that is normally pigmented and responsive to light, and an uninterrupted retinal pattern with a pecten in a normal position.

The ophthalmoscope should always be used in clinical examination but constriction of the pupil can render examination of the fundus difficult. Of more general value are tests on response to stimulation and pupillar reflexes when a pinpoint source of light is used in a darkened room.

Direct ophthalmoscopy is most often employed but indirect ophthalmoscopy has some practical advantages. Redig and Ackermann (2000) pointed out that if ocular examination is performed as part of a general examination, under general anaesthesia, no further mydriasis is required. Where this is not the case, topical non-depolarising muscle relaxants such as vecuronium can prove valuable in providing mydriasis in some species (Mikaelian *et al.*, 1994).

Korbel *et al.* (2000) investigated the use of fluorescein angiography (FAG) in raptors and suggested that the technique might help in the detection of 'subtle hemorrhages of the pecten and choroid, atrophy of vessels and the retinal pigment epithelium as well as retinal detachments and other diseases of the fundus'.

Infectious diseases affecting the conjunctiva and cornea are discussed in Chapter 6.

The eyes of raptors are prone to injury and such conditions as corneal ulceration and intra-ocular haemorrhage are common. Various forms of trauma are usually responsible. Surrounding structures may also be affected. The practice of 'seeling' the eyes of falcons by sewing their eyelids together is still sometimes carried out as an aid to training in the Middle East, and imported birds may be found to have small scars on their lids as a result.

Blindness can occur following a traumatic injury. Total blindness is usually relatively easy to diagnose on the basis of clinical signs and the total absence of a pupillary reflex. Partial loss of sight is less easily detected although slow or only partial pupillary reflexes and excessively dilated pupils are usually a feature. Examination of the internal chambers of the eye will sometimes reveal a blood clot and/or opacity. Visual function can be assessed in non-anaesthetised patients using a hand to (a) test the bird's ability to track movement and, (b) determine response to a threat. Redig and Ackermann (2000)

also advocated test-flying in a corridor with a perch at each end and testing each eye, in turn, by covering the other with a soft gauze pad.

Whether or not a captive bird could be deemed normal on ophthalmic examination very much exercised Casey Wood. After examining hundreds of eyes, he determined that many captive birds had posterior segment (chorioretinal) lesions. What effect these might have on visual acuity remains unclear.

The whole question of whether or not a totally blind raptor should be euthanased or, on the other hand, a partially sighted bird released, is a difficult one and opinions differ. The wider issue of assessment of birds prior to release or translocation is covered elsewhere.

Cataracts (Plate 25) were reported in birds of prey by Arnall and Keymer (1975) and were said to occur primarily in old age. In a survey of non-domesticated birds from the Zoological Society of London, Keymer (1977b) recorded more cataracts in the Falconiformes than in any order of birds but, interestingly, none was seen in the Strigiformes. They will possibly be reported more frequently now that birds of prey are living longer in captivity and because veterinarians are more aware of the need to examine the eyes of birds. Boydell and Forbes (1996) described lens opacity in raptors as a 'common finding'. Ocular opacity, which occurs often after traumatic injury, should not be mistaken for cataract; it usually involves disruption of the whole eye and the lens is not affected *per se*.

Neoplasms affecting the eye appear not to be common: Forbes *et al.* (2000a) reported only two cases, both melanomata. In one bird, enucleation was carried out.

The nematode *Cyathostoma* may be found in the orbit and adjacent locations (Simpson & Harris, 1992): it does not usually appear to be pathogenic but can possibly cause damage to the eyelid. Likewise, ticks and sticktight fleas can cause peri-orbital swelling, characterised by oedema and sometimes haemorrhage.

Treatment of ocular disorders can be medical or surgical, or a combination of both. Important conditions needing attention are corneal wounds (warranting surgical repair), penetrating wounds or inflammatory disease (requiring mydriasis, flushing and antimicrobial treatment), cataract (surgical removal) and severe chronic ophthalmic changes (enucleation).

Retinopathies will be detected by ophthalmoscopy but treatment is not usually feasible (Boydell & Forbes, 1996). Aguilar *et al.* (1993) reported surgical synechiotomy in a bald eagle.

The conical shape of many owls' eyes renders enucleation difficult but Murphy *et al.* (1983) reported a method that made use of the aural aperture, included in the lateral canthotomy, through which the eye could be removed.

There is very little information on diseases of the other special senses of birds of prey. Otitis is discussed in Chapter 6. Many veterinarians fail to examine (in some cases even to find) the ears of raptors. There has been considerable research on the hearing of owls, largely on account of the asymmetry of the organs (Norberg, 1977), some of it likely to provide useful groundwork for future studies on aural pathology.

CARDIOVASCULAR CONDITIONS

Cardiovascular conditions of raptors have been described, both in live birds and *post mortem* (Keymer, 1972). I have identified and reported elsewhere a number of clinical manifestations, amongst them an unusual case of circulatory failure in a redheaded merlin, endocarditis and hydropericardium. Oedema has often been seen, including pulmonary oedema associated with hydropericardium and oedema of the head and feet following mechanical obstruction. 'Shock', which can be due to impaired cardiac function, is discussed later.

As part of a *post-mortem* survey Dr Ariela Pomerance and I examined the hearts of many birds of prey, both macroscopically and histopathologically and devised what has proved to be a valuable way of sectioning hearts for both gross and histological examination – a transverse section across the great vessels and a longitudinal section through the whole heart (Cooper & Pomerance, 1982). Our findings included myofibrillar degeneration, focal myocarditis, atheromatosis, a thrombus in an epicardial vein

and pericarditis. In few of these was the lesion considered contributory to death and we were not able to associate them with clinical signs of disease. The exceptions were severe atheromatosis, which killed an eagle, and a hawk eagle, and an acute purulent pericarditis which, together with pneumonia, was considered the cause of death in a kestrel. Our findings suggest that while clinical signs of cardiovascular disease are either rare, or difficult to detect, in birds of prey, their occurrence in *post-mortem* material is not uncommon. Further work is needed to ascertain the significance of heart lesions in a clinical context.

Clinical investigation of cardiovascular conditions has been much facilitated by use of electrocardiography (ECG). A useful review was by Burtnick and Degernes (1993) who used ECG on 59 convalescing raptors: they obtained useful data on different species. Thirty years ago Wingfield and DeYoung (1972) employed ECG when treating eagles with orthopaedic conditions and also described the use of a Doppler flow probe to detect arterial blood flow. Lumeij, in his 1987 thesis, included a chapter on electrocardiography and although this dealt mainly with racing pigeons, it is relevant to raptors. Modern portable machines, especially those that can record rapid heartrate, are invaluable in work with birds of prey.

The cardiovascular system is sensitive to changes brought about by anaesthetic agents and a number of these have been investigated – for example, the effect of ketamine–xylazine (Raffe *et al.*, 1993).

The finding of arteriosclerosis and atheromatosis in raptors is not unexpected, these conditions having been first recorded over 50 years ago (Fox, 1920). Finlayson (1964) examined birds from the Zoological Society of London collection and found that there was a higher percentage of atherosclerosis in the Falconiformes than in any other Order. A number of raptors with arterial lesions, in some cases associated with myocardial degeneration, are included in the book *Comparative Atherosclerosis* (Roberts & Straus, 1965), including a free-living kite. Clinical diagnosis of such conditions is very difficult although the indications are that an overweight, under-exercised bird is most likely to be at risk. Typical atherosclerotic lesions are found at *post-mortem* examination (Plate 23) and, if the cause of death, are usually associated with pulmonary and visceral congestion.

Heart lesions may be due to other causes. Infections can result in pericarditis, epicarditis, myocarditis or endocarditis; although bacteria usually are involved, *Aspergillus fumigatus* will also produce such lesions. Sometimes focal myocarditis is seen on histopathological examination of birds that have died of other causes. In visceral gout the pericardium, and sometimes the epicardium, become coated with urates. Cardiac pathology can also be a feature of some poisons; for example Koeman *et al.* (1971) described changes in the muscle fibres of kestrels experimentally poisoned with a methyl mercury compound. Neoplasms can occasionally involve or originate from the heart: a rhabdomyosarcoma involving the myocardium of a vulture was amongst the series reviewed by Forbes *et al.* (2000a).

A condition known as 'apoplexy' has long been recognised in cagebirds and Arnall and Keymer (1975) described its possible aetiology. In a classical case the bird suddenly struggles, coughs up blood and dies within a minute. No treatment is likely to be of any avail and there are no obvious predisposing factors. In their book *Falconry in the British Isles* Salvin and Brodrick (1855) made the interesting observation that 'apoplexy' was 'fatal to nine-tenths of the merlins and sparrow-hawks trained every season'. Unfortunately they gave no description and it is possible that they were describing nervous 'fits' – but I personally doubt this since in the same book they also referred to 'epilepsy'.

A condition resembling 'stroke' is recognised in raptors, particularly old birds, and is probably cardiovascular in origin. The affected bird suddenly collapses or falls off its perch and shows weakness and incoordination. It usually recovers within a few hours (sometimes within minutes) but may remain partly paralysed or unsteady on its feet. Occasionally birds are comatose and die within 12 hours. Differential diagnoses include 'night fright' (see Chapter 5) and poisoning (see Chapter 10).

There are scattered reports of cardiovascular 'accidents' in birds of prey; for example, an owl died at the London Zoo from 'rupture of the left auricle and haemopericardium' (Hamerton, 1938, 1939). Green (1979) stated that acute cardiovascular failure may occur in birds if they are not able to adapt to stressors. Stress is discussed later on in this chapter under 'shock and stress'.

Embolism and thrombosis occur in birds and, as in other species, can follow trauma (see Chapter 5). Vasculitis can be a feature of many conditions and was, for example, seen in a central nervous system disease described in free-living Nankeen kestrels in Australia (Raidal & Jaensch, 2000).

Ischaemia of the feet or legs can occur following trauma or frostbite and is discussed in Chapter 5. In a paper on frostbite in captive birds Wallach and Flieg (1969) reported that some severely affected individuals developed valvular vegetative endocarditis.

URINARY TRACT CONDITIONS

Diseases of the urinary tract are not uncommon but in the past were often only diagnosed *post mortem*. It is of interest to note that as long ago as 1923 Fox found nephritis to be more common in the Falconiformes than in any other order of birds and there are many examples of renal disease in raptors in the Pathologists' Reports at the Zoological Society of London. A valuable overview of renal pathology was by Siller (1981).

There has been some work on diagnostic tests in birds, and blood uric acid values can now be readily measured, even on small quantities of blood. Lumeij (2000) wrote a useful review of renal physiology of birds of prey and emphasised that renal function disorders can usually only be diagnosed on blood analysis when 70% of kidney function is lost. Early diagnosis requires improved urine analysis, diagnostic imaging and biopsies.

The cloaca is a key anatomical feature of birds and is subject to a range of infectious and non-infectious diseases. It can harbour organisms, mainly microparasites, that may be transmitted to other birds during copulation (Poini & Wilkes, 2000). Impaction of the cloaca is seen, especially in birds that have been recumbent for some time, but the condition may also occur 'spontaneously'. Clinical signs include soiling of the vent region and the passing of blood in the mutes. Some cases may show paralysis of the legs. The largest cloacal calculus I have seen was 6 cm in diameter and consisted of uric acid and ammonium urate; it caused the death of a goshawk and histological examination revealed cloacitis and severe nephrosis. All cloacal calculi should be submitted for analysis; usually they consist of ammonium urate, which is a normal waste product in birds, but may contain traces of other minerals, such as apatite.

A diagnosis of a cloacal calculus may be confirmed by radiography or by digital exploration of the cloaca. For the latter, the finger, preferably in a finger stall, must be well lubricated with liquid paraffin (mineral oil) or surgical lubricant. Following such examination small calculi may be voided spontaneously; larger ones will need to be removed.

The pathogenesis of visceral gout remains unclear. Siller (1981) divided causes in the domestic fowl into (a) nephrotoxic, and (b) obstructive. Ward and Slaughter (1968) implicated an unbalanced diet as the cause of one case, in a Cooper's hawk. Wallach (1970) attributed both visceral and articular gout to an excess of dietary protein, and the role of this (and, incidentally, of starvation) in raising blood uric acid levels in chickens was demonstrated long ago by Okumura and Tasaki (1969). Halliwell *et al.* (1973) listed other possible causes including vitamin A deficiency and neoplasia and distinguished between primary uricaemia, where excess uric acid is produced, and secondary uricaemia due to impaired blood clearance by the kidneys. Deprivation of water is well recognised as a cause of visceral gout in reptiles and it is probable that a similar situation applies in birds. In this context it is important to remember that a raptor derives much of its water from its food and thus may become dehydrated if anorectic, especially if this is linked with fluid loss due to injury or exposure to high ambient temperatures.

There are no specific clinical signs in raptors with kidney disease or even visceral gout, although birds that drink excessively or have unusual droppings are suspect (see Appendix V). Lawton (2000) emphasised, however, the importance of careful inspection of the droppings during clinical examination. Renal endoscopy and biopsy are increasingly of use in diagnosis (Murray & Taylor, 1999).

Histopathological lesions are common in the kidneys of raptors but it can be difficult to be sure of their significance. Interstitial nephritis is seen relatively frequently in birds that have died of other causes but it may also be a primary condition. For example, a laughing falcon that I examined died of kidney disease associated with *E. coli*. On histological examination there was a severe interstitial nephritis in which eosinophils predominated. Other pathological lesions seen commonly in kidneys, although not necessarily a cause of death, include calcification, glomerular lesions, cystic dilatation of renal tubules and tubular degeneration.

Neoplasms involving the kidney have been described in raptors but Forbes *et al.* (2000a) suggested that one at least of these cases (Cooper, 1978b) was more likely to have been an adrenal tumour, with local or metastatic spread to both kidneys.

IMMUNOLOGICAL DISORDERS

Despite the prominent role played by the domestic fowl in our understanding of the immune response – particularly lymphocyte function – remarkably little information exists on normal and abnormal immune function in non-domesticated birds. Earlier texts alluded to conditions that might have an underlying immunological basis. Thus, Arnall (1969) listed 'allergy and anaphylaxis' amongst respiratory diseases of pigeons and he and Keymer (Arnall & Keymer, 1975) discussed the possible part played by allergy, anaphylaxis and hypersensitivity in cagebirds. In both publications, however, the absence of any reliable data on the subject is emphasised.

'Asthma' is occasionally seen, characterised by a short (less than 30 minute) period of dyspnoea or hyperpnoea that usually rapidly resolves. It may or may not have an immunological basis.

Surprisingly little progress has been made in our understanding of the immune process of birds of prey. Lawler and Redig (1984) examined the response to foreign red blood cells of the red-tailed hawk and great horned owl and Satterfield and O'Rourke (1981), Oaks (1993) and Remple and Al-Ashbal (1993) discussed the possible role of immune mechanisms in bumblefoot. In recent years it has become fashionable – perhaps with reason – to attribute 'new' diseases to impaired immunocompetence but the basis of such claims is often doubtful.

Evaluating immune function is not easy in wild animals (Kennedy-Stoskopf, 1997). The histological (and electronmicroscopical) appearance of lymphoid tissues may provide some clue – I have, for example, frequently seen lymphoid depletion in spleens and lymphoid necrosis in the bursa of Fabricius of raptors, often associated with intercurrent infections. Immunoglobulin assays, on blood, may also be helpful but, all in all, the subject is unresearched and needs attention.

Immune function in birds can be adversely influenced by many factors, including nutrition, intercurrent disease and 'stress'. Toxic chemicals can also exert an effect on the immune system of birds, even at sublethal levels (Spalding *et al.*, 2000a,b).

The role of humoral and cellular defence mechanisms in birds of prey may be very significant. For example, it has been suggested that the apparent failure of rabies virus to establish itself in birds may be due to the rapidity with which immunity develops, including antibodies bound to the central nervous system (Gough & Jorgensen, 1976). The work by Jorgenson *et al.* (1976) in which antibody titres to rabies virus in a great horned owl rose following corticosteroid administration would help to support this. Host–parasite relations play a key part in the health of birds (see Chapter 6) but much remains to be learned.

I have been unable to trace any substantiated records of truly immunological disease in birds of prey. However, if one includes reactions to foreign antigens (hypersensitivity) under this heading there are some conditions worthy of note. For example, unexplained swellings of the head, which usually resolve spontaneously within 48 hours, are probably due to bites of mosquitoes or other arthropods. Tick bites can produce severe oedema and haemorrhage, but not always (Forbes, 1993). Bee sting can kill birds of prey and is discussed in Chapter 6. Adverse reactions to drugs such as procaine, are covered in

Chapters 4 and 12. Havelka (1983) stated that birds of prey may be 'allergic' to metal rings but my own view, based upon examination of similar cases, is that the skin lesions associated with these rings are due to trauma.

There is a clear need for research into the role of allergy in birds and this may be hastened by a recent report (Colombini *et al.*, 2000) that described the development of a protocol for intradermal skin testing in parrots and recommends a site, volume of injection and optimal reading time for such tests.

I have not diagnosed anaphylactic shock in birds of prey. It could be a problem if the use of hyperimmune serum ever became prevalent, as suggested in the past (Cooper, 1975d).

Amyloid deposits are sometimes detected *post mortem* or when histological sections are stained with Congo red. McKinney (2000) reported an increased incidence of amyloidosis in falcons in the Middle East associated with chronic conditions such as bumblefoot, unresolved trichomoniasis and aspergillosis. He described a number of clinical signs – rapid weight loss with normal appetite, green discoloration of mutes, exercise intolerance and (interestingly) abnormal moult. Diagnosis is based on detection of elevated bile acid values and endoscopic detection of a green-tinged swollen liver with a wax-like appearance, followed by examination of a biopsy. McKinney concluded his article by suggesting that some low grade cases of amyloidosis may go undetected and that either liver biopsy or appropriate blood tests may need to form part of health monitoring of such birds in future.

NEOPLASIA

Until recently only a few neoplasms had been reported in birds of prey (Halliwell & Graham, 1978b: Cooper, 1978b, 1985b). Earlier reports, notably by Fox (1923), Jennings (1959), Blackmore (1965) and Keymer (1972), had contributed small numbers of cases. In the 1970s to 1980s the literature included a renal carcinoma in an augur buzzard (Wadsworth & Jones, 1980), an adenocarcinoma in a buzzard (Cooper, 1978b), a mixed cell tumour in a Seychelles kestrel (Cooper *et al.*, 1978), an oviduct adenocarcinoma in a Mauritius kestrel (Cooper, 1979c) and a mesothelioma in a ferruginous hawk (Cooper & Pugsley, 1984).

A mini-review in the 1990s (Cooper *et al.*, 1993b) included the announcement of a further four cases and the assumption continued that neoplasms were indeed rare in the Falconiformes and Strigiformes. However, following an extensive survey and questionnaire, Forbes *et al.* (2000a) were able to publish information on 122 neoplasms of 39 types in 44 species (93 falconiforms, 7 strigiforms). Sixty-eight per cent were captive, 32% in free-living birds. The authors emphasised the importance of histological examination by an experienced avian pathologist. A number of tumours in the series of Forbes *et al.* (2000a) are referred to elsewhere in this book.

Some lesions that may or may not be true neoplasms are discussed here. Papillomatosis is seen from time to time. I have removed proliferative lesions from the feet and eyelids of (falconiform) species which on histological examination have proved to be benign papillomata. Eyelid lesions in one such case occurred following severe traumatic damage to the bird's head in an aviary; hypertrophy of the cere was another feature of the case (see Chapter 4).

Some stomatitis lesions show marked epithelial proliferation with dysplastic changes but I do not believe that these are neoplastic; possibly they are associated with trauma or chronic inflammation.

Xanthomas and xanthogranulomata are not true neoplasms but sometimes masquerade as such. Thus, for example, a periosseous xanthogranuloma in a great horned owl was described by Raynor *et al.* (1999): the lesions consisted of firm swellings along the long bones and proliferation of periosseous tissues. Interestingly, the bird was free-living – a fledgling, taken to a rehabilitation centre. Other lesions may also be mistaken for neoplasms, at least initially. Stone *et al.* (1999) described synovial chondromatosis in 14 raptors, mainly owls, admitted over a 3-year period: these birds showed extensive joint lesions.

Neoplasms are far more prevalent in raptors than was previously thought. They are amongst the conditions that are likely to be recognised more frequently as birds are kept for longer in captivity.

Diagnosis depends upon prompt and detailed investigation of proliferative (and other) lesions that may be neoplastic (Plate 26) and this should include cytology and histopathology (see Chapter 4) as well as microbiology. Radiography is of value in both clinical and *post-mortem* cases; in the latter it can help to throw light on the extent and severity of the lesion (Fig. 13.7). Touch preparations of suspect lesions can sometimes provide a rapid diagnosis – and can be performed under practice conditions – but the choice of stain may influence accuracy as suggested by work on mammals (Magalhaes *et al.*, 2000). At the present time there is no one specific treatment for neoplasms: Forbes *et al.* (2000a) pointed out that much depends upon the location, identity and behaviour of the tumour. Treatment of neoplasms currently relies largely on surgery but chemotherapy and radiation therapy are gaining popularity and some apparently good results are reported. As Forbes *et al.* (2000a) stated 'this is a rapidly developing field'.

SHOCK AND STRESS

These two terms are listed here together because they are often confused.

The term 'shock' should really only be applied in cases where there are changes associated with circulatory (cardiovascular) failure, and the prevention and treatment of such conditions is discussed in Chapter 4.

Shock can result from a number of factors including trauma (especially physical damage which produces haemorrhage but also irradiation, electrocution and burning) certain infections which produce a septicaemia (e.g. pasteurellosis), infections which result in anaemia (e.g. malaria), cardiac damage and anaphylaxis. Less common causes of shock are severe pain, trauma to the peritoneum and other sensitive structures during surgery and certain drug toxicities. Dorrestein (2000) divided causes of shock in birds as follows: hypovolaemic, cardiogenic and vasogenic, but he stressed that the ultimate result of each was a circulatory compromise.

Shock produces its pathological effects by reducing the blood and oxygen supply to areas of the

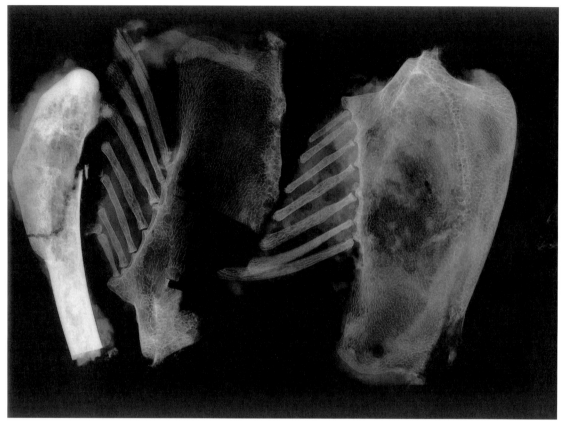

Fig. 13.7 Dissection and radiographic examination of lesions can assist in understanding the pathogenesis of disease. These tissues are from a ferruginous hawk that died from a mesothelioma: involvement of bone has resulted in a pathological fracture.

body. This effect may be produced by a reduction in the circulating blood volume, by direct action on the cardiovascular system by endotoxins or by cardiac damage. As a result cells die, metabolites are not removed and acidosis occurs. Shock also predisposes birds to disease and increases their susceptibility to chilling and freezing.

At *post-mortem* examination the carcass is dehydrated and there may be pulmonary congestion and oedema and, in some cases, a degree of hydropericardium. There may be anaemia (in the case of haemorrhage) or haemoconcentration.

The term 'stress' is one which is frequently quoted in work with wild animals but, like shock, is rarely carefully defined. 'Stressors' can cause 'stress' in an animal resulting in increased susceptibility to

disease or, in certain cases, death. According to Selye (1950) there is a 'general adaptation syndrome' (GAS) which evolves in response to stress, the three stages of the syndrome being the 'alarm reaction' the 'stage of resistance' and the 'stage of exhaustion'. All three stages can damage the body but the animal is usually able to overcome the alarm reaction and it is only when the stress is prolonged and severe that it may prove fatal.

Von Faber (1964) discussed the aetiology of stress in poultry and drew attention to the changes seen in the pituitary and adrenal glands, lymphoid tissues and blood. He listed a number of 'stressors' which may produce the general adaptation syndrome in poultry and these include fatigue, excess cold or heat, starvation, crowding or restraint. He also discussed the use of vitamins, antibiotics, hormones and tranquillisers in countering stress. There has been a considerable amount of subsequent work in the fowl, for example by Freeman (1976) and it appears that the first (alarm) stage is characterised by the release of such chemicals as glucagon, adrenaline and noradrenaline into the circulation. The adrenal cortex is stimulated via the hypothalamus and pituitary.

The significance of this to work with birds of prey is uncertain and far more research is needed. For example, what part might stress play in preventing apparently healthy birds from breeding in captivity? What role does it have in predisposition to such diseases as aspergillosis? Is it linked to immunosuppression? Can the response of a bird of prey to stressors be modified by the use of drugs, such as antibiotics, as has been suggested in the chicken? What effect does lack of stressors have? As Freeman and Manning (1976) pointed out, the subject is still little understood in the fowl, and it is likely to be a long time before we have much data on most non-domesticated birds. In the interim I think it is reasonable to assume that, while regular exposure to stressors is probably both normal and desirable, excess or prolonged stress in captive birds is likely to prove deleterious.

Diagnosis of stress is not easy. The temperament of some birds may suggest that in captivity they are 'stressed' but such behaviour can be normal for that species: one only has to observe the differences between, for example, a sparrow-hawk and a buzzard. Some clinical signs may indicate an inability to cope with stressors. In the case of free-living birds, non-invasive measurements of faecal steroids show promise as indicators of physiological stress – certainly in the Northern spotted owl (Wasser *et al.*, 1996). Care has to be taken when studying the influence of stressors in birds of prey: for example Al-Ankari (1998) warned, following research on the effect of blood sampling in saker falcons on plasma corticosterone, that progesterone measurements should be taken into account as the two were usually related. Hauska and Redig (1997) suggested that mild heterophilia without severe toxic changes and/or lymphopenia might indicate stress in raptors.

Practical recommendations for reducing stress include the avoidance of excess heat and cold, good management, adequate nutrition and prompt attention to disease. Unnecessary disturbance should be avoided and the construction of aviaries and other enclosures should take into consideration the species and temperament of the bird. For example, stress can be minimised by using higher aviaries and reducing unnecessary stimulation. In this respect one may have to strike a balance between disturbing the birds and a build-up of potential pathogens since regular cleaning of an aviary, while advisable in terms of disease prevention, may cause considerable disturbance to the inmates. Useful information about housing captive raptors was provided by Arent and Martell (1996) and Redig and Ackermann (2000) who included drawings of mews, breeding chambers and weathering areas. They and Heidenreich (1997) suggested minimum dimensions for such structures.

Green (1979) has pointed out that acute cardiovascular failure may occur in birds if they do not have time to adapt to the first (alarm) stage of the general adaptation syndrome. He emphasised the need to reduce trauma associated with anaesthesia, including careful positioning of the patient and 'neural shock' which may result from stretched nervous plexuses. These factors are discussed in more detail in Chapter 12.

Some birds appear to be suffering from 'stress' on account of a previous prolonged period of poor management, intercurrent disease or chronic injury. Such birds often have lustreless, brittle plumage, pale rather dry legs and fail to put on weight. Laboratory investigation may show a depressed PCV and/or haemoglobin values and both endo- and ectoparasite numbers may be higher than would be expected. Such birds show no obvious immediate response to treatment but will often gradually improve in condition following better management, a varied diet and vitamins. Some cases, however, continue to deteriorate and either die or have to be killed on humanitarian grounds. At *post-mortem* examination they appear in poor condition and are often anaemic, with varying degrees of hydropericardium. Histopathological examination sometimes reveals chronic inflammatory cell infiltration of the kidneys and liver but not, in my experience, other lesions that might help to support a diagnosis of stress.

The adrenal glands in some cases may appear enlarged *post mortem* and histological examinations have occasionally shown changes such as haemorrhage and excessive vacuolation of cortical cells. Further work is needed on this subject and reference ('normal') material is needed, as well as data on weights and measurements of adrenal glands. There has long been interest in the avian adrenal gland, for example, Chiasson *et al.* (1973) reported atrophy of the adrenal in poultry following the use of the anaesthetic agent ketamine hydrochloride. It is not known whether a similar situation applies in other birds.

Ulceration of the alimentary tract, which (if one extrapolates from mammals) may be associated with stress, is seen only rarely in birds of prey.

Other stress-related conditions are recognised. For example a rise in body temperature – so-called 'handling (stress) hyperthermia' – is a feature of certain avian species (Maloney & Gray, 1998). A condition which is equally relevant under 'Musculoskeletal conditions' is exertional rhabdomyolysis, also called 'capture myopathy', 'overstraining disease' and a variety of other terms. This is well recognised in mammals, but in birds it has mainly been diagnosed in flamingoes (Phoenicopteridae), where the clinical signs are leg paralysis following capture, and ducks (Anatidae), where affected birds go off their legs (Victoria Roberts, pers. comm.). The pathology of the condition is complex but is characterised by muscle necrosis and myoglobinuria. I have seen myofibrillar degeneration and myositis in birds of prey but not, so far as I am aware, changes that might be indicative of 'captive myopathy'.

Physiological assessment of rehabilitated birds prior to release is wise if stress-associated problems are to be minimised. Chaplin *et al.* (1993) used blood lactate values to assess fitness.

Clearly, much more is to be learned about stress in birds of prey. This could be a large and lengthy study. What are stressors to one species may not be so in another: as the *Lancet* (24 February 1990) pointed out, 'Investigators, however, have found no

way of coping with the fact that one man's stress is another man's stimulus'.

ENDOCRINAL CONDITIONS

There are relatively few endocrinological disturbances recognised in birds of prey other than inflammatory lesions, such as pancreatitis, and hyperparathyroidism associated with osteodystrophy. A few neoplasms have been reported – in thyroid and adrenal – and were included in the review by Forbes *et al.* (2000a). Possibly, as with other 'rare' conditions, some endocrinological diseases go unrecognised.

There has been interest in the avian pancreas since the 1890s and, as is mentioned in Chapter 12, the early work even included pancreatectomies in birds of prey. In contrast to other birds, this operation resulted in hyperglycaemia. Spontaneous diabetes mellitus was recorded in an adult red-tailed hawk by Wallner-Pendleton *et al.* (1993) who claimed that it was 'the first report of spontaneously occurring diabetes mellitus in a raptor': this may or may not be true (one would have to do a multilingual literature search to be sure) but I have certainly not diagnosed it myself. Pancreatic lesions were reported as a feature of chlamydiosis in a red-tailed hawk (Mirande *et al.*, 1992).

As was mentioned earlier, feather development is closely related to thyroid function and routine *post-mortem* examination of thyroid glands, especially from birds that clinically show poor or abnormal plumage, might prove rewarding. The only lesions of note that I have detected in the thyroid have been cysts which were possibly developmental in origin. Hamerton (1935) reported acute thyroiditis in an Eleonora's falcon.

The effect of photoperiod on raptors is related to the endocrine system. Birds kept at latitudes that are different from those in the wild, or under conditions of artificial lighting, may need extra illumination to encourage reproductive activity. It may be possible to induce extra breeding seasons by the use of appropriate lighting patterns; this might also influence the moult, as discussed earlier.

Lumeij (1987) included a chapter on endocrinology in his thesis and discussed, for example, the effect of adrenocorticotrophic hormone on plasma corticosterone concentrations and clinical evaluation of thyroid function. Lumeij primarily used racing pigeons in his studies but many of his findings are applicable to other species of bird.

PSYCHOLOGICAL DISTURBANCES

A useful early review of psychological disturbances in birds of prey was given by Jones (1981). In Chapter 3 Paolo Zucca discusses the importance of environmental stimulation and suggests that 'birds of prey have no less need of proper behavioural therapy than do other species'.

In recent years there has been great interest in ethology, the study of animal behaviour, and such research has extended to birds of prey. Particular interest has been shown in the behaviour patterns relating to courtship and breeding; valuable work has been done using captive falconiform and strigiform birds, together with studies on free-living species.

Imprinting has attracted particular attention and was first described in anseriform birds by Lorenz (1935). Imprinted birds are usually ones that have been hand-reared in isolation, away from the company of the same species; as a result they become imprinted on humans. Man is accepted first as a parent, then as a social companion and finally as a sexual partner. In the case of falcons, according to Redig and Ackermann (2000), hand-rearing up to about 7 days of age does not result in imprinting.

Some birds of prey remain imprinted for life but in other cases hand-reared birds have finally mated successfully with their own species. Imprinted birds can be used for artificial insemination, as described by Berry (1972) and Boyd *et al.* (1977). Imprinting can have profound effects, both positive and negative, on captive-breeding programmes and is very relevant to whether or not birds can be returned to the wild or retained for future propagation.

The whole subject is a complex one, which is perhaps not strictly within the realms of 'disease' but

is mentioned here since imprinting is, strictly, an aberration of normal behaviour that can have undesirable side effects. Recently there has been interest in alternative methods of rearing young birds so that they become imprinted but do not exhibit most of the undesirable traits of traditional imprints, such as aggression and screaming. Techniques for producing imprinted accipiters were described by McDermott (1998): his book should be read by all those with an interest in ethology as well as practising falconers.

There is need for more long-term research on the behaviour of captive birds of prey, especially those bred in captivity. It would be interesting to see what effect 'domestication' (captive breeding for several generations coupled with selection for certain traits) has had on behaviour. Similar work has already been performed on quail, chickens and ducks.

Differences in behaviour patterns have long been recognised by falconers, for example between birds taken as 'eyasses' (nestlings), 'haggards' (adults) and 'passagers' (subadults). An example is the description given of Beatrice in Shakespeare's *Much Ado about Nothing*:

'She is too disdainful.
I know her spirits are as coy and wild
as haggards of the rock.'

Likewise, different species vary in temperament and this is again referred to by Shakespeare (in *The Taming of the Shrew*)

'That is, to watch her, as we watch these kites
That bate, and beat, and will not be obedient.'

Changes in behaviour can be a useful early clue to the presence of disease. The failure of a falconer's bird to perform well is often the first indication of ill-health. Likewise, unexpected docility in a bird that is usually rather wild and unmanageable should be regarded with suspicion. This is why good record-keeping is so important and why investigation of perceived ill-health in raptors should be preceded by careful observation (see Chapter 4).

Variations in individual temperament are worthy of comment. While probably often due to genetic factors, poor management may be contributory. Some captive birds are extremely nervous and this may be reflected in 'shivering', poor feathering, damaged cere and rather loose mutes. Such birds are often difficult patients and, unlike those of a more placid nature – which will possibly even permit intramuscular injections to be administered while on the fist – will usually need to be cast for the most minor procedures. Temperament may well play an important part in predisposition to disease and must be borne in mind whenever case histories are considered. Highly-strung birds should be restrained as infrequently as possible since repeated contact with humans can reinforce 'neurotic' conditions. There is also the danger of injury during capture and a tendency to lose condition rapidly on account of excess physical activity.

One aspect of behaviour that appears to have attracted little interest in raptors is that of sleep. Work on the domestic fowl has shown that sleep in this species is closely related to the light/dark cycle and less clearly defined than in mammals (Howard, 1972) but there has been no detailed investigation of the role of sleep in the normal metabolism of the bird. Such studies could be of great interest in birds of prey, especially those used for falconry, whose performance might be influenced by disturbed rest. Hawks differ considerably in their tendency to sleep, some appearing to need to do so far more than others.

A number of behavioural disturbances have been noted in captive birds of prey, of which self-mutilation is perhaps the most significant. The disease 'aggresteyne' was first described in *The Boke of St Albans* (Berners, 1486) and undoubtedly referred to such mutilations (Fig. 13.8).

This condition is still occasionally seen. Some raptors peck their own or other birds' feathers (Chitty, 2000b) and, according to Malley and Whitbread (1996), Harris' hawks used for public display are particularly prone to this vice. Self-mutilation of digits and patagium also occurs. Some birds peck at sutures or at exposed wounds and in instances may damage themselves so badly that euthanasia is necessary. In milder cases the use of darkness (hooding or subdued light) or application of an 'Elizabethan collar' round the neck may prove an effective deterrent. Proprietary products, usually in the form of aerosols, are used to discourage feather pecking in poultry but I have no experience of their use in raptors – nor of behaviour-modifying drugs.

Interaction between raptors of the same or different species can also be an important problem. Some species are relatively peaceable while others will kill one another readily. There is tremendous variation between species and individuals and the degree of aggression may relate to different times of the year. Some species can usually be mixed but care must always be taken. Females may kill males, or less commonly, vice versa. If one of a pair has an old injury this may result in its being less able to fend for itself.

Prevention of fighting and aggression is based on

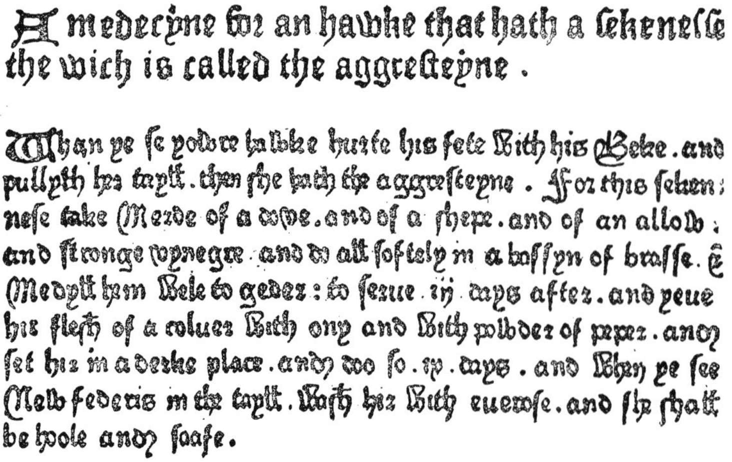
A medecyne for an hawke that hath a sekenesse the wich is called the aggresteyne.

When ye se youre hawke hurte his fete with his beke. and pullyth hys tayll. then she hath the aggresteyne. For this seken-nese take Merde of a cowe. and of a shepe. and of an allow; and stronge vynegre. and do all softely in a bassyn of brasse. & Medyll hym wele to geder: to serue .iij. dayes after. and yeue his flesh of a colver with ony and with powder of peper. and set hir in a derke place. and do so .ix. dayes. and when ye see New federis in the tayll. wash hir with euewyse. and she shall be hole and saafe.

Fig. 13.8 The 'aggrestyne', recognised in hawks trained for falconry, five hundred years ago. From the *Boke of St Albans* (1486).

managemental factors (see also Chapter 5). Whenever birds are kept together in an aviary there should be ample opportunity for them to avoid each other, especially by the provision of vegetation and other forms of cover. If one raptor is particularly aggressive it should not have another bird placed in its enclosure. An injured male bird should not normally be put with an intact female, which is larger. If mixing does have to be carried out the dominant bird should first be removed and only re-introduced 7–10 days after the newcomer. If there is any doubt about the response of a bird to others it should be introduced to them cautiously and kept under careful scrutiny. Other techniques that can be used include the initial tethering of a dominant bird in order to restrict its activity but this must be undertaken with great care.

The possible role of circadian rhythms should be mentioned. Daily cycles in body metabolism have already been recorded for raptors and can be related to their day or night-time activity (Gatehouse & Markham, 1970). Changes in circadian rhythm following, for example, disease or transportation may therefore result in behavioural abnormalities.

A feature of breeding behaviour is that some birds may appear clinically unwell; this particularly applies following copulation and prior to egg-laying when, as has been emphasised before (Cooper, 1977), a female bird may look ruffled and depressed, with eyes glazed or half-closed. The bird's abdomen can appear swollen and the mutes tend to be larger than normal. This combination of features has been termed 'egg-laying lethargy'.

The extent to which certain behavioural patterns are inbuilt is very relevant to the release of birds of prey. Thus, Bennett and Routh (2000), in a study of hand-reared tawny owls, were able to show that hunting in that species was instinctive and that young owls in their series did not appear to be at a disadvantage when compared with 'wild' juveniles. In their view the welfare of the birds was not compromised.

Avian behaviour is now a specialised subject and many veterinarians, especially in the USA (Welle, 2000) incorporate 'behavioural services' into their (mainly psittacine) avian practice. Whether this will be extended to raptors remains to be seen.

REPRODUCTIVE DISORDERS AND CAPTIVE-BREEDING

The great advances in captive-breeding, including artificial insemination, since the 1970s have led to the production of many species and interesting hybrids (Heidenreich, 1997) but have also resulted in concern over reproductive abnormalities, particularly the failure of some birds to breed in captivity. Interestingly, many hybrids are fertile and as a result second and third generation combinations have been produced. Heidenreich (1997) discussed this in some detail and provided a useful list of species and references.

A useful resumé of captive-breeding was presented by Redig and Ackermann (2000) while practical aspects were detailed by Weaver and Cade (1983) and Heidenreich (1997). Normal reproduction will not be discussed here.

With the developments in captive-breeding reproductive disorders are seen and recorded more frequently (Cooper, 1977, 1988). In an important early study, Keymer (1980) reported disorders of the female reproductive tract in 2 out of 41 falconiform birds and 4 out of 38 strigiforms: conditions seen were obstruction of oviduct or cloaca, oophoropathy and presence of a functional right ovary. The last of these is normal in many of the Falconiformes but not generally a feature of owls.

Egg material is not uncommonly passed *per cloacam* and may be associated with an infection of the reproductive tract. Cases of oviductitis and egg peritonitis have also been diagnosed *post mortem*, usually associated with *E. coli* or other Gram-negative bacteria, but in one interesting case, a rare Mauritius kestrel, a *Streptococcus* sp. was involved.

Egg-binding (impaction) can occur – an early report of this was of an eagle owl that died at the London Zoo (Hamerton, 1935) – and this must always be a differential diagnosis in birds that show abdominal discomfort or straining. Treatment should be as in smaller birds (see Appendix IX) – warmth, a lubricant such as liquid paraffin (mineral oil), and, if necessary, surgery.

A useful review of 'breeding problems' was provided by Best (1996). Failure to breed in captivity may be due to a number of factors, amongst them failure to sex the birds properly, incompatible pairs and birds that are too immature for breeding. Generally speaking, the larger the bird the slower its maturation. Best discussed the role of husbandry, behavioural abnormalities, skeletal and cloacal disease and ovarian/oviduct disorders in the failure of raptors to reproduce successfully.

Investigation of reproductive disorders can include laparoscopy and the taking of biopsies. Transcutaneous sonography can be used to detect pathological changes in gonads or kidneys and has the advantage of being both non-invasive and safe (Krautwald & Trinkhaus, 2000).

Whenever birds of prey are examined *post mortem* the size and activity of the gonads should be noted and histological sections prepared. Much remains to be learned about reproductive physiology in birds of prey and 'scoring' changes seen in histological sections, such as extent of pigmentation, spermatogenesis and seminiferous tubule : interstitium ratio, can help in building a database as well as in assessing individual cases. Occasionally an unusual lesion is noted in gonadal tissue; for example, the protozoon *Leucocytozoon* (Peirce & Cooper, 1977a).

Although not a 'disease', the accurate sexing of raptors is relevant to reproductive and behavioural health of captive birds and is sometimes required when working with free-living birds. In some species there is distinct sexual dimorphism in the plumage and no problem is likely to occur. In others, however, the only tangible difference may be one of size and here overlap can occur so that one is uncertain as to whether the bird in question is a large male or a small female!

A useful early review of the methods available for sexing was provided by Fry (1983): these included faecal steroid analysis (Czekala & Lasley, 1977; Stavy *et al.*, 1979). Subsequently many other techniques have been explored, with varying degrees of success, including ultrasonography (Hildebrandt *et al.*, 1995). Haematological and blood biochemical studies have not, generally, proved helpful in sex determination (Hoefle *et al.*, 2000).

Chromosomal investigation (karyotyping) has much to commend it and is relatively inexpensive (Stock & Worthen, 1980). However, at the time of writing such techniques are not readily available.

Exciting developments involving the use of polymerase chain reaction are leading to its use in, for example, Spanish imperial eagles (Griffiths *et al.*, 1996; Norris-Caneda & Elliott, 1998; Wink *et al.*, 1998; Hoefle *et al.*, 2000).

There is little doubt that minimally invasive methods will find increasing favour. In the meantime, sex determination by endoscopy (laparoscopy) remains a reliable and widely used technique although, being an invasive procedure, it is not without its critics. It has been used in one form or another for at least 60 years (see Chapter 12). Jones *et al.* (1984) reported on fibreoptic endoscopy in over 1000 birds of 144 different species, including 62 falconiform and 96 strigiform raptors. I have generally used either a human arthroscope or a rigid cystoscope, but in the field and in poorer countries where resources are limited I have found the American 'Focuscope' (Medical Diagnostic Services, USA) of value in sexing as well as being a useful diagnostic instrument.

Despite involving entry into the body cavity, laparoscopy is a relatively safe procedure: nearly 20 years ago Smith (1983) reported a death rate of only 0.4% in a series of over 2000 birds and now, especially with safer anaesthesia and more sophisticated light-weight instruments, the figure is probably even lower. The possibility that tissue damage associated with laparoscopy might cause problems in egg laying was raised by Frankenhuis and Kappert (1980) but does not appear to have been substantiated in practice.

More use might be made of cloacal examination in order to distinguish the different anatomy. Alternatively Hamerstrom and Skinner (1971) described 'cloacal sexing' of birds by inducing them to prolapse their cloaca. Ejaculation of semen will follow in the male and, with experience, this can be distinguished from urates. In the female prolapsing reveals the rosette-like opening to the oviduct. Unfortunately this technique also has to be carried out in the breeding season.

The possibility of venereal spread of disease has attracted little attention, although I have alluded to it as a possibility in previous editions of this book. A recent paper (Poini & Wilks, 2000) reviewed the sexual transmission of some pathogens in birds and, as a result of studies (in Australia) postulated that spread of organisms by mating *does* occur and may even be significant in terms of the success or otherwise of polygamy.

GENETIC AND DEVELOPMENTAL DISORDERS

There is an old Gaelic saying that 'All birds cannot be noble falcons, neither can all men be great men.' This serves as a useful reminder that there is inevitable biological variation between individuals of the same species. Those who study, keep, breed or train birds of prey should not assume that differences in size, plumage, temperament or ability are necessarily due to some organic disease. Nor should veterinary surgeons be tempted to try anabolic steroids or other 'growth promoting' drugs unless there is a clear clinical indication for such therapy.

Little is yet known of the genetics of birds of prey though it is to be hoped that the current intensive work on captive-breeding will result in greater understanding of the subject. In view of the shortage of breeding stock there has as yet been only limited opportunity for conscious selection of certain traits in birds of prey, but this will inevitably occur. It is important that the subject is approached scientifically if undesirable characteristics are not to be perpetuated, although it should be noted that considerable controversy exists as to whether one should select traits that are advantageous in the wild (such as fear of humans) or in captivity (such as tameness). The important consideration is, of course, whether offspring are to be released or retained, although even this is a gross over-simplification since many other factors also have to be taken into account.

Inbreeding may be of relevance to the conservation of raptors in the wild since, once a population is small, the inbreeding coefficient increases and, *inter alia*, susceptibility to disease may be enhanced. This may, for example, be the case with the Mauritius kestrel (Cooper *et al.*, 1981). The possible role of inbreeding in the 'fatty liver-kidney syndrome of merlins' (Cooper & Forbes, 1983; Forbes & Cooper, 1993) (Plate 22) is also of interest.

Insofar as developmental abnormalities are concerned, I have examined cases of hydrocephalus in captive-bred peregrines (Fig. 13.9) and received reports of a number of other conditions. Cade (1980) described a 'drooping alula' syndrome in captive-bred peregrines but this may have been nutritional rather than genetic in aetiology. Two cases of developmental abnormalities in birds in the wild in Britain have been reported (Cooper, 1984c) – a peregrine that had duplication of a hind toe, extra vestigial digits and unilateral bowing of radius and ulna (Fig. 13.10a,b), and a merlin with syndactyly – but others have gone unrecorded. The possibility of an increased incidence of such abnormalities because of the population 'bottle-neck' that occurred in raptors in Britain and elsewhere in the 1960s should be explored. In this context it should be noted that vestigial wing claws (see Chapter 3) are a feature of a few species including the great grey owl (Nero & Loch, 1984) and that supernumerary digits on the legs of a yellow-billed kite in Africa were described by Brooke (1975).

A short article in *The Times* (October 1981) reported a golden eagle with 'two pairs of claws on each leg' but I have been unable to trace any further information on this bird.

Fluctuating asymmetry (FA) – small deviations from morphological symmetry – can be a feature of inbreeding in birds as in other species (Brown,

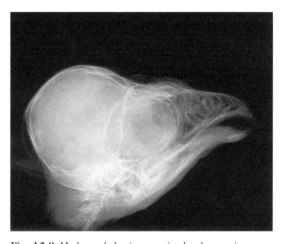

Fig. 13.9 Hydrocephalus in a captive-bred peregrine chick. Note the pronounced swelling of the skull.

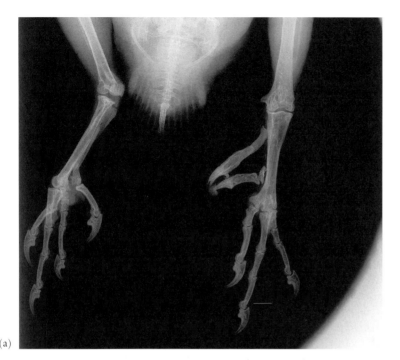

(a)

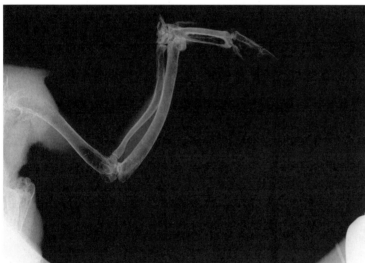

(b)

Fig. 13.10 Developmental abnormalities in a peregrine: (a) duplication of digit 1 on a foot; (b) excessive bowing of radius and ulna on one wing only.

1996). Recording of FA is important, whether dealing with live or dead birds and should become part of standard clinical and *post-mortem* procedures.

The hybridisation of species has been criticised in some circles and at the time of writing has prompted heated debate in falconry circles (Robinson, 1999; Webster, 1999) and in a Position Statement by the International Association for Falconry and Conservation of Birds of Prey (IAF, 2000). There are scientific arguments for the production of such hybrids in captivity in order to learn more of such subjects as behavioural genetics and taxonomy of the various species. Many hybrids are fertile and as a result second and third generation combinations have been produced (Heidenreich, 1997). Interestingly, there are suggestions that some diseases may be a result of hybridisation – a strange condition of the feathers in one bird about which I was recently consulted, for example – but as yet there appears to be no proof of this.

There is often confusion over the terminology used when discussing genetic and developmental abnormalities. The word 'genetic' implies some disturbance of the genes and this may be due to a mutation or to detrimental genes acquired from the parents at conception. A 'congenital' abnormality is one present at birth and it may or may not be genetic in origin. An 'inherited' disease is a genetic condition that is transmitted to a bird from one or both of its parents or, through them, from a previous ancestor; it may be passed to a subsequent generation. A 'developmental abnormality' is one that occurs during the process of growth and development and this includes the period within the egg. It will be apparent that there can be considerable overlap between the terms used above. For example, an owl that has no tail when it hatches from the egg has a congenital abnormality which is developmental in character. The condition may or may not be due to a genetic abnormality and if it is, the condition might or might not have been inherited.

There are still very few published data on abnormalities in birds of prey. Much work has been carried out on poultry, pigeons and (to a lesser extent) certain cagebirds and some of this is likely to prove relevant to raptors (Buckley, 1969).

Although plumage changes, such as albinism, melanism and erythrism are recognised in birds of prey (Brown & Amadon, 1968), other abnormalities are either rare or undiagnosed as mentioned under 'Endocrinal conditions'.

Lesions are not infrequently seen on histopathological examination that are probably developmental in origin, an example being fluid-filled cysts in the thyroid gland. Some clinical conditions also appear to be developmental – bent keels, for example – but whether they are genetic in origin is open to question.

Other congenital abnormalities in captive birds are reported verbally but, alas, are not documented nor is material submitted for professional examination. For example, in 1977 I was told that a pair of lanners had produced five youngsters, three of which were lacking a cloaca.

It is clearly important that abnormalities and traits noted in both free-living and captive-bred birds are fully documented.

EMBRYONIC DEATH AND PROBLEMS AFFECTING THE NESTLING ('NEONATAL DISEASES')

Developments in the captive-breeding of birds of prey opened up a whole new spectrum of problems and challenges. The subject was reviewed in a paper presented at the Second World Conference on Breeding Endangered Species in Captivity (Cooper, 1977). Captive-breeding of raptors has sometimes been described as an art, rather than a science, and it certainly seems to be true that some people have better results than others, even when using apparently identical methods.

In contrast to the situation three decades ago, captive-breeding is now an accepted and important aspect of raptor management that can contribute much to conservation and research. Indeed, Cade (1982) pointed out that the expertise now available in this field means that no raptor species need ever become extinct. However, despite the successes, problems remain – amongst them the diagnosis and treatment/prevention of so-called 'neonatal diseases'.

Despite extensive work on the embryology and causes of embryonic death in the domestic fowl and quail and certain other species, there is still little information on the subject in birds of prey. It is vital that those who breed birds of prey in captivity keep comprehensive records and submit unhatched eggs and dead chicks for *post-mortem* examination (*see* Chapter 4); only in this way will substantial progress be made. Studies on captive birds should be accompanied by research on free-living raptors: thus, for example, Houston *et al.* (1993) carried out an interesting and useful survey of unhatched eggs in raptor nests in Saskatchewan, Canada.

The pathological examination of eggs is of great importance (see Chapter 4 and Appendix III) and even apparently normal infertile eggs should be collected and stored for investigation so that baseline data on external appearance, size and thickness can be established (Plate 27). Methods of investigation of eggs were described earlier (1993c). Papers of relevance on raptor eggs include those by Jenkins (1984), Pattee *et al.* (1984) and Bird *et al.* (1984). The last of these described the normal embryonic development of the American kestrel and refers to similar work on the pariah kite by Desai and Malhotra (1980). There is no doubt that comparable studies are needed on many other raptor species. Until this is done interpretation of findings in eggs

which have failed to hatch will continue to prove difficult. Likewise, photographic records of the appearance of eggs that have been candled can be of great value in order to improve interpretation of changes during incubation (Delany *et al.*, 1999). Radiographic investigation of eggs prior to their being opened will also yield useful information that should be documented (Fig. 13.11).

Failure to hatch is common and is usually due to the eggs being infertile. Many factors can lead to infertility of the eggs as discussed in an early paper on the problems of captive breeding of birds of prey by Mendelssohn and Marder (1970). Amongst the factors involved are behavioural problems in the adults, such as imprinting or nervousness, which may result in a degree of courtship but not culminate in mating. The birds may be too young or too

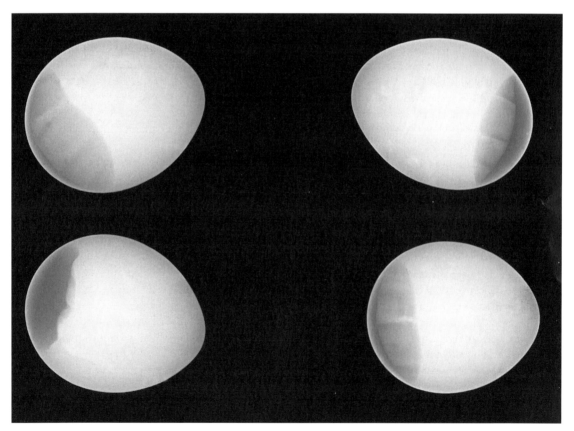

Fig. 13.11 Radiographic appearance of eggs of a peregrine. These are infertile and beginning to deteriorate: gas is visible. Such examination, coupled with candling, can be useful prior to opening eggs, especially in legal cases.

old. Alternatively, the aviary may be unsuitable or there is so much disturbance that mating never takes place. Birds may be physically incapable of copulating – for example, because of an injury. Conversely, the *absence* of humans may be responsible for the failure of partially imprinted birds to copulate.

These and other problems have been discussed by a number of authors. It is also possible that an individual bird is of low fertility or even sterile; this is often difficult to ascertain in view of the other factors which may have complicated the picture. However, it is not unreasonable to assume that a bird that has had a reproductive disorder, or is nutritionally deficient, or perhaps is a hybrid, may show reduced fertility.

Obesity is probably an important cause of poor fertility since many captive raptors are grossly overfed. It is also possible that excessive use of a male bird for breeding may lead to reduced fertility but I have been unable to trace any information on this in raptors. There has been some limited work on the onset and duration of fertility in female birds of prey; for example Berry (1972) and Bird and Buckland (1976) reported 4 and 8.1 days for goshawks and American kestrels respectively. Stimulation of sexual behaviour in the male prairie falcon was attempted by intramuscular injection of testosterone propionate (2.5–5.0 mg) (Boyd *et al.*, 1977) but in their discussion the authors questioned its value. Testosterone implants were subsequently used by others, including colleagues in Britain but the results were not always good and some male goshawks became sexually aggressive (N.H. Harcourt-Brown pers. comm.). Implants and injections did not appear to be effective in other species.

Various other factors can be involved in low fertility in galliform birds and are possible causes in birds of prey. Examples are poisons, unsatisfactory lighting patterns, lethal or sublethal genes, extremes of temperatures, use of certain drugs and poor artificial insemination techniques.

Examination of semen samples is discussed briefly in Chapter 4. Birds of low fertility may show sperm abnormalities, such as swollen heads or kinked tails, or the motility may be poor. The latter can be a feature of old samples and therefore a second specimen should be obtained and examined as soon as possible after collection.

Eggs are sometimes soft and abnormal in shape. It is important that such features are recorded since they may indicate disease or immaturity in the hen or be signs of an inadequate diet. Various factors may result in thin eggshells and some of these were discussed (as differential diagnoses for pesticide poisoning) by Ratcliffe (1970); more detailed data are available from poultry textbooks. The possible role of heat stress is mentioned in Chapter 5.

Fertile eggs may fail to hatch for a variety of reasons. They can be damaged by the hen bird or by rough handling. They may become infected with bacteria or fungi. There may be embryonic mortality on account of dietary deficiencies in the female bird (see Chapter 10). Most important of all, the eggs may become chilled on account of neglect by the hen bird or, more commonly, because the incubator is at fault. An incorrect temperature and/or relative humidity can easily result in embryonic death, and the latter is often a contributory factor in cases of 'dead-in-shell' (Plate 28). Genetic features probably also play a part in the failure of eggs to hatch but, as was emphasised earlier, information is lacking.

Infection of eggs may occur on account of poor hygiene in breeding quarters. Heintzelman (1971) discussed the possible role of bacteria-contaminated nestboxes in embryonic death of free-living and captive American kestrels, and Porter and Wiemeyer (1970) suggested that a number of organisms, amongst them *Proteus* spp., might cause such mortality. Far too little work has been done on this subject, another reason for ensuring that unhatched eggs are examined pathologically. Appendix VI lists some findings in eggs and their possible significance.

Prevention of the above problems is not easy, but some simple guidelines may help. Eggs should always be handled with extreme care so as not to damage the embryo or other contents. Hygiene is vital since pathogenic organisms may enter an egg through the pores in the shell. The use of protective clothing, especially gloves, is recommended and incubators should be fumigated between batches or at the end of a season. Incubator technique is particularly important and the novice is strongly advised to seek advice before embarking on artificial incubation of eggs. The hen bird which is sitting on eggs must be exposed to as little disturbance as possible.

Some eggs begin to hatch but the chick is unable to emerge and will, unless assisted, die in the shell. In such cases the relative humidity (which is often at fault) should be increased and careful efforts can be made to help remove the chick. Small portions of the shell should be chipped away until the chick is free but special care must be taken not to cause haemorrhage; if this occurs the procedure is being carried out too early. Incubation requirements depend upon the ecology of the bird, and the reader who requires further information on this subject is referred to the paper by Drent (1970). For example, some species such as the gyrfalcon, which nests where the ambient humidity is low, can tolerate a lower humidity than others. An oedematous chick or an unabsorbed yolk sac may be an indicator of too *high* a humidity although the latter is often also a manifestation of other managemental problems.

Although information on incubation and allied matters is gradually being amassed, those who breed raptors can still learn much from contact with the poultry industry. Many techniques for domestic birds – for instance hatchery hygiene methods – can be applied to birds of prey and publications such as *International Hatchery Practice* contain relevant articles and advice.

The newly hatched chick is susceptible to a number of diseases, many of which have been mentioned elsewhere in the book. 'Neonatology' is rapidly developing into a discipline in work with psittacine birds and a similar situation may evolve with raptors. A useful review of the husbandry of young raptors and the diseases to which they can succumb was provided by Butterworth and Harcourt-Brown (1996).

In the case of some infectious diseases the chick may be protected for a certain length of time by maternal antibodies acquired from its yolk sac; this might be an argument in future for the use of appropriate vaccines in breeding stock. Probiotics can also probably play a part in protecting chicks from pathogenic bacteria and, in theory at least, are preferable to the use of antibiotics: Forbes (1996b) recommended them for hand-reared birds of prey. The principles of 'competitive exclusion' are discussed (see Chapter 4) and were reviewed by Mead (2000).

Infectious diseases of importance in neonates include bacterial hepatitis and septicaemia. Older birds, especially merlins, may develop coccidiosis. These are all discussed elsewhere in the book.

It is particularly important to remember the young bird's susceptibility to hypothermia; it *must* be kept warm. It can be maintained at incubator temperature for the first 48 hours; thereafter it should be kept at a constant temperature of 32–35°C for the first week. As a general rule the larger the bird the lower the temperature needed but if in doubt it is best to adjust the temperature according to the reaction of the birds. Chicks that are too hot pant and those that are too cold appear hunched and shiver. Accommodation which provides a temperature gradient is probably best; the chick can then move to its preferred temperature.

Failure of retraction of the yolk sac can prove fatal. Small protrusions usually resolve spontaneously but larger ones may need amputation or surgical placement into the body cavity.

The chick is also prone to traumatic injuries, and greenstick fractures and subcutaneous emphysema commonly occur. Young chicks must be handled with the greatest care, especially when being weighed or examined.

Nutritional disorders can occur, ranging from an impacted crop or transient diarrhoea to osteodystrophy (Fig. 10.3). Hypoglycaemia will occur in young birds that do not receive food every few hours.

Confinement on a slippery surface may result in splayed legs which, without treatment, can lead to irreversible damage. The bird should be put on a rougher surface or in a bowl (padded) and a figure-of-eight bandage can be tied temporarily around the legs in order to adduct them.

Contact with other chicks and reducing the temperature to encourage huddling and reduce further splaying were recommended by Butterworth and Harcourt-Brown (1996).

The key to the hand-reared young bird is for it to be treated as an individual and given as much personal attention as possible so that problems can be either prevented or diagnosed and treated promptly.

Many of the problems associated with captive-breeding are related to health and veterinary care. Much remains to be learned and a vital part of this is that detailed records are kept. In this respect the requirement in Britain (under the Wildlife and Countryside Act, 1981) for certain captive raptors to be ringed and registered has meant that 'keepers' of such birds have been obliged to maintain records of their birds and breeding results. Some of these data are, already, being made available for scientific study. Computerised records have much to commend them – preferably using an internationally recognised database – and can have the added advantage of increased confidentiality. Whatever method is used, the plea made by Prestwich, in the preface to his book *Records of Birds of Prey Bred in Captivity* (1955) remains valid nearly half a century later:

'The compiler . . . would impress on breeders the importance of recording *all* their results in one of the recognised avicultural or ornithological journals.'

'NEW' INFECTIOUS DISEASES

As emphasised in Chapter 6, many pathogens and diseases of raptors are known today that were not recorded even two decades ago (Cooper, 1993a). Some probably existed but were not recognised. Others may, possibly, be truly 'new' diseases – for example, the presumptive virus that has been postulated as the cause of decline of vultures in India (Cunningham, 2000), and is discussed further in this section. Emerging diseases of wildlife present a substantial threat to biodiversity and human health (Daszak *et al.*, 2000), and those involving birds of prey may serve as important indicators of environmental change and/or spread of pathogens.

A key part of understanding 'emerging' diseases is to have reliable information about host:parasite relations and how these can be influenced by different factors. Remarkably few data exist on the host: parasite relations of birds of prey. Even the 'normal' flora and fauna of most raptorial species have not been studied: as Philips (2000) pointed out in a recent review, 'The mite fauna of most falconiform and strigiform species is completely unknown'. Until more information is available – on micro-parasites and macroparasites *and* on how raptors respond to them – biologists and veterinarians will continue to face difficulties in elucidating the causes of outbreaks of infectious disease in these birds.

At the time of writing a decline in vultures, mainly of the genus *Gyps*, especially in India but possibly also further afield, is attracting concern (Parry-Jones, 2001). Prakash (1999) working in the Keoladeo National Park, Bharatpur, Rajasthan, India reported a sharp decline over a decade – a drop of 96% in the population of white-backed vultures and 97% of long-billed vultures. Various causes have been postulated including a reduction in food supply, fewer nesting sites, increased homozygosity, calcium deficiency, pesticide or other poisoning and 'disease'. The last of these is taken to mean 'infectious disease' but no data were given by Prakash to support this claim and the clinical signs described could be non-specific: amongst his recommendations were that 'pathological studies should be initiated immediately'.

In a paper at the Pan African Ornithological Congress (PAOC) in Uganda, Virani *et al.* (2000) presented the hypothesis that an 'infectious disease factor' (sic) might be responsible and argued that if this was the case, *Gyps* species in Europe, the Middle East and Africa might be at risk. As a result surveillance and monitoring of vultures in East Africa has already started, and a workshop on the subject has been organised in Uganda (Cooper *et al.*, 2001).

The incident above has focused attention on unexpected population declines of raptors and the many factors that might, singly or in combination, lead to such 'crashes'. At the same time, it has illustrated how badly prepared is the scientific community to deal effectively and cooperatively with such crises. Even methods of investigation appear not to have been coordinated, and consultation with relevant specialists has been selective, partly because of political sensitivities. There is a clear need for an internationally agreed strategy and a useful starting point would probably be the protocols and other information published by the International Council for Bird Preservation (now BirdLife International) in its technical publication *Disease and Threatened Birds* (Cooper, 1989a). Disease modelling may prove to be an important feature of investigating epizootics, perhaps using a VORTEX computer simulation model as employed in population viability analyses on various species (see, for example, Seal & Lacy, 1989).

Episodes of mortality and morbidity in free-living birds of prey require a systematic, interdisciplinary and 'forensic' approach. Only in that way will all relevant data be collected and practicable methods of control, treatment or prevention be instigated.

Diseases in Wild (Free-living) Bird Populations

CONTRIBUTED BY I. NEWTON

In this chapter, I attempt to review some of what we know about the effects of infectious disease on wild (free-living) bird populations. This is a somewhat different proposition from assessing effects on individuals, which may, because of disease, suffer reduced breeding success or survival. For disease to reduce a population level, it must affect a substantial proportion of individuals, and at least some of the mortality it inflicts in a given period must be additive to other mortality and not simply 'compensatory', replacing other forms of death.

While we can construct a long list of the disease agents known to have affected individual raptors, or individual raptor broods, we are far from being able to assess the effects (if any) of these diseases on raptor population levels. What we can do, however, is to examine disease impacts on other bird populations which have been better studied, and draw conclusions which might be more generally applicable, and hence relevant to raptors. Throughout this chapter, I shall use the term 'disease' to cover only a clinically abnormal state resulting from parasite (macro/microparasite) infection and not to encompass the effects of other degenerative and metabolic disorders, nutrient deficiencies and toxic chemical effects (see Chapters 5 and 13).

The important point about parasitic diseases is that they are infectious, passing 'horizontally' from one individual to another (via direct contact or vectors), or 'vertically' from parent to offspring.

Because, in general, parasites are transmitted more efficiently at high than low host population densities, they can act on host populations in a density-dependent manner, affecting an increasing proportion of individual hosts as host numbers rise, and thereby helping to regulate host numbers. In this way, infectious disease could hold the host population in balance, and in some cases below the level it would achieve in the absence of disease.

One problem in assessing disease impacts on wild populations is that diseases are often associated with other conditions. For example, individuals weakened by starvation might become vulnerable to disease, as might those that for some reason are crowded together. On the other hand, individuals that lose part of their daily food intake to internal parasites may be more prone to the effects of food shortage than other individuals that are free of parasites. Disease is thus increasingly seen as a response, not only to parasite infection, but to the overall condition of the host. This makes it hard to separate the effects of disease from the food shortage or other environmental conditions that might favour it, and means that deaths from disease are often unlikely to be completely additive to other mortality. Interactions between disease and predation are also likely: disease may predispose certain individuals to predation, which may in turn reduce the spread of disease.

These various interactions mean that the

independent effects of many parasites on host populations can be properly assessed only by experiment. Only recently, however, have biologists attempted to remove parasites from wild (free-living) populations by use of chemicals, enabling effects on host numbers to be examined. This has been done by use of pesticides which destroy the parasite vectors (Kissam *et al.*, 1975), by drugs or other chemicals which destroy the parasites themselves (Hudson, 1986; Chapman & George, 1991), or by vaccination which reduces the impacts of the parasites on individual hosts (Hudson & Dobson, 1991). Most manipulations that have involved birds have been concerned more with the effects of parasites on individual survival and breeding success than on population levels. However, natural experiments, involving the accidental introduction of a disease or disease vector to a new area, have occurred from time to time, sometimes with devastating effects on the local bird life, as explained later.

THE PARASITES

The parasitic mode of life is so prevalent in nature that parasites probably outnumber hosts, both in species and in individuals. The reasons are fairly obvious, in that most types of parasites are small (some very small), and many different types of parasites can live in association with a single host. This great plethora of pathogenic organisms fall naturally into two groups, namely microparasites (viruses, bacteria, fungi, protozoa) and macroparasites (helminth worms, arthropods) (Anderson & May, 1979a,b). The former are characterised by their small size, short life-cycles, and high rates of reproduction within individual hosts. With few exceptions, the duration of infection is short relative to the lifespan of the hosts. Some microparasites are transmitted by direct contact between host individuals, and others through vectors, such as blood-sucking ticks and mosquitoes (see Chapter 7). Hosts that survive infection usually develop some immunity to subsequent infections.

In contrast to microparasites, most macroparasites are visible to the naked eye. Internal ones, such as helminth worms, do not multiply directly within a host, but produce infective stages which usually pass out of the host before transmission to another host. They are relatively long-lived and usually produce only a limited immune response, so that their infections tend to persist, with hosts accumulating parasites through life or continually being reinfected.

Parasitic worms almost always have clumped distributions, being found in small numbers in most host individuals and in large numbers in a few. This is important because the effects of such parasites on individual hosts typically depend on the total burden of worms, and not simply on whether or not the host is infected. The death of only a few hosts (those with heavy burdens) can lead in turn to the loss of a large number of worms. This process tends to limit the impact of macroparasites on host populations. In some circumstances, however, especially if the free-living infective stages are long-lived, helminth worms can induce recurrent epidemics (epizootics) that spread through a host population with devastating effects similar to those observed for microparasites. Why certain individuals in a population acquire heavy parasite loads, while others do not, may depend on behaviour, diet, body condition, age and genetic predisposition, as well as on chance.

The variety of parasitic worms found in different bird species depends on diet (which influences infection risk), life span (which affects the time for accumulation), social behaviour (which influences transmission), migratory habits (which affects the number of sites visited), body size (larger having more) and habitat (aquatic species having more) (Gregory *et al.*, 1991). Most waterbirds support a diverse community of such parasites, with large numbers of individuals per host. Some parasite species may be present in almost every individual in a population, while others are present in only a small proportion.

In contrast to macroparasite worms, which live within the host body, parasitic arthropods mostly live on the outside. Such ectoparasites include various lice (Mallophaga), mites and ticks (Acarina), flies (Diptera), fleas (Siphonaptera) and bugs (Hemiptera) (see Chapter 7). They mostly feed on blood, causing tissue damage and anaemia, as well as allergic responses and bacterial infections. In large numbers, they can thus weaken and sometimes kill their hosts. Ectoparasites themselves do not normally cause heavy mortality, except in the nestlings of some species, including raptors, but they can be important in transmitting microparasites. This is especially true of some ticks which can attach themselves to several hosts in succession.

Some ectoparasites are transmitted from host to host at times of physical contact, but most can move from environment to host. As with internal macroparasites, therefore, transmission of ectoparasites depends on both parasite and host density and behaviour, as well as on other factors. Because the immune response is at best limited, birds suffer from permanent infection with ectoparasites or from continual reinfection.

It is also useful to distinguish specialist (host-specific) parasites from generalists, which can have more than one definitive host species. For specialists, the rate of spread is influenced by the density of the host, so that the infection rate can show density-dependence (or delayed density-dependence), leading to predictable interactions between parasite and host populations. Because the two are coupled in a closed system, the host must usually attain a certain density (or contact rate) before the parasite can persist and spread, and a disease tends to become self-limiting before it can annihilate a population. For generalist parasites, however, total numbers are influenced by all their host species, so that a particular vulnerable host might be affected more severely than expected from its numbers alone. In extreme cases, the numbers of a vulnerable host species may be kept at a low level through the persistence of a 'reservoir of infection' in alternative hosts living in the same area (rabies in various carnivores being an obvious example). The level of infection in the vulnerable host is not then density-dependent with respect to that specific host, but with respect to the sum total of all potential host species in the area concerned. Whereas it is difficult for a specialist parasite to drive its host species to extinction (because the parasite population itself declines as host densities fall), a generalist could in theory extinguish one or more host species locally or globally so long as its population density was maintained by other, more robust, hosts. Examples are given below.

Certain host species are more vulnerable to particular generalist parasites than others, either because they are infected more easily or because they are more susceptible to the effects of an infection once acquired. In the initial infection, as expected, colonial and flocking species are at greater risk than solitary ones. In the shallow lakes of Texas, the bacterial disease avian cholera has occurred in waterfowl mainly after summer droughts, when the wintering birds are unusually crowded. During an outbreak in January–March 1950, one bird in every 2500 died each day, up to 0.3% of the ducks being fatally affected at one time (Petrides & Bryant, 1951). The smaller species, such as green-winged teal (*Anas carolinensis*), lesser scaup (*Aythya affinis*) and ruddy duck (*Oxyura jamaicensis*), suffered more than the larger ones. Teal, for instance, were 22 times more likely to die than mallard *Anas platyrhynchos*. Variation in susceptibility, once infected, has been shown in various Hawaiian birds with respect to avian malaria due to *Plasmodium relictum* (Table 14.1); in different crane species with respect to the arbovirus equine encephalitis (Dein *et al.*, 1986), in different pigeon species with respect to pigeon herpesvirus (Snyder *et al.*, 1985), in different grouse species with respect to the viral disease louping ill (Reid *et al.*, 1980), and in various waterfowl species with respect to avian cholera (Rosen & Bischoff, 1949; Petrides & Bryant, 1951; Vaught *et al.*, 1967) and viral duck plague (Spieker, cited in Wobeser, 1981). There are many other examples of different susceptibility among zoo animals, and in extreme cases, the same pathogen may be wholly innocuous to one species but fatal to a closely related one from another part of the world.

The impact of any pathogen on a population also depends on whether the pathogen influences mortality or fecundity. If individuals infected with a host-specific pathogen soon die, their swift removal from the population limits the spread of the pathogen. But if infected individuals do not die, but merely fail to reproduce, the pathogen can spread widely, lowering reproduction in enough individuals to cause population decline. An example of this process, involving a strongyle parasite in red grouse *Lagopus*

Table 14.1 Survival among various Hawaiian birds experimentally infected with avian malaria *Plasmodium relictum*.

	Endemic					Introduced		
	Laysan finch Telespyza cantans	Apapane Himatione sanguinea	Iiwi Vestiaria coccinea	Mauna Kea Amakihi Hemignathus virens	Mauna Loa Amakihi Hemignathus virens	Red-billed leiothrix Leiothrix lutea	Japanese white-eye Zosterops japonicus	Canary Serinus canaria
Number infected	5	5	5	6	5	5	5	5
Number died	5	2	3	4	1	0	0	0

The Laysan finch *Telespyza cantans* endemic to the Pacific island of Laysan had never been exposed to malaria, the endemic Hawaiian species had been exposed for less than 100 years, while the introduced species had had a long evolutionary association with the disease. All birds had the malarial parasites in their blood, but the only deaths occurred among endemic birds. From van Riper *et al.* (1986).

l. scoticus, is given under 'Cyclic fluctuations in host numbers', later in this chapter.

BREEDING SUCCESS

Parasites can reduce the breeding success of birds either by lowering the body condition of adults, or by lowering the body condition and survival of the chicks. In most bird species chick deaths from parasitism seem few or non-existent, and assume nowhere near the importance of predation. In certain species, however, deaths from parasitism are a major cause of reduced breeding output. Most studies have concerned ectoparasites, which can reach high infestations in species that use the same nest sites year after year, like many raptors, or in colonies close to other pairs (Rothschild & Clay, 1952). Some ectoparasites can survive for months or even years in sheltered nest sites, breeding each time the sites are occupied, and building up substantial populations over a period of years. They can cause nest desertions, reductions in chick growth and survival, as well as other effects (Newton, 1998).

Ectoparasites are a major cause of nest desertion and chick mortality in various species of swallows and in colonial seabirds can sometimes lead to nest desertions on a large scale. For example, some 5000 sooty tern (*Sterna fuscata*) pairs out of a colony of 40 000 pairs abandoned eggs and chicks in response to an infestation of ticks (*Ornithodoros capennnis*) (Feare, 1976). Some examples of parasite effects on raptor breeding are given in Table 14.2.

Examination of unhatched eggs and dead chicks from frequently used nest holes and nest boxes has often revealed heavy bacterial contamination, as found, for example, in house sparrows (*Passer domesticus*) and Eurasian tree sparrows (*Passer montanus*), (Pinowski *et al.*, 1988), as well as in unhatched eggs from American kestrels (Barnard, 1989). In some such species, bacterial infections may thus contribute to reduced hatching success and chick survival.

As mentioned above, parasites can also affect bird reproduction through effects on adults. In Tengmalm's Owl, high levels of *Leucocytozoon* blood parasites in the females were associated with reduced clutch size, but only in years of poor food supply; no such association was apparent in years of abundant food (Korpimäki *et al.*, 1993). Following an outbreak among mourning doves (*Zenaida macroura*) of trichomoniasis (caused by a protozoan parasite *Trichomonas*), many birds died, but some of those that recovered did not breed; the males examined had under-sized testes and the females showed

Table 14.2 Effects of parasites on the breeding of various raptor species.

Host species	Parasite species	Reduction in breeding performance	Location	Source
Prairie falcon *Falco mexicanus*	Tick, probably *Ornithodoros concanensis*	Chick survival (65%)	Colorado	Webster, 1944
Sharp-shinned hawk *Accipiter striatus*	Bot-fly *Philornis* sp.	Chick survival (33%)	Puerto Rico	Delannoy & Cruz, 1991
Goshawk *Accipiter gentilis*	Protozoon *Trichomonas gallinae*	Chick survival (slight)	Britain	Cooper & Petty, 1988
Red-tailed hawk *Buteo jamaicensis*	Fly *Eusimulium clarum*	Chick survival (24%)	California	Fitch *et al.*, 1946
Golden eagle *Aquila chrysaetos*	Protozoon *Trichomonas gallinae*	Chick survival (3%)	Idaho	Beecham & Kochert, 1975
Tengmalm's owl *Aegolius funereus*	Haematozoon *Leucocytozoon ziemanni*	Clutch size (ca 20%)	Finland	Korpimäki *et al.*, 1993

no sign of egg development (Haugen, 1952). Despite these instances, parasitism is clearly a much less widespread cause of breeding failure among birds than is predation.

ADULT MORTALITY

Studies of adult mortality in birds have given similar results to those on breeding success, that is: in most species parasites and disease seem to be a minor cause of deaths, but in some species they are of over-riding importance (Itamies *et al.*, 1980; Dobson & May, 1991). In waterfowl, for example, diseases probably account for a larger proportion of non-hunting mortality than any other cause of death (Bellrose, 1980).

Studies of diseases in full-grown birds typically rely on the *post-mortem* examination of carcasses. Some studies result from specific epizootics, and serve mainly to confirm the cause, while others result from more general surveys intended to assess the relative frequency of different mortality causes in particular bird species. The latter need to be treated with caution (Table 14.3). For one thing, such surveys depend on birds found dead by people, which are unlikely to represent a random cross-

section of deaths. Secondly, the proportion of deaths attributable to parasites varies according to the thoroughness of the examination procedure; many studies do not test for microparasites, especially viruses. On this aspect, greater collaboration between biologists and veterinarians would help (see Chapter 1). Thirdly, if predators are present, they may remove and eat many heavily parasitised individuals before they die, further reducing the perceived importance of parasites (for examples of predators selectively removing parasitised individuals from a population, both among birds and among other animals, see van Dobben, 1952; Holmes & Bethel, 1972; Vaughan & Coble, 1975; Temple, 1987). Lastly, even if a large proportion of deaths is attributable to parasitic disease, this seldom tells us anything conclusive about the effects of disease on population levels, because of possible interactions with other mortality factors. The mere presence of parasites in a carcass does not necessarily imply that they were the primary cause of death. In addition, potentially pathogenic organisms have frequently been detected in the digestive tracts of birds, which otherwise appear healthy (for an example in raptors see Cooper *et al.*, 1986). Others, such as the anthrax bacterium (*Bacillus anthracis*) did not survive passage through the gut of a white-backed vulture

Table 14.3 Causes of mortality as determined by *post-mortem* analyses of birds found dead.

Species	Region (years)	Numbers examined	Diagnosed causes of death (%)							Source
			Starvation[1]	Predation[2]	Disease[3]	Accident/ trauma[4]	Poisoning[5]	Shot or trapped[6]	Other[7]	
Various species[a]	Britain (1952–59)	1000	–	–	28[b]	33	10	–	21	Jennings, 1961
Various species[a]	Britain (1960–62)	583	–	–	155[b]	84	205	–	139[c]	Macdonald, 1962, 1963
Various songbirds	USA (1989)	152	–	–	12	26[d]	25	–	37	Okoniewski & Novesky, 1993
Long-eared owl *Asio otus*	Britain (1963–95)	123	18	–	4	61	8	3	5	Wyllie et al., 1996
Great horned owl *Bubo virginianus*	USA (1975–93)	132	32	–	4	33	8	9	13	Franson & Little, 1996
Tawny owl *Strix aluco*	Britain (<1978)	172	18	–	–	–	–	–	82[e]	Hirons et al., 1979
Barn owl *Tyto alba*	Britain (1963–89)	627	20	+	3	54	9	2	11	Newton et al., 1991
Pheasant *Phasianus colchicus*	Wisconsin (1955–58)	226	–	42	–	1	–	29	28[f]	Burger, 1964

Species	Location (years)	Sample								Source
Bald eagle *Haliaeetus leucocephalus*	USA (1966–81)	692	6	–	8	31	11	38	15	Reichel *et al.*, 1984[8]
Red-tailed hawk *Buteo jamaicensis*	USA (1975–92)	163	20	–	13	18	15	1	–	Franson *et al.*, 1996
Sparrow-hawk *Accipiter nisus*	Britain (1962–97)	1781	18	2	2	66	3	4	5	Newton *et al.*, 1999b
Kestrel *Falco tinnunculus*	Britain (1962–97)	1483	40	1	5	36	8	2	8	Newton *et al.*, 1999a
Kestrel *Falco tinnunculus*	Britain (1966–80)	92	48	–	10	5	23	–	14	Keymer *et al.*, 1981
Various raptors	USA (1972–77)	850	–	–	8	34	–	38	–	Redig, 1978
Mute swan	England (1979–85)	260	–	–	10	24	46	5	15	Birkhead, 1982;
Cygnus olor	Scotland (1980–86)	147	–	–	17	21	14	9	39	Sears, 1988; Spray & Milne, 1988
Whooper swan *Cygnus cygnus*	Scotland (1981–86)	57	–	–	2	28	47	11	12	Spray & Milne, 1988

+ = less than 1%.

[1] Emaciated and no other obvious cause. [2] Includes birds scavenged. [3] Includes infectious diseases and other disorders; not all diseases, notably viruses, were checked for in all studies. [4] Includes collision, road casualties, drowning, electrocution. [5] Mostly by pesticides, also lead in some species, and entirely lead in swans. [6] Includes oiled swans. [7] The last of 7 papers published during 1969–84 from which the results here are taken. [a] Most commonly examined birds were thrushes, finches, tits, starlings, sparrows, pigeons and gulls. [b] Includes 85 large parasites, 70 infections, excluding viral. [c] Called adverse environmental factors, including oiling, degenerative diseases and unknown. [d] Includes some predation. [e] No other cause of death examined other than starvation. [f] Shock, died within 3 days of release.

Gyps africanus, but the more resistant spores may have done so (Houston & Cooper, 1975).

Nor is it safe to infer much about the impact of macroparasites from the numbers found in individual hosts (Toft, 1991). Because most macroparasites that kill their hosts also kill themselves, the more virulent the parasite, the lower the mean number of parasites expected per host, or the lower the proportion of hosts infected at one time. So the presence of few parasites or diseased individuals in a host population could mean that the parasites are a trivial cause of mortality, or that the parasites are so virulent that they are continually removing hosts (and themselves) from the population.

Experiments have proved more revealing than *post-mortem* studies about the effects of parasites on adult birds. For example, chewing lice (Mallophaga – see Chapter 7) eat the feathers of birds and can therefore affect insulation. They are normally kept at low numbers by preening, but can be removed completely by fumigating birds, enabling their effects to be assessed. Among feral pigeons in captivity, louse-infested birds had higher metabolic rates than cleaned ones, presumably in response to greater heat loss through their damaged plumage, and in the wild fumigated pigeons showed higher overwinter survival than sham-fumigated ones (Booth *et al.*, 1993).

ANTI-PARASITE BEHAVIOUR

To counter the effects of ectoparasites, birds have well developed anti-parasite behaviour (Møller, 1989). Parasite numbers are reduced partly by direct removal from the plumage and nest, by routine preening, bathing and dust-bathing, or by anting in which the plumage is treated with formic acid (Simmons, 1966). Nest sanitation also helps, including removal of faecal sacs, ejection of faeces over the nest rim and frequent renovation of nest material (Bucher, 1988). The nest lining used by some birds may reduce parasite loads, as several favoured plant materials have repellent or pesticidal properties (Clark & Mason, 1985). Some tropical birds nest near wasps and bees which, among other benefits, help to reduce the risk from parasitic flies. More-

over, some species prone to nest parasitism by cuckoos or cowbirds have various behaviours, from mobbing to egg rejection, to reduce the risk. Some species can distinguish clean from tick-infested nest sites, and prefer to mate with clean rather than parasitised mates (Clayton, 1990). In fact, one theory of mate choice in birds states that individuals select mates on the basis of genetic disease resistance by scrutiny of the very characters (such as plumage condition) that reflect health and vigour (Hamilton & Zuk, 1982). Individual birds that were genetically prone to parasite effects would then never look as good as individuals that could resist these effects, and so different birds would thereby infallibly advertise their genetic qualities through their plumage.

EFFECTS OF PARASITES ON POPULATIONS

Most bird species can be counted most easily when they are breeding, because they are conspicuous then, and tied for long periods to specific locations where they rest. Knowledge of population changes in many bird species, from year to year or from place to place, is based entirely on counts of breeding numbers, or on indices of breeding numbers, such as displaying males, or nests. On biological grounds, it could also be argued that counts of breeding numbers are the most appropriate measure of population size to take. For it is at the start of the breeding season that numbers reach their annual low, and it is upon breeders that future additions to the population depend. On this basis, in assessing the effect of disease or any other limiting factor, the key question is whether, if that factor were absent, breeding numbers would be any higher. In the case of parasites, the answer to this question is sometimes no and sometimes yes.

At the population level, parasites can cause a number of outcomes: (1) no obvious effects on host breeding numbers; (2) a permanent lowering of host numbers below what would otherwise occur; (3) regular fluctuations in host numbers; (4) irregular fluctuations in host numbers, associated with periodic epidemics (epizootics); or (5) declines to extinction. The circumstances that might produce these various patterns have been elucidated by mathematical modelling (Anderson & May, 1978; May & Anderson, 1978), and can be illustrated by particular case histories from the field, as described below.

No obvious effects on host breeding numbers

This is probably a common situation, but the evidence is indirect: namely, that all bird species that have been studied harbour some parasites, yet in many species deaths from parasitism or disease are almost unknown, in either chicks or adults. In some recent studies, for example, protozoan blood parasites were found to have no obvious effects on the body condition, survival or breeding success of various passerines and raptors (Peirce & Marquiss, 1983; Bennett *et al.*, 1988, 1993b; Ashford *et al.*, 1990; Weatherhead & Bennett, 1991, 1992; Tella *et al.*, 1996), so at the levels found, could not have affected their population levels. Possibly these parasites might not always be so benign if the hosts were exposed to other debilitating influences at the same time, but the studies concerned produced no evidence for this view. Secondly, despite harbouring parasites, many bird species are known to be limited in breeding numbers primarily by other factors, such as food supply, nest sites or predation (Newton, 1980, 1998); they often show territorial behaviour which leads to the exclusion of a surplus of non-breeders (Newton, 1992). Any mortality they might suffer from parasites is seemingly trivial in the limitation of breeding numbers. Thirdly, many generalist parasites have been introduced into island avifaunas along with introduced birds, yet only rarely have they been implicated in population declines of their new hosts.

Lowering of host breeding numbers

Mathematical models have revealed how a parasite–host interaction might lead to a stable equilibrium, in which the infection rate remains constant. If the parasite kills hosts in a density-dependent manner, the host population could be regulated at a level lower than might occur in the absence of the parasite. To my knowledge, no such stable, closely coupled interactions between a specialist parasite

and its host have yet been described from birds, but they may well exist. However, one example of population limitation by a generalist parasite involves the louping ill flavi-virus, which affects the central nervous system of red grouse (*Lagopus l. scoticus*) and other animals. The virus occurs patchily in the British uplands and is transmitted between hosts by the sheep tick (*Ixodes ricinus*). Although the ticks may feed on a wide range of hosts, only sheep and red grouse are known to produce viraemias (virus in the blood) which exceed the threshold necessary for efficient transmission (Reid *et al.*, 1978; Duncan *et al.*, 1979). Thus louping ill is usually considered as a two-host one-vector system. The mortality that occurs in red grouse in areas where louping ill is endemic (enzootic) is sufficient to reduce grouse stocks to low densities, but continuing infection of the grouse is dependent on the presence both of sheep or other alternative hosts and of ticks as vectors.

Although louping ill will kill adult grouse, its main effect is on chicks. In an experimental study of captive birds, Reid (1975) found that 78% of 37 experimentally infected juveniles developed clinical signs of weakness and died in 6 days. Comparative studies on wild grouse in northern England indicated that, in areas with ticks and louping ill, chick survival was about half the level found in areas with ticks and no louping ill, or in areas with neither ticks nor louping ill (Hudson & Dobson, 1991). In areas where ticks were abundant, 84% of adult grouse had antibodies to louping ill, indicating previous infection (Reid *et al.*, 1978).

Red grouse may be susceptible to louping ill because they have not been exposed to this or a similar viral disease during their evolution. Perhaps the virus has only recently been introduced to their moorland habitat, presumably in sheep (Reid *et al.*, 1980). After vaccination, sheep no longer act as a reservoir host, which in areas with no other host, provides a means of eradicating the disease from both sheep and grouse.

Cyclic fluctuations in host numbers

Both micro- and macroparasites can induce oscillations in host abundance, through acting in a delayed density-dependent manner. This works as follows: as host numbers rise, parasitic infection grows, until enough hosts are infected to cause a crash in host numbers. Host densities are then below the level needed for efficient parasite transmission, which allows the host population to increase again, and the cycle to repeat itself, with the parasite remaining throughout one step behind the host. At any one stage, therefore, host mortality is related not to host density at the time, but to density at an earlier stage in the cycle, hence the term delayed density dependence.

The best studied example of such a cycle interaction concerns the red grouse as affected by the disease strongylosis, caused by a nematode worm *Trichostrongylus tenuis* (Lovat, 1911; Hudson *et al.*, 1992a,b). In its moorland habitat, the red grouse is the only host for this parasite. In some areas, the worms are found in the gut caeca of nearly every grouse examined, often causing little harm, but when present in large numbers they weaken and sometimes kill the host. The eggs of the parasite pass out of the gut with the caecal faeces. The larvae hatch and, after some development, they climb to the tips of heather plants, which form the main food of red grouse. In this way they pass from one grouse to another. Active larvae can usually be found on the heather plants from June to September, when the worm numbers in grouse increase. By the end of the year the ingested larvae do not develop into the adult stage, but remain arrested within the grouse, developing into adults in the following spring (Shaw, 1988). The adult worms themselves are long-lived, probably as long as the grouse, so infection is cumulative. The infection intensifies year by year as the numbers of grouse rise, until eventually the population crashes, with a consequent reduction in the numbers of the parasite. Population cycles in red grouse are thus thought to be produced by the effects of nematode parasitism acting mainly on the fecundity and survival of the grouse in a delayed density-dependent manner.

The impact of these parasites on the bodyweight, breeding and survival of grouse was examined in field experiments conducted over several years (Hudson, 1986; Hudson *et al.*, 1992b). The basic techniques were to catch grouse at random and to treat half the birds with an anthelminthic to reduce worm burdens and the remaining birds with water as a control and then to monitor their subsequent performance. All the birds were marked so that they could be individually identified. Overwinter weight gain was greater in treated birds than in control birds, as was subsequent clutch size, hatching success and chick survival. Replication of the experiment in several other areas gave similar results, confirming that parasitism had a major influence on grouse breeding success. Moreover, in the main study area, treated birds were significantly more likely to survive from spring and be shot in the following autumn, and less likely to be found dead in the interim, than were untreated birds. Grouse found dead on the study area in spring generally had high parasite burdens.

The experiment clearly showed that parasites reduced the productivity and survival of individual grouse. On its own, it could not show whether parasitism affected population levels, rather than merely influencing which individuals succumbed in a population ultimately limited by other factors. Another experiment was needed for this, in which large proportions of the grouse on a moor were caught each year and treated with an anthelminthic. Their numbers did not crash as expected, but in unprecedented manner they remained high for several years until the end of the experiment. Meanwhile, grouse numbers on nearby moors, which had previously fluctuated in phase with those on the experimental moor, continued to cycle as before. This experiment therefore showed that strongyle parasites were responsible for causing regular crashes in grouse numbers, and that without the parasite, grouse numbers could maintain a high and stable level (Hudson *et al.*, 1998).

This experimental work also provided evidence for a link between parasitism and predation (Hudson, 1986; Hudson & Dobson, 1991; Hudson *et al.*, 1992b). On several moors, grouse killed by foxes (*Vulpes vulpes*) and other predators had higher worm burdens than grouse that survived through the summer, to be shot in autumn. During incubation, hen grouse are thought to produce less scent than usual, making it harder for mammalian predators to find their nests. The scent probably arises from the caecum which stops producing caecal faeces at that time. Wild hens that were dosed with an anthelminthic to reduce their worm burdens were found less often (15% of finds) by trained dogs hunting by scent than undosed hens (85% of finds). In contrast, for human observers hunting by sight, the figures were 45% and 55%. It seemed that, compared with treated hens, heavily parasitised hens emitted more scent, making them more vulnerable to predation. If this was so, parasitism was the predisposing factor to death by predation. Parasites might also reduce the competitive ability of individual grouse, for birds without territories generally had higher worm burdens than those with territories (Jenkins *et al.*, 1963).

Grouse disease may only have reached the importance it has in Britain because of predator control, which allows the grouse to achieve densities at which parasite transmission is enhanced. Thus, in recent studies, the presence of many heavily parasitised birds in the population was associated with a scarcity of predators. Mathematical modelling revealed how predators, by selectively removing the most infected grouse, could allow an increase in grouse density: they effectively blocked the regulatory role of the parasites, and stopped the cycle in grouse numbers (Hudson *et al.*, 1992b). Even if predation merely reduced the post-breeding density of the grouse, it could greatly hamper the spread of the parasite. Low levels of predation were sufficient to achieve this effect in the model, but at higher levels, predation was itself enough to reduce grouse density to an even lower average level, despite the scarcity of parasites.

Population cycles involving strongylosis are known among red grouse chiefly on wetter, western moors. On drier moors parasite numbers are too low to kill many grouse. This has been attributed to poorer survival of the free-living stages of the parasite on drier moors, for in the laboratory their survival depends on humidity as well as on temperature. On drier moors, therefore, grouse numbers may cycle from some different cause or may simply fluctuate irregularly. One feature of parasite involvement is the marked crashes in numbers, so that the population typically falls from peak to trough in 1–2 years. Elsewhere the cycles are longer and more

symmetrical, as both the rise and fall in grouse numbers take place progressively over several years. Clearly, although parasites might contribute to cycles in some areas, they are not responsible for cycles in all areas. It remains possible that their main effect is to induce crashes at high density, and thereby shorten a cycle that would still occur, but with longer periodicity, from different causes. This research on the grouse–nematode relationship is one of the few examples where the combination of field observations and experiments, coupled with the use of mathematical models, has indicated that pathogens can have a significant impact on the population dynamics of an avian host, in this case contributing to regular cycles in grouse abundance.

Irregular fluctuations in host numbers

Irregular declines in the numbers of some birds are caused by periodic outbreaks of parasitic diseases, which kill large numbers of individuals in successive single events. Such epizootics have been recorded in a wide range of bird species, but particularly in waterfowl which are often crowded in large concentrations, facilitating transmission. The most important of such diseases include duck plague and avian cholera.

Duck plague results from a herpesvirus infection, also called duck virus enteritis (DVE), which is found throughout the northern hemisphere, usually in domestic ducks. Strains of the virus vary in virulence, and not all waterfowl are equally susceptible. The virus attacks the vascular system, usually causing death within 14 days of infection (Wobeser 1981). The chief clinical signs include haemorrhages throughout the body and diphtheritic membranes on the oesophagus and elsewhere. Infected birds excrete the virus, so transmission occurs through contact between individuals or with a contaminated environment. The virus can remain latent in carrier birds for up to 4 years before they begin to excrete it again at times of stress (Burgess *et al.*, 1979). The first recorded epizootic in wild waterfowl occurred during the 1972–73 winter, when a single outbreak killed an estimated 42% of the 100 000 mallard (*Anas platyrhynchos*) wintering at the Lake Andes National Wildlife Refuge in South Dakota (Friend

& Pearson, 1973). Mortality peaked at 1000 birds per day in late January, when the population was concentrated on a limited area of open water. At the same time, only 3% of 9000 geese were affected, probably because they fed away from the contaminated water on land nearby.

Avian cholera (or pasteurellosis) is caused by the bacterium *Pasteurella multocida*. It is a highly infectious disease capable of killing birds within 4–6 hours after infection, though 4–9 days is more common. Typically, the birds die in good condition, but with small haemorrhages on the body surface and pinpoint lesions on the liver, heart and other organs. Transmission is primarily by inhalation or ingestion of the bacterium. The disease has been recorded in more than 100 bird species, but waterfowl are again its most obvious victims (Botzler, 1991). More than 60000 birds died at the Muleshoe Refuge in Texas during 1956–57 (Jensen & Williams, 1964), and an estimated 70000 died in California in 1965–66 (Rosen, 1971). Even larger outbreaks, involving diving ducks, occurred in Chesapeake Bay in 1970 and 1978 (Montgomery *et al.*, 1979). During an outbreak in California, affecting mainly American coots (*Fulica americana*), the disease spread to waterfowl and rodents, resulting in deaths of owls and hen harriers (Rosen & Morse, 1972).

In general, mortality of single individuals (or small groups) from avian cholera, are reported frequently, from a wide variety of locations. Epizootics occur only where waterfowl are concentrated, as on refuges, and typically begin in one host species (usually a common one), then spread to other species using the same area. They may be related to water quality (especially organic content) and other environmental conditions (Botzler, 1991).

Epidemics (epizootics) involving macroparasites have also occurred among waterfowl. On the Baltic Islands of Finland, eider duck (*Somateria mollissima*) numbers increased between 1920 and 1930, but in the breeding season of 1931 many females and young died from infection with the acanthocephaline worm *Polymorphus boschadis*. The numbers of eiders then rose again, reaching their former level by 1933–34. They were then reduced by a second epidemic in 1935, which continued less

severely for the next 3 years, by which time breeding numbers were only two-thirds and in some places only one-third of what they had been (Lampio, 1946; Grenquist, 1951).

Waterfowl are also often infected with cestodes (tapeworms), as well as with trematodes which have molluscs as intermediate hosts. Of the 475 trematode species identified in waterfowl, only 32 have been found to cause pathological changes or death (McDonald, 1969). As an example, dabbling ducks have often died on the St Lawrence river marshes in Canada during summer, as a result of infection with the trematode *Cyathocotyle bushiensis* (Gibson *et al.*, 1972). Heavy burdens were acquired by the ducks feeding day after day on infected snails, resulting in severe caecal damage. Of the 264 species of cestodes found in waterfowl, none is normally fatal, except when infestation is so great as to block the gut (Grenquist *et al.*, 1972; Persson, 1974), or when coupled with malnutrition or other debilitation, accounting in one instance for the deaths of about 50 mute swans (*Cygnus olor*) (Jennings *et al.*, 1961).

Psittacine birds also seem susceptible to epizootics which kill large proportions of local populations at one time, again associated with their gregarious habits. In Australia, sulphur-crested cockatoos (*Cacatua galerita*) in one flock of 120 birds showed more than 80% mortality in a 12-month period, and crimson rosellas (*Platycercus elegans*) in a flock of 20 birds showed 50% mortality in a 20-month period, in both cases resulting from a virus-associated disease (McOrist, 1989).

Many other epizootics among wild birds have been recorded, with examples from among game birds, pigeons, gulls, petrels and others. One example, in the southeastern United States in 1950–51 involved the deaths of many thousands of mourning doves *Zenaida macroura* from trichomoniasis (Stabler & Herman, 1951; Haugen, 1952), a disease which can also be passed on to raptors (see Cooper & Petty (1988) for examples of the disease in nestling Northern goshawks which are presumed to have eaten pigeons). In many of these species, however, study of other limiting factors suggests that disease cannot be more than sporadically important. Similarly, in some species subject to long-term study in particular localities, numbers suddenly and markedly declined, only to recover again in subsequent years (e.g. an unprecedented 70% decline in a Florida scrub jay (*Aphelocoma coerulescens*) population, (Woolfenden & Fitzpatrick (1991)). Although no disease was identified, epidemics were suspected.

Our understanding of what precipitates irregular epizootics is poor, but not all follow the same pattern. Some result from an unexplained appearance of a particular disease agent, others from a disease agent that becomes fatal only when the birds are exposed to some other stress such as food shortage, or crowding or other conditions that facilitate transmission. Thus, some diseases that are not serious in the wild can kill many captive birds kept at high density in the same place for long periods. An example from poultry is Newcastle disease, caused by a paramyxovirus. Yet other epizootics have been attributed to a genetic change in a disease organism itself: to the evolution of a new virulent strain, or of a strain that can switch from one host species to another previously unsuited to it. Whatever their origin, most epizootics tend to be sporadic, affecting birds in different localities in different years, but some have spread widely, with devastating impacts on overall population levels, as for myxomatosis in rabbits (*Oryctolagus cuniculus*).

Mass mortality caused by natural toxins

Other forms of mass mortality occur in birds from time to time, as a result of toxins produced by micro-organisms. The well known 'duck sickness' or botulism is a form of paralytic food-poisoning caused by a neurotoxin from the bacillus *Clostridium botulinum* (Kalmbach & Gunderson, 1934; Sciple, 1953). The anaerobic *Clostridium* is almost ubiquitous in nature, found in most parts of the world, and persisting in spore form for years; it grows well on organic matter in shallow stagnant waters or mud during warm weather. Deaths from botulism have been noted in about 70 bird species in 21 families, but mostly in waterfowl and gulls. The chief clinical feature is a flaccid paralysis which prevents the birds from flying. Often the wings droop, the head sags to one side (hence the term 'limber neck') and the eyelids may become encrusted. Birds die from respiratory failure or from drowning and may appear in good condition with no internal lesions (Locke & Friend, 1987). In the corpses of poisoned birds *Clostridium* multiplies, and the toxin concentrates. These corpses may be eaten by raptors, which may in turn be affected, although turkey vultures (*Cathartes aura*) have shown unusual resistance (Kalmbach, 1939a) (see Chapter 6). Outbreaks end when temperatures cool, when birds leave the site or switch to other foods, when flies stop breeding, or when water levels stabilise (Wobeser, 1981).

Although botulism is not infectious, its effects can be spectacular. An estimated million birds died from botulism at a lake in Oregon in 1925, 1–3 million at Great Salt Lake in Utah in 1929, and 250 000 at the northern end of Great Salt Lake in 1932, and 250 000 (25%) out of two million birds on Tulare Lake in California in 1938–41. Many other outbreaks have involved smaller numbers of birds (Manuwal, 1967; Smith *et al.*, 1983), but totalled over wide areas or over a period of years they can be substantial, for example the 4–5 million waterfowl deaths attributed to botulism in the United States in 1952 (Smith, 1975).

The impact of botulism can be so substantial that after each severe outbreak the populations concerned could take several years to recover their numbers. Frequent outbreaks could thus cause populations to remain for much of the time below the level that would otherwise occur.

Decline to extinction

Like other animals, birds may have little resistance to a pathogen with which they have had no previous contact. A disease may reach new areas as a result of natural spread of the parasite or its vectors, or through inadvertent introduction by humans. In this context, alien diseases may have contributed to the decline in the numbers of certain endemic landbirds on oceanic islands, restricting the distribution of some and annihilating others. The best documented examples are from Hawaii, where the release of mosquitoes around 1820 (supposedly by a spiteful ship captain) led to the establishment in the local bird population of avian malaria and avian pox

(Warner, 1968). These parasites are only mildly virulent to the introduced birds from other parts of the world, with which the pathogens have had long evolutionary associations. But they often kill both chicks and adults of the native Hawaiian birds, which have only recently become exposed to these diseases and have little or no natural resistance. The evidence is strongest for avian malaria caused by *Plasmodium relictum capistranoae*, which, at low and medium elevations where mosquitoes occur, is readily transmitted from introduced to native birds (van Riper *et al.*, 1986). This has led to great reductions in the distributions and numbers of many endemic bird species, which are now mainly restricted to high or dry areas where mosquitoes are scarce or absent. Parts of the islands below 1500 metres, where mosquitoes are commonest, are now occupied almost entirely by resistant introduced bird species. In addition, the extinction of roughly half the indigenous landbirds of the Hawaiian Islands since their discovery by Europeans in 1778 has been attributed mainly to these two introduced diseases (Warner, 1968).

Deductions from field observations were supported by experiments in which various Hawaiian birds in captivity were inoculated with malaria. Many individuals of the endemic species died, whereas all the introduced ones survived (Table 14.1). All of the experimental birds had malarial parasites in their blood and those that died were found to have extremely high numbers, but no other obvious parasites or diseases. In a survey of the occurrence of malarial *Plasmodium* in various bird species trapped or found dead, the infection rate of different species ranged from 0 to 29% (van Riper *et al.*, 1986). Interestingly, birds struck by cars had a significantly higher prevalence of malaria than did birds caught in mist nets. Debilitation resulting from the disease may thus have increased the likelihood of deaths from another cause. Similarly, more birds than expected had both pox and malaria than had one or other disease alone. This could have been because infection with one disease lowered resistance to another, or because such twin-infected birds had received greater attention from mosquitoes, which transmit both.

Although the evidence is largely correlative, it appears that both the elevational distributions of the native birds and their relative abundances in different habitats are influenced to a major extent by the malarial parasite. Because the species differ in their susceptibility to both diseases, the extent of this influence varies among species. The introduced species, being largely resistant to both diseases, are distributed independently of them and reach greatest densities in the lowland forests where food is most abundant. Levels of parasitism are not the only factor influencing the distributions and numbers of Hawaiian birds, however, as habitat changes and introduced predators are also involved. Introduced diseases have been found among the birds of other oceanic islands (see Peirce *et al.*, 1977; Peirce, 1979 for Mascarenes; Harmon *et al.*, 1987 for Galapagos), and have been suggested as a contributory cause of extinctions of endemic birds, but without compelling evidence.

As with all host–parasite associations, the long-term survival of a declining host species could depend on whether it can achieve some new lower level of stability (as could happen if parasitism were density-dependent), or alternatively evolve some measure of resistance before it dies out.

DISEASES IN ENDANGERED SPECIES

In widespread populations, disease often comes in a shifting pattern of local outbreaks, influenced partly by local conditions, including host densities. Particular localities might lose their populations temporarily, only to be recolonised subsequently by unaffected individuals from elsewhere. But as the distribution of many bird populations becomes ever more reduced through human action, and ever more restricted to reserves, the chances of an epizootic wiping out an entire species become greater. Experience with the black-footed ferret *Musteta migripes*, in which canine distemper killed 70% of the last known population in North America (Thorne & Williams, 1988), illustrates two epidemiological features that are common to endangered species. First, because such species have small populations, they are themselves unlikely to sustain infections of virulent pathogens, acquiring them only from other more common host species. Secondly, because most individuals in the population are never exposed to a pathogen, there is little acquired immunity. In these circumstances, when an epizootic does occur, it can kill a large proportion of individuals. The reduction of any small population through disease, whether in the wild or in captivity, can have the additional effect of genetic impoverishment (because some genotypes are eliminated altogether), with the risk that the population is less able to withstand the next disease. Increasingly, the question will arise whether we should aim to preserve endangered species in natural association with their parasites and pathogens, or whether we should try to keep them – like people in developed countries – unnaturally free from infectious diseases (May, 1988). The latter will almost certainly be necessary to get some rare species through the bottleneck of low numbers.

One frequent effect of bringing endangered species into zoos or other such facilities is to increase their population density, thereby increasing the efficiency of disease transmission. Another common effect in such facilities is to bring species from different parts of the world together so that some are exposed to new diseases (Cooper, 1989a). This is a frequent cause of mortality in captive parrots, as susceptible and resistant carrier species come into contact. Many infectious agents have been implicated in parrot deaths, including viruses, bacteria, fungi and protozoa (Gaskin, 1989). In several other bird species, captive stocks maintained for conservation reasons have been heavily reduced in numbers and genetic variance by disease outbreaks, often caught through contact with other more resistant species housed on the same site. For example, some rare Mauritius pink pigeons (*Columba mayeri*) died in Albuquerque Zoo because of a *Herpesvirus* transmitted to them by foster doves (*Columba livia*) (Snyder *et al.*, 1985). Other potential dangers come from the release of captive individuals which can ferry novel pathogens back to wild populations that lack immunity (Cooper, 1989a; Wilson *et al.*, 1994), and from the translocation of infected wild individuals from one locality to another, a process which could extend the range of a pathogen.

In addition, the threat of new diseases is ever present. Soon after people began to domesticate wild animals, they unwittingly shared with them the mix of pathogens from which new potent diseases evolved. Thus measles is thought to have evolved from rinderpest or canine distemper, and influenza from ancient pig diseases. One way in which new viral diseases arise occurs when, within the same animal, two different viruses invade the same cell, and during propagation, exchange genetic material with one another in a process akin to hybridisation. They can then produce a new virus which, in some instances, might be more virulent than either parent form, or able to infect a new host resistant to both parental forms. Moreover, the production of different strains of virus by a mixture of mutations and selection can occur on a timescale that is faster than that in which any host species can evolve resistance.

Other emerging diseases may not be new, just old diseases that suddenly find conditions right for them, so can suddenly leap from obscurity to prominence (see also Chapter 13). What is certain is that the increasing scale of movement of people around the globe, and the associated trade in wildlife and wildlife products, will result in bird and other animal populations being increasingly brought into contact with new pathogens or old pathogens in new settings (Ashton & Cooper, 1989). Two of the current major killing diseases of waterfowl in North America, avian cholera and duck plague, may have originally come from domestic poultry imported to the continent. Both diseases were first identified in poultry in the 1880s, and in wild duck populations in 1944 (avian cholera) and 1979 (duck plague) (Baldassarre & Bolen, 1994). As an example of the reverse situation, of imported wild birds infecting domestic ones, the catastrophic epizootic of Newcastle Disease that hit the California poultry industry in 1971 was clearly linked to the importation of parrots from South America. In this outbreak, nine million birds were destroyed as part of the control programme (Lancaster & Alexander, 1975).

Other conservation problems have arisen from domestic animals acting as reservoirs of infection for more vulnerable wild species. A high mortality occurred in monkeys (*Presbytis entellus* and *Macaca radiata*) after cattle were introduced into forest in

India (Boshell, 1969). The cattle increased the numbers of a biting tick and hence the rate of infection of the flavi-virus causing Kysanur Forest Disease. On the reciprocal view, agriculturists often view wildlife as a reservoir of infection for domestic stock; and a programme of badger (*Meles meles*) control in parts of Britain was aimed at reducing the incidence of tuberculosis in cattle.

CONCLUDING REMARKS

With so few case histories, it is impossible to guess at the full ecological significance of parasites in bird populations. Existing information would suggest that, in most bird species, parasites cause little mortality among adults or young and are much less prevalent as a major limiting factor for breeding numbers than are predation or food shortage. Many species might experience the occasional epidemic, after which their numbers take several years to recover fully, and among waterfowl in some parts of North America epizootics might be so frequent as to assume the role of main limiting factor. These incidents are likely to increase in future as human impacts on habitat force ever greater numbers of waterfowl to concentrate on refuges, or remain there for longer periods. The disease louping ill can depress red grouse (*Lagopus l. scoticus*) populations in some areas and strongylosis is involved in the cyclic fluctuations of red grouse numbers in other areas. The present level of both diseases is a result of human action in increasing the numbers of alternative hosts (louping ill), or in decreasing the numbers of predators (strongylosis), and thereby increasing the densities of grouse to a level at which parasitic transmission is high. Moreover, while ectoparasites can reduce the breeding output of some raptors and other birds, this does not necessarily reduce the subsequent breeding numbers, especially as such species are often limited by shortage of food or nest sites.

Owing to infectious disease often being associated with other stress factors (stressors), such as starvation or crowding, which might predispose to it, much of the mortality it causes is not necessarily additive to other mortality. Moreover, the effects of

one parasite species might well vary according to the number of other parasites the host contains, with multiple infections having greater impact than single infections, an aspect largely unexplored. The immune system of birds can also be suppressed by certain pollutants, increasing susceptibility to disease. For example, mallard experimentally dosed with PCBs, DDT, dieldrin or selenium showed reduced resistance to a duck hepatitis virus (Friend & Trainer, 1969; Whiteley, 1989), while mallard exposed to petroleum oil had decreased resistance to the avian cholera bacterium *Pasteurella multocida*.

Disease organisms are also likely to have marked effects on the evolution and genetic make-up of host populations (Price, 1980). Throughout history, many animal and plant species have been continually afflicted with devastating disease outbreaks, leading to selection for disease resistance, and in extreme cases which left few survivors, leading to marked reductions in genetic variance. The importance of maintaining genetic diversity with respect to disease defence is indicated by certain natural populations which have reduced genetic variability and apparent increased vulnerability to infectious disease (O'Brien & Evermann, 1988).

In this chapter, I have been concerned primarily with the effects of disease on bird numbers, but disease organisms could also restrict bird distributions, preventing certain species from occupying large areas of otherwise suitable habitat. We would normally have no way of knowing this, except in special circumstances, as on Hawaii.

From the foregoing, what can we infer about the likely effects of parasitic diseases on raptor populations? Only a small proportion of raptor species (such as lesser kestrels and certain *Gyps* vultures) live in dense colonies in which disease could easily spread through a population, but again I know of no recorded instances. The possibility that the decline of *Gyps* vultures in India might be linked to an infectious agent is discussed briefly in Chapter 13. In most raptor species, individuals live solitary lives, coming into close contact with another (usually single) individual chiefly in the breeding season. A few other, normally solitary species, come together only on migration, notably in communal roosts. Hence, the scope for disease to spread 'horizontally' through raptor populations is extremely limited. On the other hand, some raptors, notably falcons and owls, use the same enclosed nest sites year after year, which enables certain ectoparasites to persist at the sites, ready to infect each year's occupants and their chicks. Heavy parasite loads on peregrines and prairie falcons have caused substantial chick mortality in some areas, reducing the breeding output of the population, but with no obvious effect on subsequent breeding numbers. Heavy infestations with ectoparasites are less frequent in raptors that use the same stick nests year after year, but such species often have more than one nest in their territory, and the use of alternate nests in different years may help to break the build-up in parasite numbers.

It is from close contact with their prey that raptors are likely to pick up many generalist parasites. The occurrence of 'frounce' (trichomoniasis) in Northern goshawks and other raptors can be attributed to direct infection from affected pigeons in which the disease is common, and many ticks and other external parasites must jump ship from prey to predator. To all such parasites, bird-eating raptors are likely to be most susceptible, for while many external parasites of birds can live on other birds, parasites of other animals cannot usually transfer to birds. In picking up ticks and other blood-feeding parasites from their prey, raptors could be vulnerable to any microparasites that the blood-suckers transmit.

Raptors could also pick up parasitic worms from the bodies of their prey. In those species of raptors examined, parasitic worms were found in only a small proportion of individuals examined (Newton *et al.*, 1999b). Infections could be greater in fish-eating species, such as osprey, but I know of no relevant studies. While we cannot exclude the possibility that parasitic diseases might occasionally limit raptor numbers in particular areas, there are no documented examples. On the other hand, there is abundant evidence for effects of other limiting factors, such as food supply, nest sites and pesticides (Newton, 1979). In other words, it seems that, while individual raptors frequently suffer from parasite infections, and chick survival is sometimes reduced, the effects of parasites are not usually suf-ficiently prevalent or severe to limit breeding densities.

As stressed at the outset, the best way to assess reliably the impact of parasites is to remove them in some way, and measure the response in the host population. Now that such work has started on wild populations by use of pesticides or drugs, the doors are open to further experimental work which should improve our understanding of disease impacts. There is an obvious need for experiments that examine the effects of parasites on populations and not merely on individual survival and breeding success. Those involving strongyle worm removal from red grouse are a step in this direction (Hudson *et al.*, 1992b, 1998).

SUMMARY

In understanding interactions between parasites and their hosts, a useful distinction to make is between microparasites (viruses, bacteria, fungi and protozoa) and macroparasites (helminths and arthropod ectoparasites). Microparasites are responsible for most recorded epizootics which periodically cause large-scale reductions in bird numbers. Macroparasites occur more often as persistent infections which reduce breeding or survival rates, but in a few species cause sudden and massive reductions in numbers.

Parasites can have the following main effects on bird breeding densities, depending on circumstances: (1) cause no obvious change (e.g. various species with certain blood-parasites); (2) hold breeding density below the level that could otherwise occur (e.g. red grouse with louping ill); (3) cause periodic massive reductions in numbers, either regular (e.g. red grouse with strongyle worms) or irregular (e.g. waterfowl with avian cholera); and (4) cause decline to extinction (e.g. some Hawaiian bird species with avian pox and malaria). While individual raptors often suffer from parasite infections, and chick survival is sometimes reduced, effects are not usually prevalent or severe enough to reduce breeding densities.

Some major impacts have occurred when bird species, mainly through human action, have come into contact with generalist parasites to which they have no natural resistance. Species can be driven to low densities or even extinction by parasites that are maintained at high densities by alternative, non-susceptible hosts. The role of parasites in bird population dynamics can change with changes in the density of (1) the host and parasite species them-selves; (2) alternative host species; and (3) any necessary vector species, all of which influence the ease of transmission. They can also alter with changes in other environmental conditions which affect infection and transmission rates. The impact of diseases on wild bird populations could increase in the future, as a result of various human activities.

Discussion and Conclusions

'Enough, if something from our hands have power to live, and act, and serve the future hour.'

William Wordsworth

So what has been achieved as a result of studies on the health and diseases of birds of prey? What have we learned from 30 years of unprecedented research on raptors in the wild and in captivity? How much remains to be done?

First of all, my own investigations and those of others have demonstrated that in many respects the veterinary care of birds of prey in captivity does not differ markedly from that of other members of the class Aves. Most of the infectious and non-infectious causes of morbidity and mortality are those that are also associated with disease and death in such species as parrots, pigeons, thrushes and finches – even domestic poultry. Clinical techniques applicable to other orders of birds can usually be used safely and effectively in raptors, as can most laboratory investigations.

Some of the conditions seen in captive birds of prey relate to the management of these species. Thus, hawks kept for falconry appear to be particularly susceptible to bumblefoot, to certain types of fractures and to poisoning acquired from items provided as food. The apparent prevalence of other conditions often reflects their importance to those who keep the birds; for example, damage to plumage is likely to be considered more relevant by a falconer, who is flying his hawk and hoping to catch quarry, than it is to an aviculturist whose raptors spend most of their time in an aviary. The latter will, however, show greater concern about the possibility of a reproductive disorder or small numbers of ecto-parasites than will a rehabilitator whose prime aim is to return birds to the wild.

That said, it is becoming clear that certain diseases are either specific to, or particularly prevalent in, certain species or genera of raptors. In a few instances there are important differences in susceptibility between the Falconiformes and the Strigiformes. Such findings are beginning to vindicate the point that I made in my 1978 edition when I postulated, 'It is not unreasonable to assume that, in the course of time, some specific diseases of the barn owl, merlin and other raptorial birds will also be recognised.' This is now proving to be the case. Publications on medical conditions and care of, for example, the California condor (Stringfield, 1998; Ensley, 1999), bearded vulture (Scope & Frey, 2000) and Mauritius kestrel (Dutton et al., 2000) have appeared and others on individual species will surely follow. Diseases that seem (at present) to be confined to certain types of bird of prey include a fatty liver-kidney syndrome of merlins (Forbes & Cooper, 1993) while other conditions, for example aspergillosis, are more prevalent in some species than others.

As was pointed out earlier, the continued appearance of checklists or reviews relating to, for example, mites (Philips, 2000) and ecto- and endoparasites (Taft, 2000), are reminders of how little is still known about the 'normal' fauna and flora of most

235

raptors, even their conspicuous macroparasites. Far less, of course, is documented on their microparasites. The bacteria and fungi that inhabit the skin, buccal cavity and intestinal tract of some raptor species have been studied but the picture is far from complete and as a result it can prove difficult to interpret bacteriological findings when disease or death is being investigated. Virtually nothing is known about the part played by viruses as inhabitants of clinically healthy birds of prey. Far, far, more work is needed on this subject, and the studies could be greatly enhanced if they were performed in free-living as well as in captive birds. The value of research on 'normal' raptors, caught on migration or as part of ringing (banding) programmes, has been emphasised in foregoing chapters and is intentionally repeated here. Such investigations should, whenever possible, include the collection of blood and other tissue samples because, again, so relatively little is known of what is and what is not 'within normal limits' for a given species. The collection and analysis of these forms the basis of health monitoring (see Chapter 4 and Appendices VII and VIII) and will play an important part in improving our ability to interpret findings in free-living, as well as captive, birds. It is vital, however, that tried and tested protocols for sampling, transportation and processing of specimens are developed and used on an international basis. Likewise, databases should be established and made available to all. At present technical methods used in different locations differ substantially and information on birds of prey remains scattered and not always easily accessible. Free and open exchange is vital if knowledge about raptor health is to be disseminated and real progress is to be made. In this vein the World Wide Web, via the internet, provides many (not all) with a means of gaining access to data in addition to conventional sources such as books and papers.

Disease is a dynamic process and it is not surprising that 'new' diseases have emerged and some 'old' ones seem to have disappeared. In the case of captive raptors, factors that may contribute to the emergence of a 'new' condition include intensification of management, whereby certain organisms such as *Caryospora*, may flourish and then cause ill-health (Papazahariadou *et al.*, 2001). Free-living raptors

may, likewise, be affected by organisms that either build up in numbers in nest sites or are introduced during badly planned translocation programmes – although, as pointed out by Ian Newton in Chapter 14, proven instances of such occurrences in birds of prey are rare.

My own study of raptor medicine and pathology over nearly four decades has never been full-time and has usually had to be fitted into a busy work programme. Much of it has been unpaid and unfunded. However, during that period, I have striven to improve our knowledge of the diseases of these birds and have drawn up proposals as to how best the health of captive and free-living raptors might be monitored and enhanced. Throughout, I have found it fruitful to maintain close co-operation with others, especially zoologists, field ornithologists, aviculturists, falconers and naturalists. Benefits have clearly accrued from such collaboration. It has, in particular, yielded information that has enhanced the health of birds in captivity, not only those kept for falconry, captive-breeding and display, but also raptors in rehabilitation centres and in conservation programmes – for instance, the Mauritius kestrel.

Although we still have much to learn about the health and diseases of birds of prey, the opportunities to do so have never been better. Falconiformes and Strigiformes continue to command much attention from both scientists and lay persons. Free-living raptors are at the top of various food chains and as such are not only particularly prone to poisoning (see Chapters 1 and 11) but also can be susceptible to infectious diseases acquired from their prey (see Chapter 14). Few people now doubt the value and importance of scientific studies on the ecology and status of free-living birds and veterinary involvement in such projects is increasingly being sought, especially where questions are being asked about health or disease (Greenwood, 1996). As I know from my own experiences, such collaboration between biologists, veterinarians and others can only be beneficial (Cooper, 1993a).

As stressed elsewhere, the past three decades have seen the appearance of many publications on bird of prey medicine and pathology – not only scientific papers in journals but also 'popular' articles in magazines and newsletters intended for birdkeepers, rehabilitators and falconers. Such literature has helped those concerned with raptors to approach the subject of health and disease scientifically and methodically. The majority of publications have, however, originated from Europe and North America, with small numbers from Australasia, the Middle East and other richer parts of the world. And yet, it is often in the poorer countries that birds of prey are most at risk and where information and help are most needed. It is imperative that there is closer international liaison if such gaps are to be bridged – hence my plea earlier for free and open exchange of information.

In 1978 I stated that 'the whole field of bird of prey medicine is expanding and it is reasonable to assume that the next 10 years will see dramatic developments in such fields as clinical chemistry, anaesthesia, surgery and pathology. Those involved in raptor medicine are likely to become more specialised in their various disciplines and it is probable that future editions of this book will include contributions by experts in different fields.' Those words have proved prophetic. Laboratory and clinical techniques advanced dramatically during that decade and this trend has continued exponentially since. Specialisation in avian medicine is now possible through such bodies as the (British) Royal College of Veterinary Surgeons (RCVS), the European College of Avian Medicine and Surgery (ECAMS) and the American Board of Veterinary Practitioners (ABVP). Short courses and workshops for veterinarians are popular in many countries and these often cover, or include, specific sessions on birds of prey. There are increasing numbers of clinicians, anaesthetists, surgeons and pathologists with knowledge and experience of avian veterinary science.

What of the future? Are advances comparable to those that have occurred since 1970 likely to take place? What changes will we see insofar as captive raptors are concerned? To what extent might the present emphasis on treatment of the individual sick or injured bird be replaced by greater attention to health monitoring and preventive medicine and by work on free-living raptors?

No-one can be sure but scientific research on raptors will almost certainly assume increasing importance with 'evidence-based', peer-reviewed, data replacing what are still often anecdotal accounts or subjective opinions. Much of the research will, as now, be centred on clinical and *post-mortem* studies of naturally occurring diseases but experimental work is very likely also to contribute and this may take several forms.

Developments in captive-breeding, coupled with gene technology, might result in the production of strains of birds of prey that are, amongst other things, resistant to certain disorders. Improved techniques of artificial insemination may result in the recognition of venereally transmitted diseases or, conversely, the procedure may find new acceptance as a means of *preventing* the spread of pathogens by minimising direct contact between birds.

It can be argued that experimental work using raptors or other birds as laboratory 'models' is essential if many of the queries relating to raptor health and disease are to be elucidated and, for example, new vaccines are to be developed and tested (Remple, 2001). The production of germ-free or gnotobiotic birds could facilitate the study of infectious disease and of 'normal' anatomy and physiology. Such experimental work is likely to receive a mixed reception, since there is considerable public concern in some countries over the use of live animals in research. Those who carry out such studies must therefore ensure that the investigations cannot satisfactorily be performed by using a non-sentient system and that due attention is paid to the care and well-being of the birds involved.

The welfare of all captive raptors is likely to attract increasing interest and concern in the future. In recent years even such standard procedures as the tethering of falconers' hawks have come under scrutiny. A research project on the welfare of captive raptors was carried out in Britain, at the University of Kent (Cromie & Nicholls, 1995), and some useful recommendations emerged, particularly in respect of management methods. These recommendations, amongst other things, dissuaded the (British) Royal Society for the Prevention of Cruelty to Animals from seeking a ban on falconry, and led, instead, to the development of guidelines to address welfare issues (see Appendix XI).

The now well recognised role of birds of prey as

important indicators of 'ecosystem health' means that research on these species in the wild is likely to become more prevalent and more necessary. Long-term studies will assume increasing importance, with particular reference to distribution, breeding success and population change. The status of most raptors will need constant surveillance, especially in the context of alterations in land use and agricultural practice. However, such work will not be confined to rural locations: some species of birds of prey are already prevalent in, and depend upon, cities while others are in the process of becoming 'urbanised'. This relatively new field of urban wildlife conservation was discussed at an International Symposium, held in Arizona, USA, in 1999 and the conclusions were that certain animals, including raptors, will prove to be valuable environmental sentinels in such situations. At the same time, however, new 'raptor–human conflicts' may emerge, some relating to the possible carriage and transmission by birds of prey of pathogenic organisms.

Interest in raptors and their biology, including their health, seems unlikely to wane in this 'post-pesticide era'. On the contrary, the subject may increase in importance and involve people from many disciplines in various parts of the world. Birds of prey may have been associated with humans for centuries and great advances may have been made over the past 30 years, but much remains to be learned of their health, diseases and causes of death. If the raptor biologist and the veterinarian are to work together productively, they must have ready access to data on these species. So too must all those who bear responsibility for these birds in captivity – falconers, zoo staff, researchers, rehabilitators and aviculturists. It is hoped that this book will continue to play a role in meeting those demands.

Appendices

List of Species of Raptor

The English and scientific names below are based, in part, upon *A Complete Checklist of the Birds of the World* by Richard Howard and Alick Moore (1994). They comprise the birds of prey to which reference or allusion is made in the text of the book – sometimes with English names given as used by the author of cited papers or contributors to this volume.

Scientific names of other, non-avian, taxa appear in the text, not in the list.

Subspecies are not usually differentiated in this book. Thus, for example, the European black kite (*Milvus migrans migrans*) and the African (yellow-billed) kite (*Milvus migrans parasitus*) are both listed as 'Black kite' (*Milvus migrans*).

In this list, as in the text, a traditional method of differentiation of 'raptors' into Falconiformes and Strigiformes is followed. The transfer of falconiform species to the order Ciconiiformes, as advocated by Proctor and Lynch (1993), is at present under discussion by ornithologists.

English name	Scientific name
FALCONIFORMES	
Turkey vulture	*Cathartes aura*
Californian condor	*Gymnogyps californianus*
King vulture	*Sarcorhamphus papa*
Andean condor	*Vultur gryphus*
Osprey	*Pandion haliaetus*
Black-shouldered kite	*Elanus caeruleus*
Mississippi kite	*Ictinia missippiensis*
Black kite	*Milvus migrans*
Red kite	*Milvus milvus*
African fish eagle	*Haliaeetus vocifer*
(American) bald eagle	*Haliaeetus leucocephalus*
White-tailed sea eagle	*Haliaeetus albicilla*
Steller's sea eagle	*Haliaeetus pelagicus*
Black (cinereous) vulture	*Aegypius monachus*
Lappet-faced vulture	*Aegypius (Torgos) tracheliotus*
Hooded vulture	*Necrosyrtes monachus*
Eurasian (griffon) vulture	*Gyps fulvus*
Cape (griffon) vulture	*Gyps coprotheres*
African white-backed vulture	*Gyps africanus*
White-rumped vulture	*Gyps bengalensis*
Long-billed vulture	*Gyps indicus*
Eurasian griffon	*Gyps fulvus*
Egyptian vulture	*Neophron percnopterus*
Lammergeier	*Gypaetus barbatus*
Bateleur	*Terathopius ecaudatus*
Dark chanting goshawk	*Melierax metabates*
Pale chanting goshawk	*Melierax canorus*
Gabar goshawk	*Melierax gabar*
African harrier-hawk	*Polyboroides typus*
Hen (Northern) harrier	*Circus cyaneus*
Western marsh-harrier	*Circus aeruginasus*
African goshawk	*Accipiter tachiro*
Shikra	*Accipiter badius*
Northern (Eurasian) sparrow-hawk	*Accipiter nisus*
Sharp-shinned hawk	*Accipiter striatus*
Great (Black goshawk) sparrow-hawk	*Accipiter melanoleucus*
Cooper's hawk	*Accipiter cooperii*
Northern goshawk	*Accipiter gentilis*
Harris' hawk	*Parabuteo unicinctus*

English name	Scientific name
FALCONIFORMES	
Swainson's hawk	*Buteo swainsoni*
Red-tailed hawk	*Buteo jamaicensis*
Ferruginous hawk	*Buteo regalis*
Eurasian buzzard	*Buteo buteo*
Rough-legged hawk	*Buteo lagopus*
Augur buzzard	*Buteo rufofuscus*
Harpy eagle	*Harpia harpyja*
Philippine eagle	*Pithecophaga jefferyi*
Tawny eagle	*Aquila rapax*
Steppe eagle	*Aquila nipalensis*
Imperial eagle	*Aquila heliaca*
Wahlberg's eagle	*Hieraaetus wahlbergi*
Golden eagle	*Aquila chrysaetos*
African hawk eagle	*Hieraaetus fasciatus*
Martial eagle	*Hieraaetus bellicosus*
Secretary bird	*Sagittarius serpentarius*
Common caracara	*Polyborus plancus*
Laughing falcon	*Herpetotheres cachinnans*
Collared falconet	*Microhierax caerulescens*
Lesser kestrel	*Falco naumanni*
American kestrel	*Falco sparverius*
Common (Eurasian) kestrel	*Falco tinnunculus*
Mauritius kestrel	*Falco punctatus*
Red-headed (necked) falcon	*Falco chicquera*
Merlin	*Falco columbarius*
Seychelles kestrel	*Falco araea*
Nankeen (Australian) kestrel	*Falco cenchroides*
Northern (Eurasian) hobby	*Falco subbuteo*
Aplomado falcon	*Falco femoralis*
Eleonora's falcon	*Falco eleonorae*
Lanner falcon	*Falco biarmicus*
Prairie falcon	*Falco mexicanus*
Lagger (laggar) falcon	*Falco jugger*
Saker falcon	*Falco cherrug*
Gyr falcon (gyrfalcon)	*Falco rusticolus*
Peregrine	*Falco peregrinus*
Barbary falcon	*Falco pelegrinoides*
STRIGIFORMES	
Barn owl	*Tyto alba*
Spectacled owl	*Pulsatrix perspicillata*
Great horned owl	*Bubo virginianus*
Northern (Eurasian) eagle owl	*Bubo bubo*
Spotted eagle owl	*Bubo africanus*
Verreaux's eagle owl	*Bubo lacteus*
Malay fish owl	*Bubo ketupu*
Snowy owl	*Nyctea scandiaca*
African wood owl	*Strix woodfordii*
(Eurasian) tawny owl	*Strix aluco*
Spotted owl	*Strix occidentalis*
Great grey owl	*Strix nebulosa*
Barred owl	*Strix varia*
Red-chested owlet	*Glaucidium tephronotum*
Little owl	*Athene noctua*
Tengmalm's (boreal) owl	*Aegolius funereus*
Saw-whet owl	*Aegolius acadicus*
Long-eared owl	*Asia otus*
Short-eared owl	*Asio flammeus*
African Marsh owl	*Asio capensis*

Clinical Examination Forms, including Questionnaire

SUGGESTED QUESTIONNAIRE FOR HISTORY AND REASONS FOR PRESENTATION

Name and contact details of person presenting the bird(s) ....
....
Species (if known) .... Age (if known) ....
Sex (if known) .... Time in possession of person presenting the bird ....
Origin: *Wild (free-living) casualty/Captive bird

IF A WILD CASUALTY:
Date and time of recovery .... Location of recovery (with grid reference if available) ....
Circumstances of recovery (including any relevant observations at the time and, if available, weight of the bird when found) ....
....
Summary of action taken at the time ....
Summary of any treatment/care given, including food, fluids, medicines ....
....
Continue below where appropriate

IF A CAPTIVE BIRD:
Origin: *Captive-bred/Purchased/Permanent casualty/Other   If Other, give details ....
Other birds kept at same premises ....
Management: *In aviary/Trained/Other   If Other, give details ....
Summary of management system ....
....
Diet .... Supplements ....
Source and storage of diet (food) ....
Reason for presenting the bird(s) ....
Clinical signs ('symptoms') observed – give details ....
....
....
Specific comments on feeding ....
Specific comments on muting (defaecation) ....
Specific comments on casting ....
Any treatment given ....
Comments on factors that may (or may not) be relevant to the bird's present ill-health (e.g. changes in management, disease in other birds on the premises) ....
....
....
Other information that may be relevant (if appropriate add photographs, drawings of bird, aviary, etc.) ....
....
....

Name .... Signature .... Date .... Time ....

* delete/complete as appropriate

CLINICAL EXAMINATION FORM

BACKGROUND

Species (common* and scientific name) .... Age .... Sex ....

Presented by:

Name .... Contact details ....

....

Questionnaire completed[†] YES/NO (if YES, refer to the questionnaire; if NO, clinician to complete relevant parts of the questionnaire)

History of bird ....

Clinical history ....

....

FINDINGS

Weight (mass) .... Measurements ....

How presented (in box/on fist, etc.) ....

Distant observation possible[†] YES/NO

If YES, (bird unaware) observations (use checklist if necessary) ....

....

If NO, (bird aware) observations ....

Handling and restraint: [†]Unanaesthetised/Anaesthetised/Hooded/Unhooded/Other

If OTHER, please give details ....

General findings ....

Specific findings: (List under parts of the body (e.g. head) or organ system (e.g. respiratory system) or, if preferred, under clinical techniques (e.g. auscultation, endoscopy))

Samples taken for laboratory investigation:

(List under specimens (e.g. faeces, swab) or investigative techniques (e.g. cytology, bacteriology) or a combination of both)

Provisional diagnosis/conclusions ....

Final diagnosis/conclusions ....

Follow-up work needed ....

Name .... Signature .... Date .... Time ....

* in non-Anglophone countries this may be in a language other than English

[†] delete/complete as appropriate

Post-mortem *and Egg/Embryo* *Protocol and Examination* *Form*

POST-MORTEM EXAMINATION FORM

Species .... Reference No. ....

Date of Submission .... Origin ....

Relevant history/circumstances of death:

Request – diagnosis (cause of death/ill-health), health monitoring, forensic investigation/research/other

Any special requirements re techniques to be followed, fate of body/samples

Submitted by .... Date ....

Received by .... Date ....

Measurements: Carpus tarsus other   Bodyweight (Mass)

Condition score: Obese or fat/good/fair or thin/poor

State of preservation: Good/fair/poor/marked autolysis   A number ('score')
                                                                     can be used for these
Storage since death: Refrigerator/ambient temperature/frozed/fixed

---

EXTERNAL OBSERVATIONS, including preen gland, state of moult, ectoparasites, skin condition, lesions etc.

MACROSCOPIC EVALUATION ON OPENING THE BODY, including position and appearance of organs, lesions etc.

ALIMENTARY SYSTEM

MUSCULOSKELETAL

CARDIOVASCULAR

RESPIRATORY   This section can be expanded, as necessary –
                                             subheadings can be inserted, including
URINARY   checklist of organs and tissues

REPRODUCTIVE

LYMPHOID (including bursa)

NERVOUS

OTHER
SAMPLES TAKEN

....	Bact	Paras	Hist	DNA	Cytology	Other (e.g. serology)
....	Bact	Paras	Hist	DNA	Cytology	Other (e.g. serology)
....	Bact	Paras	Hist	DNA	Cytology	Other (e.g. serology)
....	Bact	Paras	Hist	DNA	Cytology	Other (e.g. serology)
....	Bact	Paras	Hist	DNA	Cytology	Other (e.g. serology)
....	Bact	Paras	Hist	DNA	Cytology	Other (e.g. serology)
....	Bact	Paras	Hist	DNA	Cytology	Other (e.g. serology)

LABORATORY FINDINGS

Date: .... Initials: .... Reported to whom: ....

PRELIMINARY REPORT (based on gross findings and immediate laboratory results, e.g. cytology)

Reported to .... Date .... Time ....

FINAL REPORT (based on all available information)

FATE OF CARCASS/TISSUES
destroyed/frozen/fixed in formalin (other)/retained for Reference Collection/sent elsewhere

PM examination performed by: .... Date .... Time ....
Reported by: .... Date ....

EXAMINATION OF UNHATCHED EGGS–PROTOCOL

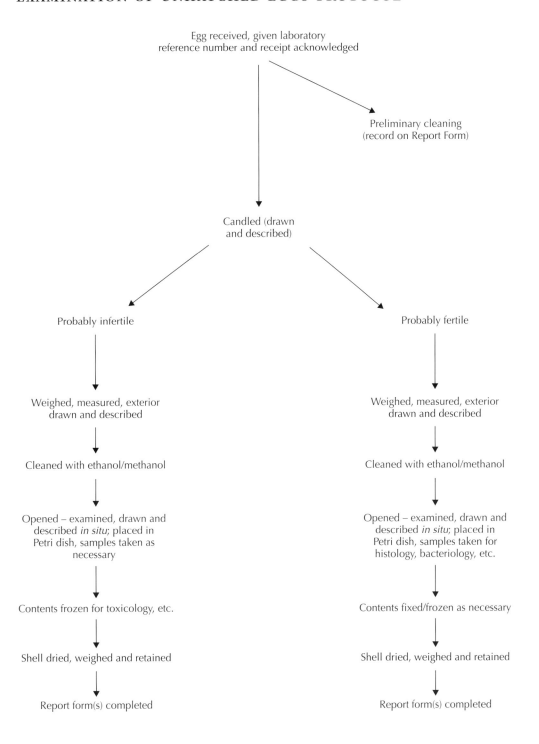

EXAMINATION OF EGGS/EMBRYOS–REPORT FORM

Reference number:
Received: (date) .... (by) ....
Receipt acknowledged by: .... Date ....
Method of packing/wrappings:
History:

EGG/EMBRYO EXAMINATION
(to be completed for each specimen)

Species: (Common name) .... (Scientific name) ....
Owner/Origin: ....
Weight of whole unopened egg: .... Length: .... Width: ....
External appearance (see Fig. 1)
Appearance on candling (see Fig. 2)
        Embryo
        Air cell
        Blood vessels
        Fluids

Fig. 1   Fig. 2

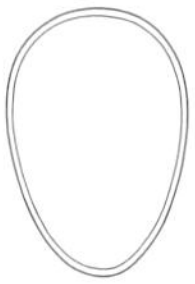

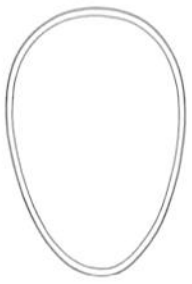

Appearance when opened (see Fig. 3)
Contents:

Fig. 3

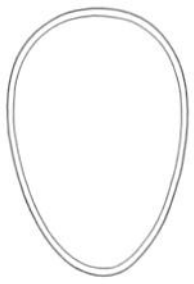

Embryo: Length (crown-rump)
           Amniotic cavity
           Allantoic cavity
           Yolk sac
Other comments:

Microbiology:

Histopathology:

Other tests:

Samples sent elsewhere:

Weight of dried eggshell: .... Thickness (measurement or index): ....
Samples stored
COMMENTS

Date: .... Signature: .... Name: ....

Cytology and Blood Smear Report Forms

CYTOLOGY REPORT

Species ....

Reference ....

History/Background ....

....

....

Sample submitted ....

Date and time of collection ....

Stain(s) and number of preparation(s) ....

....

General comments on preparation(s) ....

....

Cell Types	Numbers (+/++/+++)	Features	Comments

Other findings ....

....

....

Summary or interpretation of findings ....

....

....

Advice or action (if appropriate) ....

....

Name:.. Signature: .... Date: ....

REPORT ON BLOOD SMEARS

Species .... Reference ....
History/Background ....
Dates .... Comments ....

No.	Quality		Parasites	Abnormalities	Blood cells or counts	Comments
	Smear	Stain				

P = poor   M = moderate   G = good   NPS = no parasites found   A = artefact
1–3 = grades   ± = subgrade
Polychromatophilic index of 1–5% assumed normal

Key to Major Clinical Diagnoses

Locality	Clinical sign or lesion	Possible diagnoses
Head	Wounds	Trauma, infection, neoplasm
	Swelling	Trauma, pox, sinusitis, insect or tick bite, stomatitis, e.g. trichomoniasis, abscess, neoplasia
	Rhythmical distension of soft tissue in front of eyes	Upper respiratory infection (sinusitis) or physical obstruction, *Cyathostoma*
	Ocular lesions	Trauma, conjunctivitis, ophthalmitis, vitamin A deficiency, pox, cataract, chlamydiosis (chamydophilosis)
	Eyes closing	A common sign of any serious or debilitating condition. A sign of many diseases including (sometimes) tuberculosis.
	Sneezing	Rhinitis, sinusitis, irritation by dust or chemicals, *Cyathostoma*
	Nasal discharge	Rhinitis, sinusitis, chlamydiosis, tick reaction
	Blockage of nares	Rhinitis, sinusitis, rhinoliths, as above
	Nasal haemorrhage	Trauma or hypertensive (?) rupture of blood vessels. Tick bite reaction
	Pale mucous membranes	Blood loss, anaemia, 'shock'
	Blue mucous membranes	Cyanosis, normal colour for some species, e.g. merlins. Commonest cause is pulmonary aspergillosis
	Mouth lesions	Trichomoniasis, capillariasis, pox, owl herpes virus infection, candidiasis, stomatitis, especially *Pseudomonas*. Foreign bodies, e.g. material wrapped around tongue. Vitamin A deficiency
	Fluid from mouth	Capillariasis or other mouth lesions, some types of poisoning
	Blood from mouth	As for nasal haemorrhage (above)
	Damp feathers on side of head	Otitis (bacterial or myiasis), trauma, conjunctivitis, corneal lesions

Locality	Clinical sign or lesion	Possible diagnoses
	Head on one side	Otitis, trauma, encephalitis or other nervous disease (including lead poisoning and Newcastle disease (ND))
	Head hanging low	Blindness, lead poisoning, cervical trauma
	Blindness (complete or partial)	Trauma, poisoning (especially) chlorinated hydrocarbons and lead), vitamin A deficiency
	Voice change	Respiratory disease, syngamiasis, starvation, several other conditions. Most commonly syringeal aspergillosis
Wings	Wounds	Trauma, infection, predation, neoplasia
	Wing hanging or paralysed	Fracture, dislocation tendonitis/arthritis, traumatic damage to joint (shoulder/elbow carpus), nerve, tendon or ligament, osteodystrophy, irritant injection in pectoral muscles. *Salmonella* septic arthritis. Wing tip oedema (WTO)
	Blood on feathers	Compound fracture, skin wound, damaged young (blood) feathers
	Swellings	Fracture, abscess, granuloma, tuberculosis, bursitis, WTO, neoplasia especially fibrosarcoma
	Missing or drooping feathers	Moulting, feather abnormalities, gangrene. (See also 'Absence of feathers' under 'Legs', and 'Feather loss on abdomen' under 'Body', and 'Feathers')
Legs	Swelling or displacement	Osteodystrophy, rickets, fracture, dislocation, bursitis, abscess, granuloma, tuberculosis, oedema, osteopetrosis, neoplasia especially squamous cell carcinoma
	Wounds	Trauma, poor fitting jesses, bites from prey or predators
	Paralysed	Spinal trauma, internal lesions, egg-laying, vitamin deficiency, Marek's disease?, lead poisoning, spinal aspergillosis, spinal abscess
	Absence of feathers	Ectoparasites, feather abnormality, possibly an underlying hormonal or metabolic disorder. Liver or kidney failure
	Hocks held straight, not bent	A general sign of ill-health
Feet	Swelling	Bumblefoot, articular gout, arthritis, trauma, jesses or ring too tight
	Blood	Puncture wound
	Pale in colour	Low dietary carotene
	Localised lesions	Pox, Type 1 bumblefoot, trauma, vitamin A deficiency, papillomatosis
	Paralysed	As for nervous signs, these may occur in conjunction with enteritis – lead poisoning
	Knuckling over	Nervous damage, lead poisoning

Locality	Clinical sign or lesion	Possible diagnoses
Body	Wounds	Trauma, dermatitis (various causes), neoplasia
	Swelling	Fracture, abscess, tuberculosis, swollen liver, granuloma, haematoma, obesity, neoplasia, subcutaneous emphysema, irritant injection, egg peritonitis, amyloidosis
	Abdominal distension and discomfort	Egg peritonitis, impacted cloaca, damage during insemination, other abdominal lesions, amyloidosis
	Feather loss on abdomen	Trauma, normal brood patch (female). Liver/kidney disease
	Soiling of cloaca	Enteritis, cloacitis, prolonged recumbency, cloacal calculus
	Tail bobbing	Respiratory disease, cloacal calculus
	Sternal lesion	Trauma, prolonged recumbency, genetic
	Dry, lustreless, preen gland	Preen gland dysfunction
	Swollen preen gland	Impaction, infection, neoplasia
Feathers	Missing	Moult, current or previous trauma, nutritional deficiency, metabolic disturbance, non-specific factors
	Broken	Trauma, metabolic disturbance, nutritional deficiency
	Frayed	Ectoparasites, metabolic disturbance, nutritional deficiency. Poor husbandry
General signs	Chronic weight loss	Tuberculosis, aspergillosis, various types of parasitism, neoplasia, hepatopathy
	Dyspnoea	Foreign body in upper alimentary or respiratory tract, syngamiasis, rhinitis, pneumonia, air sacculitis, aspergillosis, trichomoniasis
	Hyperpnoea	Overheating, septicaemia, pneumonia, air sacculitis, anaemia. Inhaled toxin
	Excessive drinking	Tuberculosis, renal disease, other infections, dehydration, egg-laying
	Anorexia	Overweight, several infectious diseases, food unpalatable, pain or trauma to mouth or gastro-intestinal tract
	Dysphagia	Pellet not cast, foreign body, any condition affecting buccal cavity or causing dyspnoea. Unaccustomed to food type offered
	Flicking of food	Stomatitis and certain other conditions, food unpalatable, Commonly crop infection

Locality	Clinical sign or lesion	Possible diagnoses
	Regurgitation and/or vomition	Oesophageal capillariasis or other crop lesion, gastritis, air sacculitis. May also occur under stressful conditions, including travel. Occurs with some drugs if food in crop/proventriculus
	Wet, foetid casting	As for regurgitation
	Failure to cast, or delay in casting	A sign of many diseases (see text). Also associated with overfeeding and dry food and lead poisoning
	Diarrhoea	Bacterial yeast or parasitic infection of intestine, cloacitis, low roughage diet, air sacculitis, unsuitable food, non-specific factors (e.g. chilling)
	Poorly formed mutes	Enteritis (bacterial/parasitic), cloacitis, egg-laying
	Excessive (voluminous) mutes	Malabsorption, fermentation in gut, 'stress'
	Dry mutes (and/or reduced volume)	Dehydration or obstruction
	Green mutes	Low food intake, hepatitis or blood breakdown
	Clay-coloured faeces	Malabsorption
	Yellow faeces	Renal disease, hepatic disease (especially toxic damage, e.g. lead poisoning), previous administration of certain drugs (e.g. 2-amino-5-nitrothiazole, B vitamins)
	Mutes containing undigested food	Malabsorption, decreased gut transit time, 'stress'
	Dysentery (fresh blood)	Trauma, cloacal calculus, cloacitis, constipation (straining), parasites. Adenovirus infection
	Dysentery (partly digested blood)	Coccidiosis, capillariasis, other causes of haemorrhage in upper tract, bruising (including surgery)
	Excess urinary portion	Renal disease, polydipsia
	Unabsorbed yolk sac (chicks)	Chilling or other environmental stressor
	Nervous signs	Poisoning (especially insecticidal or lead), vitamin B1 deficiency, hypocalcaemia, hypoglycaemia, bacterial otitis or encephalitis, trauma, Newcastle disease, hyperglycaemia, chlamydiosis (chlamydophilosis)
	Trembling	Nervous temperament, various nervous diseases
	Hunched posture	A general sign of ill-health, spinal kyphosis
	Poor flight performance	Low condition, calcium deficiency, hepatopathy, hypoglycaemia. Any serious illness or lack of exercise

Key to Major (Gross) Post-mortem Diagnoses including Findings in Eggs

KEY TO MAJOR (GROSS) POST-MORTEM DIAGNOSES

Locality	Lesion	Possible diagnoses
External	As in previous Appendix	As in previous Appendix
Subcutis	Haemorrhage especially in head, neck region	Tick bite, trauma
Pectoral muscle changes	Haemorrhage, swelling, reduction in size, lesions	Trauma, intramuscular injections, disuse atrophy, *Sarcocystis*
Internal		
Body cavity	Inflammation Caseous lesions	Peritonitis, septicaemia, foreign body penetration. Aspergillosis, tuberculosis, nocardiosis, neoplasia
	Haemorrhage	Trauma, euthanasia by intraperitoneal injection, electrocution, poisoning, 'apoplexy'
	Pale colour, watery blood	Anaemia
	Bright pink colour	Carbon monoxide poisoning
	Hyperaemia of organs	Septicaemia, poisoning
	Internal swellings	Haematoma, abscess, neoplasia, tuberculosis, aspergillosis, egg in oviduct or body cavity
	Congestion of organs	Congestive cardiac failure
	White deposits on serosae and elsewhere	Visceral gout, intraperitoneal barbiturate, neoplasia post-mortem mould if necropsy delayed
Respiratory tract	Inflammation	Rhinitis, bronchitis, air sacculitis, pneumonia, sinusitis
	Clouding or thickening of air sacs	Post-mortem degeneration, air sacculitis, fat deposition in air sacs
	Nematodes	*Cyathastoma*, *Syngamus* or *Serratospiculum* infestation
	Lesions in lung or air sacs	Pneumonia, air sacculitis, aspergillosis, inhalation pneumonia, abscess (extension from fractured rib), trauma, neoplasia

Locality	Lesion	Possible diagnoses
	Pulmonary congestion	Pneumonia, hypostatic congestion, congestive cardiac failure
	Black or dark material in lungs or air sacs	Anthracosis, silicosis, inhalation of certain drugs
	Haemorrhage/oedema	Various infectious diseases, cardiovascular failure, polytetrafluoroethylene (PTFE) poisoning
Alimentary tract	Inflammation	Enteritis of bacterial or other aetiology
	Nematodes Cestodes Trematodes Acanthocephalans	Helminthiasis (various species)
	Haemorrhages	Coccidiosis, capillariasis, poisoning, electrocution
	Green material	Low food intake, lead poisoning
	Stones and fibrous material in gizzard	Impacted gizzard, presence of rangle, inanition, lead poisoning
	Constipation	Impacted cloaca, high roughage diet, mechanical lesion of intestinal tract, e.g. intussusception
Cardiovascular system	Flabby heart Oedema Hydropericardium	Anaemia or other circulatory disturbance, developmental abnormality
	Lesions of pericardium	Pericarditis, septicaemia, visceral gout
	Lesions of myocardium	Myocarditis (acute or chronic), *Leucocytozoon*
	Lesions of endocardium	Atheromatosis, endocarditis
	Lesions of blood vessels	Vasculitis, atheromatosis, arteriosclerosis
Liver	Foci	Tuberculosis, aspergillosis, yersiniosis, viral hepatitis, other infections, neoplasia
	Other parenchymal lesions	Septicaemia, viral hepatitis, trauma, neoplasia, fatty change, amyloidosis, *Leucocytozoon*
	Capsular lesions	Septicaemia, air sacculitis, chlamydiosis, aspergillosis, visceral gout
Kidney	White foci	Urate aggregates – dehydration, renal failure; yersiniosis, other infections
	Swollen	Nephritis, nephrosis, gout, fatty change, amyloidosis, neoplasia

Locality	Lesion	Possible diagnoses
Cloaca	Distended	Cloacal calculus
	Wall thickened or inflamed	Cloacitis
	Fresh blood	Cloacal calculus, cloacitis, constipation (straining) or traumatic injury (e.g. associated with artificial insemination). Intussusception
Adrenal glands	Enlarged	Adrenal hypertrophy, infection, 'stress'?
Nervous system	Lesions on nerves	Tuberculosis, aspergillosis, trauma, Marek's disease?
	Congestion of brain and meninges	Nervous disease, infection, trauma, bird in abnormal position before or at death
Locomotory system	Muscle atrophy	Lack of use of muscle, starvation
	Pale muscles	Anaemia, possibly parasite (e.g. *Sarcocystis*) lesions
	Soft, pliable, bones	Young bird, osteodystrophy (metabolic bone disease)
	Multiple fractures	Osteodystrophy, trauma, neoplasia
	Swelling of bones or joints	Arthritis, osteitis, healing fracture, neoplasia
	Longitudinal twisting of long bones	Osteodystrophy
	Intraosseous haemorrhages of skull	Agonal, trauma
	Pale bone marrow	Anaemia
	Bright pink bone marrow	Carbon monoxide poisoning

SOME FINDINGS IN EGGS AND THEIR POSSIBLE SIGNIFICANCE

Finding	*Possible interpretation(s)*
Infertile egg	Parent birds not of same species; of one sex; one or both immature; incompatible; incapable (e.g. because of physical injury) of courtship or copulation, one or both infertile from infectious causes
Soft-shelled, thin-shelled or abnormal egg (infertile or fertile)	Calcium deficiency; oviduct abnormality or old age (hen bird). Elevated levels of chlorinated hydrocarbon insecticides
Profuse growth of bacteria from contents of infertile egg	Contamination in nest/incubator. Prolonged/poor storage
Profuse growth of bacteria from contents of fertile egg; more than one species of organism, not recognised avian pathogens	As above
One (possibly two) organisms in pure culture, recognised avian pathogens	Embryonic death possibly due to infection
Dead embryo, late incubation, no evidence of infection, unusual position in egg	Death possibly due to inability to hatch (malpositioning)
Dead embryo, no evidence of infection or malpositioning. Abnormalities, e.g. hydrocephalus, duplication of digits	Death possibly due to genetic or other factor causing abnormality
Dead embryo, no evidence of infection, malpositioning or abnormalities	Incorrect incubation temperature or relative humidity, faulty turning in incubator, prolonged/poor storage; infection; nutritional deficiency
Embryo dead-in-shell at hatching stage	Low relative humidity prior to hatching, trauma (e.g. human interference)
Chlorinated hydrocarbon insecticides, heavy metals or other chemicals in egg contents or egg shell	Infertility/death of embryo, possibly due to poisons *OR* elevated values indicative of high environmental pollution

The Principles of Health Monitoring, with Particular Reference to the Movement of Raptors

'Diseases are easier prevented than cured: everyone therefore that intends to keep Hawks should be well advised in the first place how to preserve them from Sickness and Maladies, which is of greater concern than to cure them when distempered.'

Richard Blome

(Adapted in part from a paper presented by John E. Cooper at the Middle East Falcon Research Group Specialist Workshop, Abu Dhabi, United Arab Emirates, November 1995.)

INTRODUCTION

This paper is concerned with the health monitoring of birds of prey with special, but not exclusive, reference to those destined for movement from one place to another. Such movement is increasingly being used as a tool in species' conservation (Gipps, 1991) but there are those who question its wisdom (Conant, 1988) and many concerns have been expressed over the dangers that it may present in terms of spread of pathogens (Cooper & Greenwood, 1981a,b; Cooper, 1989a; Castle & Christansen, 1990; Wolff & Seal, 1993).

First, it is important to be familiar with the accepted definitions relating to movement of live animals (IUCN Position Statement on the Translocation of Living Organisms, 1987):

'Introduction' – the intentional or accidental dispersal by human agency of a living organism outside its historically known range.

'Reintroduction' – the intentional movement of an organism into part of its native range from which it has disappeared or become extirpated in historic times as a result of human activities or natural catastrophe.

'Restocking' – the movement of numbers of plants or animals with the intention of building up the number of individuals of that species in an original habitat.

'Translocation' – the captive transport and release of free-ranging wild animals, moving them from one part of their historic range to a different location, but one where the species occurs at present or has historically occurred naturally.

Other definitions that are particularly relevant to health monitoring are:

'Health' – freedom from disease; bodily and mentally vigorous.

'Disease' – any impairment of normal physiological function affecting all or part of an organism.

'Infection' – the presence of an organism that is capable of causing disease.

The principles of health monitoring are the same regardless of whether the birds are to be moved or (for example) to be monitored as part of other activities such as studies on migration (Cooper, 1989b) or routine management of captive collections.

CONSIDERATIONS WHEN BIRDS OF PREY ARE MOVED

The following are the important questions that have to be asked before movement of a raptor takes place:

(1) Are there factors relating to the health of the raptor that may affect its survival or well-being in its new environment?
For example:

Presence of infectious agents (with or without clinical disease)
Presence of non-infectious disease e.g. injuries, developmental abnormalities
Undesirable genetic traits
Undesirable psychological (behavioural) traits
Other deleterious features of the bird's 'fitness'.

(2) Are any of these factors likely also to affect other species or the environment in to which the raptor is to be moved?
Examples of those that may have such an effect are:

Presence of infectious agents (with or without clinical disease)
Undesirable genetic traits
Undesirable psychological (behavioural) traits

(3) What other factors will need to be taken into account when the bird is moved?
For example:

Legal, e.g. CITES, animal health regulations, restrictions on the release of 'non-indigenous' species (Cooper, M. E., 1987)
Ethical, e.g. welfare of the bird, local cultural attitudes and traditions.

In this Appendix particular emphasis is laid upon infectious agents, the dangers that these can present when birds of prey are moved and the precautions, by employing health monitoring, that can be taken to minimise the risk of spread of such organisms.

THE ROLE AND RELEVANCE OF INFECTIOUS AGENTS

Nettles (1992) drew attention to the dangers presented by the movement of animals when he stated:

'Wildlife veterinarians are aware that each wild animal is actually a biological package that encompasses the microbiologic flora, viruses and endoparasites and ectoparasites of the animal. Therefore the moving of wild animals always holds the potential for relocation of a disease agent as well.'

Thus it is possible that a bird of prey may, during the course of being moved, disseminate or spread organisms, such as:

Macroparasites	Microparasites
Lice	Viruses
Fleas	Bacteria
Ticks	Chlamydiae (Chlamydophilae)
Hippoboscids	Rickettsiae
Leeches	Fungi
Nematodes	Algae
Cestodes	
Trematodes	
Protozoa	

In addition, many other extraneous animals, plants, eggs, seeds etc. may be transported mechanically (e.g. on the plumage or in the intestine) and subsequently shed when raptors are moved. These all come under the general heading of 'exotic organisms' and there is great concern about the effect that some are having in different parts of the world (Courtenay & Robins, 1975; Ebenhard, 1986).

Carriage of the organisms listed above may be *passive* or *active* and the organisms may or may not be associated with disease.

STEPS TO MINIMISE THE RISK OF SPREAD OF INFECTIOUS AGENTS

How can the 'biological package' of Nettles, referred to above, be rendered as harmless as possible, thus reducing the risks of organism/disease spread as a result of movement?

The answer is: by assessing and, where feasible, enhancing the health status of all birds intended to be moved.

Enhancement of health status will be considered first.

MEASURES TO ENHANCE THE HEALTH STATUS OF BIRDS INTENDED FOR MOVEMENT

The birds should be:

(1) From a reliable source that has no history of significant disease, is subject to routine veterinary attention and can be inspected

(2) Clinically healthy

(3) Subjected to rigorous health monitoring, both before and after movement

(4) Quarantined (isolated) for at least 2 weeks before movement or before introduction into their new environment

(5) Released under controlled conditions, following a standard protocol

(6) Fitted with a means of identification (e.g. microchip) and preferably also a radio or satellite transmitter

(7) Observed and followed-up (surveillance) after release – with full monitoring if the bird is recaptured alive or is found dead.

Number (3) – *health monitoring* – is the key to minimising the risk of spread of organisms and forms the basis of the remainder of this Appendix.

HEALTH MONITORING

Monitoring can be defined as the 'overall surveillance of a group or population'. The word comes from the Latin *monere*, to warn.

Health monitoring is different from diagnosis in that monitoring is primarily concerned with assessing the health status of supposedly normal birds while diagnosis relates to the detection and identification of disease in birds that are unwell. There is, however, some overlap.

The aim of monitoring is thus to ascertain as accurately as possible the health status of apparently normal birds or groups of birds and to specify (describe and quantify) this. Monitoring also provides an opportunity for the collection and recording of biological data about the individual bird, the group from which it originates or that species.

Monitoring can be carried out on:

- Live birds
- Dead birds
- The environment.

The term 'screening' is sometimes used as a synonym for 'monitoring' but strictly it refers to the situation when a group or population is monitored, using sampling rather than comprehensive examination of each individual. The term can also be used when an individual bird is monitored but only a limited number of tests is performed or only certain samples are taken.

The results of monitoring provide a 'specification (profile)' for that bird or group of birds. The reliability of the results depends upon the quality of monitoring procedures – 'quality assurance' – and a programme of 'quality control' (internal or external review and critical assessment) is advisable. 'Validation' of an investigative technique is its evaluation to determine its fitness for a particular use (OIE, 1996).

Pre-planned health monitoring programmes should be supplemented by the 'opportunistic' collection of samples – for example, when live birds have to be handled or moved (for instance, during ringing (banding)), and whenever a raptor is found dead or has to be euthanased. Any sample may provide useful information. However, it must be remembered that the minimal sample size in order to detect a particular organism, lesion or disease may be considerable. For example, from a group of 50 raptors with a 10% disease incidence 20 have to be sampled in order to give 95% confidence limits of finding one positive specimen.

Detailed information on the health monitoring of birds was first given in *Disease and Threatened Birds* (Cooper, 1989a); other relevant publications include Cooper (1987b, 1989b). The role of pathogens and disease in populations was discussed by Anderson and May (1982), Dobson and Hudson (1986), Loye and Zuk (1991a,b) and May (1988).

Protocols for clinical and *post-mortem* monitoring are given later in this appendix and in Appendices II and III.

All data must be systematically collated for analysis and interpretation. Quantitative methods should be used whenever possible including scoring systems for example, the bird's condition and histopathological findings.

Why is health monitoring of raptors important?

(1) To provide background data on the health of the individual, population or species and to obtain 'early warning' of any inconsistencies that may precede disease
(2) To reduce the risk of introducing disease or organisms into other populations of that species, or other species (see 4 below), or the environment in which they live
(3) To minimise risks to the health and welfare of the individual or species itself
(4) To protect the health of
    (a) other wild (free-living) animals
    (b) domestic animals
    (c) humans, that may come into contact with the raptor(s)
(5) To satisfy legal and ethical requirements (see Appendix XI).

How do we monitor the health of free-living and captive raptors?

(1) By analysing demographic and other records (especially free-living birds), clinical and *post-mortem* reports, and published and unpublished data
(2) By observation and examination of live birds especially when these can be captured (free-living birds) or handled (captive birds)
(3) By *post-mortem* and pathological examination of birds that die or have to be euthanased
(4) By studying and sampling the birds' environment
(5) By introducing 'sentinels' (susceptible birds or other species) to see if clinical or subclinical changes occur, or if parasites and other organisms are acquired, when the sentinels have been in proximity with the raptors or their environment (Savidge, 1986; Rocke & Brand, 1994).

(2), (3) and (4) are key features of all health monitoring programmes and follow a standard routine, as shown in Fig. AVII.1.

Action is not always necessary. *Awareness* of the situation is the important outcome: an informed decision (for example, as to whether or not a particular bird should be translocated or released) can then be made.

Important practical and ethical considerations in health monitoring

(1) Risk to the bird and to personnel, of injury, stress, infectious disease or death
(2) Cost – even basic monitoring requires funding
(3) Facilities available – especially relevant under field conditions
(4) Expertise available – some techniques require skill in, e.g. blood sampling or *post-mortem* technique
(5) Practicability – will the proposed techniques prove feasible, especially in the field?
(6) Reliability of results – this will relate to the quality and numbers of samples and how many birds can be sampled; facilities, procedures and staff; numbers of samples/sample frequency needed
(7) Legality – is the health monitoring legal? Are permits required? Does a veterinarian have to be involved? Should he/she be registered with the local authorities?
(8) Acceptability to the public and others – for example, the capture and sampling of rare birds may prompt criticism from some groups, even if permitted by law.

A cost:benefit analysis is always needed

Monitoring of live birds

Basic

Analysis of history and records
Observation and examination
(1) Presence or absence of:
    (a) clinical signs of disease
    (b) injuries or external lesions
    (c) ectoparasites.
(2) (a) bodyweight ⎤ coupled with standard
    (b) measurements ⎬ data on sex, age and
    (c) condition score ⎦ reproductive status

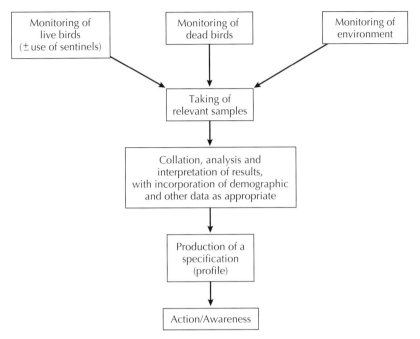

Fig. AVII.1 Health monitoring.

(3) Gross appearance of:
(a) faeces
(b) pellets (castings) – where appropriate.

Laboratory tests
(1) Presence or absence of parasites and/or abnormalities in faeces and pellets.
(2) PCV (haematocrit) and total blood protein (TP).
(3) Differential blood counts plus presence or absence of parasites or cellular abnormalities in blood smears.

Additional investigations, if personnel and facilities permit

(1) Bacteriological examination of swabs from:
(a) trachea
(b) cloaca.
(2) Blood tests – complete haematology and biochemistry.
(3) Examination of serum for specified antibodies (serology).
(4) Retention of material for DNA and other studies.

(5) Other investigations (see Fig. AVII.2).

Monitoring of dead birds

Basic

Analysis of history and records
Post-mortem examination
(1) Gross examination
(a) bodyweight ⎤ coupled with standard
(b) measurements ⎥ data on sex, age and
(c) condition score ⎦ reproductive status
(d) appearance of internal organs
(e) presence or absence of fat
(f) presence of absence of ectoparasites
(g) presence or absence of ectoparasites in alimentary or respiratory tract.
(2) Basic microscopical examination:
(a) wet preparations of faeces or gut contents
(b) cytology of any organs or tissues showing abnormality.
(3) Toxicology – submission or retention (frozen) of carcass or tissues for analysis (e.g. for chlorinated hydrocarbon pesticides, heavy metals).

263

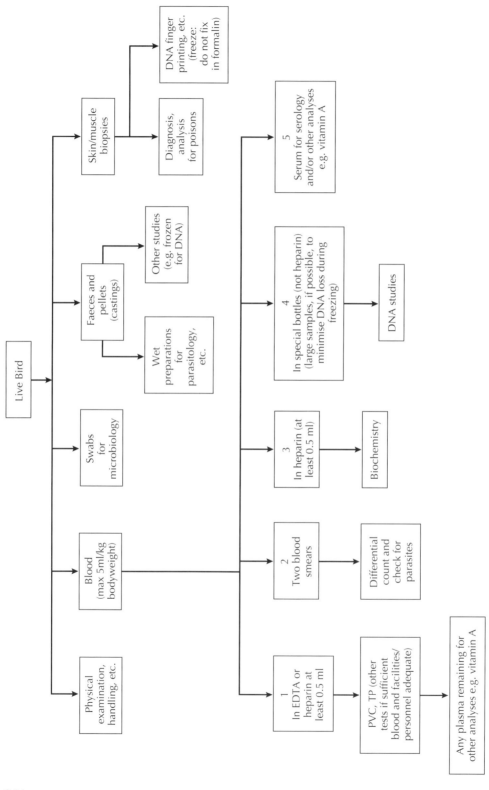

Material should be retained for retesting and reference – for example, blood smears and parasites. Serum can be stored for subsequent investigation. Any extra blood can be frozen for DNA studies.

Fig. AVII.2 Sample-taking during health monitoring of live raptors.

Additional investigations, if personnel and facilities permit

(1) Bacteriology:
  (a) heart blood
  (b) intestinal contents
  (c) any significant lesions.
(2) Histopathology:
  (a) lung, liver and kidney (plus bursa from young birds)
  (b) other organs if lesions are suspected.
(3) Submission or retention (frozen/fixed) of tissues for virology, mycoplasmology, electron-microscopy, DNA studies etc.
(4) Other investigations (see Fig. AVII.3).

Monitoring of the environment

(1) Analysis of existing data relating to the locality, e.g. climatology, geology, epizootiology (O.I.E., 1991).
(2) Health monitoring, including microbiological and toxicological investigation, of other species (captive and free-living), live and dead, in the locality.
(3) Examination and analysis of water, soil and other samples.
  Use of settle plates or other methods of assessing airborne bacteria and fungi (usually only practicable when monitoring live birds).
(4) Use of sentinel birds – options include:
  (a) using the same or other species

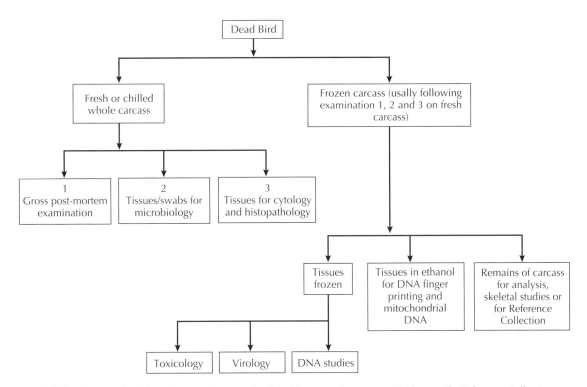

Material should be retained for reference whenever feasible (Cooper and Jones, 1986). If a specific Reference Collection exists, the carcass should be fixed in formalin other than small portions of tissue, e.g. liver, which should be *frozen* or (less satisfactory) fixed in ethanol for DNA work. Complete carcasses are sometimes used for analysis, to measure body composition, as part of assessing 'condition' (Brown, 1996).

Fig. AVII.3 Sample-taking during health monitoring of dead raptors.

(b) having immunocompetent or immuno-suppressed sentinels or a mixture of both

(c) following exposure, examining the sentinels alive, *post mortem* or both.

When translocation is planned, environmental monitoring should be carried out both *prior* to movement and *following* establishment of the birds.

Methods of environmental monitoring used in work with birds of prey are at present imprecise and urgently need refining and standardising.

CONCLUSIONS

Health monitoring is an integral part of the management of both captive and free-living raptors. It should be considered essential before individuals or groups of birds are translocated, introduced, restocked or reintroduced.

The general rules of health monitoring are as follows:

(1) Some monitoring is better than none.

(2) Plan carefully – prepare a protocol and follow it.

(3) Be prepared to be selective – a cost:benefit analysis based on a disease risk assessment is usually necessary.

(4) Standardise techniques, following recognised protocols and procedures where appropriate, and consider a system of quality control.

(5) Adhere to all relevant legislation, whether national, regional or international, and in the case of CITES, obtain necessary permits for recognisable derivatives as well as for live or dead birds (see Appendix XI).

(6) Collect and collate data systematically and quantitatively; store on standard databases (e.g. MedARKS) and deposit in record centres where these are appropriate.

(7) Analyse and interpret results carefully – especially those that are negative. Remember that failure to detect an organism is not, as suggested by some (for example, Steadman *et al.*, 1990), an indication that the organism is absent. Many factors can be responsible for 'negative' findings – for example, the failure to locate parasites in blood smears (Cooper & Anwar, 2001).

(8) Produce a written specification (profile) for the animal or population in the form of a report, certificate or 'medical passport'.

(9) Save material where possible – for re-testing, for subsequent research and to assist other scientists. Consider establishing a Reference Collection, especially when working with threatened or little known species (Cooper *et al.*, 1998).

(10) Repeat health monitoring if the bird is to be recaptured subsequently or is found dead.

(11) Disseminate results in publications and lectures: encourage others to follow similar techniques and promote the concept of standard monitoring protocols.

Minimally Invasive Health Monitoring

'The physician should know the invisible, as well as the visible.'

Paracelsus

(Adapted from an oral paper presented by John E. Cooper at the 3rd International Raptor Biomedical Conference, Midrand, South Africa, August 1998 and based on work at the Centre Vétérinaire des Volcans, B P 105, Ruhengeri, Rwanda, Central Africa 1993–95.)

INTRODUCTION

Over the past 30 years there has been an upsurge of interest in the health of free-living and captive birds of prey (raptors) of the orders Falconiformes and Strigiformes (Cooper & Greenwood, 1981a,b; Cooper, 1985a,b,c; Redig *et al.*, 1993). This has been prompted by a number of factors, including (a) concern over the decline in numbers of some species of raptor in the wild, (b) the need to monitor birds prior to introduction, reintroduction or translocation, and (c) the relative paucity of information on infection and subclinical disease available to those involved in such activities as rehabilitation and translocation and in the maintenance and breeding of raptors in captivity. Avian biologists have become more involved in studies on the health of birds for many reasons, amongst them because of the possible link between parasites and gene quality – a hypothesis that has attracted much attention over the past 15 years (Loye & Zuk, 1991a,b; Crawley, 1992).

Studies on free-living raptors may involve capture,

handling and manipulation. Biologists use such 'intervention' techniques in order to examine, mark, track or to perform experimental procedures. Veterinarians restrain and manipulate birds of prey to perform clinical examination, to take samples for laboratory investigation and to carry out medical or surgical treatment.

The monitoring of the health of free-living birds can be an important part of management programmes. It often involves 'invasive' intervention techniques, as outlined above – for example, the taking of blood and other samples for laboratory investigation. However, there are strong arguments for minimising such intervention. Restraint, examination and the taking of samples can cause stress, damage or death to individual birds and may have detrimental effects on others in the nest, colony or group. Adverse publicity, withdrawal of research licences or even prosecution can follow. Clinical and laboratory results obtained from animals that have been trapped may be erroneous. In addition to all of these, there is increasing public and professional concern about the welfare of wildlife and the ethics of invasive methods of intervention (Macdonald & Linzey, 1996; Cooper, 1998).

In this Appendix, techniques are described that can prove useful in the health monitoring of free-living raptors, but which can be considered 'minimally invasive' in so far as their effect on the birds is concerned. The methods that are advocated are based on work in Rwanda, Central Africa, when the author was Director of the Centre Vétérinaire des Volcans, 1993–95.

THE AIMS OF HEALTH MONITORING

The primary aim of health monitoring of birds of prey is to obtain data for analysis in order to ascertain whether a population shows clinical signs of disease or is subclinically affected by an infectious agent or a non-infectious factor (e.g. a toxin).

Substantial scientific information can be obtained from a bird if it is examined thoroughly, alive, and samples are taken. This, however, involves capture and restraint and the attendant disadvantages and dangers that were listed earlier. *Post-mortem* examination also yields valuable data – sometimes more than clinical investigation – but, unless the specimen is found dead, necessitates killing the bird.

Far less information can be obtained if the whole live bird is not examined and, instead, samples are collected for laboratory investigation; however, such 'minimally invasive' techniques have a significant role to play in health assessment and are likely to assume even more importance in future.

METHODS

Analysis of records

Analysis of records – for example, breeding success – can prove useful in health monitoring. While such records rarely provide a specific diagnosis, they can play a part, especially in combination with other information, in compiling a picture of the health status of a population. However, it is vital that records are reliable. There are clear advantages if those establishing demographic databases for birds of prey collaborate closely with veterinarians in order to ensure that pertinent information, of value to people in both disciplines, is being recorded in a readily retrievable form.

Observation

Observation implies that raptors are inspected from a distance, without their being touched or manipulated in any way. Often, the bird is unaware that it is being observed. Careful observation (Table AVIII.1) can provide valuable data and may even yield information that is not always available if a bird of prey is handled. This is because some subtle clinical signs, such as muscle fasciculations or mild lameness, can disappear or be imperceptible once the bird is restrained and handled. The use of a video recording has much to commend it but this is not always practicable.

Detection and interpretation of behavioural changes depend upon a sound knowledge of the species: the veterinarian involved in such work will benefit from the advice of raptor biologists.

Collection of samples

A range of samples can be collected from birds of prey and used in health monitoring. These may be collected from nests (used or unused) or from below roosts.

Examples of samples that may be collected in a minimally (or non) invasive way and which can prove useful in monitoring are given in Table AVIII.2. Samples must always be carefully and conscientiously collected and transported. Feathers, pellets and mutes from roosts should be sought early in the morning when they will be relatively fresh. Linking a sample with an individual bird can be difficult; health monitoring is often carried out on a group (flock) basis.

Feathers and eggs of birds have proved particularly amenable to analysis and examination (Peakall, 1987) and provide a good example of where there is often untapped information about health. Whenever possible, changes or abnormalities in samples should be quantified.

In addition to faeces, feathers and the like shed by live birds, carcasses of raptors may be found (e.g. below a roost) and can be examined *post mortem*. Such opportunistic specimens are often of great value and will supplement the information obtained from samples.

Table AVIII.1 Methods of health monitoring – observation.

Feature	Comments
General behaviour, including interaction with other birds of the same or different species. Success in hunting. Dispersal patterns. Response of individual birds to stimuli, e.g. sound, disturbance, vocalisation	Usually non-specific but differences may be general indicators of ill-health
Gait, flight	Abnormalities may indicate injury, weakness, poisoning, possibly certain infectious diseases (e.g. paramyxovirus infection)
Feeding, drinking, defaecation	Changes are important indicators of general health. Not easily observed in the field
Appearance of plumage including presence or absence of feathers that are soiled, damaged or bear 'fretmarks'. Preening frequency and intensity. Normal or abnormal moult	Useful indicators of health, especially when coupled with the collection of dropped feathers for laboratory examination (see Table AVIII.2)
Appearance including presence or absence of lesions, discharges, of eyes, nares, ears, etc.	Comparison of one organ (e.g. eye) with the other can prove useful: asymmetry may be significant even if no specific lesions are apparent. Careful observation, usually with binoculars, is often necessary to detect such changes

Table AVIII.2 Methods of health monitoring – samples.

Samples	Comments
Faeces/urates (mutes)	Can provide much useful information on gross and microscopical examination and can be cultured for micro-organisms. Faeces can be fixed in ethanol and frozen for subsequent investigation, including genetic (DNA) analysis
Feathers	Dropped feathers, especially during the moult, can yield information on health status. They can be examined microscopically for example, fretmarks, and analysed for (e.g.) heavy metals. Ectoparasites can be identified and counted. If follicle is present, DNA studies can be attempted
Nests	May contain feathers, faeces/urates, and ectoparasites which can be examined as above. Some feathers and other material in the nest may be from prey species – care must be taken in interpretation
Food remains, e.g. carcasses, viscera	If fresh, may provide information on feeding behaviour and possibly even permit collection of saliva for examination for parasites
Pellets (castings)	A rich source of information about the bird's diet and digestion. May contain parasites. Can be dissected (after soaking) and cultured for micro-organisms. DNA studies may prove possible
Unhatched eggs or eggshells	Can provide useful data on infectious disease, pesticides, nutrition: can be examined microscopically, cultured and chemically analysed. Material should be retained for DNA and other studies

It is important that samples are collected, handled and processed proficiently and the following rules, first put forward by Cooper (1998) and modified here, are suggested:

(1) Take any sample that is available, even if at the time it appears inadequate or of poor quality. It may not be easy or even possible to obtain another later.

(2) Collect samples hygienically and use the optimum container, swab, transport medium or fixative. Seal containers, especially bags, securely to prevent escape of parasites. Follow a standard technique that minimises error at each stage of collection.

(3) If there is likely to be a substantial delay before processing the specimen, consider carrying out some investigations (e.g. examination of wet preparations of faeces for fragile parasites) in the field. Special equipment, e.g. a battery-operated microscope, may be needed for this (Cooper & Samour, 1997).

(4) If there is insufficient material to carry out a range of tests, choose those that are most relevant. Draw up protocols to facilitate this choice. Where possible use standard investigative techniques (O.I.E., 1996).

(5) Where necessary, seek help from others with specialist knowledge or facilities. Remember that submission to another country of 'recognizable derivatives' from certain protected species may necessitate CITES permits (Cooper, M. E., 1987). While intended to protect endangered species, these requirements can prove prejudicial to *bona fide* research and health studies (Cooper, 1995).

(6) Keep careful records including, where possible, photographs of important findings.

(7) Retain surplus material so that it can be used for further tests or retrospective studies at a later date. Remember the importance of DNA studies: share samples wherever possible.

(8) Publish results and share experiences. Send copies of reports to IUCN Veterinary and Reintroductions Specialist Groups.

DISCUSSION

The monitoring of the health of wild (free-living) animals is becoming increasingly important as populations come under pressure due to habitat degradation and other adverse factors. At the same time, however, concern is being voiced over the extent to which wild species are often manipulated in order to obtain scientific information.

The capture, restraint and sampling of free-living raptors in order to investigate their health status is likely to continue. If less invasive techniques are to be promoted there is a need to improve their efficacy and value in terms of the information yielded and how this can best be interpreted and used. Methods of health monitoring could be refined and improved using captive birds of prey – for example, those kept in zoos or laboratories – and the resulting data might be of relevance to their health and welfare as well as to raptors in the wild.

Minimally invasive techniques demand a new approach by those working with free-living raptors. The ability to capture, to restrain and to take specimens such as blood from birds must be balanced with a willingness to observe, to record and to collect and examine faeces and samples. This in turn will lead to close collaboration between veterinarians, wildlife biologists, behaviourists and aviculturists. The subject is truly interdisciplinary.

ACKNOWLEDGEMENTS

I am grateful to numerous colleagues in Britain and overseas who have assisted me in my studies on raptors, in particular in the development of non-invasive or minimally invasive techniques for use in these and other species. Early work on this topic in Rwanda was cut short by the outbreak of war in 1994 but I remain indebted to those African colleagues and assistants in Kigali and Ruhengeri, some of whom died in the conflict, for helping to put ideas into practice.

Medicines and Other Agents used in Treatment, including Emergency Anaesthesia Kit and Avian Resuscitation Protocol

MEDICAL AGENTS USED FOR TREATMENT (FORMULARY)

The agents listed are either those that have been used by the author or those for which reliable data, such as published papers, are available. In the vast majority of cases, the agent listed is not licensed for use in raptors or other species of bird and therefore appropriate precautions should be taken, including completion of a consent form by the owner and, in the European Union, the 'cascade' system must be followed (see Appendix XI).

Many of the agents listed are 'prescription-only' medicines and therefore only available in some countries, such as those of Western Europe, through or on the authority of a veterinarian. Conversely, a few of the generic substances mentioned, e.g. pyrethrum powder, are easily obtained in certain (tropical) countries but no longer permitted to be used or rarely seen in the 'West'. Traditional (falconers') remedies are not specifically included in this appendix but may be mentioned in the text (and references) and a few more modern versions, e.g. sugar water, are listed.

Trade names are not given. Dosages are usually given on the basis of mg/kg per dose but the value of using allometric scaling for birds of different sizes should be remembered.

In providing this list no responsibility is taken for efficacy or safety of the products mentioned. If in doubt, the veterinarian should consult the manufacturers or refer to published reports of usage. As in other fields, the use of agents is subject to change and modification, both in practical and legal terms, and it is therefore incumbent on the reader to assess current thinking and opinion before use.

Agents are, where appropriate, listed alphabetically.

Type of agent	Dosage and route	Comments
Antibiotics		
Amikacin	15 mg/kg, bid im, 5–10 d	Bumblefoot and other bacterial infections
Amoxycillin	150 mg/kg, sid (long-acting preparation) or bid im or orally 5–7 bid	Bacterial infections
Carbenicillin	100–200 mg/kg, tid im, 5 d	*Pseudomonas* and other resistant bacteria
Cephalexin	50–100 mg/kg, tid im or orally, 5 d	Bacterial infections
Clavulanate-potentiated amoxycillin	150 mg/kg bid orally, 5–7 d	Bacterial infections. Can be nephrotoxic (Beynon *et al.*, 1996)
Clindamycin	50 mg/kg bid orally, 7–10 d	Bone and tendon infections
Cloxacillin	250 mg/kg, bid orally, 7–14 d	Bumblefoot and other infections
Potentiated sulphonamide (co-trimazine-sulphadiazine and trimethoprim)	10–60 mg/kg, bid orally, 5–7 d	Infections. Can be nephrotoxic (Beynon *et al.*, 1996)
Enrofloxacin (and marbofloxacin)	10–15 mg/kg bid im or orally, 5–7 d	Infections. Used widely in many species, many ages, but Heidenreich (1997) urged caution in use for young birds and reported possible adverse effects on moult. Bird may regurgitate/vomit food (less likely with marbofloxacin which can also stimulate appetite)
Lincomycin	50–70 mg/kg bid im or orally, 7–14 d	Bumblefoot and bone infections. Can also be given by intra-articular injection
Metronidazole	50 mg/kg, sid orally, 5–7 d	Anaerobic infections (see also Antiprotozoal)
Oxytetracycline	25–50 mg/kg tid im or orally, 5–10 d (long-acting 200 mg/kg sid, im)	Can cause muscle damage intramuscularly (Cooper, 1983)
Piperacillin	100 mg/kg, bid iv or im, 5–7 d	Bumblefoot and other infections (see Robbins *et al.*, 2000)
Procaine penicillin	Not recommended	Can be toxic
Tobramycin	5–10 mg/kg, bid iv or im, 5–7 d	Can be nephrotoxic but less so than other current aminoglycosides
Tylosin	15–30 mg/kg, bid im, 3–5 d	Mycoplasmosis and other infections
Sodium fusidate and other topical agents	As appropriate	Avoid prolonged use of topical agents without appropriate sensitivity tests. Avoid agents that include corticosteroids – response may be good but may recur or predispose to other infections, especially in 'aspergillosis-sensitive' species

The use of antibiotic-impregnated beads is discussed in the text.

Antimycotic (antifungal) agents		
Amphotericin B	1.5 mg/kg, tid iv, 5–7 d	Aspergillosis. Administer with fluids to reduce nephrotoxicity (can also be administered *per tracheam* to treat lesions in syrinx or by airsac wash). (See Gylstorff & Grimm, 1987; Redig, 1981, 1993a; and Forbes *et al.*, 1992)
	0.25–1.0 ml, sid orally, 5–7 d	

Type of agent	Dosage and route	Comments
Enilconazole (diluted 10%)	0.5 m/kg, sid *per tracheam*, 7–10 d or by nebulisation tid, 20 min	Aspergillosis – lesions in syrinx. Irritant to eyes (Heidenreich, 1997). (See Baronetzky-Mercier & Seidel, 1995)
Fluconazole	2–5 mg/kg, sid orally, 7–10 d	Aspergillosis. Parrott (1991) recommended higher dose
Flucyctosine	20–30 mg/kg, qid orally, 20–90 d	Aspergillosis. (See Redig, 1981, 1993a)
Itraconazole	10 mg/kg sid orally, 7–10 d (prophylactic) or (bid) 3–6 weeks (therapeutic)	Aspergillosis May be hepatotoxic Associated with other side effects in humans
Ketoconazole	25 mg/kg, bid im, 7–10 d	Aspergillosis. Can be hepatotoxic. Higher doses recommended by Wagner *et al.* (1991)
Miconazole	10 mg/kg, sid im, 6–12 d or nebulise tid for 10 d	See Furley and Greenwood (1982) and Gylstorff and Grimm (1987)
Nystatin	200 000–300 000 units bid orally, 7–14 d	Candidiasis
'F10'	See text	(See text)
Antiprotozoal agents	(See also Chapter 7)	
Carnidazole	25 mg/kg, once	Trichomoniasis
Chloroquine phosphate	25 mg/kg, sid im	*Plasmodium, Leucocytozoon* (See Huckabee, 2000; Heidenreich, 1997)
Clazuril	5–10 mg/kg, every third day on three occasions, orally	Coccidiosis
Potentiated sulphonamide (see earlier)	60 mg/kg, bid orally for 3 d, then a break of 2 d, then a further 3 d treatment	Coccidiosis. The dosage regime will encourage natural immunity
Metronidazole	50 mg/kg, sid orally, 5–7 d	Trichomoniasis
Pyrimethamine	0.25–0.5 mg/kg, bid orally for 30 d	Sarcocystosis, toxoplasmosis, other protozoal infections?
Toltrazuril	10 mg/kg, tid orally, on alternate days on three occasions or one dose a week for 3 weeks	Coccidiosis (See Forbes & Simpson, 1997b)
Anthelmintics	(See also Chapter 7)	
Fenbendazole	100 mg/kg, once orally 20 mg/kg, sid orally, 5–7 d 20 mg/kg, sid orally, 10–14 d	General control of nematodes Control of *Eucoleus* and *Capillaria* Control of *Serratospiculum*. Heidenreich (1997) reported that it can be toxic to vultures
Ivermectin	200 µg/kg, once, im sc surface application or orally Higher doses may be acceptable	Will also have some action against arthropod ectoparasites. Dilute with water Changes in plasma enzymes occur when high doses are administered (Lierz, 2001)
Levamisole	10–20 mg/kg, once orally or sc (or for 2 days)	Control of nematodes (*Eucoleus/Capillaria* may need larger dose). Narrow therapeutic/toxic margin. Immunostimulant?
Mebendazole	20 mg/kg daily, orally, 10–14 d	Control of *Serratospiculum* and some other nematodes. Heidenreich (1997) reported 'possibly toxic in some birds'

Type of agent	Dosage and route	Comments
Praziquantel	5–10 mg/kg, once orally or sc (higher dosages have also been reported)	Cestodiasis (a longer course will help to control trematodes) (Smith, 1996)
Pyrantel	20 mg/kg, once orally	Control of nematodes
Thiabendazole	100–200 mg/kg, bid for 10 days, orally	Control of nematodes. May interfere with egg-laying (Heidenreich, 1997)
Acaricides and insecticides	(See also Chapter 7)	
Cypermethrin (diluted 2%)	Applied to premises	Control of *Dermanyssus* and ticks in environment
Fipronil	Once on plumage/skin, repeated if necessary	General ectoparasiticide. May cause drying of feathers: do not use on flight feathers
Permethrin	On plumage, repeated as necessary	Control of lice and other ectoparasites
Ivermectin	See under Anthelmintics (sc or surface application)	General ectoparasiticide. Will also have some effect against endoparasites
Malathion (diluted)	Applied to premises	Control of *Dermanyssus* and ticks in environment
Piperonyl butoxide/ pyrethrin	On plumage, repeated as necessary	Control of lice and other ectoparasites
Pyrethrum powder	On plumage, repeated as necessary	Control of lice and other ectoparasites
Flowers of sulphur	As above	An old-fashioned and mild – but very safe – way of controlling lice and other ectoparasites
Anaesthetics agents, tranquillisers, etc.		
Diazepam	0.5–1.0 mg/kg, tid iv or im	To control nervous diseases ('fits'). Reactions vary
Midazolam	As diazepam	As diazepam. Water-soluble: therefore can be easily mixed with ketamine. Less irritant, shorter acting than diazepam
Isoflurane	4–5% induction, 2–2.5% maintenance	Inhalation agent. Relatively safe. (See Fitzgerald & Blais, 1993)
Sevoflurane/desflurane	See Chapter 12	See text
Ketamine	5–10 mg/kg, im, repeated as necessary (larger doses, 50–100 mg/kg as bait – see text)	Sedative *per se* or, in combination with other agents, an anaesthetic – still useful under conditions where inhalation anaesthesia is impracticable
Analgesics		
Tiletamine/zolazepam	40–80 mg/kg, orally, 10–20 mg/kg, im	Not licensed for use in Britain but available elsewhere. See Zenker and Janovsky (1998)
Medetomidine	100–300 µg/kg, im	Combined with ketamine for anaesthesia. Can be reversed
Carprophen	1–2 mg/kg, bid, im iv orally	See Huckabee (2000)
Flunixin	2–10 mg/kg, sid im, for up to 5 d	Useful in arthritis. May cause regurgitation (Dorrestein, 2000)
Ketoprofen	1 mg/kg sid, im, for up to 10 days	As above
Lignocaine (2% diluted ×5 in saline)	0.5 ml/kg – local infiltration	Use with caution, especially in small birds (see text)

Type of agent	Dosage and route	Comments
Meloxicam	0.1–0.2 mg/kg, sid im or orally	Useful in arthritis and other inflammatory/ painful conditions
Antidotes to poisons		
Atropine	0.1 mg/kg, repeated every 3–4 hours, im or iv	Anticholinesterase, e.g. organophosphate poisoning. Not recommended by Heidenreich (1997)
D-penicillamine	55 mg/kg, bid orally, 7–14 d	Heavy metal poisoning
Pralidoxime chloride	100 mg/kg, repeated once after 6–12 hours	See atropine above
Sodium calcium edetate	10–40 mg/kg, bid for 5–10 d, iv or im	Heavy metal poisoning
Hormones and similar agents		
Dexamethasone	2 mg/kg, sid for 1–2 d	Anti-inflammatory. Treatment of shock. Avoid prolonged use of this and other steroids
Prednisolone	0.5–1.0 mg/kg, once, im	Anti-inflammatory
	2–4 mg/kg, once iv or im	Shock
Oxytocin	3–5 IU/kg, im	Egg-binding
Prostaglandin gel	As necessary	Egg-binding
Thyroxine	See text	Induction of moult (see text)
Levothyroxine sodium	Up to 1 mg/kg, orally for 14 d	Described by Heidenreich (1997) who added 'can have negative side effects'
Nutritional/metabolic therapy		
B-vitamin complex	Orally as necessary	Non-specific deficiencies
Biotin	50 μg/kg, daily for up to 30 d, orally	Non-specific deficiencies. May aid beak and talon regrowth
Calcium borogluconate (10%)	1–5 ml (100–500 mg)/kg, once sc or (slowly) iv	Hypocalcaemia (including 'fits'), egg-binding
Dextrose solution (10%)	Up to 10 mg/kg orally, repeated	Hypoglycaemia, 'energy deficiency'
Dextrose solution (50%)	1–2 ml (500–1000 mg)/kg, once, iv slowly	Hypoglycaemia, 'energy deficiency'
EFAs (essential fatty acids)	As appropriate, orally	Dermatitis – if atopy suspected
Iron dextran	10 mg/kg, once, im	Iron deficiency anaemia
Selenium/vitamin E	As necessary	See Beynon et al. (1996)
Thiamine	10–50 mg/kg, sid for as long as necessary, orally	Thiamine deficiency (including 'fits')
Vitamin A	Up to 20 000 IU/kg weekly, im	Hypovitaminosis A and to stimulate epithelial regeneration, e.g. bumblefoot
Antiseptics, disinfectants and wound-cleaning preparations		
Gentian violet/crystal violet	Applied topically as necessary to wounds	Cheap, visible. Readily available in poorer countries
Tincture of iodine	As above	As above
Povidone–iodine	Applied topically to wounds. Wash off within 5 min	To clean open wounds

Type of agent	Dosage and route	Comments
Saline (1–2%)	As for povidone–iodine	As for povidone–iodine
Washing soda (2–5%)	For buildings and surfaces (e.g. post-mortem table)	Cheap and effective. Wash off after use
Household bleach	As for washing soda	As for washing soda
Ethanol or methanol (70%)	As required – for instruments	Will evaporate
Glutaraldehyde	As per manufacturers' instructions – for endoscopes etc.	Toxic
'F10'	See text	See text

Many commercial disinfectants are available in different parts of the world. Use disinfectants as per manufacturers' instructions. Hot water/steam are valuable for disinfection/sterilisation. Surfaces should be cleaned before disinfection.

Miscellaneous

Barium sulphate	1–5 mg/kg, once or repeated, orally	Radio-opaque contrast medium. Also protects mucosa in enteritis cases
Doxapram	10 mg/kg, once iv or on to mucosa	Respiratory stimulant
Frusemide	1.5 mg/kg, tid or qid, im	Diuretic
Isoxsuprine	5–10 mg/kg, sid orally for up to 30 d	To improve circulation in, e.g. wing tip oedema
Liquid paraffin (mineral oil)	Up to 5 ml/kg orally or *per cloacam*	Purgative and to lubricate cloacal impaction
Magnesium sulphate	0.25–1.0 g/kg, sid, for 1–2 d orally	Purgative, to increase gut motility, e.g. in lead poisoning
Magnesium sulphate (5%, 10% or 20%)	As necessary, iv	Emergency chemical euthanasia following bird's loss of consciousness (do not use magnesium sulphate alone)
Propentofylline	5 mg/kg, bid orally for up to 30 d	See isoxsuprine above
Dextrose saline	Up to 4% daily, sc or orally or 15 ml/kg, tid qid, iv	Fluid replacement
Lactated Ringer's solution	As for dextrose saline	As above – preferable to dextrose saline
Sucrose in water (5%)	Up to 5 ml/kg, orally repeated as necessary	A mild purgative, may stimulate appetite
Salt (NaCl) solution (5%)	Up to 20 ml/kg, orally, repeated as necessary	Emetic. Provide water *ad libitum* after use
Kaolin (or kaolin/bismuth) suspension	Up to 15 ml/kg, orally, repeated as necessary	Antidiarrhoeal. Avoid mixtures that contain morphine
Pancreatic extracts and/or trypsin solution	Topical	Irrigation of bumblefoot and other lesions where cellular debris persists (Can also be used to predigest food that is used to hand-rear vulture chicks – see Heidenreich (1997))
Metoclopramide	2 mg/kg, tid, iv	To increase gut motility
Cisapride	0.25 mg/kg, tid, orally	To increase gut motility
Activated charcoal	2–10 mg/kg, as necessary, orally	Antidiarrhoeal, adsorbs toxins

sid = once daily, bid = twice daily, tid = thrice daily, qid = four times daily, d = day, im = intramuscular, iv = intravenous, sc = subcutaneous.

EMERGENCY ANAESTHESIA KIT

Each kit contains

Number	Item
1	4.0 mm diameter endotracheal tube (sterile for air sac intubation)
5	Sterile scalpel blades
5	1 ml syringe
5	2.5 ml syringe
2	24 G iv catheters
2	22 G iv catheters
4	23 G butterfly catheters
4	25 G butterfly catheters
5	23 G needles
5	25 G needles
5	27 G needles
5	Cotton wool balls
2	Cotton buds
0	
1 bottle	Doxopram (drops)
1 bottle	Doxopram (injection)
1 bottle	Adrenaline
1 bottle	Bicarbonate

If you use items for dealing with an emergency, please ensure that they are replaced immediately.

(Reproduced with permission of Dr Tom Bailey, MRCVS of the National Avian Research Center, UAE)

AVIAN RESUSCITATION PROTOCOL

- Airway
- Breathing
- Circulation
- Drugs.

Respiratory arrest

- Remove bird from anaesthesia system
- Check glottis and intubate if not already done. If this is not possible, place an airsac tube
- 'Sternal massage' – lightly press chest to induce fresh air intake
- Flush anaesthetic machine and administer oxygen by positive pressure if breathing motions are not initiated through endotracheal or airsac tube
- Administer doxopram 10 mg/kg iv or use drops on the mucosa of the oropharynx
- Consider bicarbonate therapy – 1 mEq/kg iv.

Cardiac arrest

- Remove bird from anaesthesia
- Sternal massage
- Adrenaline – 0.1 mg/kg iv
- Cardiac massage.

(Reproduced with permission of Dr Tom Bailey, MRCVS of the National Avian Research Center, UAE)

Field Work, Field Kits and Portable Equipment, and Field Post-mortem *Technique*

FIELD KITS AND PORTABLE EQUIPMENT

A paradox of raptor (and other) medicine is that veterinarians practising in Western Europe, North America and other richer countries usually have access to modern equipment and refined technology for their patients while their counterparts in poorer or more isolated parts of the world, who are often working with much rarer species, are subject to the vagaries of unreliable communications, electricity and water supplies. As a result, there can be a dichotomy between standards of clinical and laboratory work and results in 'Western' practice and those of veterinarians (and biologists) working with threatened birds, especially in tropical and subtropical areas.

Similar difficulties can face those who are doing projects in wealthier countries, but in isolated areas such as islands or forests where even the collection of good samples (for example, for health monitoring) can be problematic, let alone the performance of tests or treatment.

In this appendix, the role and deployment of field kits and portable equipment are briefly reviewed.

Needs

The veterinarian or raptor biologist who is working in isolated localities will, when selecting equipment, need to consider the following:

(1) Will it be independent, when necessary, of mains electricity and piped water? These are luxuries that are often either not available at all in isolated areas or subject to cuts and failures.

(2) How portable is it? Will it contribute substantially to the weight (mass) of a load that will probably need to be carried by hand (perhaps on the head!), often for long periods?

(3) How sturdy is its construction? Will it tolerate transportation and the knocks, jars and other insults that this may entail? How will it resist environmental conditions that may range from a hot, dry desert to a cold, wet rainforest?

(4) What is the cost? Budgets for work in isolated areas are usually small and the purchase of expensive equipment is often not a realistic option. This is not always the case, however: in certain countries of the world, such as the Gulf States of Arabia, veterinarians are often able to use expensive equipment even in the desert, and some field projects elsewhere are sufficiently well funded to permit quality rather than the price to be the main criterion when choosing veterinary instruments.

It follows, therefore, that one must carry out a cost:benefit analysis. A great deal depends upon the duration of the project. For example, it may be possible to use slightly less robust equipment for a 1–2 week field project than for an ongoing programme that lasts months or years. Each case has to be assessed on its merits.

The other important consideration relates to the use to which the equipment will be put. Portable field kits can be used (a) for clinical work (diagnosis or health monitoring), (b) for *post-mortem* work (diagnostic or health monitoring), or (c) for laboratory diagnostic work, utilising samples from either live or dead birds or both. In this appendix the emphasis is on (a) and (c).

Features of field kits

As explained above, field kits should be (1) independent of electricity and piped water supplies, (2) portable and, (3) durable. In addition, especially when working in poorer areas, or on a restricted budget, it may be necessary for them to be (4) relatively inexpensive.

The first of these is usually achieved by (a) capitalising on advances in electronic and optical technology and (b) minimal use of water, or ability to use local supplies e.g. from rivers or rain. Insofar as (a) is concerned, this often means utilising miniaturised, battery-powered equipment (Cooper, 1985b) and high quality lenses but it must not be forgotten that direct solar illumination can be used – for example, by the simple expedient of attaching a mirror to a microscope.

Portability depends upon size, mass and, to a limited extent, shape. Size can often be reduced by (for example) using one eyepiece for a microscope instead of two, or by employing an optical system that reduces the distance between lenses. Mass is minimised by using modern plastics and lightweight metals, such as aluminium, rather than brass or steel.

Durability is relative but is usually related to the structure of the instrument itself – for example, some plastics are more rugged than others – or how well it can be protected from trauma by using (for example) foam rubber or other materials as liners.

A careful balance has to be struck between making equipment inexpensive and maintaining standards. Costs can often be reduced very simply without compromising quality. For example, when working in Rwanda I successfully used local bamboo to make spatulae and utilised plastic film pots as containers for specimens.

Field kits need to be carefully and securely packed. Although portable kits are available for human medical use, they appear not yet to be produced for veterinary purposes and certainly not for raptor work! A rucksack ('backpack') would appear to be suitable since it is relatively easy to carry, but is not satisfactory *per se* as a container. It is preferable to use one of the luggage-type packing cases that are marketed for photographic or endoscopic equipment. Failing that, an all-purpose box of the type designed to carry tools or fishing gear can be employed (Frye *et al.*, 2001).

The size and shape of the container are also important. It needs to be readily transported in the field (probably in a rucksack or on a porter's head) but at the same time should easily be stowed in the overhead luggage rack of a plane or bus.

All items within the container need to be individually protected against falls and vibration. Closed-cell polyurethane foam liners are ideal and are usually an integral part of the luggage-type packing cases referred to above. Extra insulation – and absorptive material in case spillage occurs – can be added.

Field kits should be secured with a lockable padlock. They should also bear warning stickers and the name of the owner. Notices should be in local languages as well as in English and line drawings may help to explain the importance and purpose of the field kit to people who may not be able to read, such as baggage handlers.

Care must be taken that the kit does not contain drugs or other items that may not, by law, be transported from one country to another. A list of contents should always be available for inspection – again, in local languages as well as in English where this is appropriate. A stethoscope, placed in a prominent place, is often useful in terms of impressing and enhancing relations with Customs authorities and security staff!

Contents

The detailed contents of a field kit for raptor work will depend upon the location and the type of investigations being carried out. However, the following items are recommended as basic elements for clinical and laboratory work and they include many of the pieces of equipment that are likely to be used for other purposes:

Clinical Diagnostic Kit

Stethoscope (lightweight)

Auriscope (otoscope) (lightweight)
Ophthalmoscope (lightweight)
Rigid endoscope (battery-operated)
Pen torch (flashlight)
Spare bulbs and batteries
Syringes and needles (disposable)
At least one boilable, re-usable, syringe and needle
Empty soft drinks cans, appropriately labelled, as 'sharps boxes' for used needles, etc.
Selected drugs (medicines)
Cotton wool
Dressings
Suture material
Basic surgical ('cut-down') set
Cautery (battery-operated)
Clippers
Spring balance(s)
Tape measure or ruler
Hoods or cloth bags
Gloves – surgical and for handling
Small towel
Oesophageal and other tubes
Mouth gag/wooden spatulae
Aluminium foil
Sampling equipment for laboratory work (from the Laboratory Diagnostic Kit)

Laboratory Diagnostic Kit

Microscope (battery-operated and/or with mirror attachment)
Pre-cleaned, frosted microscope slides and slide-box or tray
Worm-egg counting slide
Coverslips
Lens tissues
Pencil for labelling microscope slides (or diamond-tipped pen)
Saline, saturated NaCl solution and other reagents for parasitology
Fixatives – methanol, formalin
Selected stains for cytology
Lightweight (plastic) staining jar
Urine and blood chemistry test strips
Hand-held refractometer
Transport medium for bacteria, viruses, mycoplasmas and *Trichomonas*

Small vacuum flask
Scalpel, scissors, forceps, artery forceps (haemostats)
Post-mortem equipment where appropriate
Plastic (film) pots for specimens
Plus, items from Clinical Diagnostic Kit as necessary

Recommended Items in all Kits

Voice-activated microcassette tape-recorder
Hand-held, palm-top computer
Pencils, pens, papers
Plastic metric ruler
Callipers and micrometer
Elastic bands, string, adhesive tape
Self-sealing plastic bags
Small screwdriver and pliers
Emergency pack – business cards, emergency contact list, protocols for snakebite (etc.), emergency drugs and antidotes, foreign language phrase books.

An item that proves invaluable in the field but is rarely mentioned in reports is a lightweight folding umbrella! This can be used primarily for protection from the sun, snow and other elements but in addition can be utilised for collection of rainwater and even for such purposes as catching invertebrates and other small animals when 'beating' undergrowth as part of environmental monitoring!

It is worth noting that some items on the list such as the tape-recorder and palm-top computer are not only lightweight but also easily and rapidly hidden. This can be important in war-torn countries or where there is political sensitivity about strangers, especially if they appear to be for noting and storing information. It is a sad fact that some of the world's rarest and least well studied species inhabit areas of unrest.

Discussion

Many of those who work with raptors live in countries, or work in regions, where facilities are minimal and financial and logistic considerations dictate that equipment must be cheap, relatively independent of electricity and other services and easily transported. The kits described in this appendix will help to raise the standards of raptor work – whether diagnostic or for the purpose of health monitoring – in such circumstances.

FIELD *POST-MORTEM* EXAMINATIONS – GENERAL

If unexpected deaths occur in a population of endangered or threatened birds – or even in common species on a large scale – every effort should be made to ascertain the cause. There is still relatively little known about causes of mortality and morbidity in free-living raptors, and material from species that are rare or restricted in distribution should never be wasted. Many factors, ranging from poisons and parasites to stress and starvation, can be involved in mortality episodes in the wild and an accurate diagnosis may necessitate various tests on different tissues and samples.

These guidelines are intended to assist those who may have to deal with dead birds and who have little experience of veterinary pathology.

General points

If death occurs:

(1) Obtain as much information as possible about the local circumstances of the death(s) and clinical history. **TAKE DETAILED NOTES.**

(2) If possible seek advice (for example from a veterinary laboratory or experienced avian pathologist) before embarking upon any examinations yourself. If a competent person is available in the near vicinity submit carcasses to him/her for investigation; if it is possible to send specimens to someone elsewhere (for example overseas by air) consider doing so. See list of laboratories in Cooper (1989a).

(3) Pending examination, carcasses or tissues should be chilled (refrigerator temperature) **BUT NOT FROZEN** – although freezing preserves specimens, it damages tissues and can make certain investigations (e.g. histology) very difficult. Freeze only if there is likely to

be a delay of 7 days or more before examination is carried out.

If you have to carry out a *post-mortem* examination yourself or advise on procedures:

(1) Always follow strict hygienic precautions. In particular, it is wise to wear rubber gloves. Boil or disinfect instruments after use.

(2) Keep detailed records. Preferably one person should carry out the examination while another writes. Report systematically everything you see, even if it has to be in nontechnical language. Try to have a camera available so that specific features can be photographed, or make sketches – even rough diagrams can be useful.

(3) Be prepared to take tissue samples and store fresh, and in formalin for all organ systems. Ensure that material (fresh/frozen tissues or blood) is retained for DNA studies. Also, if practicable in the field, be prepared to take swabs for microbiology from tissues showing lesions. One cannot take too many samples.

Specific points – birds of prey

(1) Before commencing an examination, investigate the bird externally for signs of injury, including fractures and parasites. Check the legs for metal rings (bands) or other identification marks. Describe the plumage, paying particular attention to signs of damage or moulting. Examine the skin of the belly to see if it is red and swollen – possibly indicative of a brood-patch. Try to age the bird: at least ascertain whether it is immature, subadult or adult. Weigh the whole carcass. Take other measurements, e.g. carpus, tarsal length.

Check any bags or containers (that enclosed the bird) for parasites or other material e.g. castings.

(2) Dampen the plumage with warm water (preferably containing a disinfectant soap solu-

tion) so as to facilitate *post-mortem* examination and to reduce airborne infection.

(3) Open the body cavity by cutting into the abdomen and lifting the sternum and examine all organs *in situ* before disturbing; record any abnormalities, e.g. growths, or swellings attached to an organ, possible ruptures, haemorrhage etc. Having removed or displaced liver and gut, sex the bird from the presence of testes or ovary and comment on their size and condition (hardly visible, obvious, oviduct containing egg, etc.). If in doubt sketch what you see. Make measurements where possible.

(4) Take small (1 cm cubes or less) of any tissues that appear abnormal plus major organs: lung, liver and kidney and place (fix) them in 10% formalin for subsequent histological examination. If formalin is not available, use 70% ethanol or methanol (methylated spirits or high-proof liquor will do in an emergency). Ensure that the volume of fixative is at least ten times as great as that of the tissue.

(5) Remove the heart and store fresh at refrigerator temperature (usually +4°C) for later bacteriological examination. If this is not possible or after culture has been performed, fix the heart in formalin or alcohol as above.

(6) Open parts of the gastro-intestinal tract carefully. See if there is food in the stomach (and/or crop if present): retain the food in ethanol/methanol, formalin or deep-freeze it for subsequent analysis. Search the tract for worms or other parasites; preserve them in formalin or alcohol. If possible, examine a sample of intestinal contents under a microscope for evidence of parasite eggs or protozoa. Refrigerate some gut contents for subsequent parasitological and bacteriological examination; if the latter is not possible, add a few drops of formalin or alcohol to preserve eggs and retain the specimen. Similarly, examine the trachea or preserve it whole in formalin or ethanol.

(7) When the points above have been carried out, wrap the whole carcass in at least one plastic bag and ensure it is well labelled (write in pencil or permanent marker and tie to specimen) and freeze it at as low a temperature as possible for subsequent toxicological and virological examination.

(8) After examination do not discard anything. Retain feathers, skin, pellets (castings) and stomach contents. These can all be frozen for reference at a later date.

(9) If pathological samples have to be sent by post or transported elsewhere ensure that they are properly packed. Postal and Customs Regulations must be consulted. Endangered species legislation (CITES) may be applicable even if the sample is small and has been fixed. Fresh (non-fixed) pathological material may only be imported into certain countries (e.g. Britain) under licence; this is usually issued by the relevant Agriculture Department and is completely independent of any CITES requirements.

For more information about transporting samples see Appendix XI.

Comments

The above notes are for guidance only. Variations in the protocol may be necessary, depending upon the circumstances.

Those who work with rare or isolated species should anticipate potential problems and at an early stage establish contact with either a local laboratory/veterinary pathologist or an experienced person elsewhere. Materials that may be needed (e.g. formalin) should be kept in stock.

Reference should be made also to *Disease and Threatened Birds* (Cooper, 1989a).

A BASIC *POST-MORTEM* TECHNIQUE FOR USE IN THE FIELD

(1) *External*
Weigh and measure (use standard techniques).

Identify the species and attempt to age and sex.

Examine externally (including all orifices) – record any parasites, lesions or abnormalities. Retain samples, fixed or fresh, as necessary.

Check important structures e.g. preen gland.

Photograph if possible.

(2) *Internal*

Open carcass – examine internal organs.

Record any lesions or abnormalities and whether alimentary tract contains food.

Check important structures e.g. bursa

Retain samples, fixed or fresh, as necessary.

Photograph if possible

(3) *Immediate investigations*

Open portions of intestines and look with naked eye or hand lens for parasites.

Make two wet preparations in saline and examine for parasites, food items and other material under the microscope.

Do 'touch preparations' (impression smears) of liver and any organs showing abnormalities, stain immediately and examine.

(4) *Longer term investigations*

Preserve in formalin or other fixative: lung, liver, kidney plus any abnormality.

Preserve other samples as appropriate (see Specific points – birds of prey)

(5) *Retention of carcass*

Save remains of the bird – if possible – either in, fridge, frozen or fixed in formalin.

General guidelines are to retain specimens in fridge (+4°C) for up to 7 days, frozen/fixed thereafter. Remember that samples for DNA studies should be either frozen or fixed in methanol, not in formalin (see Appendix VII).

Record in a diary as well as on a *post-mortem* sheet how the carcass and samples have been saved and include a reminder that they may need to be processed/discarded at a later date.

Some key rules

- Even (especially) if protective clothing and appropriate equipment are not available, practise strict hygiene (a 'clean:dirty' technique) at all times. In particular, do not contaminate paperwork and the outside of specimen containers.
- Keep written records of all findings plus (if possible) tape-recordings and/or photographs.
- If in doubt, retain material for further investigation later.

Legislation and Codes of Practice Relevant to Working with Raptors

M. E. COOPER LLB, FLS

'None shall bear any Hawk of English Breed, called Eyass, Goshawk, Tassel, Lanner, Lanneret or Falcon, in Pain to forfeit the same to the King.'
'He who brings any Eyass-Hawk from beyond the Sea, shall have a Certificate under the Customer's Seal where he lands; or if out of Scotland, then under the Seal of the Lord Warden of his Lieutenant, certifying that she is a foreign Hawk, upon Pain of forfeiting the Hawk.'
Statute of Henry VII, dated 1496 (Stat. 11 Hen. 7 c. 17)
The Laws Concerning Game, William Nelson 5th edition 1753

INTRODUCTION

The veterinary care and biological knowledge of birds of prey have reached new levels in the twenty-first century. Many species are scarce or threatened in the wild and are highly prized and valued in captivity. The provision of veterinary care for such species is no longer a novelty and veterinarians working with raptors have developed it into a speciality in its own right.

The science and skills of veterinary care can be complemented by a knowledge or understanding of the law relating to birds of prey both in their free-living state and in captivity. A knowledge of both these subjects is important because they are often inter-linked and it is in the transition from wild to captive that the law is most under pressure. It is important for the veterinarian, biologist, conservationist and the bird of prey keeper to be conversant with the law on birds of prey. It will enable them to ensure not only that their own activities are carried out within the law but also that they are in a position to pass on that information to others.

LEVELS OF LAW

In a book on the veterinary aspects of birds of prey there are a variety of fields of law that are applicable in addition to that relating to raptors as such (Cooper, ME, 1987, 1993; Wilson, 1989; McKean, 1993). Most of this legislation is produced on a national basis and therefore varies from one country to another both as to content and in respect of how (and how effectively) it is implemented and enforced.

There is some legislation that applies on an international basis in compliance with global or regional treaties. To a large extent this is also put into effect by individual countries by way of their national laws. In the case of the European Union (EU), some of its legislation (Regulations) takes direct effect in the law of the Member States while others (Directives) have to be implemented by Member States. Consequently there will be common provisions in the 15 States of the EU. This does not necessarily mean that all laws are the same in the EU countries – for they are entitled to enact stricter measures than the minimum required by the EU legislation.

Many countries that have a federal constitution have different tiers of legislation. Thus, some provisions are made at provincial level and others at federal (national) level. In the case of provincial legislation (as in Canada, the USA, Australia, India, Switzerland and Germany, for example) individual provinces (other terms may be state, canton, land, etc.) may have separate (and differing) laws in any given field. In addition, countries may be at different stages of development of their law on a particular subject.

In a book that is intended for an international readership it may be useful to indicate which fields of law are most relevant and to give some indication of its content. The reader will then be able to identify a chosen aspect of law within any particular jurisdiction. Thus, most countries have conservation, veterinary or animal health laws; however, the detailed provisions may vary and these can be ascertained within the relevant country. Since this book has a strong British influence, there is some reference to its legislation, guidance and relevant literature although it is too complex to be treated in detail.

DEFINITIONS

It is extremely important to take note of the definitions provided in animal legislation. Only very rarely does any particular law apply to all animals. It is more likely that it will be restricted to certain species or categories of animal. While there may be similarity in certain kinds of law, the detailed content is likely to vary from one country or one province to another. It is important, therefore, to obtain and to read carefully any legislation that is being used and to ensure that it is up-to-date.

It is also important that those seeking to use or to apply the law should ensure that they have the latest version. It is common for laws to be amended or replaced. Books cannot deal with future changes in the law so recourse must be had to legal advisors, specialist legal encyclopaedias and literature and, of course, to the actual legislation to ensure that information is accurate before acting upon it. Increasingly, information and legislation is available via the internet from government, treaty and other websites.

GUIDELINES, STANDARDS, CODES OF PRACTICE

Primary legislation (acts, statutes, ordinances) may be supplemented by subsidiary provisions such as rules, regulations, guidelines, standards or codes of practice. They are made under the authority of a statute but are more flexible and easier to amend. They may be enforceable by penalties or they may be available as supporting evidence in a prosecution under the primary legislation.

There are also non-statutory provisions that are made and observed on a voluntary basis in order to maintain standards. These can range from obligations as members of a profession, of a club or other group to the adoption of standards (codes of practice) for a sport. They are increasingly applicable to work on free-living birds of prey where public, sometimes official, concern about welfare and other matters has prompted researchers to draw up protocols that include ethical guidelines. This approach is likely to become increasingly prevalent and can have particular merit in special or unusual situations where self-regulation is appropriate. Examples from Britain include BFSSFC (undated), HB/BFSS (1997) and BWRC (undated) and from the USA, Oring (1988); IUCN/SSC (undated) provides an example of guidelines produced on an international basis.

LAW SPECIFIC TO BIRDS OF PREY

The relevant legislation can be divided between that relating to:

- Free-living birds of prey
- Captive birds of prey

There is, of course, overlap in the circumstances and the application of the law but, generally speaking, the provisions are primarily directed at one or other of these categories but may become applicable to birds in the other category.

Free-living birds of prey

The wide range of international laws that provide protection for birds of prey are summarised in the Table below.

International protection

Level of legislation	Legislation	Comments
	Wildlife and species protection	
Global See: Wijnstekers (1995); van Heijnsbergen (1997)	Convention on International Trade in Endangered Species of Wild Fauna and Flora (CITES)	International movement of listed species is controlled (see EU CITES Regulation under Regional)
	Convention on the Conservation of Migratory Species of Wild Animals (Bonn Convention/CMS)	Parties are required to make agreements for the conservation of migratory species listed in Appendix I (2 species of birds of prey are included) or II (including most Falconiformes) to the Convention
	Convention on Biological Diversity (CBD)	Encourages Parties to regulate the use of genetic resources and ensure the fair distribution of benefits. National laws may affect research in, and captive-breeding of, raptors, especially in developing countries
Regional European Union (EU)	EU Birds Directive	Prescribes protection measures and protected species of birds
	EU CITES Regulation	Implements CITES in the EU
USA and other countries	Migratory Bird Treaty Acts (USA)	Agreements between the USA, Canada, Mexico, Japan, Britain regarding the protection of migratory species
National	Legislation made in individual countries for wildlife protection in general	Species protection
	Protection of individual species	Bald Eagle Protection Act (USA), Philippines Eagle Owl Act (Philippines)
Habitat protection Global	Convention on Wetlands of International Importance especially as Waterfowl Habitat (Ramsar)	Encourages Parties to nominate and protect wetland sites. These may also be of benefit to raptors
	Convention Concerning Protection of the World Cultural and National Heritage (World Heritage)	Encourages Parties to nominate and protect sites of outstanding natural beauty. Includes some areas of importance to wildlife
Regional EU	Habitats Directive	Prescribes protection measures for habitat, including that important to wildlife
National	Legislation made in individual countries for the protection of habitat	Restrictions on the use of designated areas

National Species Protection

Legislation varies from country to country but the core provisions that are likely to be found in such wildlife laws can be summarised as follows:

- It is illegal to kill, injure or take any adult, young or egg either of any wild bird or, as in some laws, of any bird listed in the legislation.

- Provisions may also make it illegal to disturb birds at the nest during the breeding season or to destroy a nest in use.

- Hunting and trapping (or, at least, the use of indiscriminate or cruel) methods are proscribed or restricted. There are hunting seasons for certain species, such as some waterfowl.

- Trade in all, or specified, species is prohibited or restricted, for example, to captive-bred specimens. This is likely to include exchange or barter and the advertisement, transportation or possession for the purposes of trade. Importation and exportation may be dealt with in the species legislation or in separate provisions for the implementation of CITES.

- Possession of an illegally acquired protected species may also be an offence.

- There may be additional restrictions or extra penalties for more rare species.

- Certain *prima facie* illegal activities may be permitted under licence. These may include: taking for authorised purposes (e.g. scientific, captive breeding, educational or conservation reasons); other purposes might be ringing (banding), trapping or killing for the control of pest species.

- In some countries provision is specifically made to allow birds to be taken and kept for rehabilitation. Permits may variously be required for the taking (rescue), rehabilitation and release stages.

- Falconry is treated in a variety of ways. In some countries (such as Norway) it is prohibited, or it is regulated (USA, Germany) or is allowed

without specific restrictions for the sport (UK). There may, however, be provisions that affect falconry, since some of the general restrictions regarding, for example, species protection or hunting and trapping, may affect the sport or the recovery of lost birds.

- Penalties for breaking species protection laws are likely to include fines, imprisonment, confiscation of equipment used in the course of committing an offence, loss of licence or disqualification from holding one.

- The legal provisions regarding birds of prey are complex; guidance on the British law is available, particularly in respect of those that are protected by larger penalties for offences, that must be ringed and registered if kept in captivity and the provisions therefor.

National Habitat Protection

Protected areas have numerous titles such as biosphere reserves, national parks, game parks, game reserves, nature reserves (and, in the UK, sites of special scientific interest).

These normally provide protection (of various grades) for the designated area which often includes species' protection at defined levels depending on the use allowed. Thus, a national park may totally protect habitat and species but it may have adjacent land (e.g. a buffer zone) in which activities such as grazing or controlled hunting is allowed).

Birds of prey in captivity

The law relating to birds of prey in captivity is largely regulated at national or sub-national level, although EU legislation has an impact on its member countries, and CITES (see below) is applied by the many parties to the Convention. The relevant legislation is summarised in the table below.

Birds of prey in captivity

Type of legislation	*Comments*
Authorisation	
Zoos Travelling entertainment Flying displays Keeping, breeding Rehabilitation Sale in pet shops	Licensing is often required for this type of activity. Licences may be issued by national, provincial or local authority, and the legislation and type of licence varies from country to country.
Research	Research that may cause animals pain or distress is very strictly regulated in some countries and may extend to birds of prey both in captivity and in the wild. There may be strict licensing and ethical review processes. Veterinary supervision may be required. Record-keeping and inspection may also be a significant feature.
Welfare	
Cruelty	Many countries have laws that make the cruel treatment of animals illegal. This may be overt acts of cruelty such as beating or it may be more general, causing unnecessary suffering. The precise situations and types of animals and the anti-cruelty and enforcement provisions vary considerably.
During transportation	Some countries also have legislation specifically relating to the transport of animals and this may extend to birds.
Guidelines	Airlines usually require birds to be transported in compliance with the International Air Transport Association (IATA) Regulations (IATA, annual). The transport (by any method) of CITES species should comply with the CITES Guidelines (CITES, 1980) on transport.
EU Directive	While these two codes are not law as such, the EU Directive relating to the transport of animals makes it mandatory to comply with them. EU member countries must have legislation requiring that birds are transported without being caused injury or unnecessary suffering in appropriate containers and environmental conditions.
Animal health (disease control)	
In-country	Animal health (disease control) laws provide powers to control outbreaks of infectious diseases. Chlamydiosis and Newcastle disease (for example) controls may be applied to birds in captivity.
Importation	There are often controls applied to birds when they are imported. Import licences, veterinary health certificates and quarantine or isolation may be required.
Trade	
International	Most provisions regarding trade reflect CITES requirements.
National (in-country)	Trade in birds of prey may be controlled and permits required. This will depend on the species, whether it is captive-bred or taken from the wild (the latter is usually forbidden in the case of endangered species) and the purpose for which it is traded.

Type of legislation	Comments
Import and export	(Cooper, ME, 1989)
National wildlife laws	Some countries require an additional permit to take an indigenous species abroad because such animals are the property of its government or because there is control of genetic resources through legislation related to the Convention on Biodiversity. In the latter case, royalties may also become payable.
National animal health laws CITES Welfare in transport	See under Animal health, Trade and Welfare (above).
Customs and sales tax	May be applied to imports of birds that have a commercial value.
Samples	
Animal health and CITES laws apply	See under Animal health and Trade.
Postal regulations (national/ international)	There are special provisions for the packaging and mailing of pathological material.
Access to land	The landowner's permission is normally required before people enter land for activities with birds of prey such as falconry, research, rehabilitation, or the protection of breeding birds.

THE CONVENTION ON INTERNATIONAL TRADE IN ENDANGERED SPECIES (CITES)

The Convention on International Trade in Endangered Species of Wild Fauna and Flora (CITES) has a substantial impact on the commercial use of birds of prey. While this is largely related to international aspects as opposed to national legal controls, it also has an effect, in the EU, on their use on a national basis.

The title to the Convention also suggests very strongly that it relates to trade. However, this is only partly true and although those familiar with CITES use the term 'trade', it is well recognised that it applies to any international movement of species listed on the Appendices to the Treaty. It has been referred to in one Resolution passed by the Parties as 'cross-border movement'. This is easier to understand and, although CITES does not apply to provincial borders in countries with a federal constitution and to movement within the EU, the intent is there to refer to any international movement of CITES species, whether or not for commercial purposes.

The Convention requires permits to be obtained to authorise the international movement of any CITES species, i.e. those listed in Appendices I, II or III to the Convention. These can be summarised briefly as follows:

APPENDIX I — Species currently threatened with extinction and affected by trade

APPENDIX II — Species likely to become threatened unless trade is subject to regulation; to protect other species at risk from trade

APPENDIX III — Species listed by individual countries to safeguard a population in their country

The grant of import and export permits to authorise international movement must satisfy the requirements of the Convention, summarised as follows:

APPENDIX I: Export permit to be granted only if:

(1) not detrimental to the survival of the species
(2) not obtained in breach of national conservation laws
(3) a live animal will be prepared and shipped to

minimise risk of injury, damage to health or cruel treatment

(4) an import permit has been granted by destination country

Import permit to be granted only if:

(1) purpose is not detrimental to the survival of the species
(2) recipient can suitably house and care for live animal
(3) not to be used for primarily commercial purpose

APPENDIX II: Export permit to be granted only if (1), (2), (3) above (for Appendix I export permits) are satisfied.

While the Convention does not stipulate an import permit for Appendix II specimens, many countries do in fact, for enforcement and other reasons, require importation to be authorised by a permit.

Appendix II permits are used to monitor the trade of species that are thought to be at risk from commercial use. In addition, captive-bred specimens of Appendix I species can be traded and moved under Appendix II permits.

The Convention applies not only to whole live animals but also to dead ones and any parts and derivatives of CITES species. This is of particular relevance to those who need to send overseas veterinary samples that have been taken for reasons such as the diagnosis of disease or injury, for the monitoring of healthy birds or for identification or for use as evidence in law enforcement. All these items, if identifiable in any way as having been taken from CITES species, require permits to authorise their international movement, just as do live specimens of the species. There is a proposal to provide some form of expedited permit procedure for specimens from Appendix I species but this is likely to be limited to samples that are being moved for non-commercial and strictly conservation purposes. It is currently being formulated and will be considered at the Conference of the Parties in 2002 (Cooper, ME, 2000a).

Additional matters for EU countries:

- The EU CITES Regulations include in the Annexes not only all Convention species listed but also many more. In addition they give Appendix I status (by listing them in Annex A) to many Appendix II species.

- The EU Regulations and some other countries require an import permit for Appendix II species and, indeed, the EU provisions on permits and those of other countries are considerably more complex that the Treaty itself.

- The EU CITES Regulations include, over and above the Treaty provisions, a restriction on the purchase, sale, display or use for commercial purposes, of Annex A species within the EU. Thus, a permit is required for public exhibition (e.g. by zoos, other collections, by rehabilitation centres and for flying displays) or for the use in captive-breeding projects of the parent stock even though they are not to be sold. It is a condition of sale of permits that the specimen sold is permanently identified by a microchip. There are now standards for the placing of microchips in specific places in the body according to species (Anon, 1999). There are a few circumstances in which an alternative form of marking is allowed.

Enforcement is left by both the Convention and the EU Regulations to the national laws of individual countries.

Implementation of the EU Regulations is complicated and advice should be sought from the relevant country. Extensive guidance literature is provided in Britain and other countries, usually by the government department responsible for the environment or from other literature (such as Garbe (1989, 1993), Wijnstekers (1995), DETR (1996, 1998) and EC/TE/WWF (1998)) and from relevant government and institutional internet websites.

VETERINARY LEGISLATION

Legislation regulating the practice of veterinary medicine is found in most countries. Typical provisions are set out below.

Right to practise

Only registered veterinarians may practise 'veterinary surgery'. There may be exceptions that allow para-veterinary professionals to carry out specified veterinary activities, sometimes under supervision. These may include veterinary nurses, practitioners of complementary therapies, the owner or for the provision of emergency first aid. The precise scope of such exceptions varies from one country to another.

Species

The veterinary legislation usually applies to the treatment of birds but in some countries there is no restriction (in the veterinary law) on who is allowed to provide medical care for wildlife; likewise, some laws still do not apply to treatment given free-of-charge. Wild bird rehabilitators are subject to permits, training and inspection in some countries.

Procedures restricted to veterinarians

'Veterinary surgery' generally includes diagnosis, treatment and surgery. There may be exceptions.

Matters often restricted to veterinarians

Health certification, quarantine supervision, care of research animals and inspection of permitees' premises and birds are generally restricted to veterinarians.

Law enforcement investigation

Veterinarians may have responsibilities in respect of these activities.

Medicines

Many medicinal products are restricted as to production, supply and administration. Pharmaceutical laws allow only veterinarians or pharmacists to supply specified veterinary drugs; administration must be by or in accordance with the instructions of a veterinarian. The EU legislation requires the veterinarian to prescribe only veterinary medicines that are approved for the species and problem that has been diagnosed in an animal. In the case of raptors, there may be occasions when there are no drugs of choice that are approved for use in birds. In such situations the veterinarian must follow the 'cascade' in the choice of drug. In Britain the veterinarian is required to inform the client of this and is recommended to obtain the client's consent in writing (BVA, 2000; RCVS, 2000).

Professional discipline and liability

Veterinarians are subject to the ethical codes imposed by the veterinary legislation and professional body. A veterinarian must also practise to a standard that is expected of members of the profession. If a veterinarian fails to do this, a client who has suffered loss as a result, may be able to recover damages in civil law, from the former for professional negligence (malpractice) (Cooper, ME, 1987; Wilson, 1989; McKean, 1993; RCVS, 2000).

Other relevant legislation.

Area covered by legislation	Comments
Employment Occupational health and safety laws Precautions against accidents	These require high standards of protection for workers including safe working practices and equipment, protective clothing. Risk assessments and local rules for specific situations may be required. These are also useful procedures to apply in any situation where there is no such law or it is inadequate. Guidelines, codes of practice and 'local rules' are often drawn up for individual situations
Liability for accidents at work	Independently of the above, there may be civil law liability for causing accidents (see immediately below)

291

Area covered by legislation	Comments
Civil law liability e.g.: 　Negligence 　Nuisance 　Strict liability for animals 　Escape of animals 　Professional negligence	Liability in the civil law (in which individuals or bodies sue for compensation (damages)) for death, injury or loss caused by another – under these categories of civil law or in some countries in accordance with rights provided under a code of civil law
Forensic work 　Law enforcement 　Evidence 　Expert witness	These activities are regulated by primary legislation, statutory rules or court procedure

OTHER RELATED ISSUES

Rehabilitation

Rehabilitation has three stages, each of which may have legal implications:

- *Rescue*: This is likely to involve taking a sick or injured raptor from the wild for treatment and care. There must be provision in the species protection law to allow this or authorisation must be obtained.
- *Rehabilitation*: Permission may be required to keep the bird; veterinary or other laws may regulate who may care for or treat the bird; welfare laws apply while the bird is in captivity and may even extend to its release.
- *Release*: An assessment of its fitness for release may be necessary to justify a decision to release or to retain in captivity in accordance with the law (Cooper *et al.*, 1980). It may be necessary to balance a requirement to return the bird to the wild with the welfare implications of releasing it. A veterinarian may be asked to give an opinion or certificate in such a case.

Alien species

There is considerable concern regarding the intentional release of non-indigenous species into the wild and this may be prohibited by law. It should be taken into consideration when flying, breeding or keeping imported raptors.

Research

Raptors may be used in scientific research in the laboratory and in the field. Much of this work may require authorisation in many countries, particularly where this includes work that is invasive or is likely to cause pain or distress (Dolan, 2000). Veterinary supervision may also be required. Ethical guidelines may apply to research, including fieldwork (see Oring, 1988).

Even when such authorisation is not necessary, government (usually the science or education department) permits may be required to carry out any form of research. Permits may also be required to authorise the study, taking or use of wildlife and for access to protected areas or private land.

Live prey

The use of live prey either as food or for training captive raptors is often considered to be an ethical or welfare issue in that it may cause suffering in the animals presented as live prey. This may constitute an offence under cruelty legislation. It is, therefore, advisable to make an assessment of the circumstances leading to the need to feed or use live prey and to weigh up the welfare considerations for the bird and the proposed prey and to be able to justify the line of action adopted.

292

Microchipping and other marking methods

Legislation may require the marking of birds of prey, particularly where trade or other commercial use is involved.

CITES Recommendation Conf. 8.13 (Rev.) recommends the use of microchip transponders for the permanent marking of CITES species and that the sites used should be those advised by the IUCN/SSC Conservation Breeding Specialist Group (CBSG).

The EU CITES Regulations require the marking of captive-bred Annex A birds with an individually numbered closed ring or, where this is not possible (due to the physical or behavioural properties of the specimen concerned), with a uniquely numbered microchip transponder (DETR, 1998; Wellstead, 1998). All other CITES birds that are to be sold or used or displayed for commercial purposes must be marked with a microchip unless this is not possible.

Details of the microchip must be recorded on permits and certificates and the marking must be undertaken with regard to humane care and wellbeing and natural behaviour of the bird.

Various sites have been recommended for the implantation according to several organisations. These are set out in Anon (1999). In most cases the left pectoral muscle is recommended but the Federation of Zoological Gardens of Great Britain and Ireland add the left thigh, and the CBSG advise:

- Large (>1.5 kg and/or long-legged): dorsally at juncture of neck and body

- Medium to small (<1.5 kg): left pectoral muscle
- All New World and Old World vultures: base of neck
- All other Falconiformes: left pectoral muscle

Ethical issues

There are numerous ethical issues regarding birds of prey from those relating to the practice of falconry to maintaining raptors in captivity and for exhibition. Guidelines and codes of practice are used to indicate and encourage good practice for matters such as raptor flying demonstrations (HB/BFSS, 1997), rehabilitation (BWRC, undated), welfare and husbandry, re-introductions to the wild (IUCN/SSC undated), research (Dolan, 2000) and for zoos (DETR, 2000a; Macdonald & Charlton, 1999). In the case of, for example, animal research and zoological collections, an ethical committee is often established to review particular issues and proposed research and other activities.

CONCLUSION

The wildlife conservation legislation has critical implications for anyone associated with birds of prey, the veterinary laws affect the care and treatment of raptors, and a variety of other legal requirements also have to be taken into consideration. Such provisions are detailed, complex and vary from country to country – this appendix provides an introduction to the basic principles relevant to birds of prey in health and disease.

References and Further Reading

It should be noted that some of the publications listed were subsequently reprinted or appeared in several editions. The edition referred to is the one used during the compilation of this book.

Ackerman, N., Isaza, R., Greiner, E. & Berry, C. (1992) Pneumocolon associated with *Serratospiculum amaculata* in a bald eagle. *Veterinary Radiology and Ultrasound*, **33**(4), 351–355.

Aguilar, R.F. & Redig, P.T. (1995) Diagnosis and treatment of avian aspergillosis. In: *Kirk's Current Veterinary Therapy XII* (eds J.D. Bonagura & R.W. Kirk). W. B. Saunders, PA, USA.

Aguilar, R.F., Shaw, D.P., Dubey, J.P. & Redig, P.T. (1991) *Sarcocystis*-associated encephalitis in an immature Northern goshawk (*Accipiter gentilis atricapillus*). *Journal of Zoo and Wildlife Medicine*, **22**, 466–469.

Aguilar, R.F., Smith, V.E., Ogburn, P. & Redig, P.T. (1995) Arrhythmias associated with isoflurane anesthesia in bald eagles (*Haliaeetus leucocephalus*). *Journal of Zoo and Wildlife Medicine*, **26**(4), 508–516.

Aguilar, R.F., Stiles, J., Bistner, S.I. & Redig, P.T. (1993) Surgical synechiotomy in an adult bald eagle (*Haliaeetus leucocephalus*). *Journal of Zoo and Wildlife Medicine*, **24**(1), 63–67.

Akaki, C. & Duke, G.E. (1998) Egestion of chitin in pellets of American kestrels and Eastern screech owls. *Journal of Raptor Research*, **32**(4), 286–289.

Al-Ankari, A.S. (1998) Relationship between gonadal steroids and corticosterone during blood sampling in saker falcons. *Journal of Wildlife Diseases*, **34**(3), 653–655.

Allen, M. (1980) *Falconry in Arabia*. Orbis, London, UK.

Anderson, R.M. & May, R.M. (1978) Regulation and stability of host–parasite population interactions: 1. Regulatory processes. *Journal of Animal Ecology*, **47**, 219–249.

Anderson, R.M. & May, R.M. (1979a) Population biology of infectious diseases. Part 1. *Nature*, **280**, 361–367.

Anderson, R.M. & May, R.M. (1979b) Population biology of infectious diseases. *Nature*, **280**, 361–367; 455–461.

Anderson, R.M. & May, R.M. (1982) *The Population Biology of Infectious Diseases*. Springer-Verlag, Berlin, Germany.

André, J-P. (1999) Affections de la peau, des productions cornées et des plumes. *Le Point Vétérinaire*, **30**, 119–120.

Andreu de Lapíere, E. (1999) *Vade-Mecum Pour Les Animaux Exotiques de Campagnie*. Edition Med Com, Paris, France.

Andrew, W. & Hickman, C.P. (1974) *Histology of the Vertebrates*. The C V Mosby Company, St Louis, MO, USA.

Anon (1953) Encephalitis in short-wings. *The Falconer*, **11**, 28–30.

Anon (1977) The function of fever. *Lancet* ii, 178.

Anon (1983) Nematodes found in the orbital sinuses of a kestrel (*Falco tinnunculus*). *Veterinary Record*, **112**, 24.

Anon (1988) *Units, Symbols and Abbreviations*. Royal Society of Medicine Services, London, UK.

Anon (1995) Relieving pain in wild birds of prey. *Animal News* (Morris Animal Foundation) **II**, 1; 3.

Anon (1997) *ISIS Physiological Data Reference Values Volume 1, Herps Birds*. International Species Information System and the American Association of Zoo Veterinarians, MN, USA.

Anon (1999) Guidelines for microchip transmission sites in exotic species. *Journal of Small Animal Practice*, **40**, 201.

Anon (2000a) Help research road deaths. *Peregrine* (Newsletter of the Hawk and Owl Trust), 2.

Anon (2000b) VLA Surveillance Report. *Veterinary Record*, **147**, 562.

Anon (2001) Raptors. *Veterinary Record*, **148**, 68.

Antillon, A., Scott, M.L., Krook, L. & Wasserman, R.H. (1977) Metabolic response of laying hens to different dietary levels of calcium, phosphorus and vitamin D3. *Cornell Veterinarian*, **67**, 413–444.

Apinis, A.E. & Pugh, G.J.F. (1967) Thermophilous fungi of birds' nests. *Mycopathologia et Mycologia applicata*, **33**, 1–9.

Applebee, K.A. & Cooper, J.E. (1989) An anaesthetic or euthanasia chamber for small animals. *Animal Technology*, **40**, 39–43.

Appleby, B.M., Anwar, M.A. & Petty, S.J. (1999) Short-term and long-term effects of food supply on parasite burdens in Tawny Owls, *Strix aluco. Functional Ecology*, **13**, 315–321.

Arent, L.R. & Martell, M. (1996) *Care and Management of Captive Raptors*. The Raptor Center, University of Minnesota, USA.

Arnall, L. (1969) Diseases of the respiratory system. In: *Diseases of Cage and Aviary Birds* (ed. M.L. Petrak). Lea and Febiger, PA, USA.

Arnall, L. & Keymer, I.F. (1975) *Bird Diseases*. Baillière Tindall, London, UK.

Asakura, S., Nakagawa, S., Masui, M. & Yasuda, J. (1962) Immunological studies of aspergillosis in birds. *Mycopathologia et Mycologia Applicata*, **18**, 249–256.

Ashford, R.W., Wyllie, I. & Newton, I. (1990) *Leucocytozoon toddi* in British Sparrowhawks *Accipiter nisus*: observations on the dynamics of infection. *Journal of Natural History*, **24**, 1101–1107.

Ashton, W.L.G. & Cooper, J.E. (1989) Exclusion, elimination and control of avian pathogens. In: *Disease and Threatened Birds* (ed. J.E. Cooper), pp. 31–38. International Council for Bird Preservation, Cambridge, UK.

Ault, S.J. (1984) Electroretinograms and retinal structure of the eastern screech owl (*Otus asio*) and great horned owl (*Bubo virginianus*). *Raptor Research*, **18**, 62–66.

Avicultural Society (1977) *Register of non-domesticated birds bred under controlled conditions in Britain during 1976*. Coordinated by B. Sayers, Chelmsford, Essex, UK.

Aye, P.P., Morishita, T.Y. & Angrick, E.J. (1998) Virulence of raptor-origin *Pasteurella multocida* in domestic chickens. *Avian Diseases*, **43**, 279–285.

Bain, O. & Mawson, P.M. (1981) On some oviparous filarial nematodes mainly from Australian birds. *Records of the South Australian Museum*, **18**(13), 265–284.

Bain, O. & Vassiliades, G. (1969) Cycle évolutif d'un Dicheilonematinae, *Serratospiculum tendo*, filaire parasite du falcon. *Annales de Parasitologie Humaine et Comparée*, **44**, 595–604.

Baker, J.R. (1977) The results of post-mortem examination of 132 wild birds. *British Veterinary Journal*, **133**, 327–333.

Balasch, J., Musquera, S., Palacios, L., Jimenez, M. &

Palomeque, J. (1976) Comparative hematology of some falconiforms. *Condor*, **78**, 258–259.

Baldassarre, G.A. & Bolen, E.G. (1994) *Waterfowl Ecology and Management*. Wiley, New York, USA.

Bang, B. & Cobb, S. (1968) The size of the olfactory bulb in 108 species of birds. *Auk*, **85**, 55–61.

Barnard, P. (1989) Faecal bacteria in unhatched eggs of box-nesting Kestrels (*Falco sparverius*). In: *Disease and Threatened Birds* (ed. J.E. Cooper). International Council for Bird Preservation, Cambridge, UK.

Baronetzky-Mercier, A. & Seidel, B. (1995) Greifvögel und Eulen. In: *Krankheiten der Zoo- und Wildtiere* (eds C. Gabrisch & P. Zwart). Blackwell-Wissenschaftsverlag, Berlin, Germany.

Bartholomew, G.A. & Cade, T.J. (1957) The body temperature of the American kestrel, *Falco sparverius. Wilson Bulletin*, **69**, 149–154.

Barton, N.W. & Houston, D.C. (1993) A comparison of digestive efficiency in birds of prey. *Ibis*, **135**, 363–371.

Barton, N.W. & Houston, D.C. (1994) Morphological adaptation of the digestive tract in relation to feeding ecology in raptors. *Journal of Zoology*, London **232**, 133–150.

Barton, N.W. & Houston, D.C. (1996) Factors influencing the size of some internal organs in raptors. *Journal of Raptor Research*, **30**(4), 219–223.

Barus, V. & Sergejeva, T.P. (1989a) Capillariids parasitic in birds in the Palearctic region (1) genus *Capillaria. Acta Scientiarum Naturalium Academiae Scientiarum Bohemoslovacae Brno*, **23**(3), 1–50.

Barus, V. & Sergejeva, T.P. (1989b) Capillariids parasitic in birds in the Palearctic region (2) genera *Eucoleus* and *Echinocoleus. Acta Scientiarum Naturalium Academiae Scientiarum Bohemoslovacae Brno*, **23**(6), 1–47.

Barus, V. & Sergejeva, T.P. (1990) Capillariids parasitic in birds in the Palearctic region (3) genus *Baruscapillaria. Acta Scientiarum Naturalium Academiae Scientiarum Bohemoslovacae Brno*, **24**(10), 1–53.

de Bastyai, L. (1968) *Hunting Bird from a Wild Bird*. Pelham Books, London, UK.

Bauck, L.A. & Haigh, J.C. (1984) Toxicity of gentamicin in great horned owls (*Bubo virginianus*). *Journal of Zoo and Wildlife Medicine*, **15**, 62–66.

Bauer, H.W. (1985) *The primary structure of the hemoglobins from adult condor* (Vultur gryphus). *New aspects on the relationship of the Cathartiformes (New World vultures) to the Accipitriformes (hawks) and Ciconiiformes (storks)*. Dissertation, University of Munich, Germany.

Baumel, J.J., King, A.S., Breazile, J.E., Evans, H.E. & Vanden-Berge, J.C. (1993) *Handbook of Avian Anatomy: Nomina Anatomica Avium*, 2nd edn. Nuttall Ornithological Club, Harvard University, MA, USA.

Baumgartner, R., Hatt, J.M. & Isenbügel, E. (1994) Fractures in birds of prey – diagnosis, management and prognosis. *Proceedings, 1ˢᵗ European Conference of the Wildlife Disease Association (European Section)*, **14**.

Bean, J.R. & Hudson, R.H. (1976) Acute oral toxicity and tissue residues of thallium sulphate in golden eagles, *Aquila chrysaetos. Bulletin of Environmental Toxicology*, **15**, 118–121.

Beaulieu, D. (1992) La trichomonase chez les oiseaux de proie. *Chronique Vétérinaire*, **4**(1), 10.

Beebe, F. & Webster, H. (1964) *North American Falconry and Hunting Hawks*. World Press, Denver, CO, USA.

Beebe, F.L. (1976) *Hawks, Falcons and Falconry*. Hancock House Publishers Ltd, British Columbia, Canada.

Beecham, J.J. & Kochert, M.N. (1975) Breeding biology of the Golden Eagle in southwestern Idaho. *Wilson Bulletin*, **87**, 506–513.

Beguin, J. (1983) *Report on the chemical control of voles.* Department of Agriculture of the Republic and Canton of Neuchâtel, Switzerland.

Belant, J.L. & Seamans, T.W. (1999) Alpha-chloralose immobilization of rock doves in Ohio. *Journal of Wildlife Diseases*, **35**(2), 239–242.

Bell, A.A. & Murton, R.K. (1977) *Dieldrin residues in carcases of kestrels and barn owls.* Institute of Terrestrial Ecology, Annual Report 1976, 22–25, Cambridge, UK.

Bellairs, A. d'A. & Jenkin, C.R. (1960) The skeleton of birds. In: *Biology and Comparative Physiology of Birds* (ed. A.J. Marshall). Academic Press, New York, USA.

Bellrose, F.C. (1980) *Ducks, Geese and Swans of North America*. Stackpole Books, Harrisburg, PA, USA.

Bennett, G.F. (1970) *Trypanosoma avium* Danilewsky in the avian host. *Canadian Journal of Zoology*, **48**, 803–807.

Bennett, G.F., Bishop, M.A. & Peirce, M.A. (1993a) Checklist of the avian species of *Plasmodium* Marchiafava and Celli, 1885 (Apicomplexa) and their distribution by avian family Wallacean life zones. *Systematic Parasitology*, **26**, 171–179.

Bennett, G.F., Caines, J.R. & Bishop, M.A. (1988) Influence of blood parasites on the body mass of passeriform birds. *Journal of Wildlife Diseases*, **24**, 339–343.

Bennett, G.F., Garnham, P.C.C. & Fallis, A.M. (1965) On the status of the genera *Leucocytozoon* Ziemann, 1898, and *Haemoproteus* Kruse, 1890 (Haemosporidia: Leucocytozoidae and Haemoproteidae). *Canadian Journal of Zoology*, **43**, 927–932.

Bennett, G.F., Peirce, M.A. & Ashford, R.W. (1993b) Avian hematozoa: mortality and pathogenicity. *Journal of Natural History*, **27**, 993–1001.

Bennett, G.F., Whiteway, M. & Woodworth-Lynas, C.B. (1982) *A host–parasite catalogue of the avian haematozoa*. Occasional Papers in Biology, No. 5, Memorial University of Newfoundland, Canada.

Bennett, J.A. & Routh, A.D. (2000) Post-release survival of hand-reared tawny owls (*Strix aluco*). *Animal Welfare*, **9**, 317–321.

Bennett, P.M., Gascoyne, S.C., Hart, M.G., Kirkwood, J.K. & Hawkey, C.M. (1991) Development of LYNX: a computer application for disease diagnosis and health monitoring in wild mammals, birds and reptiles. *Veterinary Record*, **128**, 496–499.

Benson, W.W., Pharoah, B. & Miller, P. (1974) Lead poisoning in a bird of prey. *Bulletin of Environmental Contamination and Toxicology*, **11**, 105–108.

Berg, W., Johnels, A., Sjöstrand, B. & Westermark, T. (1966) Mercury content in feathers of Swedish birds from the past 100 years. *Oikos*, **17**, 71–83.

Bergmann, H.H. (1987) *Die Biologie des Vogels. Eine Exemplarische Einführung in Bau, Funktion und Lebensweise*. Aula Verlag, Wiesbaden, Germany.

Berners, Dame Juliana (1486) *The Boke of St Albans*. Printed at St Albans by the Schoolmaster Printer. Reprinted with Introduction by William Blades. Elliott Stock, (1881), London, UK.

Berry, R.B. (1972) Reproduction by artificial insemination in captive American goshawks. *Journal of Wildlife Management*, **36**, 1283–1288.

Bert, E. (1619) *An Approved Treatise of Hawkes and Hawking*. Richard Moore. Reprinted in 1891 and again in 1969 by Bernard Quaritch Ltd, London, UK.

Bertran, J. & Margalida, A. (1997) Griffon vultures (*Gyps fulvus*) ingesting bones at the ossuaries of bearded vultures (*Gypaetus barbatus*). *Journal of Raptor Research*, **31**(3), 287–288.

Best, R. (1996) Breeding problems. In: *Manual of Raptors, Pigeons and Waterfowl* (eds P.H. Beynon, N.A. Forbes & N. Harcourt-Brown). BSAVA, Cheltenham, UK.

Beyerbach, U. (1980) Kennzeichnung und Identifikation von Greifvögeln. *Der Praktische Tierarzt*, **61**, 936–940.

Beynon, P.H., Forbes, N.A. & Harcourt-Brown, N.H. (1996) *Manual of Raptors, Pigeons and Waterfowl*. British Small Animal Veterinary Association, Cheltenham, UK.

BFSSFC (undated) *British Field Sports Society Falconry Committee and the Hawk Board Code of Welfare and Husbandry of Birds of Prey and Owls*. British Field Sports Society, London, UK.

Bibby, C. (1999) Making the most of birds as environmental indicators. In: *Proceedings of the 22nd*

International Ornithological Congress (eds N.J. Adams & R.H. Slotow), Durban, South Africa. *Ostrich*, **70**(1), 81–88.

Bicknell, E.J., Greichus, A., Greichus, Y.A., Bury, R.J. & Knudtson, W.U. (1971) Diagnosis and treatment of aspergillosis in captive cormorants. *Sabouraudia*, **9**, 119–122.

Bigland, C.H. (1966) Common diseases of non-commercial and pet birds. *Canadian Veterinary Journal*, **7**, 252–259.

Bigland, C.H., Liu, S-K. & Perry, M.L. (1964) Five cases of *Serratospiculum amaculata* (Nematoda: Filaroidea) infection in prairie falcons (*Falco mexicanus*). *Avian Diseases*, **8**, 412–419.

Bilo, D., Best, G., Schönenberger, I. & Nachtigall, W. (1972) Zur Methode der Halothan-Inhalationsnarkose bei Vögeln (Taube und Wellensittich). *Journal of Comparative Physiology*, **79**, 137–152.

Bingman, V.P., Riteers, L.V., Strasser, R. & Gagliardo, A. (1998) Neuroethology of avian navigation. In: *Animal Cognition in Nature* (eds R.P. Balda, I.M. Pepperberg & A.C. Kamil). Academic Press, London, UK.

Bini, P.P., Floris, B., Nuvole, P., Pau, S. & Zedda, M.T. (1989) Caratteristiched ematologiche ed ematochimiche del gabbiona reale (*Larus argentatus*) e della poiana comune (*Buteo buteo*). *Bollotin Societi Italia Biologia Sperimentia*, **65**, 831–837.

Bird, D.M. & Buckland, R.B. (1976) The onset and duration of fertility in the American kestrel. *Canadian Journal of Zoology*, **54**, 1395–1397.

Bird, D.M. & Ho, S.K. (1976) Nutritive values of whole-animal diets for captive birds of prey. *Raptor Research*, **10**, 45–49.

Bird, D.M. & Lague, P.C. (1975) Treatment of bumble-foot by radiotherapy. *Hawk Chalk*, **XV**, 57–60.

Bird, D.M., Goutier, J. & Montpetit, V. (1984) Embryonic growth of American Kestrels. *The Auk*, **101**, 392–396.

Bird, D.M., Lague, P.C. & Buckland, R.B. (1976) Artificial insemination versus natural mating in captive American kestrels. *Canadian Journal of Zoology*, **54**, 1183–1191.

Birkhead, M. (1982) Causes of mortality in the Mute Swan on the River Thames. *Journal of Zoology, London*, **198**, 15–25.

Bishop, M.A. & Bennett, G.F. (1992) *Host-parasite catalogue of the avian haematozoa (Supplement 1) and bibliography of the avian blood-inhabiting haematozoa (Supplement 2)*. Occasional Papers in Biology, No. 15, Memorial University of Newfoundland, Canada.

Blackmore, D.K. (1965) *The pattern of disease in budgerigars: a study in comparative pathology*. PhD thesis, London, UK.

Blackmore, D.K. & Gallagher, G.L. (1964) An outbreak of erysipelas in captive wild birds and mammals. *Veterinary Record*, **76**, 1161–1164.

Blackmore, D.K. & Keymer, I.F. (1969) Cutaneous diseases of wild birds, in Britain. *British Birds*, **62**, 316–331.

Blaine, G. (1936) *Falconry*. Reprinted in 1976 by Neville Spearman Ltd, London, UK.

Blanco, G., Gajon, A., Doval, G. & Martinez, F.J. (1998) Absence of blood parasites in griffon vultures from Spain. *Journal of Wildlife Diseases*, **34**(3), 640–643.

Blancou, J. & Rajaonarison, J. (1972) Note sue le rôle vecteur des rapaces dans la propagation de certaines maladies bactériennes. *Revue d'élevage et de médicine vétérinaire des pays tropicaux*, **25**, 187–189.

Blome, R. (1686) *The Gentleman's Recreation*. Printed by S Roycroft, London, UK.

Blood, D.C. & Studdert, V.P. (1988) *Saunders Comprehensive Veterinary Dictionary*. W. B. Saunders, London, UK.

Blundell, A. (1990) *Health monitoring of prey items – a precautionary step*. Study in partial fulfilment of the Diploma in the Management of Endangered Species, University of Kent, Canterbury, UK.

Blus, L.J. (1996) DDT, DDD and DDE in birds. In: *Environmental Contaminants in Wildlife* (eds W.N. Beyer, G.H. Heinz & A.W. Redmon-Norwood). The Society of Environmental Toxicology and Chemistry (SETAC), Boca Raton, FL, USA.

Boal, C.W. & Mannan, R.W. (1999) Comparative breeding ecology of Cooper's hawks in urban and exurban areas of southeastern Arizona. *Journal of Wildlife Management*, **63**(1), 77–84.

Boal, C.W., Hudelson, K.S., Mannan, R.W. & Estabrook, T.S. (1998a) Hematology and hematozoa of adult and nestling hawks in Arizona. *Journal of Raptor Research*, **32**(4), 281–285.

Boal, C.W., Mannan, R.W. & Hudelson, K.S. (1998b) Trichomoniasis in Cooper's hawks from Arizona. *Journal of Wildlife Diseases*, **34**(3), 590–593.

Board, R.G., Tullett, S.G. & Perrott, H.R. (1977) An arbitrary classification of the pore systems in avian eggshells. *Journal of Zoology, London*, **182**, 251–265.

Bock, W.J. (1974) The avian skeletomuscular system. In: *Avian Biology*, Vol. VI (eds D.S. Farmer & S.R. King). Academic Press, London and New York.

Bogue, G. (1980) Treating endoparasites and ectoparasites in birds of prey. *Methods: The Journal of Animal Health Technology*, **3**(4), 10–13.

Bölske, G. & Mörner, T. (1981) Case report – isolation of a *Mycoplasma* sp. from three buzzards (*Buteo* spp.). *Avian Diseases*, **26**, 406–411.

Bolte, A.L., Meurer, J. & Kaleta, E.F. (1999) Avian host spectrum of avipoxviruses. *Avian Pathology*, **28**(5), 415–432.

Bonath, K. (1972a) Zur Inhalationsnarkose von Hühnern, Tauben, Enten und anderen Vögeln mit Halothan und Äther und deren Wirkung auf Blutdruck, Herz-, Atemfrequenz und Körpertemperatur. *Zentralblatt für Veterinärmedizin*, **19**, 639–660.

Bonath, K. (1972b) Inhalations-, Injektions- und Lokalanaesthesie der Vögel. *Sonderdruck aus Verhandlungsbericht des XIV Internationalen Symposiums über die Erkrankungen der Zootiere*. Akademie-Verlag, Berlin, Germany.

Bonham, A., Beresford, N. & Smith, J. (2000) Working in the Chernobyl zone. *NERC News*, Autumn 2000, 20–21.

Bonser, R.H.C. (1996) The mechanical properties of feather keratin. *Journal of Zoology, London*, **239**, 477–484.

Booth, D.T., Clayton, D.H. & Block, B.A. (1993) Experimental demonstration of the energetic cost of parasitism in wild hosts. *Proceedings of the Royal Society*, **B 253**, 125–129.

Borst, G.H.A., Zwart, P., Mullink, H.W.M.A. & Vroege, C. (1976) Bone structures in avian and mammalian lungs. *Veterinary Pathology*, **13**, 98–103.

Borzio, F. (1973) Ketamine hydrochloride as an anesthetic for wild fowl. *Veterinary Medicine/Small Animal Clinician*, **68**, 1364–1365.

Boshell, M.J. (1969) Kysanur forest disease: ecological considerations. *American Journal of Tropical Medicine and Hygiene*, **18**, 65–80.

Böttcher, M. (1982) Erfahrungen mit der diagnostischen endoskopie beim vogel. *Tierärztl. Prax*, **10**, 183–188.

Botzler, R.G. (1991) Epizootiology of avian cholera in wildfowl. *Journal of Wildlife Diseases*, **27**, 367–395.

Bougerol, C. (1967) *Essai sur la Pathologie des Oiseaux de Chasse au Vol*. Alfort, France.

Boughton, D.C. (1988) Dircadoduodian rhythms in avian coccidia. *Transactions of the American Microscopical Society*, **107**, 329–344.

Bowerman, W.W., IV, Evans, E.D., Giesy, J.P. & Postupalsky, S. (1994) Using feathers to assess risk of mercury and selenium to bald eagle reproduction in the Great Lakes region. *Archives of Environmental Contamination and Toxicology*, **27**, 294–298.

Boyd, L. (1977) Hybridization of falcons by artificial insemination. *Symposium of the Zoological Society of London*, September, 1977.

Boyd, L.L., Boyd, N.S. & Dobler, F.C. (1977) Reproduction of prairie falcons by artificial insemination. *Journal of Wildlife Management*, **41**, 266–271.

Boydell, I.P. & Forbes, N.A. (1996) Diseases of the head (including the eyes). In: *Manual of Raptors, Pigeons and Waterfowl* (eds P.H. Beynon, N.A. Forbes & N.H. Harcourt-Brown). British Small Animal Veterinary Association, Cheltenham, UK.

Brearley, M.J., Cooper, J.E. & Sullivan, M. (1991) *Colour Atlas of Small Animal Endoscopy*. Wolfe, London, UK.

Bright, P.R. (2000) GIS: a tool for protecting the health of wild bird populations. *Proceedings of the Association of Avian Veterinarians*, 181–183.

Brisbin, I.L. (1970) A determination of live-weight caloric conversion factors for laboratory mice. *Ecology*, **51**, 541–544.

Brisbin, L. & Wagner, C.K. (1970) Some health problems associated with the maintenance of American kestrels, *Falco sparverius*, in captivity. *International Zoo Yearbook*, **10**, 29–30.

Britten, M.W., Kennedy, P.L. & Ambrose, S.K. (1999) Performance and accuracy evaluation of small satellite transmitters. *Journal of Wildlife Management*, **63**(4), 1349–1358.

Brooke, R.K. (1975) A pathological yellow-billed kite. *Honeyguide*, **82**, 39.

Brown, C.J. & Bruton, A.G. (1991) Plumage colour and feather structure of the bearded vulture (*Gypaetus barbatus*). *Journal of Zoology, London*, **223**, 627–640.

Brown, L.H. (1976a) *British Birds of Prey*. Collins, London, UK.

Brown, L.H. (1976b) *Birds of Prey; Their Biology and Ecology*. Hamlyn, London, UK.

Brown, L. & Amadon, D. (1968) *Eagles, Hawks and Falcons of the World*. Country Life Books, Hamlyn House, Middlesex, UK.

Brown, L. & Amadon, D. (1989) *Eagles, Hawks and Falcons of the World*. The Wellfleet Press, Secacus, NJ, USA.

Brown, M.E. (1996) Assessing body condition in birds. In: *Current Ornithology*, Volume 13 (eds V. Nolan & E.D. Ketterson). Plenum Press, New York, USA.

Bruce, D.W., McIlroy, S.G. & Goodall, E.A. (1990) Epidemiology of a contact dermatitis of broilers. *Avian Pathology*, **19**, 523–537.

Bruggers, R.L., Jaeger, M.M., Keith, J.O., Hegdal, P.L., Bourassa, J.B., Latigo, A.A. & Gillis, J.N. (1989) Impact of fenthion on nontarget birds during Quelea control in Kenya. *Wildlife Society Bulletin*, **17**, 149–160.

Bucher, E.H. (1988) Do birds use biological control against nest parasites? *Parasitology Today*, **4**, 1–3.

Bucke, D. & Mawdesley-Thomas, L.E. (1974) Tuberculosis in a barn owl (*Tyto alba*). *Veterinary Record*, **95**, 373.

Buckley, P.A. (1969) Genetics. In: *Diseases of Cage and Aviary Birds* (ed. M.L. Petrak). Lea & Febiger, PA, USA.

Burckardt, D. (1988) UV Vision: a bird's eye view of feathers. *Journal of Comparative Physiology*, **164**, 787–796.

Burger, G.V. (1964) Survival of Ring-necked Pheasants released on a Wisconsin shooting preserve. *Journal of Wildlife Management*, **28**, 711–721.

Burgess, E.C., Ossa, J. & Yuill, T.M. (1979) Duck plague: a carrier state in waterfowl. *Avian Diseases*, **24**, 940–949.

Burnett, C. (1998) *Adelard of Bath, Conversations with his Nephew*. Cambridge Medieval Classics, Cambridge, UK.

Burtnick, N.L. & Degernes, L.A. (1993) Electrocardiography on fifty-nine anesthetized convalescing raptors. In: *Raptor Biomedicine* (eds P.T. Redig, J.E. Cooper, J.D. Remple & D.B. Hunter). University of Minnesota Press, USA.

Burton, R. (1991) *Birds Flight*. Eddison Sadd Editions Limited, London, UK.

Burtscher, H. (1965) Die virusbedingte Hepatosplenitis infectiosa strigorum. I Mitteilung: Morphologische Untersuchungen. *Pathologia Veterinaria*, **2**, 227–255.

Burtscher, M. & Sibalin, M. (1975) Herpesvirus striges: host spectrum and distribution in infected owls. *Journal of Wildlife Diseases*, **11**, 164–169.

Busch, D.A., de Graw, W.A. & Clampitt, N.C. (1978) Effects of handling–disturbance stress on heartrate in the ferruginous hawk (*Buteo regalis*). *Raptor Research*, **12**, 122–125.

Busch, D.E., de Graw, W.A. & Clampitt, N.C. (1984) Biotelemetered daily heart rate cycles in the red-tailed hawk (*Buteo jamaicensis*). *Raptor Research*, **18**, 74–77.

Bush, M. (1981) Diagnostic avian laparoscopy. In: *Recent Advances in the Study of Raptor Diseases* (eds J.E. Cooper & A.G. Greenwood). Chiron Publications, Keighley, Yorkshire, UK.

Butterworth, G. & Harcourt-Brown, N.H. (1996) Neonatal husbandry and related diseases. In: *Manual of Raptors, Pigeons and Waterfowl* (eds P.H. Beynon, N.A. Forbes & N.H. Harcourt-Brown). British Small Animal Veterinary Association, Cheltenham, UK.

Butynski, T. (1995) Myiasis in two free-living crowned eagles. *Journal of African Raptor Biology*, **10**(2), 49–50.

BVA (2000) *BVA Code of Practice on Medicines*. British Veterinary Association, London, UK.

BWRC (undated) *Guidelines for Wildlife Rehabilitation Units*. British Wildlife Rehabilitation Council, Horsham, W. Sussex, UK.

Cade, T.J. (1968) The gyrfalcon and falconry. *Living Bird*, 7, 237–240.

Cade, T.J. (1975) *Captive Breeding – the 1975 Season*. The Peregrine Fund, Laboratory of Ornithology, Cornell University, USA.

Cade, T.J. (1980) The husbandry of falcons for return to the wild. *International Zoo Yearbook 3*, **20**, 23–35.

Cade, T.J. (1982) *Falcons of the World*. Collins Sons & Co., London, UK.

Cade, T.J., Enderson, J.H., Thelander, C.G. & White, C.M. (1988) *Peregrine Falcon Populations: Their Management and Recovery*. The Peregrine Fund Inc., Boise, ID, USA.

Cadle, D.R. & Martin, G.R. (1976) Metomidate as sole anaesthetic agent in tawny owls. *Veterinary Record*, **98**, 91–92.

Calder, W.A. & Schmidt-Nielsen, K. (1968) Panting and blood carbon dioxide in birds. *American Journal of Physiology*, **215**, 477–482.

Calnek, B.W., Barnes, H.J., Beard, C.W., Reid, W.M. & Yoder, H.W. (1991) *Diseases of Poultry*, 9th edn. Wolfe, London, UK.

Campbell, J.A. (1934) Some observations relative to ailments of inmates in a zoological collection. *Journal of the American Veterinary Medical Association*, **84**, 711–739.

Campbell, T.W. (1984) Diagnostic cytology in avian medicine. *Veterinary Clinics of North America*, **14**, 317–344.

Campbell, T.W. (1993) Cytodiagnosis in raptor medicine. In: *Raptor Biomedicine* (eds P.T. Redig, J.E. Cooper, J.D. Remple & D.B. Hunter). University of Minnesota Press, USA.

Carpenter, J.W., Mashima, T.Y. & Rupiper, D.J. (2001) *Exotic Animal Formulary*, 2nd edn. W.B. Saunders, PA, USA.

Castle, M.D. & Christansen, B.M. (1990) Hematozoa of wild turkeys from the mid-western United States: translocation of wild turkeys and its potential role in the introduction of *Plasmodium kempi*. *Journal of Wildlife Diseases*, **26**(2), 180–185.

Cawthorn, R.J. (1993) Cyst-forming coccidia of raptors: Significant pathogens or not? In: *Raptor Biomedicine* (eds P.T. Redig, J.E. Cooper, J.D. Remple & D.B. Hunter). University of Minnesota Press, Minneapolis, MN, USA.

Cerna, Z. & Louckova, M. (1977) *Microtus arvalis*, the intermediate host of a coccidian from the kestrel (*Falco tinnunculus*). *Vestnik Ceskoslov enske Spolecnosti Zoologicke*, **XLI**, 1–4.

Chaplin, S.B., Mueller, L.R. & Degernes, L.A. (1993) Physiological assessment of rehabilitated raptors prior to release. In: *Raptor Biomedicine* (eds P.T. Redig, J.E. Cooper, J.D. Remple & D.B. Hunter). University of Minnesota Press, MN, USA.

Chapman, B.R. & George, J.E. (1991) The effects of ectoparasites on Cliff Swallow growth and survival. In: *Bird–Parasite Interactions* (eds J.E. Loye & M. Zuk). University Press, Oxford, UK.

Chastel, C., Guiguen, C., Castel, O. & Beaucournu, J.C. (1991) Pathological effects, vector role and new hosts of *Ixodes pari* equals *Ixodes frontalis* Acari, Ixodoidea, Ixodidae. *Annales de Parasitologie Humaine et Comparée*, **66**(1), 27–32.

Cheng, T.C. (1986) *General Parasitology*, 2nd edn. Academic Press, FL, USA.

Chiasson, R.B., Egge, A.S. & Lynch, B. (1973) The effect of ketalar on the adrenal gland of young white leghorn cockerels. *Poultry Science*, **52**, 1014–1018.

Chitty, J.R. (2000a) Use of Vet Bio SIST in bumblefoot management. *Proceedings of the Association of Avian Veterinarians*, 109–111.

Chitty, J.R. (2000b) Feather chewing and split keel in a raptor. *Proceedings of the Association of Avian Veterinarians*, 489–491.

Cho, B.R. & Kenzy, S.G. (1975) Virologic and serologic studies of zoo birds for Marek's disease virus infection. *Infection and Immunity*, **11**, 809–814.

Christian-Franson, J. & Little, S.E. (1996) Diagnostic findings in 132 great horned owls. *Journal of Raptor Research*, **30**(1), 1–6.

Christian-Franson, J., Galbreath, E.J., Wiemeyer, S.N. & Abell, J.M. (1994) *Erysipelothrix rhusiopathiae* infection in a captive bald eagle (*Haliaeetus leucocephalus*). *Journal of Zoo and Wildlife Medicine*, **25**(3), 446–448.

Chu, H.P., Trow, E.W., Greenwood, A.G., Jennings, A.R. & Keymer, I.F. (1976) Isolation of Newcastle disease virus from birds of prey. *Avian Pathology*, **5**, 227–233.

Chubb, K. (1982) A case of right cranial nerve paralysis in a red-tailed hawk. *Ontario Field Biologist*, **36**, 96.

CITES (1980) *Guidelines for Transport and Preparation for Shipment of Live Wild Animals and Plants*. International Union for Conservation of Nature, Gland, Switzerland.

Clark, L. & Mason, J.R. (1985) Use of nest material as insecticidal and antipathogenic agents by the European Starling. *Oecologia*, **67**, 169–176.

Clark, W., Duffy, K., Gorney, E., McGrady, M. & Schultz, C. (1988) Supernumarary primaries and rectrices in some Eurasian and North American raptors. *Journal of Raptor Research*, **22**(2), 53–58.

Clark, W.S. (1981) A modified dho-gaza trap for use at a raptor banding station. *Journal of Wildlife Management*, **45**(4), 1043–1044.

Clark, W.S. (1995) Capture and banding of migrant raptors. *Israel Journal of Zoology*, **41**, 237–242.

Clark, W.S. & Gorney, E. (1987) Oil contamination of raptors migrating along the Red Sea. *Environmental Pollution*, **46**, 307–313.

Clarke, A. (1977) Contamination of peregrine falcons (*Falco peregrinus*) with fulmar stomach oil. *Journal of Zoology, London*, **181**, 11–20.

Clausen, B. & Gudmundsson, F. (1981) Causes of mortality among free-ranging gyrfalcons in Iceland. *Journal of Wildlife Diseases*, **17**(1), 105–109.

Clausen, B. & Karlog, O. (1977) Thallium loading in owls and other birds of prey in Denmark. *Nordisk Veterinaermedicin*, **29**, 227–231.

Clay, T. & Price, R.D. (1970) A new genus and species of the *Menoponidae(Mallophaga)* from the African Swallowtailed Kite. *Journal of Medical Entomology*, 7, 119–121.

Clayton, D.H. (1990) Mate choice in experimentally parasitised rock doves: lousy males. *American Zoologist*, **30**, 251–262.

Clayton, N.C. & Lee, W.D. (1999) Memory and the hippocampus in food-storing birds. In: *Animal Cognition in Nature* (eds R.P. Balda, I.M. Pepperberg & A.C. Kamil). Academic Press, London, UK.

Clum, N.J., Fitzpatrick, M.P. & Dierenfeld, E.S. (1997) Nutrient content of five species of domestic animals commonly fed to captive raptors. *Journal of Raptor Research*, **31**(3), 267–272.

Clyde, V.L. & Paul-Murphy, J. (2000) Avian analgesia. In: *Kirk's Current Veterinary Therapy XIII Small Animal Practice* (ed. J.D. Bonagura). W.B. Saunders, PA and London.

Coatney, G.R. & West, E. (1937) Some notes on the effect of atrebrine on the gametocytes of the genus *Leucocytozoon. Journal of Parasitology*, **23**, 227–228.

Cobb, S. (1960) Observations on the comparative anatomy of the avian brain. *Perspectives in Biology and Medicine*, **3**, 383–408.

Coles, B.H. (1984) Some considerations when nursing birds in veterinary premises. *Journal of Small Animal Practice*, **25**, 275–288.

Coles, B.H. (1997) *Avian Medicine and Surgery*. Blackwell Scientific Publications, London, UK.

Colombini, S., Foil, C.S., Hosgood, G. & Tully, T.N. (2000) Intradermal skin testing in Hispaniolan parrots (*Amazona ventralis*). *Veterinary Dermatology*, **11**, 271–276.

Comben, N. (1969) The early English printed literature on the diseases of poultry and other birds. *The Veterinarian*, **6**, 17–25.

Conant, S. (1988) Saving endangered species by translocation. Are we tinkering with evolution? *BioScience*, **38**(4), 254–257.

Cooke, A.S., Bell, A.A. & Haas, M.B. (1982) *Predatory Birds, Pesticides and Pollution*. Institute of Terrestrial Ecology, Cambridge, UK.

Cooper, J.E. (1965) Death of a trained falcon attributed to chlorinated hydrocarbon poisoning. *The Falconer*, **4**, 230–232.

Cooper, J.E. (1968a) The trained falcon in health and disease. *Journal of Small Animal Practice*, **9**, 559–566.

Cooper, J.E. (1968b) Diseases of hawks. *The Falconer*, **V**, 55–57.

Cooper, J.E. (1968c) Tuberculosis in birds of prey. *Veterinary Record*, **82**, 61.

Cooper, J.E. (1969a) Oesophageal capillariasis in captive falcons. *Veterinary Record*, **84**, 634–636.

Cooper, J.E. (1969b) Some diseases of birds of prey. *Veterinary Record*, **84**, 454–457.

Cooper, J.E. (1969c) Two cases of pox in recently imported peregrine falcons (*Falco peregrinus*). *Veterinary Record*, **85**, 683–684.

Cooper, J.E. (1970a) Diseases of birds of prey. *Annual Report of the Hawk Trust*, **1**, 22–31.

Cooper, J.E. (1970b) Use of the hypnotic agent 'Methoxymol' in birds of prey. *Veterinary Record*, **87**, 751–752.

Cooper, J.E. (1971) First aid and preventive medicine for hawks. *The Falconer*, **V**, 299–304.

Cooper, J.E. (1972a) Feather conditions of birds of prey. *Journal of the North American Falconers' Association*, **XI**, 39–44.

Cooper, J.E. (1972b) Possible vaccination against aspergillosis. *Raptor Research*, **6**, 105.

Cooper, J.E. (1972c) Some haematological data for birds of prey. *Raptor Research*, **6**, 133–136.

Cooper, J.E. (1973a) Health and disease. In: *A Hawk for the Bush* (ed. J.G. Mavrogordato), 2nd edn. Neville Spearman, London, UK.

Cooper, J.E. (1973b) Blood parasites from a red-chested owlet *Glaucidium tephronotum*. *Bulletin of British Ornithologists' Club*, **93**, 25–26.

Cooper, J.E. (1973c) Post-mortem findings in East African birds of prey. *Journal of Wildlife Diseases*, **9**, 368–375.

Cooper, J.E. (1974a) Metomidate anaesthesia of some birds of prey for laparotomy and sexing. *Veterinary Record*, **94**, 437–440.

Cooper, J.E. (1974b) Trichlorphon as a safe insecticide for use on birds of prey. *Veterinary Record*, **94**, 455.

Cooper, J.E. (1974c) Current work on raptor diseases in Kenya, East Africa. *Raptor Research*, **8**, 1–5.

Cooper, J.E. (1975a) First aid and veterinary treatment of wild birds. *Journal of Small Animal Practice*, **16**, 579–591.

Cooper, J.E. (1975b) Haematological investigations in East African birds of prey. *Journal of Wildlife Diseases*, **11**, 389–394.

Cooper, J.E. (1975c) The role of vaccination in the maintenance of captive birds of prey. *Raptor Research*, **9**, 21–26.

Cooper, J.E. (1975d) Osteodystrophy in birds of prey. *Veterinary Record*, **97**, 307.

Cooper, J.E. (1976a) Health and diseases of hawks. *International Conference on Falconry and Conservation*, Abu Dhabi, 10–18 December, 1976.

Cooper, J.E. (1976b) Clinical conditions of East African birds of prey. *Tropical Animal Health and Production*, **8**, 203–211.

Cooper, J.E. (1977) Veterinary problems of captive breeding and possible reintroduction of birds of prey. *International Zoo Yearbook*, **17**, 32–38.

Cooper, J.E. (1978a) *Veterinary Aspects of Captive Birds of Prey*. The Standfast Press, Saul, Gloucestershire, UK.

Cooper, J.E. (1978b) An adenocarcinoma in a buzzard (*Buteo buteo*). *Avian Pathology*, **7**, 29–34.

Cooper, J.E. (1978c) Preventive medicine in birds of prey. In: *Zoo and Wild Animal Medicine* (ed. M.E. Fowler). W.B. Saunders, PA, USA.

Cooper, J.E. (1979a) The history of hawk medicine. *Veterinary History*, **NSI**, 11–18.

Cooper, J.E. (1979b) Veterinary care of birds. *Animal Regulation Studies*, **2**, 21–29.

Cooper, J.E. (1979c) An oviduct adenocarcinoma in a Mauritius kestrel (*Falco punctatus*). *Avian Pathology*, **8**, 187–191.

Cooper, J.E. (1980a) Medicine and diseases of birds of prey. *Annual Proceedings of the American Association of Zoo Veterinarians*, Washington DC, USA, 73–75.

Cooper, J.E. (1980b) Diseases of the sparrow-hawk (*Accipiter nisus*). *The Falconer*, **VII**, 252–256.

Cooper, J.E. (1980c) Surgery of the foot of falcons: a historic operation. *Annals of the Royal College of Surgeons of England*, **62**, 445–448.

Cooper, J.E. (1980d) Additional observations on the intertarsal joint of the African harrier hawk (*Polyboroides typus*). *Ibis*, **122**, 94–98.

Cooper, J.E. (1982a) A historical review of goshawk training and disease. In: *Understanding the Goshawk* (eds R.E. Kenward & I. Lindsay). International Association for Falconry and Conservation of Birds of Prey, Oxford, UK.

Cooper, J.E. (1982b) Some aspects of John Hunter's work on the diseases of birds of prey. *Annals of the Royal College of Surgeons of England*, **64**, 345–347.

Cooper, J.E. (1983) Pathological studies on the effects of intramuscular injections in the starling (*Sturnus vulgaris*). *Sonderdruck aus Verhandbericht des 25 Internationalen Symposiums über die Erkrankungen der Zootiere*. Wien, Akademie-Verlag, Germany.

Cooper, J.E. (1984a) The conservation and captive management of raptors: an overview. *International Zoo Yearbook*, **23**, 1–7.

Cooper, J.E. (1984b) Avian anaesthesia. *Veterinary Record*, **114**, 283.

Cooper, J.E. (1984c) Developmental abnormalities in two British falcons (*Falco* spp.). *Avian Pathology*, **13**, 639–645.

Cooper, J.E. (1985a) Diagnostic techniques in birds. *The Veterinary Annual*, **25**, 236–244.

Cooper, J.E. (1985b) *Veterinary Aspects of Captive Birds of Prey*. Standfast Press, Gloucester, UK.

Cooper, J.E. (1985c) Preventive medicine in birds of prey. In: *Zoo and Wild Animal Medicine* (ed. M.E. Fowler), 2nd edn. W.B. Saunders, PA, USA.

Cooper, J.E. (1987a) Raptor care and rehabilitation: precedents, progress and potential. *Journal of Raptor Research*, **21**(1), 21–26.

Cooper, J.E. (1987b) Pathological studies on avian pododermatitis (bumblefoot). *Sonderdruck aus Verhandlungsbericht des 29 Internationalen Symposiums über die Erkrankungen der Zootiere*. Akademie-Verlag, Germany.

Cooper, J.E. (1987c) Pathology. In: *Raptor Management Techniques Manual* (eds B.A.G. Pendleton, B.A. Millsap, K.W. Cline & D.M. Bird). National Wildlife Federation, Washington DC, USA.

Cooper, J.E. (1988) Reproductive disorders in birds of prey. *Veterinary Annual*, **28**, 129–135.

Cooper, J.E. (1989a) *Disease and Threatened Birds*. ICBP Technical Publication No. 10. International Council for Bird Preservation (now Bird Life International), Cambridge, UK.

Cooper, J.E. (1989b) The importance of health monitoring of migrating raptors. In: *Raptors in the Modern World* (eds B.-U. Meyburg & R.D. Chancellor). World Working Group on Birds of Prey, Berlin, London and Paris.

Cooper, J.E. (1990) Birds and zoonoses. *Ibis*, **132**, 181–191.

Cooper, J.E. (1993a) The need for closer collaboration between biologists and veterinarians in research on raptors. In: *Raptor Biomedicine* (eds P.T. Redig, J.E. Cooper, J.D. Remple & D.B. Hunter). University of Minnesota Press, USA.

Cooper, J.E. (1993b) Pathological studies on the barn owl. In: *Raptor Biomedicine* (eds P.T. Redig, J.E. Cooper, J.D. Remple & D.B. Hunter). University of Minnesota Press, USA.

Cooper, J.E. (1993c) Pathological studies on eggs and embryos. In: *Raptor Biomedicine* (eds P.T. Redig, J.E. Cooper, J.D. Remple & D.B. Hunter). University of Minnesota Press, USA.

Cooper, J.E. (1993d) Historical survey of disease in birds. *Journal of Zoo and Wildlife Medicine*, **24**(3), 256–264.

Cooper, J.E. (1993e) Infectious and parasitic diseases of raptors. In: *Zoo and Wild Animal Medicine. Current Therapy 3* (ed. M.E. Fowler). W.B. Saunders, PA, USA.

Cooper, J.E. (1994) Biopsy techniques. *Seminars in Avian and Exotic Pet Medicine*, **3**(3), 161–165.

Cooper, J.E. (1995) Permit problems. *New Scientist*, (**149**); 53.

Cooper, J.E. (1996a) Introduction. In: *Manual of Raptors, Pigeons and Waterfowl* (eds P.H. Beynon, N.A. Forbes & N.H. Harcourt-Brown). British Small Animal Veterinary Association, Cheltenham, UK.

Cooper, J.E. (1996b) Physical injury. In: *Non Infectious Diseases of Wildlife* (eds A. Fairbrother, L.N. Locke & G.L. Hoff). Iowa State University Press, USA.

Cooper, J.E. (1996c) Fits, incoordination and coma. In: *Manual of Raptors, Pigeons and Waterfowl* (eds P.H. Beynon, N.A. Forbes & N. Harcourt-Brown). BSAVA, Cheltenham, UK.

Cooper, J.E. (1996d) A preen gland abnormality in a free-living white-headed vulture (*Aegypius occipitalis*). *Journal of Raptor Research*, **30**(1), 45.

Cooper, J.E. (1998) Minimally invasive health monitoring of wildlife. *Animal Welfare*, 7, 35–44.

Cooper, J.E. & Al-Timimi, F. (1986) A simple restraining device for birds. *Avian/Exotic Practice*, **3**, 5–7.

Cooper, J.E. & Anwar, A. (2001) Blood parasites of birds: a plea for more cautious terminology. *Ibis*, **143**, 149–150.

Cooper, J.E. & Cooper, M.E. (1998) Forensic veterinary medicine. *Seminars in Avian and Exotic Pet Medicine*, 7(4).

Cooper, J.E. & Eley, J.T. (eds) (1979) *First Aid and Care of Wild Birds*. David & Charles, Newton Abbot, UK.

Cooper, J.E. & Forbes, N. (1983) A fatty liver–kidney syndrome of merlins. *Veterinary Record*, **112**, 182–183.

Cooper, J.E. & Forbes, N.A. (1986) Studies on morbidity and mortality in the merlin (*Falco columbarius*). *Veterinary Record*, **118**, 232–235.

Cooper, J.E. & Frank, L. (1973) Use of the steroid anaesthetic CT 1341 in birds. *Veterinary Record*, **92**, 474–479.

Cooper, J.E. & Gibson, L.W. (1983) Injuries associated with rings. *Veterinary Record*, **113**, 224.

Cooper, J.E. & Greenwood, A.G. (1981a) *Recent Advances in the Study of Raptor Diseases*. Chiron Publications, Keighley, Yorkshire, UK.

Cooper, J.E. & Greenwood, A.G. (1981b) Conclusions. In: *Recent Advances in the Study of Raptor Diseases* (eds J.E. Cooper & A.G. Greenwood). Chiron Publications, Keighley, Yorkshire, UK.

Cooper, J.E. & Houston, D.C. (1972) Lesions in the crop of vultures associated with bot fly larvae. *Transactions of the Royal Society of Tropical Medicine and Hygiene*, **66**, 515–516.

Cooper, J.E. & Jones, C.G. (1986) A Reference Collection of Endangered Mascarene Specimens. *The Linnean*, **2**(3), 32–37.

Cooper, J.E. & Kreel, L. (1976) Radiological examination of birds: report of a small series. *Journal of Small Animal Practice*, **17**, 799–808.

Cooper, J.E. & Mbassa, G.K. (1994) Domestic fowl as a possible source of pathogens for wild birds in Africa. *Veterinary Record*, **134**, 532.

Cooper, J.E. & Mellau, L.S.B. (1992) Sticktight fleas (*Echidnophaga gallinacea*) on birds. *Veterinary Record*, **130**, 108.

Cooper, J.E. & Needham, J.R. (1976) An investigation into the prevalence of *S. aureus* on avian feet. *Veterinary Record*, **98**, 172–174.

Cooper, J.E. & Needham, J.R. (1981) The starling (*Sturnus vulgaris*) as an experimental model for staphylococcal infection of the avian foot. *Avian Pathology*, **10**, 273–279.

Cooper, J.E. & Petty, S.J. (1988) Trichomoniasis in free-living goshawks (*Accipiter gentilis gentilis*) from Great Britain. *Journal of Wildlife Diseases*, **24**(1), 80–87.

Cooper, J.E. & Pomerance, A. (1982) Cardiac lesions in birds of prey. *Journal of Comparative Pathology*, **92**, 161–168.

Cooper, J.E. & Pugsley, S.L. (1984) A mesothelioma in a ferruginous hawk (*Buteo regalis*). *Avian Pathology*, **13**, 797–801.

Cooper, J.E. & Redig, P.T. (1975) Unexpected reactions to the use of CT 1341 by red-tailed hawks. *Veterinary Record*, **97**, 352.

Cooper, J.E. & Samour, J.H. (1997) Portable and field equipment for avian veterinary work. *Proceedings of the European Committee of the Association of Avian Veterinarians*, London, 19–24 May 1997.

Cooper, J.E. & West, C.D. (1988) Radiological studies on endangered Mascarene fauna. *Oryx*, **22**, 18–24.

Cooper, J.E., Dranzoa, C. & Cooper, M.E. (2001) Vultures in decline? Methods of study and investigation. *Proceedings of a workshop at Makerere University, Uganda*.

Cooper, J.E., Dutton, C.J. & Allchurch, A.K. (1998) Reference collections: their importance and relevance to modern zoo management and conservation biology. *Dodo, Journal of the Wildlife Preservation Trusts*, **34**, 159–166.

Cooper, J.E., Gibson, L. & Jones, C.G. (1980a) The assessment of health in casualty birds of prey intended for release. *Veterinary Record*, **10**, 340–341.

Cooper, J.E., Gorney-Labinger, E. & Ion, F. (1993a) Parasitological and other studies on migrating raptors. In: *Raptor Biomedicine* (eds P.T. Redig, J.E. Cooper, J.D. Remple & D.B. Hunter). University of Minnesota Press, USA.

Cooper, J.E., Gschmeissner, S. & Ion, F. (1989) The laboratory investigation of feathers. *Proceedings of 2nd European Symposium on Avian Medicine and Surgery*, Utrecht, The Netherlands. (Dutch translation in *DierenArt Vetenschappeligke Praktigkgenekte Informatie*, **4**, 102–110.)

Cooper, J.E., Jones, C.G. & Owadally, A.W. (1981) Morbidity and mortality in the Mauritius kestrel (*Falco punctatus*). In: *Recent Advances in the Study of Raptor Diseases* (eds J.E. Cooper & A.G. Greenwood). Chiron Publications, Keighley, Yorkshire, UK.

Cooper, J.E., Needham, J.R. & Fox, N.C. (1986) Bacteriological haematological and clinical chemical studies on the Mauritius kestrel (*Falco punctatus*). *Avian Pathology*, **15**, 349–356.

Cooper, J.E., Redig, P.T. & Burnham, W. (1980b) Bacterial isolates from the pharynx and cloaca of the peregrine falcon (*Falco peregrinus*) and gyrfalcon (*F. rusticolus*). *Raptor Research*, **14**, 6–9.

Cooper, J.E., Watson, J. & Payne, L.N. (1978) A mixed cell tumour in a Seychelles kestrel (*Falco araea*). *Avian Pathology*, **7**, 651–658.

Cooper, J.E., Wilkens, W. & Lawrence, K. (1993b) Four cases of neoplasia in birds of prey. In: *Raptor Biomedicine* (eds P.T. Redig, J.E. Cooper, J.D.

Remple & D.B. Hunter). University of Minnesota Press, USA.

Cooper, M.E. (1987) *An Introduction to Animal Law.* Academic Press, London and New York.

Cooper, M.E. (1989) Legal considerations in the movement and submission of avian samples. In: *Disease and Threatened Birds* (ed. J.E. Cooper). International Council for Bird Preservation, Cambridge, UK.

Cooper, M.E. (1993) Legal implications for the management of infectious disease in captive breeding and re-introduction programs. *Journal of Zoo and Wildlife Medicine*, **24**(3), 296–303.

Cooper, M.E. (2000a) Legal considerations in the international movement of diagnostic and research samples from raptors – conference resolution. In: *Raptor Biomedicine III* (eds J.T. Lumeij, J.D. Remple, P.T. Redig, M. Lierz & J.E. Cooper). Zoological Education Network, Lake Worth, FL, USA.

Cooper, M.E. (2000b) Ethical considerations in wildlife health. In: *Wildlife Health in Conservation.* Department of Conservation. Publication No. 204 Veterinary Continuing Education, Massey University, New Zealand.

Cooper, R.A., Molan, P.C. & Harding, K.G. (1999) Antibacterial activity of honey against strains of *Staphylococcus aureus* from infected wounds. *Journal of the Royal Society of Medicine*, **92**, 283–285.

Couch, J.R. & Ferguson, T.M. (1975) Nutrition and embryonic development in the domestic fowl. *Proceedings of the Nutrition Society*, **34**, 1–3.

Courtenay, W.R. & Robins, C.R. (1975) Exotic organisms: an unsolved, complex problem. *BioScience*, **25**(6), 306–313.

Courts, S.E. (1995) *Dietary Manual. Descriptions of the Feeding Regimes Currently in Use.* The Jersey Wildlife Preservation Trust, Jersey, British Isles.

Cowan, M.L., Clark, S.K., Grundy, H.C. & Chisholm, E.M. (2000) Surgical management of *Mycobacterium avium* intracellulare infection in children. *Journal of the Royal Society of Medicine*, **93**, 536–537.

Cowan, S.T. & Steel, K.J. (1975) *Manual for the Identification of Medical Bacteria.* Cambridge University Press, Cambridge, UK.

Cox, H. & Lascelles, G. (1892) *Coursing and Falconry.* The Badminton Library, Longmans, Green & Co., London.

Craig, T.H. & Powers, L.R. (1976) Raptor mortality due to drowning in a livestock watering tank. *Condor*, **78**, 412.

Crawley, M.J. (1992) *Natural Enemies. The Population Biology of Predators, Parasites and Diseases.* Blackwell Scientific Publications, London, UK.

Crawley, R.R., Ernst, J.V. & Milton, J.L. (1982) *Sarcocystis* in a bald eagle (*Haliaeetus leucocephalus*). *Journal of Wildlife Diseases*, **18**, 253–255.

Cribb, P.H. & Haigh, J.C. (1977) Anaesthetic for avian species. *Veterinary Record*, **100**, 472–473.

Crisp, E. (1854) Filaria in the heart of a peregrine falcon (*F. peregrinus*). *Transactions of the Pathological Society of London*, **5**, 345.

Crissey, S.D., Silfka, M.S. & Lintzenich, B.A. (1999) Whole body cholesterol, fat, and fatty acid concentrations of mice (*Mus domesticus*) used as a food source. *Journal of Zoo and Wildlife Medicine*, **30**(2), 222–227.

Crocoll, S. & Parker, J.W. (1981) *Protocalliphora* infestation in broad-winged hawks. *Wilson Bulletin*, **93**, 110.

Cromie, R.L. & Nicholls, M.K. (1995) *The welfare and conservation aspects of keeping birds of prey in captivity.* Report to the RSPCA, Horsham, W. Sussex, UK.

Croxall, J.P. (1979) In: *First Aid and Care of Wild Birds* (eds J.E. Cooper & J.T. Eley). David & Charles, Newton Abbot, UK.

Csermely, D. (2000) Rehabilitation of birds of prey and their survival after release. A review. In: *Raptor Biomedicine III* (eds J.T. Lumeij, J.D. Remple, P.T. Redig, M. Lierz & J.E. Cooper). Zoological Education Network, Lake Worth, FL, USA.

Cummings, J.H., Duke, G.E. & Jegers, A.A. (1976) Corrosion of bone by solutions simulating raptor gastric juice. *Raptor Research*, **10**, 55–57.

Cunningham, A. (2000) Vulture die off – India. *Newsletter of the European Association of Zoo and Wildlife Veterinarians*, **2**, 15.

Czekala, N.M. & Lasley, B.L. (1977) A technical note on sex determination in monomorphic birds using faecal steroid analysis. *International Zoo Yearbook*, **17**, 209–211.

Daghir, N.J. (1975) Studies on poultry by-product meals in broiler and layer rations. *World's Poultry Science Journal*, **31**, 200–211.

Dahlhausen, B., Lindstrom, J.G. & Radabaugh, C.S. (2000) The use of terbinafine hydrochloride in the treatment of avian fungal disease. *Proceedings of the Association of Avian Veterinarians*, 35–39.

Danielsson, B. (1977) *Cynegetic Anglica I. William Twiti: The Art of Hunting 1327.* Almquist and Wiksell International, Stockholm, Sweden.

Daoust, P-Y., Wadowska, D., Kibenge, F., Campagnoli, R.P., Latimer, K.S. & Ritchie, B.W. (2000) Proliferative pododermatitis associated with virus-like particles in a Northern gannet. *Journal of Wildlife Diseases*, **36**(2), 378–382.

Daszak, P., Cunningham, A.A. & Hyatt, A.D. (2000)

Emerging infectious diseases of wildlife – threats to bio-diversity and human health. *Science*, **287**, 443–449.

Davidson, M. (1997) Ocular consequences of trauma in raptors. *Seminars in Avian and Exotic Pet Medicine*, **6**, 121–130.

Davies, R.A.G. & Randall, R.M. (1989) Historical and geographical patterns in eggshell thickness of African fish eagles *Haliaeetus vocifer*, in relation to pesticide use within southern Africa. In: *Raptors in the Modern World* (eds B.U. Meyburg & R.D. Chancellor). World Working Group on Birds of Prey, Berlin, Germany.

Davis, T.A.W. (1975) Food of the kestrel in winter and early spring. *Bird Study*, **22**, 85–91.

Dawson, R.D. & Bartolotti, G.R. (1997) Are avian hematocrits indicative of condition? American kestrels as a model. *Journal of Wildlife Management*, **61**, 1297–1306.

Dawson, R.D. & Bartolotti, G.R. (2000) Reproductive success of American kestrels: the role of prey abundance and weather. *The Condor*, **102**(4), 814–822.

Dedrick, M.L. (1965) Notes on a strigeid trematode – an intestinal parasite of a prairie falcon. *Journal of the North American Falconers' Association*, **4**, 12–14.

Degernes, L.A. & Redig, P.T. (1993) Soft-tissue wound management in avian patients. In: *Raptor Biomedicine* (eds P.T. Redig, J.E. Cooper, J.D. Remple & D.B. Hunter). University of Minnesota Press, MN, USA.

Dein, F.J., Carpenter, J.W., Clark, C.G., Montali, R.J., Crabbs, C.L., Tsai, T.F. & Docherty, D.E. (1986) Mortality of captive whooping cranes caused by eastern equine encephalitis virus. *Journal of the American Veterinary Medical Association*, **189**, 1006–1010.

Delannoy, C.A. & Cruz, A. (1991) *Philornis* parasitism and nestling survival of the Puerto Rican sharp-shinned Hawk. In: *Bird–Parasite Interactions* (eds J.E. Loye & M. Zuk). Oxford University Press, UK.

Delany, M.E., Tell, L.A., Millam, J.R. & Preisler, D.M. (1999) Photographic candling analysis of the embryonic development of orange-winged Amazon parrots (*Amazona amazonica*). *Journal of Avian Medicine and Surgery*, **13**, 116–123.

Delogu, M. (1993) Il ripristino strutturale dell'omero negli uccelli mediante R.G.T. e tecniche di fissazione esterna ed interna associate. *Atti della Società Italiana delle Scienze Veterinarie*, **XLVII**, 2349–2353.

Delogu, M. & Zucca, P. (1999) *Serratospiculum amaculata*: indagine epidemiologica in uccelli rapaci e prima segnalazione in Italia. In: *Atti del XXXVII Convegno della Società Italiana di Patologia Aviare, La Selezione Veterinaria*, 8–9: 687–691.

Desai, J.H. & Malhotra, A.K. (1980) Embryonic

development of pariah kite *Milvus migrans govinda*. *Journal of the Yamishina Institute of Ornithology*, **12**, 82–86.

DETR (1996) *Wildlife Crime: A Guide to Wildlife Law Enforcement in the UK*. The Stationery Office, London, UK.

DETR (1997) *Wildlife Inspectors' Seminar Report*. Department of the Environment, Transport and the Regions, Bristol, UK.

DETR (1998) *A Guide to the European Wildlife Trade Regulations*. Department of the Environment, Transport and the Regions, Bristol, UK.

DETR (2000a) *Secretary of State's Standards of Modern Zoo Practice*. Department of the Environment, Transport and the Regions, Bristol, UK.

DETR (2000b) *Birds of Prey and EC Regulations* (Leaflet). Department of the Environment, Transport and the Regions, Bristol, UK.

Devriese, L.A. & Devos, A.H. (1975) Suppressive effects of antibiotics on experimentally inoculated *Staphylococcus aureus* populations on the skin of poultry. *Avian Pathology*, **4**, 295–302.

Dierenfeld, E.S., Sandfort, C.E. & Satterfield, W.C. (1989) Influence of diet on plasma vitamin E in captive peregrine falcons. *Journal of Wildlife Management*, **53**, 160–164.

Dieter, M.P. (1973) *Sex Determination of Eagles, Owls and Herons by Analysing Plasma Steroid Hormones*. Special Scientific Report, No. 167. US Fish and Wildlife Service, Washington DC, USA.

Disbrey, B.D. & Rack, J.H. (1970) *Histological Laboratory Methods*. Livingstone, Edinburgh, UK.

Divers, S.J. & Cooper, J.E. (2000) Reptile hepatic lipidosis. *Seminars in Avian and Exotic Pet Medicine*, **9**(3), 153–164.

van Dobben, W.H. (1952) The food of the cormorants in the Netherlands. *Ardea*, **40**, 1–63.

Dobson, A.P. & Hudson, P.J. (1986) Parasites, disease and the structure of ecological communities. *TREE*, **1**(1), 11–14.

Dobson, A.P. & May, R.M. (1991) Parasites, cuckoos and avian population dynamics. In: *Bird Population Studies* (eds C.M. Perrins, J.-D. Lebreton & G.J.M. Hirons). Oxford University Press, UK.

Dolan, K. (2000) *Laboratory Animal Law*. Blackwell Science, Oxford, UK.

Dorrestein, G.M. (1996) Principles of therapy. In: *Manual of Raptors, Pigeons and Waterfowl* (eds P.H. Beynon, N.A. Forbes & N.H. Harcourt-Brown). BSAVA, Cheltenham, UK.

Dorrestein, G.M. (2000) Nursing the sick bird. In: *Avian*

Medicine (eds T.N. Tully, M.P.C. Lawton & G.M. Dorrestein). Butterworth-Heinemann, Oxford, UK.

Döttlinger (1995) Influence of diet on haematological parameters in captive peregrine falcons (*Falco peregrinus*). Cited by Heidenreich (1997).

Douthwaite, R.J. (1992) Effects of DDT on the Fish Eagle *Haliaeetus vocifer* population of Lake Kariba in Zimbabwe. *Ibis*, **134**, 250–258.

Drent, R. (1970) Adaptive aspects of the physiology of incubation. *Proceedings of the XV International Ornithological Congress*, 258–280.

Dresser, P.J., Wimsatt, J. & Burkhard, M.J. (1999) Effects of isoflurane anesthesia on hematological and plasma biochemical values of American kestrels (*Falco sparverius*). *Journal of Avian Medicine and Surgery*, **13**(3), 173–179.

Dubey, J.P., Porter, S.L., Hattel, A.L., *et al.* (1991) *Sarcocystis*-associated clinical encephalitis in a golden eagle (*Aquila chrysaetos*). *Journal of Zoo and Wildlife Medicine*, **22**, 233–236.

Dubey, J.P., Porter, S.I., Tseng, F., Shen, S.K. & Thulliez, P. (1992) Induced toxoplasmosis in owls. *Journal of Zoo and Wildlife Medicine*, **23**, 98–102.

Du Bose, R.T. (1972) Rabies. In: *Diseases of Poultry* (eds M.S. Hofstad *et al.*), 6th edn. Iowa State University Press, USA.

Duckett, J.E. (1984) Barn owls (*Tyto alba)* and the 'second generation' rat-baits utilised in oil palm plantations in Peninsular Malaysia. *Planter, Kuala Lumpur*, **60**, 3–11.

Duke, G.E. (1987) Gastrointestinal physiology and nutrition. In: *Raptor Management Techniques Manual* (eds G.B.A. Pendleton, B.A. Millsap, K.W. Cline & D.M. Bird). Institute for Wildlife Research, National Wildlife Federation, Scientific and Technical Series No. 10, Washington DC, USA.

Duke, G.E., Ciganek, J.G. & Evanson, O.A. (1973) Food consumption and energy, water and nitrogen budgets in captive great-horned owls (*Bubo virginianus*). *Comparative Biochemistry and Physiology*, **44A**, 283–292.

Duke, G.E., Jegers, A.A., Loff, G. & Evanson, O.A. (1975) Gastric digestion in some raptors. *Comparative Biochemistry and Physiology*, **50A**, 649–656.

Dukes, T.W. & Fox, G.A. (1983) Blindness associated with retinal dysplasia in a prairie falcon, *Falcon mexicanus*. *Journal of Wildlife Diseases*, **19**, 66–69.

Duncan, J.S., Reid, H.W., Moss, R., Philips, J.D.P. & Watson, A. (1979) Ticks, louping ill and red grouse on moors in Speyside, Scotland. *Journal of Wildlife Management*, **42**, 500–505.

Durant, A.J. (1953) Removing the vocal cords of fowl.

Journal of the American Veterinary Medical Association, **122**, 14–17.

Dutton, C.J., Cooper, J.E. & Allchurch, A.F. (2000) The pathology and diseases of the Mauritius kestrel (*Falco punctatus*). In: *Raptor Biomedicine III* (eds J.T. Lumeij, J.D. Remple, P.T. Redig, M. Lierz & J.E. Cooper). Zoological Education Network, Lake Worth, FL, USA.

Duxbury, J.M. (1998) *An Application of Stable Isotope Ecology to the Study of Raptor Diets*. MS Thesis, University of Alberta, Canada.

Dykstra, M.J., Loomis, M., Reininger, K., Zombeck, D. & Faucette, T. (1997) A comparison of sampling methods for airborne fungal spores during an outbreak of aspergillosis in the forest aviary of the North Carolina Zoological Park. *Journal of Zoo and Wildlife Medicine*, **28**(4), 454–463.

Eastham, C.P., Nicholls, M.K. & Fox, N.C. (2001) *Postmortem* shrinkage in large falcons. *Falco*, **17**, 9–11.

Ebedes, H. (1973) The capture of free-living vultures in the Etosha National Park with phencyclidine. *Journal of the South African Wildlife Management Association*, **3**, 105–107.

Ebenhard, T. (1986) Introduced birds and mammals and their ecological effects. *Swedish Wildlife Research*, **13**(4), 5.

EC/TE/WWF (1998) *Reference Guide to European Community Wildlife Trade Regulation*. European Commission/TRAFFIC Europe/World Wildlife Fund, Brussels, Belgium.

Elliott, J.E., Norstrom, R.J. & Smith, G.E.J. (1996) Patterns, trends and toxicological significance of chlorinated hydrocarbons and mercury contamination in bald eagle eggs from the Pacific coast of Canada, 1990–1994. *Archives of Environmental Contamination and Toxicology*, **31**, 354–367.

Elliott, R.H., Smith, E. & Bush, M. (1974) Preliminary report on hematology of birds of prey. *Journal of Zoo Animal Medicine*, **5**, 11–16.

Ellis, D.H. & Lish, J.W. (1999) Trash-caused mortality in Mongolian raptors. *Ambio*, **28**(6), 536–537.

Ellis, K.L. (1986) Bilateral bumblefoot in a wild red-tailed hawk. *Journal of Raptor Research*, **20**, 132.

Enderson, J.H. & Berthrong, M. (1980) Pseudomembranous gastritis compatible with *Clostridium* sp. in a captive peregrine falcon. *Raptor Research*, **18**, 72–74.

Ensley, P.K. (1999) Medical management of the California condor. In: *Zoo and Wild Animal Medicine Current Therapy 4* (eds M.E. Fowler & R.E. Miller). W.B. Saunders, PA, USA.

Erdélyi, K., Tenk, M. & Dán, Á. (1999) Mycoplasmosis

associated perosis type skeletal deformity in a saker falcon nestling in Hungary. *Journal of Wildlife Diseases*, **35**(3), 586–590.

Evans, H. ap (1960) *Falconry for You*. John Gifford Ltd, London, UK.

Evans, I.M., Dennis, R.H., Orr-Ewing, D.C., *et al.* (1997) The re-establishment of red kite breeding populations in Scotland and England. *British Birds*, **90**, 123–138.

Evans, L.B. & Piper, S. (1981) Bone abnormalities in the Cape vulture (*Gyps coprotheres*). *Journal of the South African Veterinary Association*, **52**, 67–68.

Evelyn, J. (1664) *The Diary of John Evelyn*. London, England.

von Faber, H. (1964) Stress and general adaptation syndrome in poultry. *World's Poultry Science Journal*, **20**, 175–182.

Fain, A. & Smiley, R.L. (1989) A new cloacarid mite (Acari, Cloacaridae) from the lungs of the great-horned owl (*Bubo virginianus*) from the USA. *International Journal of Acarology*, **15**(2), 111–116.

Farner, D.S., King, J.R. & Parkes, K.C. (1971–1985) *Avian Biology, 8*, **4**, 119–257. Academic Press, New York, USA.

Feare, C.J. (1976) Desertion and abnormal development in a colony of Sooty Terns *Sterna fuscata* infested by virus-infected ticks. *Ibis*, **118**, 112–115.

Fernie, K.J. (1998) *Effects of electric and magnetic fields on selected physiological and reproductive parameters of American kestrels*. PhD dissertation, McGill University, Montreal, Quebec, Canada.

Ferreira, D.F. (1616) *Arte da Caça de Altaneria*. Lisbon.

Ferrer, M., Garcier-Rodriguez, T., Carrillo, J.C. & Castroviejo, J. (1987) Haematocrit and blood chemistry values in captive raptors (*Gyps fulva, Buteo buteo, Milvus migrans, Aquila heliaca*). *Comparative Biochemistry and Physiology* A, **87**, 1123–1127.

Figuer, L. (1873) *La vita e i costumi degli animali – Gli uccelli*. Fratelli Treves, Milan, Italy.

Fimreite, N. & Karstad, L. (1971) Effects of dietary methyl mercury on red-tailed hawks. *Journal of Wildlife Management*, **35**, 293–300.

Fimreite, N., Fyfe, R.W. & Keith, J.A. (1970) Mercury contamination of Canadian prairie seed eaters and their avian predators. *Canadian Field-Naturalist*, **84**, 269–276.

Finlayson, R. (1964) Vascular disease in captive animals. *Symposium of the Zoological Society of London*, **11**, 99–106.

Fisher, H. (1972) The nutrition of birds. In: *Avian Biology*, Vol. II (eds D.S. Farner, J.R. King & K.C. Parkes). Academic Press, New York and London.

Fisher, S. (1957) Loss of immunizing power of staphylococcal toxin during routine toxoiding with formalin. *Nature*, **180**, 1479–1480.

Fitch, H.S., Swenson, F. & Tillotson, D.F. (1946) Behavior and food habits of the Red-tailed Hawk. *Condor*, **48**, 205–237.

Fitzgerald, G. & Blais, D. (1993) Inhalation anesthesia in birds of prey. In: *Raptor Biomedicine* (eds P.T. Redig, J.E. Cooper, J.D. Remple & D.B. Hunter). University of Minnesota Press, USA.

Fitzgerald, G. & Cooper, J.E. (1990) Preliminary studies on the use of propofol in the domestic pigeon (*Columba livia*). *Research in Veterinary Science*, **49**, 334–338.

Flecknell, P.A. & Waterman-Pearson, A. (2000) *Pain Management in Animals*. W.B. Saunders, London and Edinburgh.

Flegg, J.J.M., Glue, D.E. & Mead, C.J. (1974) Sexing birds of prey. *Veterinary Record*, **94**, 625.

Fleischer, R.C., Olson, S.L., James, H.F. & Cooper, A.C. (2000) Identification of the extinct Hawaiian eagle (*Haliaeetus*) by mt DNA sequence analysis. *The Auk*, **117**, 1051–1054.

Forbes, N.A. (1993) Pathogenicity of ticks on aviary birds. *Veterinary Record*, **133**, 532.

Forbes, N.A. (1996a) Respiratory problems. In: *Manual of Raptors, Pigeons and Waterfowl* (eds P.H. Beynon, N.A. Forbes & N.H. Harcourt-Brown). British Small Animal Veterinary Association, Cheltenham, UK.

Forbes, N.A. (1996b) Chronic weight loss, vomiting and dysphagia. In: *Manual of Raptors, Pigeons and Waterfowl* (eds P.H. Beynon, N.A. Forbes & N.H. Harcourt-Brown). British Small Animal Veterinary Association, Cheltenham, UK.

Forbes, N.A. (1997a) Disease risks with translocation of raptors into, out of and within Europe. *Journal of The British Veterinary Zoological Society*, **2**, 42–50.

Forbes, N.A. (1997b) Adenovirus infection in Mauritius kestrels (*Falco punctatus*). *Journal of Avian Medicine and Surgery*, **11**, 31–33.

Forbes, N.A. (2000) Raptor medicine. *Seminars in Avian and Exotic Pet Medicine*, **9**, 197–203.

Forbes, N.A. & Cooper, J.E. (1993) Fatty liver–kidney syndrome of merlins. In: *Raptor Biomedicine* (eds P.T. Redig, J.E. Cooper, J.D. Remple & D.B. Hunter). University of Minnesota Press, USA.

Forbes, N.A. & Flint, C.G. (2000) *Raptor Nutrition*. Campaign for Falconry, UK.

Forbes, N.A. & Fox, M.T. (2000) Control of endemic *Caryospora* species infestation of captive raptors. *Proceedings of the Association of Avian Veterinarians*, 173–179.

Forbes, N.A. & Harcourt-Brown, N.H. (1996) Miscellaneous. In: *Manual of Raptors, Pigeons and Waterfowl* (eds P.H. Beynon, N.A. Forbes & N.H. Harcourt-Brown). British Small Animal Veterinary Association, Cheltenham, UK.

Forbes, N.A. & Rees Davies, R. (2000) Practical raptor nutrition. *Proceedings of the Association of Avian Veterinarians*, 165–167.

Forbes, N.A. & Simpson, G.N. (1993) Pathogenicity of ticks on aviary birds. *Veterinary Record*, **133**(21), 532.

Forbes, N.A. & Simpson, G.N. (1997a) A review of viruses affecting raptors. *Veterinary Record*, **141**, 1320126.

Forbes, N.A. & Simpson, G.N. (1997b) *Caryospora neofalconis*: an emerging threat to captive-bred raptors in the United Kingdom. *Journal of Avian Medicine and Surgery*, **11**(2), 110–114.

Forbes, N.A., Cooper, J.E. & Higgins, R.J. (2000a) Neoplasms of birds of prey. In: *Raptor Biomedicine III* (eds J.T. Lumeij, J.D. Remple, P.T. Redig, M. Lierz & J.E. Cooper). Zoological Education Network, Lake Worth, FL, USA.

Forbes, N.A., Higston, S. & Zsivanovits, P. (2000b) Falcon herpesvirus in the UK. *Veterinary Record*, **147**, 492.

Forbes, N.A., Simpson, G.N. & Goudswaard, M.F. (1992) Diagnosis of avian aspergillosis and treatment with itraconazole. *Veterinary Record*, **130**, 519–520.

Forrester, D.J., Telford, S.R.J., Foster, G.W. & Bennett, G.F. (1994) Blood parasites of raptors in Florida. *Journal of Raptor Research*, **28**, 226–231.

Fowler, M.E. (1978) *Zoo and Wild Animal Medicine*. W.B. Saunders, PA, USA.

Fowler, M.E. (1986) Metabolic bone disease. In: *Zoo and Wild Animal Medicine* (ed. M.E. Fowler), 2nd edn. W.B. Saunders, PA, USA.

Fowler, N.G. & Hussaini, S.N. (1975) *Clostridium septicum* infection and antibiotic treatment in broiler chickens, *Veterinary Record*, **96**, 14–15.

Fox, H. (1920) Arterial sclerosis in wild animals. *American Journal of the Medical Sciences*, **49**, 821–825.

Fox, H. (1923) *Disease in Captive Wild Mammals and Birds*. J B Lippincott Co., Philadelphia and London, UK.

Fox, N. (1976) Rangle. *Raptor Research*, **10**, 61–64.

Fox, N.C. (1977) Some morphological data on the Australasian harrier (*Circus approximans gouldi*) in New Zealand. *Notornis*, **24**, 9–19.

Frank, L.G. & Cooper, J.E. (1974a) A report on the use of a pectoral muscle biopsy in the field for organochlorine residue analysis. *Raptor Research*, **8**, 33–36.

Frank, L.G. & Cooper, J.E. (1974b) Further notes on the use of CT 1341 in birds of prey. *Raptor Research*, **8**, 29–32.

Frankenhuis, M.T. & Kappert, H.J. (1980) Infertility due to surgery on body cavity in female birds – cause and prevention. *Sonderdruck aus Verhandlungsbericht, des XXII Internationalen Symposiums über die Erkrankungen der Zootiere*. Akademie-Verlag, Germany.

Franson, J.C. (1994) Parathion poisoning of Mississippi kites in Oklahoma. *Journal of Raptor Research*, **28**, 108–109.

Franson, J.C. (1996) Interpretation of tissue lead residues in birds other than wildlife. In: *Environmental Contaminants in Wildlife: Interpreting Tissue Concentrations* (eds W.N. Beyer, G.H. Heinz & A.W. Redmon-Norwood), pp. 265–279. Lewis, Boca Raton, USA.

Franson, J.C. & Little, S.E. (1996) Diagnostic findings in 132 Great Horned Owls. *Journal of Raptor Research*, **30**, 1–6.

Franson, J.C., Thomas, N.J., Smith, M.R., Robbins, A.H., Newman, S. & McCartin, P.C. (1996) A retrospective study of postmortem findings in Red-Tailed Hawks. *Journal of Raptor Research*, **30**, 7–14.

Frasca, J.S., Schwartz, D.R., Moiseff, A. & French, R.A. (1999) Feather folliculoma in a captive-bred barn owl (*Tyto alba*). *Avian Diseases*, **43**, 616–621.

Frazer, J.F.D. (1977) Growth of young vertebrates in the egg or uterus. *Journal of Zoology, London*, **183**, 189–201.

Frederick II, Emperor (1247) *De Arte Venandi cum Avibus*. Hohenstaufen, Germany.

Freeland, W.J. (1976) Pathogens and the evolution of primate sociality. *Biotropica*, **8**, 12–24.

Freeman, B.M. (1976) Stress and the domestic fowl: a physiological re-appraisal. *World's Poultry Science Journal*, **32**, 249–256.

Freeman, B.M. & Manning, A.C.C. (1976) Failure of procaine penicillin and zinc bacitracin to modify the response of the fowl to stressors. *British Poultry Science*, **17**, 285–292.

Frey, H. & Kutzer, E. (1982) Zur Diagnostik heimischer Greifvogel- und Eulenparasiten. *Der Praktische Tierarzt*, **10**, 894–902.

Frey, H. & Zink, R. (2000) Aspects of management within the European bearded vulture (*Gypaetus barbatus*) reintroduction project (F25 832/78, WWF 1657/78). In: *Raptor Biomedicine III* (eds J.T. Lumeij, J.D. Remple, P.T. Redig, M. Lierz & J.E. Cooper). Zoological Education Network, Lake Worth, FL, USA.

Friedburg, K.M. (1962) Anesthesia of parakeets and canaries. *Journal of the American Veterinary Medical Association*, **141**, 1157–1160.

Friend, M. & Pearson, G.L. (1973) Duck plague: the present situation. In: *Western Proceedings, Annual Conference Western Association* (ed. State Game and Fish Commissioners). Washington DC, USA.

Friend, M. & Trainer, D.O. (1969) Polychlorinated biphenyls: interaction with duck hepatitis virus. *Science*, **170**, 1314–1316.

Fromont, E. (1993) *Hématologie et Parasits Sanguins des Rapaces*. Thèse, Ecole Nationale Veterinaire de Lyon, France.

Fry, D.M. (1983) Techniques for sexing monomorphic vultures. In: *Vulture Biology and Management* (eds S.R. Wilbur & J.A. Jackson). University of California Press, USA.

Frye, F.L., Cooper, J.E. & Keymer, I.F. (2001) Outfitting and employing a compact field laboratory. *ZooMed, The Bulletin of the BVZS*, **1(2)**, 28–36.

Fudge, A.M. (2000) *Laboratory Medicine. Avian and Exotic Pets*. W.B. Saunders, Philadelphia and London.

Fudge, A.M. (2001) Diagnosis and treatment of avian bacterial diseases. *Seminars in Avian and Exotic Pet Medicine*, **10**(1), 3–11.

Fuller, M.R. (1975) A technique for holding and handling raptors. *Journal of Wildlife Management*, **39**, 824–825.

Fuller, M.R., Redig, P.T. & Duke, G.E. (1974) Raptor rehabilitation and conservation in Minnesota. *Raptor Research*, **8**, 11–19.

Furley, C.W. & Greenwood, A.G. (1982) Treatment of aspergillosis in raptors (Order Falconiformes) with miconazole. *Veterinary Record*, **111**, 584–585.

Furmaga, S. (1957) The helminth fauna of predatory birds (Accipitres and Striges) of the environment of Lublin. *Acta Parasitologica Polonica*, **5**, 215–297.

Furr, P.M., Cooper, J.E. & Taylor-Robinson, D. (1977) Isolation of mycoplasmas from three falcons (*Falco* spp.). *Veterinary Record*, **100**, 72–73.

Gabrisch, K. & Zwart, P. (1987) *Krankheiten der Wildtiere*. Schlütersche, Hannover, Germany.

Garbe, J.L. (1989) Wildlife law. In: *Law and Ethics of the Veterinary Profession* (ed. J.F. Wilson). Priority Press, Yardly, PA, USA.

Garbe, J.L. (1993) Wildlife jurisprudence. In: *Legal Issues Affecting Veterinary Practice* (ed. J.D. McKean). *The Veterinary Clinics of North America*, **23**(5), 1061–1070.

Garcia-Rodriguez, T., Ferrer, M., Recio, F. & Castroviego, J. (1987) Circadian rhythms of determined blood chemistry values in buzzards and eagle owls. *Comparative Biochemistry and Physiology*, **88**, 663–669.

Garnham, P.C.C. (1966) *Malarial Parasites and Other Haemosporidia*. Blackwell, Oxford, UK.

Gascoyne, S.C., Bennett, P.M., Kirkwood, J.M. &

Hawkey, C.M. (1994) Guidelines for the interpretation of laboratory findings in birds and mammals with unknown reference ranges: plasma biochemistry. *Veterinary Record*, **134**, 7–11.

Gaskin, J.M. (1989) Psittacine viral diseases: a perspective. *Journal of Zoo and Wildlife Medicine*, **20**, 249–264.

Gatehouse, S.N. & Markham, B.J. (1970) Respiratory metabolism of three species of raptor. *The Auk*, **87**, 738–741.

Gee, G.F., Carpenter, J.W. & Hensler, G.L. (1981) Species differences in hematological values of captive cranes, geese, raptors and quail. *Journal of Wildlife Management*, **45**, 463–483.

Gensbøl, B. (1992) *Guida ai rapaci diurni – d'Europa, Nord Africa e Medio Oriente*. Zanichelli, Bologna, Italy.

Gentle, M.J. (1992) Pain in birds. *Animal Welfare*, **1**, 235–247.

Gentle, M.J. & Tiltson, V.L. (2000) Nociceptors in the legs of poultry: implications for potential pain in pre-slaughtered shackling. *Animal Welfare*, **9**, 227–236.

Gentz, E.J. (1996) *Fusobacterium necrophorum* associated with bumblefoot in a wild great-horned owl. *Journal of Avian Medicine and Surgery*, **10**, 258–261.

Gerbermann, H. & Korbel, R. (1992) Findings in free-living raptors infected with Chlamydia. *VIII DVG-Tagung über Vogelkrankheiten München*, 105–124.

Gerbermann, H., Jakoby, J.R. & Kösters, J. (1990) Incidence of Chlamydia in an aviary station of birds of prey. *Journal of Veterinary Medicine*, **37**, 739–748.

Gerdessen, A. (1956) *Beitrag zur Entwicklung der Falknerei un der Falkenheilkunde*. Inaugural Dissertation Tierärztliche Hochschule, Hannover, Germany.

Gerlach, C. (1979) Differentialblutbild und Plasmaenzymuntersuchungen bei Greifvögeln im Verlaufe eines Jahres (Mai 1977 bis Mai 1978). *Der Praktische Tierarzliche*, **60**, 673–674.

Gerlach, H. (1978) Grundlagen der Blutdiagnostik bei Greifvögeln. *Der Praktische Tierarzt*, **9**, 642–650.

Gervais, J.A., Rosenberg, D.K., Fry, D.M., Trulio, L. & Sturm, K.K. (2000) Burrowing owls and agricultural pesticides: evaluation of residues and risks for three populations in California, USA. *Environmental Toxicology and Chemistry*, **19**, 337–343.

Gibson, G.G., Broughton, E. & Choquette, L.P.E. (1972) Waterfowl mortality caused by *Cyathocotyle bushiensis* Khan, 1962 (Trematoda: Cyathocotylidae), St Lawrence River, Quebec. *Canadian Journal of Zoology*, **50**, 1351–1356.

Gill, F.B. (1990) *Ornithology*. W.H. Freeman, New York, USA.

Gipps, J.H.W. (1991) *Beyond Captive Breeding: Re-*

introducing Endangered Mammals to the Wild. Oxford Science Publications, Oxford, UK.

Glees, P. (1961) *Experimental Neurology.* Clarendon Press, Oxford, UK.

Goater, C.P. & Holmes, J.C. (1997) Parasite-mediated natural selection. In: *Host–Parasite Evolution* (eds D.H. Clayton & J. Moore), pp. 9–29. Oxford University Press, Oxford, UK.

Godfrey, R.D., Fedynich, A.M. & Pence, D.B. (1987) Quantification of hematozoa in blood smears. *Journal of Wildlife Diseases,* **23**(4), 558–565.

Goldstein, M.I., Lacher, T.E., Jr., Woodbridge, B., *et al.* (1999a) Monocrotophos-induced mass mortality of Swainson's hawks in Argentina, 1995–96. *Ecotoxicology,* **8**, 201–214.

Goldstein, M.I., Lacher, T.E., Jr., Zaccagnini, M.E., Parker, M.L. & Hooper, M.J. (1999b) Monitoring and assessment of Swainson's hawks in Argentina following restrictions on monocrotophos use, 1996–97. *Ecotoxicology,* **8**, 215–224.

Goldstein, M.I., Woodbridge, B., Zaccagnini, M.E., Canavelli, S.B. & Lanusse, A. (1996) An assessment of mortality of Swainson's hawks on wintering grounds in Argentina. *Journal of Raptor Research,* **30**, 106–107.

Gomez, M.P.I., Osorio, M.R. & Maza, F.A. (1993) Parasitation of falconiform, strigiform and passeriform (Corvidae) birds by helminths in Spain. *Research and Reviews in Parasitology,* **53**(3–4), 129–135.

Gough, P.M. & Jorgensen, R.D. (1976) Rabies antibodies in sera of wild birds. *Journal of Wildlife Diseases,* **12**, 392–395.

Gough, R.E., Capna, I. & Wenery, U. (2000) Herpesviruses infections in raptors. In: *Raptor Biomedicine III* (eds J.T. Lumeij, J.D. Remple, P.T. Redig, M. Lierz & J.E. Cooper). Zoological Education Network, Lake Worth, FL, USA.

Gould, S.J. (1983) *Hen's Teeth and Horse's Toes.* W.W. Norton & Company, New York and London.

Graham, D.L. (1970) Nutrition and nutritional diseases. In: *Raptor Pathology and Nutrition. Hawk Chalk,* **IX**, 30–37.

Graham, D.L., Maré, C.J., Ward, F.P. & Peckham, M.C. (1975) Inclusion body disease (Herpesvirus infection) of falcons (IBDF). *Journal of Wildlife Diseases,* **11**, 83–91.

Graham, J.E., Larocca, R.D. & McLaughlin, S.A. (1999) Implantation of an intraocular silicone prosthesis in a great horned owl (*Bubo virginianus*). *Journal of Avian Medicine and Surgery,* **13**(2), 98–103.

Green, C.J. (1979) *Animal Anaesthesia: A Handbook.* Laboratory Animal Science Association Handbook No. 8. London, UK.

Green, R.E. (2000) An evaluation of three indices of eggshell thickness. *Ibis,* **142**, 676–679.

Green, R.G. & Shillinger, J.E. (1935) A virus disease of owls. *Journal of Immunology,* **29**, 68–69.

Greenwood, A.G. (1973) Veterinary medicine of birds of prey. *Proceedings of the 1973 British Falconers Club Conference.* Oxford, UK.

Greenwood, A.G. (1974) Sexing birds of prey. *Veterinary Record,* **95**, 69.

Greenwood, A.G. (1977) The role of disease in the ecology of British raptors. *Bird Study,* **24**, 259–265.

Greenwood, A.G. (1996) Veterinary support for *in situ* avian conservation programmes. *Bird Conservation International,* **6**, 285–292.

Greenwood, A.G. & Barnett, K.C. (1981) The investigation of visual defects in raptors. In: *Recent Advances in the Study of Raptor Diseases* (eds J.E. Cooper & A.G. Greenwood). Chiron Publications, Keighley, Yorkshire, UK.

Greenwood, A.G. & Blakemore, W.F. (1973) Pox infection in falcons. *Veterinary Record,* **93**, 468.

Greenwood, A.G. & Cooper, J.E. (1982) Herpesvirus infections in falcons. *Veterinary Record,* **111**, 514.

Greenwood, A.G., Furley, C.W. & Cooper, J.E. (1984) Intestinal trematodiasis in falcons (Order Falconiformes). *Veterinary Record,* **114**(19), 477–478.

Gregory, R.D., Keymer, A.E. & Harvey, P.H. (1991) Life history, ecology and parasite community structure in Soviet birds. *Biological Journal of the Linnean Society,* **43**, 249–262.

Greiner, E.C. & Kocan, A.A. (1977) Leucocytozoon (Haemosporidia: Leucocytozoidae) of the Falconiformes. *Canadian Journal of Zoology,* **55**, 761–770.

Greiner, E.C. & Mundy, P.J. (1979) Hematozoa from southern African vultures, with a description of *Haemoproteus janovyi* sp. n. *Journal of Parasitology,* **65**(1), 147–153.

Grenquist, P. (1951) On the recent fluctuations in numbers of waterfowl in the Finnish archipelago. *Proceedings of the International Ornithological Congress,* **10**, 494–496.

Grenquist, P., Henriksson, K. & Raites, T. (1972) On intestinal occlusion in male Eider ducks. *Suom. Riista,* **24**, 91–96.

Griffiths, R., Daan, S. & Digkstra, C. (1996) Sex identification in birds using two CHD genes. *Proceedings of the Royal Society of London, Series B,* **263**, 1251–1256.

Grifols, J. (2000) Surgical repair of a mandibular fracture with a bone defect in a bearded vulture (*Gypaetus barbatus*) using a bone graft and an external fixator device. *Proceedings of the Association of Avian Veterinarians,* 133–136.

Grimm, R.J. & Whitehouse, W.M. (1963) Pellet formation in a great horned owl: a roentgenographic study. *The Auk*, **80**, 301–306.

Grinell, G.B. (1894) Lead poisoning. *Forest and Stream*, **42**, 117–118.

Grossman, M.L. & Hamlet, J. (1965) *Birds of Prey of the World*. Cassell and Company Ltd, London, UK.

Grossman, M.L. & Hamlet, J. (1988) *Birds of Prey of the World*. Bonanza Books, New York, USA.

Günther, B.M.F. (1995) *Versuche zur Differenzierung von Herpesvirusisolaten aus verschiedenen Vogelarten durch Restriktionsendonukleasen*. Inaugural dissertation, Justus Liebig Universität, Giessen, Germany.

Gyimesi, Z.S., Stalis, I.H., Miller, J.M. & Thoen, C.O. (1999) Detection of *Mycobacterium avium* subspecies *avium* in formalin-fixed, paraffin-embedded tissues of captive exotic birds using polymerase chain reaction. *Journal of Zoo and Wildlife Medicine*, **30**(3), 348–353.

Gylstorff, I. & Grimm, F. (1987) *Vogelkrankheiten*. Verlag Eugen Ulmer, Stuttgart, Germany.

Haas, D. (1993) Clinical signs and treatment of large birds injured by electrocution. In: *Raptor Biomedicine* (eds P.T. Redig, J.E. Cooper, J.D. Remple & D.B. Hunter). University of Minnesota Press, USA.

Haigh, J.C. (1981) Anaesthesia of raptorial birds. In: *Recent Advances in the Study of Raptor Diseases* (eds J.E. Cooper & A.G. Greenwood). Chiron Publications, Keighley, Yorkshire, UK.

Halliwell, W.H. (1967) Bumblefoot in raptorial birds. *Journal of the North American Falconers' Association*, **VI**, 49–53.

Halliwell, W.H. (1971) Lesions of Marek's disease in a great horned owl. *Avian Diseases*, **15**, 49–55.

Halliwell, W.H. (1972) Avian pox in an immature red-tailed hawk. *Journal of Wildlife Diseases*, **8**, 104–105.

Halliwell, W.H. (1979) Diseases of birds of prey. *Veterinary Clinics of North America*, **9**, 541–568.

Halliwell, W.H. (1981) Serum chemistry profiles in the health and disease of birds of prey. In: *Recent Advances in the Study of Raptor Diseases* (eds J.E. Cooper & A.G. Greenwood). Chiron Publications, Keighley, Yorkshire, UK.

Halliwell, W.H. & Graham, D.L. (1978a) Bacterial diseases of birds of prey. In: *Zoo and Wild Animal Medicine* (ed. M.E. Fowler). W.B. Saunders, Philadelphia, USA.

Halliwell, W.H. & Graham, D.L. (1978b) Neoplasms in birds of prey. In: *Zoo and Wild Animal Medicine* (ed. M.E. Fowler). W.B. Saunders, Philadelphia, USA.

Halliwell, W.H., Graham, D.L. & Ward, F.P. (1973)

Nutritional diseases in birds of prey. *Journal of Zoo Animal Medicine*, **4**, 18–20.

Halloran, P.O'C. (1955) *A Bibliography of References to Diseases in Wild Mammals and Birds*. American Veterinary Medical Association, USA.

Hamerstrom, F. & Skinner, J.L. (1971) Cloacal sexing of raptors. *The Auk*, **88**, 173–174.

Hamerton, A.E. (1935) Report on the deaths in the Society's Gardens during 1934. *Proceedings of the Zoological Society of London*, **105**, 443–474.

Hamerton, A.E. (1938) Report on the deaths in the Society's Gardens during 1937. *Proceedings of the Zoological Society of London*, **108**, 489–526.

Hamerton, A.E. (1939) Review of mortality rates and report on the deaths occurring in the Society's Gardens during the year 1938. *Proceedings of the Zoological Society of London*, **109**, 281–287.

Hamerton, A.E. (1941) Report on the deaths occurring in the Society's Gardens during the years 1939–1940. *Proceedings of the Zoological Society of London*, **111**, 151–187.

Hamerton, A.E. (1943) Report on the deaths occurring in the Society's Gardens during the years 1941–1942. *Proceedings of the Zoological Society of London*, **112**, 120–137.

Hamilton, W.D. & Zuk, M. (1982) Heritable true fitness and bright birds – a role for parasites. *Science*, **218**, 384–387.

Harcourt-Brown, N. (2000) *Birds of Prey. Anatomy, Radiology and Clinical Conditions of the Pelvic Limb*. CD ROM. Zoological Education Network, Lake Worth, FL, USA.

Harcourt-Brown, N.H. (2000) Tendon repair in the pelvic limb of birds of prey. Part I Anatomical considerations. Part II Surgical techniques. In: *Raptor Biomedicine III* (eds J.T. Lumeij, J.D. Remple, P.T. Redig, M. Lierz & J.E. Cooper). Zoological Education Network, Lake Worth, FL, USA.

Harcourt-Brown, N.H. (1996a) Radiology. In: *Manual of Raptors, Pigeons and Waterfowl* (eds P.H. Beynon, N.A. Forbes & N.H. Harcourt-Brown). British Small Animal Veterinary Association, Cheltenham, UK.

Harcourt-Brown, N.H. (1996b) Foot and leg problems. In: *Manual of Raptors, Pigeons and Waterfowl* (eds P.H. Beynon, N.A. Forbes & N.H. Harcourt-Brown). British Small Animal Veterinary Association, Cheltenham, UK.

Harcourt-Brown, N.H. (1996c) Radiology/foot and leg problems. In: *Manual of Raptors, Pigeons, and Waterfowl* (eds P.H. Beynon, N.A. Forbes & N.H. Harcourt-Brown), 1st edn. British Small Animal Veterinary Association, Cheltenham, UK.

Hare, T. (1939) Notes on two diseases of hawks; capillariasis and coccidiosis. *The Falconer*, **V**, 4–7.

Harmon, W.M., Clark, W.A., Hawbecker, A.C. & Stafford, M. (1987) *Trichomonas gallinae* in columbiform birds from the Galapagos Islands. *Journal of Wildlife Diseases*, **23**, 492–494.

Harrenstien, L.A., Tell, L.A., Vulliet, R., Needham, M., Brandt, C., Brondos, A. & Stedman, B. (1998) Disposition of Enrofloxacin (Baytril®) in red-tailed hawks (*Buteo jamaicensis*) and great horned owls (*Bubo virginianus*) following a single oral, intramuscular, or intravenous dose. *Proceedings of the American Association of Zoo Veterinarians and the American Association of Wildlife Veterinarians Joint Conference.* Omaha, Nebraska, USA.

Harrison, G.J. (1984a) Feather disorders. *Veterinary Clinics of North America: Small Animal Practice*, **14**, 179–199.

Harrison, G.J. (1984b) New aspects of avian surgery. *Veterinary Clinics of North America: Small Animal Practice*, **14**, 363–380.

Harting, J.E. (1891) *Bibliotheca Accipitraria. Catalogue of Books Ancient and Modern relating to Falconry.* Reprinted in 1964 by the Holland Press, London, UK.

Harting, J.E. (1898) *Hints on the Management of Hawks and Practical Falconry.* Reprinted in 1971 by the Thames Valley Press, Maidenhead, UK.

Hartmann, B. & Güntürkün, O. (1998) Selective deficits in reversal learning after neostriatum caudolaterale lesions in pigeons: possible behavioral equivalencies to the mammalian prefrontal system. *Behavioral Brain Research*, **Nov. 96**(1–2), 125–133.

Hartwich, G. (1994) *II. Strongylida: Strongyloidea und Ancylostomatoidea. Die Tierwelt Deutschlands.* 68. Teil. Gustav Fischer Verlag, Jena, Stuttgart, Germany.

Hasholt, J. (1960) Diseases of the nervous system. In: *Diseases of Cage and Aviary Birds* (ed. M.L. Petrak). Lea & Febiger, Philadelphia, USA.

Hatt, J-M. (1995) Falke und Gepard – jagdgenossen des Menschen. *Vierteljahrsschrift der Naturforschenden Gesellschaft in Zürich*, **142**(2), 61–68.

Haugen, A.O. (1952) Trichomoniasis in Alabama mourning doves. *Journal of Wildlife Management*, **16**, 164–169.

Hauska, H. & Redig, P.T. (1997) Morphologic changes in the white hemogram of raptors. *Proceedings of the 1997 European Conference on Avian Medicine and Surgery*, 19–24 May 1997, London, UK.

Havelka, P. (1983) Registration and marking of captive birds of prey. *International Zoo Yearbook*, **23**, 125–132.

Hawkey, C.M. (1991) The value of comparative haematological studies. *Comparative Haematology International*, **1**(1), 1–9.

Hawkey, C.M. & Dennett, T.B. (1989) *A Colour Atlas of Comparative Veterinary Haematology.* Wolfe, London, UK.

Hawkey, C.M., Pugsley, S.L. & Knight, J.A. (1984) Abnormal heterophils in a king shag with aspergillosis. *Veterinary Record*, **114**, 322–324.

Hawkins, M., Wright, B.D., Tell, L.A., Pascoe, P.J. & Kass, P. (2000) Anaesthetic and cardiopulmonary effects of propofol in red-tailed hawks (*Butes jamaicensis*) and great horned owls (*Bubo virginianus*). *Proceedings of the Association of Avian Veterinarians*, 227–228.

HB/BFSS (1997) *Flying Demonstrations of Birds of Prey.* The Hawk Board, Twickenham/British Field Sports Society, London, UK.

Heckel, J., Clay-Sisson, D. & Quist, C.F. (1994) Apparent fatal snakebite in three hawks. *Journal of Wildlife Diseases*, **30**(4), 616–619.

Hegdal, P.L. & Colvin, B.A. (1988) Potential hazard to eastern screech owls and other raptors of brodifacoum bait used for vole control in orchards. *Environmental Toxicology and Chemistry*, 7, 245–260.

Hegner, R.W. (1925) *Giardia felis* n.sp. from the domestic cat and Giardias from birds. *American Journal of Hygiene*, **5**, 258–273.

Heidenreich, M. (1996) *Greifvogel, Krankheiten, Haltung, Zucht.* Blackwell Wissenschafts-Verlag, Berlin and Vienna.

Heidenreich, M. (1997) *Birds of Prey: Medicine and Management.* Blackwell, Wissenschafts-Verlag, Oxford, UK.

van Heijnsbergen, P. (1997) *International Legal Protection of Wild Fauna and Flora.* IOS Press, Amsterdam, Berlin and Oxford.

Heinrich, B. (1999) *Minds of the Raven – Investigations and Adventures with Wolf Birds.* Cliff Street Books, Harper Collins, New York, USA.

Heinrichs, M.A. (1992) *Herpesvirus – Induzierte Infektionen und Krankheiten bei nicht domestizierten. Vogelarten – eine vergleichende. Literaturstudie.* Inaugural dissertation, Justus Liebig Universität, Giessen, Germany.

Heintzelman, D.S. (1971) Observations on the role of nest box sanitation in affecting egg hatchability of wild sparrowhawks in Eastern Pennsylvania. *Raptor Research News*, **5**, 100–103.

Heinz, G.H. (1996) Mercury poisoning in wildlife. In: *Noninfectious Diseases of Wildlife* (eds A. Fairbrother, L.N. Lockie & G.L. Hoff), pp. 118–127. Iowa State Univ. Press, Ames, Iowa, USA.

Henny, C.J. & Meeker, D.L. (1981) An evaluation of blood plasma for monitoring DDE in birds of prey. *Environmental Pollution (Series A)*, **25**, 291–304.

van Heokmsbergen, P. (1997) *International Legal Protection of Wild Fauna and Flora.* IOS Press, Amsterdam, The Netherlands.

Herremans, M. (2000) The 'chaotic' flight feather moult of the steppe buzzard *Buteo buteo vulpinus. Bird Study*, **47**, 332–343.

Hickey, J.J. (1969) *Peregrine Falcon Populations: Their Biology and Decline.* University of Wisconsin Press, Madison, WI, USA.

Hickey, J.J. & Anderson, D.W. (1968) Chlorinated hydrocarbons and eggshell changes in raptorial and fish-eating birds. *Science*, **162**, 271–273.

Higgins, P.A. & Warr, G.W. (2000) *The Avian Immune Response to Infectious Diseases.* Special Issue of *Developmental and Comparative Immunology*, **24**(2).

Higuchi, K. (1976) *PCB Poisoning and Pollution.* Academic Press, New York and London.

Hildebrandt, T., Pitra, C., Sömmer, P. & Pinkowski, M. (1995) Sex identification in birds of prey by ultrasonography. *Journal of Zoo and Wildlife Medicine*, **26**, 367–376.

Hill, H.M. & Work, T.H. (1947) Protocalliphora larvae infesting nestling birds of prey. *Condor*, **49**, 74–75.

Hirons, G.J.M., Hardy, A.R. & Stanley, P.I. (1979) Starvation in young Tawny Owls. *Bird Study*, **26**, 59–63.

Hitchner, S.B., Domermuth, C.H., Purchase, H.G. & Williams, J.E. (1975) *Isolation and Identification of Avian Pathogens.* American Association of Avian Pathologists, Texas A and M University, USA.

Hodges, R.D. (1974) *The Histology of the Fowl.* Academic Press, New York and London.

Hodges, R.D. (1977) Avian haematology. In: *Comparative Clinical Haematology* (eds R.K. Archer & L.B. Jeffcott). Blackwell Scientific Publications, Oxford, UK.

Hoefle, U., Blanco, J.M., Sauer-Guerth, H. & Wink, M. (2000) Molecular sex determination in Spanish imperial eagle (*Aquila adalvert*) nestlings and sex related variation in morphometric parameters. In: *Raptor Biomedicine III* (eds J.T. Lumeij, J.D. Remple, P.T. Redig, M. Lierz & J.E. Cooper). Zoological Education Network, Lake Worth, FL, USA.

Hofbauer, H. (1997) *Beitrag zur Transkutanen Ultraschalluntersuchung des Aviären Urogenitalitraktes.* Inaugural dissertation, Justus Liebig Universität, Giessen, Germany.

Hoffman, D.J., Pattee, O.H., Wiemeyer, S.N. & Mulhern, B. (1981) Effects of lead shot ingestion on aminolevulinic acid dehydratase activity, hemoglobin concentration, and serum chemistry in bald eagles. *Journal of Wildlife Diseases*, **17**, 423–431.

Holmes, J.C. & Bethel, W.M. (1972) Modification of intermediate host behaviour by parasites. In: *Behavioural Aspects of Parasite Transmission* (eds E.U.

Canning & C.A. Wright), pp. 123–149. Academic Press, London, UK.

Holt, P.E. (1977) The use of a steroid anaesthetic in a long-eared owl (*Asio otus*). *Veterinary Record*, **101**, 118.

Holz, P. & Naisbitt, R. (2000) Fitness level as a determining factor in the survival of rehabilitated raptors released back into the wild – preliminary results. In: *Raptor Biomedicine III* (eds J.T. Lumeij, J.D. Remple, P.T. Redig, M. Lierz & J.E. Cooper). Zoological Education Network, Lake Worth, FL, USA.

Hoogstraal, H. (1972) Viruses and ticks. In: *Viruses and Invertebrates* (ed. A.J. Gibbs). North-Holland Publishing, Amsterdam, The Netherlands.

Hoogstraal, H., Oliver, R.M. & Guirgis, S.S. (1970) Larva, nymph and life cycle of *Ornithodoros (Alectorobius) muesebecki* (Ixodoidea: Argasidae), a virus-infected parasite of birds and petroleum industry employees in the Arabian Gulf. *Annals of the Entomological Society of America*, **63**, 1762–1763.

Hooimeijer, J. & Zwart, P. (1987) Eulen. In: *Krankheiten der Wildtiere* (eds K. Gabrisch & P. Zwart). Schlütersche, Hannover, Germany.

Houston, C.S., Crawford, R.D. & Oliphant, L.W. (1993) Unhatched eggs in raptor nests in Saskatchewan. In: *Raptor Biomedicine* (eds P.T. Redig, J.E. Cooper, J.D. Remple & D.B. Hunter). University of Minnesota Press, USA.

Houston, D.C. (1972) *The Ecology of Serengeti Vultures.* DPhil thesis, University of Oxford, UK.

Houston, D.C. (1978) The effect of food quality on breeding strategy in griffon vultures (*Gyps* spp). *Journal of Zoology, London*, **186**, 175–184.

Houston, D.C. & Cooper, J.E. (1973) Use of the drug metomidate to facilitate the handling of vultures. *International Zoo Yearbook*, **13**, 269–271.

Houston, D.C. & Cooper, J.E. (1975) The digestive tract of the Whiteback Griffon Vulture and its role in disease transmission among wild ungulates. *Journal of Wildlife Diseases*, **11**, 306–313.

Howald, G., Mineau, P., Elliott, J.E. & Cheng, K.M. (1999) Brodifacoum poisoning of avian scavengers during rat control on a seabird colony. *Ecotoxicology*, **8**, 429–445.

Howard, B.R. (1972) Sleep in the domestic fowl. *Proceedings of the Royal Society of Medicine*, **65**, 177–179.

Howard, R. & Moore, A. (1994) *A Complete Checklist of the Birds of the World*, 2nd edn. Academic Press, London, UK.

Huchzermeyer, F.W. & Cooper, J.E. (2000) Fibriscess, not abscess, resulting from a localised inflammatory response to infection in reptiles and birds. *Veterinary Record*, **147**, 515–517.

Huckabee, J.R. (2000) Raptor therapeutics. *Veterinary Clinics of North America: Exotic Animal Practice*, **3**(1), 91–116.

Hudson, P.J. (1986) The effect of a parasitic nematode on the breeding production of Red Grouse. *Journal of Animal Ecology*, **55**, 85–92.

Hudson, P.J. & Dobson, A.P. (1991) The direct and indirect effects of the caecal nematode *Trichostrongylus tenuis* on Red Grouse. In: *Bird–Parasite Interactions* (eds J.E. Loye & M. Zuk), pp. 49–68. University Press, Oxford, UK.

Hudson, P.J., Dobson, A.P. & Newborn, D. (1992a) Do parasites make prey vulnerable to predation? Red Grouse and parasites. *Journal of Animal Ecology*, **61**, 681–692.

Hudson, P.J., Dobson, A.P. & Newborn, D. (1998) Prevention of population cycles by parasite removal. *Science*, **282**, 2256–2258.

Hudson, P.J., Newborn, D. & Dobson, A.P. (1992b) Regulation and stability of a free-living host–parasite system, *Trichostrongylus tenuis* in Red Grouse. 1: Monitoring and parasite reduction experiments. *Journal of Animal Ecology*, **61**, 477–486.

Hume, R. (1991) *Owls World*. Dragon' World Ltd, Limpsfield, Surrey, UK.

Humphreys, P.N. (1985) Water-birds. In: *A Manual of Exotic Pets* (eds J.E. Cooper & M.F. Hutchison). British Small Animal Veterinary Association, London.

Hunter, D.B., Rohner, C. & Currie, D.C. (1997) Mortality in fledgling great horned owls from black fly *Hematophaga* and *Leucocytozoon*. *Journal of Wildlife Diseases*, **33**(3), 486–491.

Hurrell, L.H. (1967) Wild raptor casualties. *The Falconer*, **V**, 30–37.

Hurrell, L.H. (1973) On breeding the sparrow-hawk in captivity. In: *A Hawk for the Bush* (ed. J.G. Mavrogordato), 2nd edn. Neville Spearman, London, UK.

Hussong, R. (1996) *Identification of Falcons and His Hybrids by Porestructure of Eggs*. Dissertation, University of Munich, Germany.

IAF (2000) Hybrid raptors: a consideration of the issues. The International Association for Falconry. *British Falconers' Club Newsletter*, **21**, 21–22.

IATA (annual) *Live Animals Regulations*. International Air Transport Association, Montreal and Geneva.

Inge Hiebl, Kösters, J. & Braunitzer, G. (1987a) The primary structures of the major and minor hemoglobin components of adult goshawk (*Accipiter gentilis*, Accipitrinae). *Biological Chemistry Hoppe Seyler*, **368**, 333–342.

Inge Hiebl, Schneeganß, D., Grimm, F., Kösters, J. & Braunitzer, G. (1987b) The primary structures of the major and minor hemoglobin components of adult European vulture. *Biological Chemistry Hoppe Seyler*, **368**, 11–18.

Inge Hiebl, Weber, R.E., Schneeganß, D., Braunitzer, G. (1989) The primary structures and functional properties of the major and minor hemoglobin components of the adult white-headed vulture. *Biological Chemistry Hoppe Seyler*, **370**, 699–706.

Irving, L. (1955) Nocturnal decline in the temperature of birds in cold weather. *Condor*, **57**, 362–365.

Isenbügel, E. & Rübel, A. (1987) Greifvögel. In: *Krankheiten der Wildtiere* (eds K. Gabrisch & P. Zwart). Schlütersche, Hannover, Germany.

Itamies, J., Valtonen, E.T. & Feagerholm, H.P. (1980) *Polymorphus minutus* infestation in eiders and its role as a possible cause of death. *Annales Zoologici Fennici*, **17**, 185–289.

IUCN/SSC (undated) *Guidelines for Re-introductions*. International Union for Conservation of Nature and Natural Resources/Species Survival Commission Re-introductions Specialist Group, Nairobi, Kenya.

Jack, A. (1996) *Ferreira's Falconry*. A translation from the Portuguese of *Arte da Caça de Altaneria* by Diogo Fernandes Ferreira, Lisbon 1616.

Jack, T.A.M. (1977) A reply to the challenge. *Birds*, **6**, 62.

Jaksch, W. (1960) Fussballengeschwulst bei Hühnern als Folge eines Mangelfutters. *Wiener tierärztliche Monatsschrift*, **47**, 388–396.

Jansen, J.A., Van der Waerden, J.P.C.M., Gwalter, R.H. & van Rooy, S.A.B. (1999) Biological and migrational characteristics of transponders implanted into beagle dogs. *Veterinary Record*, **145**, 329–333.

Jefferies, D.J. & Prestt, I. (1966) Post-mortems of peregrines and lanners with particular reference to organochlorine residues. *British Birds*, **59**, 49–64.

Jenkins, D., Watson, A. & Miller, G.R. (1963) Population studies on Red Grouse *Lagopus lagopus scoticus* (Lath.) in north-east Scotland. *Journal of Animal Ecology*, **32**, 317–376.

Jenkins, M.A. (1984) A clutch of unusually small peregrine falcon eggs. *Raptor Research*, **18**, 151–153.

Jennings, A.R. (1959) Diseases in wild birds. Fifth Report. *Bird Study*, **6**, 19–22.

Jennings, A.R. (1961) An analysis of 1000 deaths in wild birds. *Bird Study*, **8**, 25–31.

Jennings, A.R. (1969) Tumours of free-living wild mammals and birds in Great Britain. *Symposium of the Zoological Society of London*, **24**, 273–287.

Jennings, A.R. (1961) An analysis of 1000 deaths in wild birds. *Bird Study*, **8**, 25–31.

Jennings, A.R., Soulsby, E.J.L. & Wainwright, C.B. (1961) An outbreak of disease in Mute Swans at an Essex reservoir. *Bird Study*, **8**, 19–24.

Jennings, I.B. (1996) Haematology. In: *Manual of Raptors, Pigeons and Waterfowl* (eds P.H. Beynon, N.A. Forbes & N.H. Harcourt-Brown). British Small Animal Veterinary Association, Cheltenham, UK.

Jensen, W.I. & Williams, C. (1964) Botulism and waterfowl. In: *Waterfowl Tomorrow* (ed. J.P. Linduska). Government Printing Office, Washington DC, USA.

Jesiotr, M. (1973) Treatment of aspergillosis with emetine hydrochloride. *Scandinavian Journal of Respiratory Diseases*, **54**, 326–332.

Johne, R. & Müller, H. (1998) Avian polyomavirus in wild birds: genome analysis of isolates from *Falconiformes* and *Psittaciformes*. *Archives of Virology*, **143**, 1501–1512.

Johnson, D.C., Cooper, R.S. & Osborn, J.S. (1974) Velogenic viscerotropic Newcastle disease virus isolated from mice. *Avian Diseases*, **18**, 633–634.

Johnson, I.M. (1969) Electrolyte and water balance of the red-tailed hawk, *Buteo jamaicensis*. Abstract. *American Society of Zoologists*, **9**, 587.

Jones, C.G. (1981) Abnormal and maladaptive behaviour in captive raptors. In: *Recent Advances in the Study of Raptor Diseases* (eds J.E. Cooper & A.G. Greenwood). Chiron Publications, Keighley, Yorkshire, UK.

Jones, D.M. (1977a) The occurrence of dieldrin in sawdust used as a bedding material. *Laboratory Animals*, **11**, 137.

Jones, D.M. (1977b) The sedation and anaesthesia of birds and reptiles. *Veterinary Record*, **101**, 340–342.

Jones, D.M., Samour, J.H., Knight, J.A. & Ffinch, J.M. (1984) Sex determination of monomorphic birds by fibreoptic endoscopy. *Veterinary Record*, **115**, 596–598.

Jones, M.P. & Orosz, S.E. (2000) The diagnosis of aspergillosis in birds. *Seminars in Avian and Exotic Pet Medicine*, **9**(2), 52–58.

Jones, M.P., Orosz, S.E., Cox, S.K. & Frazier, D.L. (2000) Pharmacokinetic disposition of itraconazole in red-tailed hawks (*Buteo jamaicensis*). *Journal of Avian Medicine and Surgery*, **14**(1), 15–22.

Jorgenson, R.D., Gough, P.M. & Graham, D.L. (1976) Experimental rabies in a great horned owl. *Journal of Wildlife Diseases*, **12**, 444–447.

Joseph, V. (1996) Aspergillosis, the silent killer. *Journal of Wildlife Rehabilitation*, **19**, 15–18.

Joseph, V. (2000) Aspergillosis in raptors. *Seminars in Avian and Exotic Pet Medicine*, **9**(2), 66–74.

June, G.A., Sherrod, P.S., Hammack, T.S., Amaguana, R.M. & Andrews, W.H. (1995) Relative effectiveness of selenite, cystine broth, tetrathionate broth and rappaport vassiliadis medium for the recovery of *Salmonella* from raw flesh and highly contaminated foods: precollaborative study. *Journal of American Oil Chemists Society International*, **78**, 375–380.

Kaleta, E.F. (1990) Herpesviruses of birds – a review. *Avian Pathology*, **19**, 193–211.

Kaleta, E.F. & Drüner, K. (1976) Hepatosplenitis infectiosa strigum und andere Krankheiten der Greifvögel und Eulen. *Fortschritte der Veterinärmedizin*, **25**, 173–180.

Kaliner, G. & Cooper, J.E. (1973) Dual infection of an African fish eagle with acid-fast bacilli and an *Aspergillus* sp. *Journal of Wildlife Diseases*, **9**, 51–55.

Kalmbach, E.R. (1939a) American vultures and the toxin of *Clostridium botulinum*. *Journal of the American Veterinary Medical Association*, **94**, 187–197.

Kalmbach, E.R. (1939b) Nesting success: its significance in waterfowl reproduction. *Transactions of the North American Wildlife Research Conference*, **4**, 591–604.

Kalmbach, E.R. & Gunderson, M.F. (1934) Western duck sickness, a form of botulism. *US Department of Agriculture Technical Bulletin*, **411**, 1–81.

Karstad, L. & Sileo, L. (1971) Causes of death in captive wild waterfowl in the Kortright Waterfowl Park, 1969–70. *Journal of Wildlife Diseases*, **7**, 236–241.

Keith, J.O. & Bruggers, R.L. (1998) Review of hazards to raptors from pest control in Sahelian Africa. *Journal of Raptor Research*, **32**, 151–158.

Kelly-Brook, M. & Bird, D.M. (1991) Prefreeze and post-thaw effects of glycerol and dimethylacetamide on motility and fertilizing ability of American kestrel (*Falco sparverius*) spermatozoa. *Journal of Zoo and Wildlife Medicine*, **22**(4), 453–459.

Kendall, R.J., Lacher, T.E., Jr., Bunck, C., *et al.* (1996) An ecological risk assessment of lead shot exposure in non-waterfowl avian species: upland game birds and raptors. *Environmental Toxicology and Chemistry*, **15**, 4–20.

Kennedy-Stoskopf, S. (1997) Evaluating immunodeficiency disorders in captive wild animals. In: *Zoo and Wild Animal Medicine* (eds M.E. Fowler & R.E. Miller). W.B. Saunders, Philadelphia, USA.

Kenward, R.E. (1974) Mortality and fate of trained birds of prey. *Journal of Wildlife Management*, **34**, 751–756.

Kenward, R.E. (1976) *The effect of goshawk*, Accipiter gentilis, *predation on wood pigeon*, Columba palumbus, *populations*. DPhil thesis, University of Oxford, UK.

Kenward, R.E., Marcström, V. & Karlbom, M. (1993) Causes of death in radio-tagged Northern goshawks. In:

Raptor Biomedicine (eds P.T. Redig, J.E. Cooper, J.D. Remple & D.B. Hunter). University of Minnesota Press, USA.

Kern, T.J., Murphy, C.J. & Riis, R.C. (1984) Lens extraction by phacoemulsification in two raptors. *Journal of the American Veterinary Medical Association*, **185**, 1403–1406.

Keymer, I.F. (1969) Parasitic diseases. In: *Diseases of Cage and Aviary Birds* (ed. M.L. Petrak). Lea & Febiger, PA, USA.

Keymer, I.F. (1972) Diseases of birds of prey. *Veterinary Record*, **90**, 579–594.

Keymer, I.F. (1974) Ornithosis in free-living and captive birds. *Proceedings of the Royal Society of Medicine*, **67**, 733–735.

Keymer, I.F. (1977a) Diseases of birds other than domestic poultry. In: *Poultry Diseases* (ed. R.F. Gordon). Baillière Tindall, London, UK.

Keymer, I.F. (1977b) Cataracts in birds. *Avian Pathology*, **6**, 335–341.

Keymer, I.F. (1980) Disorders of the avian female reproductive system. *Avian Pathology*, **9**, 405–519.

Keymer, I.F. & Dawson, P.S. (1971) Newcastle disease in birds of prey. *Veterinary Record*, **88**, 432.

Keymer, I.F., Fletcher, M.R. & Stanley, P.I. (1981) Causes of mortality in British kestrels (*Falco tinnunculus*). In: *Recent Advances in the Study of Raptor Diseases* (eds J.E. Cooper & A.G. Greenwood), pp. 143–151. Chiron Publications, Keighley, Yorkshire, UK.

Keymer, I.F., Rose, J.H., Beesley, W.N. & Davies, S.F.M. (1962) A survey and review of parasitic diseases of wild and game birds in Great Britain. *Veterinary Record*, **74**, 887–894.

Khan, R.A. (1965) Development of *Leucocytozoon ziemanni* (Laveran). *Journal of Parasitology*, **61**, 449–457.

Kim, E-Y., Goto, R., Iwata, H., Masuda, Y., Tanabe, S. & Fujita, S. (1999) Preliminary survey of lead poisoning of Steller's sea-eagle (*Haliaeetus pelagicus*) and white-tailed sea-eagle (*Haliaeetus albicilla*) in Hokkaido, Japan. *Environmental Toxicology and Chemistry*, **18**, 448–451.

King, A.S. & McLelland, J. (1975) *Outlines of Avian Anatomy*. Baillière Tindall, London, UK.

King, A.S. & McLelland, J. (1979) *Form and Function in Birds*, Vols 1–4. Academic Press, London, UK.

King, A.S. & McLelland, J. (1984) *Birds, their Structure and Function*. Baillière Tindall, London, UK.

Kingston, N., Remple, J.D., Burnham, W., Stabler, R.M. & McGhee, R.B. (1976) Malaria in a captively-produced F1 gyrfalcon and in two F1 peregrine falcons. *Journal of Wildlife Diseases*, **12**, 562–565.

Kirkpatrick, C.E. & Colvin, B.A. (1989) Ectoparasitic fly *Carnus hemapterus* (Diptera, Carnidae) in a nestling population of common barn owls (Strigiformes, Tytonidae). *Journal of Medical Entomology*, **26**(2), 109–112.

Kirkwood, J.K. (1979) The partition of food energy for existence in the kestrel (*Falco tinnunculus*) and the barn owl (*Tyto alba*). *Comparative Biochemistry and Physiology*, **63A**, 495–498.

Kirkwood, J.K. (1980) Energy and prey requirements of the young free-flying kestrel. *Hawk Trust Report*, **10**, 12–14.

Kirkwood, J.K. (1981) Maintenance energy requirements and rate of weight loss during starvation in birds of prey. In: *Recent Advances in the Study of Raptor Diseases* (eds J.E. Cooper & A.G. Greenwood). Chiron Publications, Keighley, Yorkshire, UK.

Kirkwood, J.K. (1983) Treatment of aspergillosis in raptors. *Veterinary Record*, **112**, 182.

Kirkwood, J.K., Cooper, J.E. & Brown, G. (1979) Some haematological data for the European kestrel (*Falco tinnunculus*). *Research in Veterinary Science*, **26**, 263–264.

Kirkwood, J.K., Cunningham, S.K., Macgregor, S.M., Thornton, S.M. & Duff, J.P. (1994) *Salmonella enteritidis* excretion by carnivorous animals fed on day-old chicks. *Veterinary Record*, **134**, 683.

Kish, F. (1970) Egg laying and incubation by American golden eagle *Aquila chrysaetos canadensis* at Topeka Zoo. *International Zoo Yearbook*, **10**, 26–29.

Kisling, V.N. (1974) A review of pesticide residues in commercial zoo feeds. *International Zoo Yearbook*, **14**, 187–189.

Kissam, J.B., Noblet, R.E. & Garris, G.I. (1975) Large scale aerial treatment of an endemic area with abate granular larvicide to control black flies (Diptera: Simulidae) and suppress *Leucocytozoon smithi* of turkeys. *Journal of Medical Entomology*, **12**, 359–362.

Knight, M. (1968) *Be a Nature Detective*. Frederick Warne, London, UK.

Knudsen, E.I. & Knudsen, P.F. (1985) Vision guides the adjustment of auditory localization in young Barn Owls. *Science*, **130**, 545–548.

Knudsen, E.I., Knudsen, P.F. & Esterly, S.D. (1982) Early auditory experience modifies sound localization in barn owls. *Nature*, **295**, 238–240.

Kocan, A.A. & Gordon, L.R. (1976) Fatal air sac infection with *Serratospiculum amaculata* in a prairie falcon. *Journal of the American Veterinary Medical Association*, **169**, 908.

Kocan, A.A., Snelling, J. & Greiner, E.C. (1977a) Some

infectious and parasitic diseases in Oklahoma raptors. *Journal of Wildlife Diseases*, **13**, 304–306.

Kocan, A.A., Potgieter, L.N.D. & Kocan, K.M. (1977b) Inclusion body disease of falcons (herpesvirus infection) in an American kestrel. *Journal of Wildlife Diseases*, **13**, 199–201.

Koeman, J.H., Garsson-Hoekstra, J., Pels, E. & de Goeij, J.J.M. (1971) Poisoning of birds of prey by methyl mercury compounds. *Mededelingen van de Faculteit Landbouwwetenschappen Rijksuniversiteit Gent*, **36**, 43–49.

Köhler, B. & Baumgart, W. (1970) Toxi-Infektionen durch *Clostridium perfringens* Typ A. *Monatshefte für Veterinärmedizin*, **25**, 348–352.

Kollias, G.V., Greiner, E.C. & Heard, E.C. (1987) The efficacy of ivermectin and praziquantel against gastrointestinal nematodes and trematodes in raptors. *Proceedings of the First International Conference on Zoological and Avian Medicine*, 408–409.

König, C. (1982) Zur systematischen Stellung der Neuweltgeier (Cathartidae). *Journal für Ornithologie*, **123**, 259–267.

Korbel, R.T. (2000) Disorders of the posterior eye segment in raptors – examination procedures and findings. In: *Raptor Biomedicine III* (eds Zoological Education Network). Zoological Education Network, Lake Worth, FL, USA.

Korbel, R.T., Nell, B., Redig, P.T., Walde, I. & Reese, S. (2000) Video fluorescein angiography in the eyes of various raptors and mammals. *Proceedings of the Association of Avian Veterinarians*, 89–95.

Korpimäki, E., Hakkarainen, H. & Bennett, G.F. (1993) Blood parasites and reproductive success of Tengmalm's Owls: detrimental effects on females but not males. *Functional Ecology*, 7, 420–426.

Kösters, J. (1974) Haltungsbedingte Krankheiten bei Greifvögeln. *Der Praktische Tierarzt liche (Supplement)*, **55**, 31–33.

Kösters, J. & Meister, B. (1982) Hämatokrit- und Hämoglobinwerte bei einigen einheimischen Greifvögeln und Eulen. *Der Praktische Tierarzliche*, **63**, 444–446.

Kostka, V. (1992) *Röntgenologische Untersuchungen am Rumpf- und Gliedmasserskelett von Zier- und Wildvögeln: Anatomische, Physiologische und Pathologische. Befunde.* Inaugural dissertation, Justus Liebig Universität, Giessen, Germany.

Kramer, J.L. & Redig, P.T. (1997) Sixteen years of lead poisoning in eagles, 1980–95: an epizootiologic view. *Journal of Raptor Research*. **31**(4), 327–332.

Krautwald, M. & Trinkhaus, K. (2000) Imaging tech-

niques. In: *Avian Medicine* (eds T.M. Tully, M. Lawton & G.M. Dorrestein). Butterworth-Heinemann, Oxford, UK.

Krautwald, M.E., Tellhelm, B., Hummel, G., Kostka, V. & Kaleta, E.F. (1992) *Atlas of Radiographic Diagnosis of Cage Birds*. Paul Parey, Berlin and Hamburg, Germany.

Krautwald-Junghanns, M-E., Kostka, V.M. & Dorsch, B. (1998) Comparative studies on the diagnostic value of conventional radiography and computed tomography in evaluating the heads of psittacine and raptorial birds. *Journal of Avian Medicine and Surgery*, **12**(3), 149–157.

Krebs, J.R., Clayton, N.S., Healy, S.D., Cristol, D.A., Patel, S.W. & Joliffe, A.R. (1996) The ecology of the brain: food-storing and the hippocampus. *Ibis*, **138**, 34–46.

Krone, O. (1996) The pygmy owl (*Glaucidium passerinum*) as new host for the rare haematozoon *Trypanosoma avium*. *Applied Parasitology*, **37**, 300–301.

Krone, O. (1998) *Endoparasiten (Faunistik, Epizootiologie, Pathogenität) bei wildlebenden Greifvögeln aus drei Gebieten Deutschlands*. Veterinary Medicine Dissertation, Freie Universität Berlin, Germany.

Krone, O. (2000) Endoparasites in free-living birds of prey from Germany. In: *Raptor Biomedicine III* (eds Zoological Education Network). Lake Worth, FL, USA.

Krone, O. & Cooper, J.E. (1999) Hairworms of birds of prey. *Veterinary Record*, **145**(4), 115.

Krone, O. & Streich, J. (2000) *Strigea falconispalumbi* in Eurasian buzzards from Germany. *Journal of Wildlife Diseases*, **36**(3), 559–561.

Krone, O., Rudolph, M., Jacob, W., *et al.* (2000a) Protozoa in the breast muscle of raptors in Germany. *Acta Protozoologica*, **39**(1), 35–42.

Kučera, J. (1981a) Blood parasites of birds in Central Europe. *Leucocytozoon*. *Folia Parasitologica*, **28**, 193–203.

Kučera, J. (1981b) Blood parasites of birds in Central Europe. *Plasmodium* and *Haemoproteus*. *Folia Parasitologica*, **28**, 303–312.

Kučera, J. (1982) Blood parasites of birds in Central Europe. *Trypanosoma*, '*Atoxoplasma*', microfilariae and other rare haematozoa. *Folia Parasitologica*, **29**, 107–113.

Lacina, D. (1999) Ectoparasite *Carnus hemapterus* influences the mass growth rate of nestlings of European kestrel (*Falco tinnunculus*). *Buteo, Supplement, Abstracts of the 3rd Eurasian Conference of the Raptor Research Foundation*, p. 29.

Lahr, J.B. & Lorah, D.A. (2000) Case study: a wing

and a prayer. *Journal of Wildlife Rehabilitation*, **23**(2), 3–6.

Lampio, T. (1946) Game diseases in Finland 1924–43. *Suomen Riista*, **1**, 93–142.

Lancaster, J.E. & Alexander, D. (1975) Newcastle disease virus and spread. *Monograph No. 11*, Canadian Department of Agriculture, Ottawa, Canada.

Langelier, K.M. (1993) Barbiturate poisoning in twenty-nine bald eagles. In: *Raptor Biomedicine* (eds P.T. Redig, J.E. Cooper, J.D. Remple & D.B. Hunter). University of Minnesota Press, USA.

Larraz, D.S. (1999) Dumps for dead livestock and the conservation of wintering red kites (*Milvus milvus*). *Journal of Raptor Research*, **33**(4), 338–340.

Latham, S. (1615) *Falconry, or the Faulcons Lure and Cure*. Printed by J B, London.

Lavigne, A.J., Bird, D.M. & Negro, J.J. (1994) Growth of hand-reared American kestrels. The effect of two different diets and feeding frequency. *Growth, Development and Aging*, **4**, 197–201.

Lavin, S., Cuenca, R., Marco, I., Verlade, R. & Vinas, L. (1992) Hematology and blood chemistry of the marsh harrier (*Circus aeruginosus*). *Comparative Biochemistry and Physiology*, **103**, 493–495.

Lavoie, M., Mikaelian, I., Sterner, M., *et al.* (1999) Respiratory nematodiasis in raptors in Quebec. *Journal of Wildlife Diseases*, **35**(2), 375–380.

Lawler, E.M. & Redig, P.T. (1984) The antibody responses to sheep red blood cells of the red-tailed hawk and great-horned owl. *Developmental and Comparative Immunology*, **8**, 733–738.

Lawrence, K. (1983) Efficacy of fenbendazole against nematodes of captive birds. *Veterinary Record*, **122**, 433–434.

Lawson, P.T. & Kittle, E.L. (1970) Induced molt. *Raptor Research News*, **4**, 138.

Lawton, M. (2000) The physical examination. In: *Avian Medicine* (eds T.M. Tully, M. Lawton & G.M. Dorrestein). Butterworth-Heinemann, Oxford.

Lawton, M.P.C. (1995) Neurological problems of exotic species. In: *Manual of Small Animal Neurology* (ed. S.J. Wheeler). BSAVA, Cheltenham, UK.

Lawton, M.P.C. (1996) Anaesthesia. In: *Manual of Raptors, Pigeons and Waterfowl* (eds P.H. Beynon, N.A. Forbes & N.H. Harcourt-Brown). BSAVA, Cheltenham, UK.

Leake, L.D. (1975) *Comparative Histology*. Academic Press, New York and London.

Leclercq, B. & Whitehead, C.C. (1988) *Leanness in Domestic Birds: Genetic, Metabolic and Hormonal Aspects*. Butterworth, London, UK.

Lee, E. (2000) Avian assessment and first aid. In: *Wildlife Health in Conservation*. Department of Conservation. Publication No. 204 Veterinary Continuing Education, Massey University, New Zealand.

Leese, A.S. (1927) *A Treatise on the One-humped Camel in Health and Disease*. Haynes and Son, Stamford, Lincolnshire, UK.

Lemahieu, P., De Vriese, L. & Bijnens, B. (1985) Feather abnormalities associated with paramyxovirus-1 pigeon variant in pigeons and chickens. *Veterinary Record*, **116**, 591.

Leonard, J.L. (1969) Clinical laboratory examinations. In: *Diseases of Cage and Aviary Birds* (ed. M.L. Petrak). Lea & Febiger, PA, USA.

Lepoutre, D.R. (1982) *Contribution à l'étude de l'hématologie, la biochimie sanguine et la pathologie infectieuse et parasitaire des rapaces européens*. Thèse, Ecole Nationale Vétérinaire de Toulouse, France.

Levine, N.D. & Campbell, G.R. (1971) A check-list of the species of the genus *Haemoproteus* (Apicomplexa: Plasmodidae). *Journal of Protozoology*, **18**, 475–484.

Lierz, M. (2000) Investigation of free-ranging raptors discovered injured or debilitated in Germany. *Proceedings of the Association of Avian Veterinarians*, 139–141.

Lierz, M. (2001) Evaluation of the dosage of ivermectin in falcons. *Veterinary Record*, **148**, 596–600.

Lierz, M. & Launay, F. (2000) Veterinary procedures for falcons re-entering the wild. *Veterinary Record*, **147**, 518–520.

Lierz, M. & Remple, D. (1997) Endoparasitenbefall bei Großfalken in Dubai. *Kleintierpraxis*, **42**, 757–768.

Lierz, M., Ibrahim, M., Runge, M., Schmidt, R. & Valentin-Weigond, P. (2000a) Mycoplasmas in captive falcons in the United Arab Emirates. *Proceedings of the Association of Avian Veterinarians*, 485–486.

Lierz, M., Schmidt, R., Brunnberg, L. & Runge, M. (2000) Isolation of *Mycoplasma meleagridis* from the free-ranging birds of prey in Germany. *Journal of Veterinary Medicine Series B – Infectious Diseases and Veterinary Public Health*, **47**(1), 63–67.

Lierz, M., Schmidt, R., Goebel, T., Ehrlein, J. & Runge, M. (2000b) Detection of *Mycoplasma* spp. in raptorial birds in Germany. In: *Raptor Biomedicine III* (eds J.T. Lumeij, J.D. Remple, P.T. Redig, M. Lierz & J.E. Cooper). Zoological Education Network, Lake Worth, FL, USA.

Lierz, M., Schuster, R., Ehrlein, J. & Göbel, T. (1998) Nachweis von *Hovorkonema variegatum* bei einem Habicht (*Accipiter gentilis*). *Kleintierpraxis*, **43**(1), 43–46.

Lincer, J.L. & Peakall, D.B. (1970) Metabolic effects of polychlorinated biphenyls in the American kestrel. *Nature*, **228**, 783–784.

Lindsay, D.S., Dubey, J.P. & Blagburn, B.L. (1991) *Toxoplasma gondii* infections in red-tailed hawks inoculated orally with tissue cysts. *Journal of Parasitology*, **77**, 322–325.

Lindsay, D.S., Smith, P.C., Hoerr, F.J. & Blagburn, B.L. (1993) Prevalence of encysted *Toxoplasma gondii* in raptors from Alabama. *Journal of Parasitology*, **79**, 870–873.

Lloyd, C.S., Thomas, G.J., MacDonald, J.W., Borland, E.D., Standring, K. & Smart, J.L. (1976) Wild bird mortality caused by botulism in Britain, 1975. *Biological Conservation*, **10**, 119–129.

Locke, L.N. & Friend, M. (1987) Avian botulism. In: *Field Guide to Wildlife Diseases. Vol. 1. General Field Procedures and Diseases of Migratory Birds* (ed. M. Friend). US Department of the Interior, Fish and Wildlife Service Resource Publication, **167**. Washington DC, USA.

Locke, L.N. & Friend, M. (1992) Lead poisoning of avian species other than waterfowl. In: *Lead Poisoning in Waterfowl* (ed. D.J. Pain), pp. 19–22. Spec. Publ. 16. Waterfowl Wetlands Research Bureau, Slimbridge, Gloucestershire, UK.

Locke, L.N., Bagley, G.E., Frickie, D.N. & Young, L.T. (1969) Lead poisoning and aspergillosis in an Andean condor. *Journal of the American Veterinary Medical Association*, **155**, 1052–1056.

Lorenz, K.Z. (1935) Der Kumpan in der Umwelt des Vogels. *Journal für Ornithologie*, **83**, 137–213, 289–413.

Lovat Lord (1911) Moor management. In: *The Grouse in Health and Disease* (ed. L. Lovat). Smith, Elder and Co., London, UK.

Loye, J.E. & Zuk, M. (1991) *Bird–Parasite Interactions. Ecology, Evolution and Behaviour.* Oxford University Press, Oxford, UK.

Lucas, A.M. & Jamroz, C. (1961) *Atlas of Avian Hematology.* US Dept of Agriculture, Washington DC, USA.

Lumeij, J.T. (1987) *A contribution to clinical investigative methods for birds, with special reference to the racing pigeon* Columba livia domestica. Thesis, Faculty of Veterinary Medicine, State University, Utrech, The Netherlands.

Lumeij, J.T. (1993) Effects of ketamine–xylazine anesthesia on adrenal function and cardiac conduction in goshawks and pigeons. In: *Raptor Biomedicine* (eds P.T. Redig, J.E. Cooper, J.D. Remple & D.B. Hunter). University of Minnesota Press, USA.

Lumeij, J.T. (1996) Biochemistry and sampling. In: *Manual of Raptors, Pigeons and Waterfowl* (eds P.H. Beynon, N.A. Forbes & N.H. Harcourt-Brown). British Small Animal Veterinary Association, Cheltenham, UK.

Lumeij, J.T. (1997) Avian clinical biochemistry. In: *Clinical Biochemistry of Domestic Animals.* Academic Press, San Diego, USA.

Lumeij, J.T. (2000) (Patho)physiology and treatment of renal disorders in birds of prey. In: *Raptor Biomedicine III* (eds J.T. Lumeij, J.D. Remple, P.T. Redig, M. Lierz & J.E. Cooper). Zoological Education Network, Lake Worth, FL, USA.

Lumeij, J.T. & van Nie, G.J. (1982) Tuberculosis in raptorial birds. Review of the literature and suggestions for clinical diagnosis and vaccination. *Tijdschrift voor Diergeneeskunde*, **107**, 573–579.

Lumeij, J.T., Remple, J.D., Redig, P.T., Lierz, M. & Cooper, J.E. (2000) *Raptor Biomedicine III.* Zoological Education Network, Lake Worth, FL, USA.

Lumeij, J.T., Sprang, E.P.M. & Redig, P.T. (1998) Further studies on allopurinol-induced hyperuricemia and visceral gout in red-tailed hawks (*Buteo jamaicensis*). *Avian Pathology*, **27**, 390–393.

Lumeij, J.T., Westerhof, I., Smit, T. & Spierenburg, T.J. (1993) Diagnosis and treatment of poisoning in raptors from the Netherlands: clinical case reports and review of 2750 post-mortem cases, 1975–1988. In: *Raptor Biomedicine* (eds P.T. Redig, J.E. Cooper, J.D. Remple & D.B. Hunter). University of Minnesota Press, USA.

Lyal, Ch.H.C. (1985) Phylogeny and classification of the Psododea with particular reference to the lice (Psocodea: Phthiraptera). *Systematic Entomology and Systematics*, **10**, 145–165.

Macdonald, A.A. & Charlton, N. (1999) *A Bibliography of References to Husbandry and Veterinary Guidelines for Animals in Zoological Collections.* Federation of Zoological Gardens of Great Britain and Ireland, London, UK.

Macdonald, D. & Linzey, A. (1996) Study and be damned? *BBC Wildlife*, 1996, 64–67.

Macdonald, J.W. (1962) Mortality in wild birds with some observations on weights. *Bird Study*, **9**, 147–167.

Macdonald, J.W. (1963) Mortality in wild birds. *Bird Study*, **10**, 91–108.

Macdonald, J.W., Randall, C.J., Moon, G.M. & Ruthven, A.D. (1983) Lead poisoning in captive birds of prey. *Veterinary Record*, **113**, 65–66.

MacGillivray, W. (1836) *Descriptions of the Rapacious Birds of Great Britain.* MacLachlan & Stewart, Edinburgh, UK.

MacLaren, N.E., Krohne, S.G., Porter, R.E., Ringle, M.J. & Lindley, D.M. (1995) *Corynebacterium* endophthalmitis, glaucoma, and scleral ossicle osteomyelitis in a great horned owl (*Bubo virginianus*). *Journal of Zoo and Wildlife Medicine*, **26**(3), 453–459.

MacPhail, R.M. (1964) A goshawk's death attributed to carbon monoxide poisoning. *The Falconer*, **IV**, 174–175.

Magalhaes, A.M. de, Ramadinha, R.R., Peixoto, P.V. & de Barros, C.S.L. (2000) (Abstract) Comparative study between cytology and histopathology in diagnosis of canine neoplasms. *Veterinary Dermatology*, **II**(Suppl 1), 41–61.

Magnino, S., Fabbi, M. & Moreno, A. (2000) Avian influenza virus (H7 serotype) in a saker falcon in Italy. *Veterinary Record*, **146**, 740.

Malley, A.D. & Whitbread, T.J. (1996) The integument. In: *Manual of Raptors, Pigeons and Waterfowl* (eds P.H. Beynon, N.A. Forbes & N.H. Harcourt-Brown). British Small Animal Veterinary Association, Cheltenham, UK.

Maloney, S.K. & Gray, D.A. (1998) Characteristics of the febrile response in Pekin ducks. *Journal of Comparative Physiology B*, **168**, 177–182.

Manilla, G. (1985) On the role of birds in the spread and circulation of tick-borne viruses. *Rivista di Parassitologia*, **II**(XLVI), 11–25.

Manuwal, D.A. (1967) Observations on a localised duck sickness in the Delta Marsh; summer 1964. *Wilson Bulletin*, **79**, 219–222.

Manvell, R.J., Wenery, U., Alexander, D.J. & Frost, K.M. (2000) Newcastle disease (PMVI) viruses in raptors. In: *Raptor Biomedicine III* (eds J.T. Lumeij, J.D. Remple, P.T. Redig, M. Lierz & J.E. Cooper). Zoological Education Network, Lake Worth, FL, USA.

Markham, G. (1631) *Country Contentments or, the Husbandmans Recreations.* London.

Markham, G. (1655) *Hungers Prevention: or the whole Art of Fowling by Water and Land.* London.

Marks, J. & Birn, K.J. (1963) Infection due to *Mycobacterium avium. British Medical Journal*, **ii**, 1503–1506.

Markus, M.B. (1974) Arthropod-borne disease as a potential factor limiting the distribution of birds. *International Journal of Parasitology*, **4**, 609–612.

Markus, M.B. & Oosthuizen, J.H. (1972) Pathogenicity of *Haemoproteus columbae. Transactions of the Royal Society of Tropical Medicine and Hygiene*, **66**, 186–187.

Marshall, A.J. (1960) *Biology and Comparative Physiology of Birds.* Academic Press, New York, USA.

Martell, M.S., Goggin, J. & Redig, P.T. (2000) Assessing rehabilitation success of raptors through band returns. In: *Raptor Biomedicine III* (eds J.T. Lumeij, J.D. Remple, P.T. Redig, M. Lierz & J.E. Cooper). Zoological Education Network, Lake Worth, FL, USA.

Martin, G.R. & Gordon, I.E. (1974a) Increment-threshold spectral sensitivity in the tawny owl (*Strix aluco*). *Vision Research*, **14**, 615–621.

Martin, G.R. & Gordon, I.E. (1974b) Visual acuity in the tawny owl (*Strix aluco*). *Vision Research*, **14**, 1393–1397.

Martin, G.R., Gordon, I.E. & Cadle, D.R. (1975) Electroretinographically determined spectral sensitivity in the tawny owl (*Strix aluco*). *Journal of Comparative and Physiological Psychology*, **89**, 72–78.

Martin, H.D., Ringdahl, C. & Scherpelz, J. (1993) Physical therapy for specific injuries in raptors. In: *Raptor Biomedicine* (eds P.T. Redig, J.E. Cooper, J.D. Remple & D.B. Hunter). University of Minnesota Press, USA.

Marzluff, J.M., Vekasy, M.S., Kochert, M.N. & Steenhoff, K. (1997) Productivity of golden eagles wearing backpack radiotransmitters. *Journal of Raptor Research*, **31**(3), 223–227.

Maschek, S. (1997) *Studies of heavy metal toxification in predatory birds, and multi-element analyses using neutron activation analyses in feathers.* Dissertation, University of Munich, Germany.

Maschek, S., Grimm, F. & Waschkowski, W. (1998) Studies of heavy metal toxification in predatory birds and multi-element analyses using neutron activation analyses in feathers. *XI.DVG-Tagung über Vogelkrankheiten, München*, 296–305.

Matthews, P.J.R. & McDiarmid, A. (1977) *Mycobacterium avium* infection in free-living hedgehogs (*Erinaceus europaeus*). *Research in Veterinary Science*, **22**, 388.

Mavrogordato, J.G. (1960) *A Hawk for the Bush*, 1st edn. F H & G Witherby, London, 2nd edn (1973). Neville Spearman, London, UK.

Mavrogordato, J.G. (1966) *A Falcon in the Field.* Knightly Vernon, London, UK.

Mawson, P.M. (1977) The genus *Microtetrameres* Travassos (Nematoda, Spirurida) in Australian birds. *Records of the South Australian Museum*, **17**(14), 239–259.

May, R.M. (1988) Conservation and disease. *Conservation Biology*, **2**, 28–30.

May, R.M. & Anderson, R.M. (1978) Regulation and stability of host–parasite interactions. II. Destabilising processes. *Journal of Animal Ecology*, **47**, 249–267.

McDermott, M. (1998) *The Imprint Accipiter*. Michael McDermott, Missouri, USA.

McDiarmid, A. (1948) The occurrence of tuberculosis in the wild wood-pigeon. *Journal of Comparative Pathology*, **58**, 128–133.

McDonald, M.E. (1969) *Catalogue of helminths of waterfowl (Anatidae)*. U.S. Bureau of Sport Fisheries and Wildlife Special Science Report, Washington DC, USA.

McDowell, E.M. & Trump, B.F. (1977) Practical fixation techniques for light and electron microscopy. *Comparative Pathology Bulletin*, **IX**, 1 and 4.

McFarland, D.C., Kenzy, S.G. & Coon, C.N. (1979) Research note – a micro-method for plasma uric acid determinations in companion birds. *Avian Diseases*, **23**, 772–774.

McGeown, D., Danbury, T.C., Waterman-Pearson, A.E. & Kestin, S.C. (1999) Effect of carprofen on lameness in broiler chickens. *Veterinary Record*, **144**, 668–671.

McGowan, C. (1991) *Dinosaurs, Spitfires and Sea Dragons*. Harvard, Cambridge, MA, USA.

McGowan, C. (1999) *A Practical Guide to Vertebrate Mechanics*. Cambridge University Press, UK.

McKean, J.D. (1993) Legal issues affecting veterinary practice. *The Veterinary Clinics of North America*, **23**(5), 1061–1070.

McKeever, K. (1987) *Care and Rehabilitation of Injured Owls*, 4th edn. W.F. Rannie, Ontario, Canada.

McKinney, P. (2000) Amyloidosis in falcons in the United Arab Emirates. *Falco*, **16**, 18.

The Royal Society (1999) *Complementary and Alternative Medicine. Response to the House of Lords*. The Royal Society, London, UK.

McOrist, S. (1989) Some diseases of free-living Australian birds. In: *Disease and Threatened Birds* (ed. J.E. Cooper). International Council for Bird Preservation, Cambridge, UK.

McOrist, S., Black, D.G., Pass, D.A., Scott, P.C. & Marshall, J. (1984) Beak and feather dystrophy in wild sulphur-crested cockatoos (*Cacatua galerita*). *Journal of Wildlife Diseases*, **2**, 120–124.

Mead, G.C. (2000) Prospects for 'competitive exclusion' treatment to control salmonellas and other food borne in pathogens in poultry. *Veterinary Journal*, **159**, 111–123.

Mearns, R. (1983) Breeding peregrines oiled by fulmars. *Bird Study*, **30**, 243–244.

MEFRG (undated) *Microchips and their uses in monitoring movements of sakers and peregrines in Asia and the Middle East*. Middle East Falcon Research Group, Abu Dhabi, UAE.

Meister, B. (1981) *Untersuchungen zur Alimentären Bleivergiftung bei Greifvögeln*. Inaugural dissertation, Universität zu Giessen, Germany.

Mendelsohn, J.M., Butler, A.C. & Sibbald, R.R. (1988) Organochlorine residues and eggshell thinning in Southern African raptors. In: *Peregrine Falcon Populations: Their Management and Recovery* (eds T.J. Cade, J.H. Enderson, C.G. Thelander & C.M. White), pp. 439–447. The Peregrine Fund Inc., Boise, ID, USA.

Mendelssohn, H. & Marder, U. (1970) Problems of reproduction in birds of prey in captivity. *International Zoo Yearbook*, **10**, 6–11.

Mendenhall, V.M. & Pank, L.F. (1980) Secondary poisoning of owls by anticoagulant rodenticides. *Wildlife Society Bulletin*, **8**, 311–315.

Mesa, C.P., Stabler, R.M. & Berthrong, M. (1961) Histopathological changes in the domestic pigeon infected with *Trichomonas gallinae* (Jones' Barn Strain). *Avian Diseases*, **5**, 48–60.

Meurer, J. (1991) *Die Pocken der Vögel: Atiologie, Wirtsspektrum und Epizootiologie. Eine veterinärhistorische Studie*. Inaugural dissertation, Justus Liebig Universität, Giessen, Germany.

Mey, E. (1997) Leben auf dem Riesenseeadler *Haliaeetus pelagicus* zwei *Degeeriella*-Arten (Insecta, Phthiraptera, Ischnocera)? Mit Anmerkungen zur Biographie Georg Wilhelm Stellers. *Ornithologischer Anzeiger* **36**, 1–18.

Mey, E. (1998) Über den Artbegriff bei Mallophagen (Insecta: Phthiraptera). *Zoologische Abhandlungen Staatliches Museum für Tierkunde Dresden* **50** (Suppl.): 77–85.

Mey, E. (2000) A new genus and species of Ischnocera (Insecta, Phthiraptera) of Chimango Caracara *Milvago chimango* from Chile with annotated checklist of chewing lice parasitizing caracaras (Aves, Falconiformes, Falconidae). *Rudolstädter Naturhistorische Schriften* **10**, 59–73.

Mey, E. (2001) A new *Craspedorrhynchus* species (Phthiraptera, Ischnocera) from Australia, with an annotated checklist of the chewing louse genus. Mitteilungen des Museums für Naturkunde Berlin, Deutsche *Entomologische Zeitschrift* **48**, 117–132.

Meyer, E.A. & Jarrell, E.L. (1982) Giardiasis. *CRC Handbook Series in Zoonoses*, Volume 1, Section 3. CRC Press, Boca Raton, FL, USA.

Michell, E.B. (1900) *The Art and Practice of Hawking*. The Holland Press, London, UK.

van Miert, A.S.J.P.A.M., van Gogh, J. & Wit, J.G. (1976) The influence of pyrogen induced fever on absorption of sulpha drugs. *Veterinary Record*, **99**, 480–481.

Mikaelian, I., Paillet, I. & Williams, D.L. (1994) Comparative use of various mydriatic drugs in kestrels (*Falco tinnunculus*). *American Journal of Veterinary Research*, **55**, 270–277.

Miller, K.J.G., Converse, K.A. & Thomas, N.J. (1998) Unexplained neurologic disease in bald eagles in Southwestern Arkansas and American coots in Arkansas, North Carolina and Georgia. *1998 Proceedings of the American Association of Zoo Veterinarians and the American Association of Wildlife Veterinarians Joint Conference*, Omaha, Nebraska, USA.

Miller, M.J.R., Ewins, P.J. & Galloway, T.D. (1997) Records of ectoparasites collected on ospreys from Ontario. *Journal of Wildlife Diseases*, **33**(2), 373–376.

Miller, M.J.R., Wayland, M.E., Dzua, E.H. & Bortolotti, G.R. (2000) Availability and ingestion of lead shot shell pellets by migrant bald eagles in Saskatchewan. *Journal of Raptor Research*, **34**(3), 167–174.

Miller, T.A. (1984) Nebulization for avian respiratory disease. *Carnation Research Digest*, 7–8.

Miller-Mundy, A. (1984) Hawking in the Hebrides. *The Falconer*, 47–51.

Mineau, P., Fletcher, M.R., Glaser, L.C., *et al.* (1999) Poisoning of raptors with organophosphorus and carbamate pesticides with emphasis on Canada, the United States and the United Kingdom. *Raptor Research*, **33**, 1–37.

Minnemann, D. & Busse, H. (1983) Longevity of birds of prey and owls at East Berlin Zoo. *International Zoo Yearbook*, **23**, 108–110.

Mirande, L.A., Howerth, E.W. & Poston, R.P. (1992) Chlamydiosis in a red-tailed hawk (*Buteo jamaicensis*). *Journal of Wildlife Diseases*, **28**, 284–287.

Moiseff, A. & Konishi, M. (1981) Neuronal and behavioural sensitivity to binaural time differences in the owl. *Journal of Neuroscience*, **1**, 40–48.

Møller, A.P. (1989) Parasites, predators and nest boxes: facts and artifacts in nest box studies of birds. *Oikos*, **56**, 421–423.

Möller, D. (1976) Arabic treatises on falconry. *Paper presented at the International Conference on Falconry and Conservation, Abu Dhabi*, 10–18 December, 1976.

Montgomery, R.D., Stein, G., Stotts, V.D. & Settle, F.H. (1979) The 1978 epornitic of avian cholera on the Chesapeake Bay. *Avian Diseases*, **23**, 966–978.

Moore, L.G. & Ronniger, P.A. (1966) Raptorial foot disease. *Journal of the North American Falconers' Association*, **V**, 29–37.

Morishita, T.Y., Lowenstine, L.J., Hirsh, D.C. & Brooks, D.L. (1997) Lesions associated with *Pasteurella multocida* infection in raptors. *Avian Diseases*, **41**, 203–213.

Morishita, T.Y., McFadzen, M.E., Mchan, R., *et al.*

(1998) Serologic survey of free-living nestling prairie falcons (*Falco mexicanus*) for selected pathogens. *Journal of Zoo and Wildlife Medicine*, **29**, 18–20.

Morris, T. (2000) Anaesthesia in the fourth dimension. Is biological scaling relevant to veterinary anaesthesia? *Veterinary Anaesthesia and Analgesia*, **27**, 2–5.

Morrow, T.L. & Glover, F.A. (undated) *Experimental studies on post-mortem changes in mallards*. Special Scientific Report Wildlife No. 134, Bureau of Sport Fisheries and Wildlife, Washington DC, USA.

Mosher, J.A. (1976) Raptor energetics; a review. *Raptor Research*, **10**, 97–107.

Müller, M.G., Wernery U. & Kösters, J. (2000) Bumblefoot and lack of exercise among wild and captive-bred falcons tested in the United Arab Emirates. *Avian Diseases*, **44**, 676–680.

Mumcuoglu, Y. & Müller, R. (1974) Parasitische Milben und Würmer als Todesursache eines Unus *Bubo bubo*. *Der Ornithologische Beobachter*, **71**, 289–292.

Munday, B.L. (1977) A species of *Sarcocystis* using owls as definitive host. *Journal of Wildlife Diseases*, **13**, 205–207.

Mundy, P. (1982) *The Comparative Biology of Southern African Vultures*. Vulture Study Group, Johannesburg, SA.

Mundy, P.J. & Foggin, C.M. (1981) Epileptiform seizures in captive African vultures. *Journal of Wildlife Diseases*, **17**, 259–265.

Mundy, P.J. & Ledger, J.A. (1976) Griffon vultures, carnivores and bones. *South African Journal of Science*, **72**, 106–110.

Munger, L.L. & McGavin, M.D. (1972a) Sequential post-mortem changes in chicken liver at 4°, 20° or 37°C. *Avian Diseases*, **16**, 587–605.

Munger, L.L. & McGavin, M.D. (1972b) Sequential post-mortem changes in chicken kidney at 4°, 20° or 37°C. *Avian Diseases*, **16**, 606–621.

Munoz, E., Molina, R. & Ferrer, D. (1999) *Babesia shortti* infection in a common kestrel (*Falco tinnunculus*) in Catalonia (north eastern Spain). *Avian Pathology*, **28**, 207–209.

Murnane, R.D., Meerdink, G., Rideout, B.A. & Anderson, M.P. (1995) Ethylene glycol toxicosis in a captive-bred released California condor (*Gymnogyps californianus*). *Journal of Zoo and Wildlife Medicine*, **26**(2), 306–310.

Murphy, C.J. (1993) Ocular lesions in birds of prey. In: *Zoo and Wild Animal Medicine, Current Therapy 3* (ed. M.E. Fowler). W.B. Saunders, PA, USA.

Murphy, C.J., Brooks, D.E., Kern, T.J. & Quesenberry, K.E. (1983) Enucleation in birds of prey. *Journal of the*

American Veterinary Medical Association, **183**, 1234–1237.

Murphy, C.J., Kern, T.J. & MacCoy, D.M. (1981) Bilateral keratopathy in a barred owl. *Journal of the American Veterinary Medical Association*, **179**, 1271–1273.

Murphy, C.J., Kern, T.J., McKeever, L. & MacCoy, D. (1982) Ocular lesions in free-living raptors. *Journal of the American Veterinary Medical Association*, **181**, 1302–1304.

Murray, M.J. & Taylor, M. (1999) Avian renal disease endoscopic applications. *Seminars in Avian and Exotic Pet Medicine*, **8**(3), 115–121.

Murza, G.L., Bortolotti, G.R. & Dawson, R.D. (2000) Handicapped American kestrels: needy or prudent foragers? *Journal of Raptor Research*, **34**(2), 137–142.

Mutlow, A. & Forbes, N. (2000) *Haemoproteus* in raptors: pathogenicity, treatment and control. *Proceedings of the Association of Avian Veterinarians*, 157–163.

Nair, M.K. (1973) The early inflammatory reaction in the fowl. *Acta Veterinaria Scandinavica Supplementum*, **42**, 1–103.

Naldo, J.L. & Samour, J.H. (2001) Ammonium chloride toxicosis: a major cause of mortality in captive saker falcons during a hunting expedition to Pakistan. *Falco*, **17**, 14–15.

Naoroji, R. (1997) Contamination in egg shells of Himalayan greyheaded eagle *Ichthyophaga nana plumbea* in Corbett National Park, India. *Journal of the Bombay Natural History Society*, **94**, 398–400.

Needham, J.R. (1974) A study of the coagulase and deoxyribonuclease tests applied to staphylococci from non-human sources. *Medical Laboratory Technology*, **31**, 141–143.

Needham, J.R. (1977) The collection of animal faeces for laboratory examination. *Journal of the Institute of Animal Technicians*, **28**, 63–66.

Needham, J.R., Kirkwood, J.K. & Cooper, J.E. (1979) A survey of the aerobic bacteria in the droppings of captive birds of prey. *Research in Veterinary Science*, **27**, 125–126.

Nelson, M.W. & Nelson, P. (1976) Power lines and birds of prey. *Idaho Wildlife Review*, March–April 1976, 1–5.

Nelson, N., Elgart, S. & Mirsky, I.A. (1942) Pancreatic diabetes in the owl. *Endocrinology*, **31**, 119–123.

Nero, R.W. & Loch, S.L. (1984) Vestigial wing claws on great gray owls, *Strix nebulosa*. *Canadian Field-Naturalist*, **98**, 45–46.

Nettles, V.F. (1992) Wildlife diseases and population medicine. *Journal of the American Veterinary Medical Association*, **200**, 648–652.

Newton, C.D. & Zeitlin, S. (1977) Avian fracture healing. *Journal of the American Veterinary Medical Association*, **170**, 620–625.

Newton, I. (1976) Raptor research and conservation during the last five years. *Canadian Field-Naturalist*, **90**, 225–227.

Newton, I. (1979) *Population Ecology of Raptors*. Poyser, Berkhamsted, UK.

Newton, I. (1980) The role of food in limiting bird numbers. *Ardea*, **68**, 11–30.

Newton, I. (1986) *The Sparrowhawk*. T & AD Poyser, London, UK.

Newton, I. (1992) Experiments on the limitation of bird numbers by territorial behaviour. *Biological Reviews*, **67**, 129–173.

Newton, I. (1998) *Population Limitation in Birds*. Academic Press, London, UK.

Newton, I. & Bogan, J. (1974) Organochlorine residues, eggshell thinning and hatching success in British sparrowhawks. *Nature*, **249**, 582–583.

Newton, I. & Haas, M.B. (1988) Pollutants in Merlin eggs and their effects on breeding. *British Birds*, **81**, 258–269.

Newton, I. & Olsen, P. (1990) *Birds of Prey*. Merehurst Press, London, UK.

Newton, I. & Wyllie, I. (1992) Effects of new rodenticides on owls. In: *The Ecology and Conservation of European Owls* (eds C.A. Galbraith, I.R. Taylor & S. Percival), UK Nature Conservation Number 5. Peterborough, UK.

Newton, I., Dale, L. & Little, B. (1999a) Trends in organochlorine and mercurial compounds in the eggs of British merlins, *Falco columbarius*. *Bird Study*, **46**, 356–362.

Newton, I., Wyllie, I. & Asher, A. (1991) Mortality causes in British Barn Owls *Tyto alba*, with a discussion of aldrin–dieldrin poisoning. *Ibis*, **133**, 162–169.

Newton, I., Wyllie, I. & Asher, A. (1993) Long-term trends in organochlorine and mercury residues in some predatory birds in Britain. *Environmental Pollution*, **79**, 143–151.

Newton, I., Wyllie, I. & Dale, L. (1997) Mortality causes in British barn owls (*Tyto alba*), based on 1101 carcasses examined during 1963–1996. In: *Biology and Conservation of Owls of the Northern Hemisphere* (eds J.R. Duncan, D.H. Johnson & T.H. Nicholls). Second International Symposium, US Department of Agriculture, MN, USA.

Newton, I., Wyllie, I. & Dale, L. (1999b) Trends in the numbers and mortality patterns of sparrowhawks (*Accipter nisus*) and kestrels (*Falco tinnunculus*) in

Britain, as revealed by carcass analyses. *Journal of Zoology*, London, **248**, 139–147.

van Nie, G.J. (1975) Mogelijke chloralose vergiftiging bij buizerds. *Tijdschrift voor Diergeneeskunde*, **100**, 1052–1053.

van Nie, G.J., Lumeij, J.T., Dorrestein, G.M., Wolvekam, W.Th.C., Zwart, P. & Stam, J.W.E. (1982) Tuberculosis in raptorial birds. Clinical cases and differential diagnosis. *Tijdschrift voor Diergeneeskunde*, **107**, 563–572.

Norberg, R.A. (1977) Occurrence and independent evolution of bilateral ear asymmetry in owls and implications on owl taxonomy. *Philosophical Transactions of the Royal Society, Series B*, Vol. 280, Number 973.

Norris-Caneda, K.H. & Elliott, J.D. (1998) Sex identification in raptors using PCR. *Journal of Raptor Research*, **32**, 278–280.

Nottebohm, F. (1989) From bird songs to neurogenesis. *Scientific American*, February, 56–61.

Nunn, G.L., Klem, D., Kimmel, T. & Merriman, T. (1976) Surplus killing and caching by American kestrels (*Falco sparverius*). *Animal Behaviour*, **24**, 759–763.

Nygård, T. & Skaare, J.U. (1998) Organochlorines and mercury in eggs of White-tailed Sea Eagles *Haliaeetus albicilla* in Norway 1974–1994. *Proceedings of the World Working Group on Birds of Prey (WWGBP) Conference on Holarctic Birds of Prey*, Badajoz, 1995, pp. 501–524.

Oaks, J.L. (1993) Immune and inflammatory responses in falcon staphylococcal pododermatitis. In: *Raptor Biomedicine* (eds P.T. Redig, J.E. Cooper, J.D. Remple & D.B. Hunter). University of Minnesota Press, USA.

O'Brien, S.J. & Evermann, J.F. (1988) Interactive influence of infectious disease and genetic diversity in natural populations. *Trends in Ecology and Evolution*, **3**, 253–259.

Odening, K. (1967) Die Lebenszyklen von *Strigea falconispalumbi* Viborg, *S. strigis* uns *S. sphaerula* (Rudolphi) (Trematoda, Strigeida) im Raum Berlin. *Zoologische Jahrbücher Abteilung für Systematik, Oekologie und Geographie der Tiere*, **94**, 1–67.

Odening, K. (1969) Obligate und additionale Wirte der Helminthen. *Angewandte Parasitologie*, **10**(1), 21–36.

Odening, K. (1998) The present state of species-systematics in *Sarcocystis* Lankester, 1882 (Protista, Sporozoa, Coccidia). *Systematic Parasitology*, **41**, 209–233.

O'Donnell, J.A., Garbett, R. & Morzenti, A. (1978) Normal fasting plasma glucose levels in some birds of prey. *Journal of Wildlife Diseases*, **14**, 479–481.

Oelgart, I.J. (1976) *Falconry and Hawking Treatises Printed in the English Language*. New Mews Press, Newburyport, MA, USA.

Ogilvie, M. (1998) Rare breeding birds in the United Kingdom in 1995. *British Birds*, **91**, 417–447.

O.I.E. (1991) *Animals, Pathogens and the Environment* (Animaux, pathologie et environment) Office International des Epizooties Scientific and Technical Review **10**(3).

O.I.E. (1996) *Manual of Standards for Diagnostic Tests and Vaccines*. Office International des Epizooties, Paris, France.

Okoniewski, J.C. & Novesky, E. (1993) Bird poisoning with cyclodienes in suburbs: links to historic use on turf. *Journal of Wildlife Management*, **57**, 630–639.

Okumura, J. & Tasaki, I. (1969) Effect of fasting, refeeding and dietary protein levels on uric acid and ammonia content of blood, liver and kidney in chickens. *Journal of Nutrition*, **97**, 316–320.

Olney, P., Schmidt, C.R. & Lint, K.C. (1970) Longevity of birds of prey and owls in captivity. *International Zoo Yearbook*, **10**, 36–37.

Olsen, J. (1990) *Caring for Birds of Prey*. Springfield, CA, USA.

Orcutt, C. (2000) Vascular access ports in exotic animals. *Proceedings of Autumn Meeting of the British Veterinary Zoological Society*, 27–29.

Oring, I.W. (1988) Ornithological guidelines for the use of wild birds in research. In: *Field Research Guidelines* (ed. F.B. Orlans). Scientists' Center for Animal Welfare, Bethesda, MA, USA.

Orosz, S., Ensley, P.K. & Haynes, C.J. (1992) *Avian Surgical Anatomy. Thoracic and Pelvic Limbs*. W.B. Saunders, PA, USA.

Orosz, S.E. (2000) Overview of aspergillosis: pathogenesis and treatment options. *Seminars in Avian and Exotic Pet Medicine*, **9**(2), 59–65.

Osche, G. (1955) Über Entwicklung, Zwischenwirt und Bau von *Porrocaecum talpae, Porrocaecum ensicaudatum* und *Habronema mansioni* (Nematoda). *Zeitschrift für Parasitenkunde*, **17**, 144–164.

Owen, M. & Cook, W.A. (1977) Variations in body weight, wing length and condition of mallard *Anas platyrhynchos platyrhynchos* and their relationship to environmental changes. *Journal of Zoology, London*, **183**, 377–395.

Pain, D.J. & Amiard-Triquet, C. (1993) Lead poisoning in raptors in France and elsewhere. *Ecotoxicology and Environmental Safety*, **25**, 183–192.

Pain, D.J., Amiard-Triquet, C., Bavoux, C., Burneleau, G., Eon, L. & Nicolau-Guillaumet, P. (1993) Lead poisoning in wild populations of Marsh harriers *Circus aeruginosus* in the Camargue and Charente-Maritime, France. *Ibis*, **135**, 379–386.

Pain, D.J., Sears, J. & Newton, I. (1995) Lead concentrations in birds of prey in Britain. *Environmental Pollution*, **87**, 173–180.

Palmer, A.C. (1976) *Introduction to Animal Neurology.* Blackwell, Oxford, UK.

Palomeque, J. & Planas, J. (1977) Dimensions of the erythrocytes of birds. *Ibis*, **119**, 533–535.

Papazahariadou, M.G., Georgiades, G.K., Komnenou, A.Th. & Ganoti, M. (2001) *Caryospora* species in a snowy owl (*Nyctea scandiaca*). *Veterinary Record*, **148**, 54–55.

Parkes, A.S. & Selye, H. (1937) The endocrine system and plumage types. I. Some effects of hypothyroidism. *Journal of Genetics*, **XXXIV**, 297–306.

Parrott, T. (1991) Clinical treatment regimes with fluconazole. *Proceedings of the Annual Meeting of the Association of Avian Veterinarians*, Chicago, IL, USA.

Parry-Jones, J. (2001) Report on the International Seminar on the Indian vulture situation September 2000. *Falco*, **17**, 12–13.

Parsons, Å.J. (1974) Condition of imported birds. *Veterinary Record*, **95**, 155.

Patt, D.I. & Patt, G.R. (1969) *Comparative Vertebrate Histology.* Harper & Row, New York, USA.

Pattee, O.H. & Franson, J.C. (1982) Short-term effects of oil ingestion on American kestrels (*Falco sparverius*). *Journal of Wildlife Diseases*, **18**, 235–241.

Pattee, O.H., Mattox, W.G. & Seegar, W.S. (1984) Twin embryos in a peregrine falcon egg. *The Condor*, **86**, 352–353.

Pattee, O.H., Wiemeyer, S.N., Mulhern, B.M., Sileo, L. & Carpenter, J.W. (1981) Experimental lead-shot poisoning in bald eagles. *Journal of Wildlife Management*, **45**, 806–810.

Paul-Murphy, J. & Ludders, J.W. (2001) Avian analgesia. *Veterinary Clinics of North America: Exotic Animal Practice*, **4**(1), 35–45.

Paulus, A. & Van Den Abeele, B. (2000) *Bibliotheca Cynegetica I.* Translation into French of the treatise *De Arte Venandi cum Avibus* by Frederick II of Hohenstaufen. Jacques Laget, Nogent-le-Roi, France.

Payne, D.N., Gibson, S.A.W. & Lewis, R. (1998) Antiseptics: a forgotten weapon in the control of antibiotic resistant bacteria in hospital and community settings? *Journal of Royal Society of Health*, **118**, 18–22.

Payne R.B. (1962) How the barn owl locates prey by hearing. *Living Bird*, 151–159.

Peakall, D.B. (1976) The peregrine falcon (*Falco peregri-*

nus) and pesticides. *Canadian Field-Naturalist*, **90**, 301–307.

Peakall, D.B. (1987) Toxicology. In: *Raptor Management Techniques* (eds B.A.G. Pendleton, B.A. Millsap, K.W. Cline & D.M. Bird). National Wildlife Federation, Washington DC, USA.

Peakall, D.B. (1993) DDE-induced eggshell thinning: an environmental detective story. *Environmental Reviews*, **1**, 13–20.

Peakall, D.B. (1996) Dieldrin and other cyclodiene pesticides in wildlife. In: *Environmental Contaminants in Wildlife* (eds W.N. Beyer, G.H. Heinz & A.W. Redmon-Norwood), pp. 73–98. Lewis Publishers, Boca Raton, FL, USA.

Peakall, D.B. & Carter, N. (1997) Decreases in farmland birds and agricultural practices; a huge ecotoxicological experiment. *Toxicology and Environmental News*, **4**, 162–163.

Peakall, D.B. & Kiff, L.F. (1988) DDE contamination in Peregrines and American Kestrels and its effect on reproduction. In: *Peregrine Falcon Populations: Their Management and Recovery* (eds T.J. Cade, J.H. Enderson, C.G. Thelander & C.M. White). The Peregrine Fund Inc., Boise, ID, USA.

Pearson, R. (1972) *The Avian Brain.* Academic Press, New York and London.

Peckham, M.C. (1972) Poisons and toxins. In: *Diseases of Poultry* (eds M.S. Hofstad *et al.*). Iowa State University Press, USA.

Peckham, M.C. (1975) Herpesviruses of pigeons, owls and falcons. In: *Isolation and Identification of Avian Pathogens* (eds S.B. Hitchner *et al.*). American Association of Avian Pathologists, Texas A & M University, USA.

Peirce, M.A. (1979) Some additional observations on haematozoa of birds in the Mascarene islands. *Bulletin of the British Ornithologists Club*, **99**, 68–71.

Peirce, M.A. (1981) Current knowledge of the haematozoa of raptors. In: *Recent Advances in the Study of Raptor Diseases* (eds J.E. Cooper & A.G. Greenwood). Chiron Publications, Keighley, Yorkshire, UK.

Peirce, M.A. (1989) The significance of avian haematozoa in conservation strategies. In: *Diseases and Threatened Birds* (ed. J.E. Cooper). International Council for Bird Preservation, Technical Publication, No. 10, Cambridge, UK.

Peirce, M.A. & Cooper, J.E. (1977a) Haematozoa of birds of prey in Great Britain. *Veterinary Record*, **100**, 493.

Peirce, M.A. & Cooper, J.E. (1977b) Haematozoa of East African birds. V. Blood parasites of birds of prey. *East African Wildlife Journal*, **15**, 213–216.

Peirce, M.A. & Mead, C.J. (1977) Haematozoa of British birds. II. Blood parasites of birds from Hertfordshire. *Journal of Natural History*, **11**, 597–600.

Peirce, M.A. & Marquiss, M. (1983) Haematozoa of British birds. VII. Haematozoa of raptors in Scotland with a description of *Haemoproteus nisi* sp. nov. from the Sparrowhawk (*Accipiter nisus*). *Journal of Natural History*, **17**, 813–821.

Peirce, M.A., Bennett, G.F. & Bishop, M. (1990) The haemoproteids of the avian order Falconiformes. *Journal of Natural History*, **24**, 1091–1100.

Peirce, M.A., Cheke, A.S. & Cheke, R.A. (1977) A survey of blood parasites of birds in the Mascarene Islands, Indian Ocean, with descriptions of two new species and taxonomic discussions. *Ibis*, **119**, 451–461.

Peirce, M.A., Greenwood, A.G. & Cooper, J.E. (1983) Haematozoa of raptors and other birds from Britain, Spain and the United Arab Emirates. *Avian Pathology*, **12**, 443–446.

Pellérdy, L.P. (1974) *Coccidia and Coccidiosis*. Verlag Paul Parey, Berlin and Hamburg, Germany.

Pence, D.B. & Casto, S.D. (1976) Nasal mites of the subfamily Speleognathinae (Ereynetidae) from birds in Texas, USA. *Journal of Parasitology*, **62**(3), 466–469.

Pendleton, B.A.G., Millsap, B.A., Cline, K.W. & Bird, D.M. (eds) (1987) *Raptor Management Techniques Manual*. National Wildlife Federation, Washington DC, USA.

Pepler, D. & Oettlé, E.E. (1992) *Trichomonas gallinae* in wild raptors on the Cape Peninsula. *South African Journal of Wildlife Research*, **22**(3), 87–88.

Pepperberg, I.M. (1998) Talking with Alex: logic and speech in parrots. In: *Exploring Intelligence – Scientific American*, **9**(4), 60–66.

Pérez, J.M., Extremera, A.L. & Ruiz, I. (1994) Bacteriological study of the feathers and lice of captive common buzzards (*Buteo buteo*). *Avian Pathology*, **23**, 163–168.

Pérez, J.M., Ruiz-Martínez, I. & Cooper, J.E. (1996) Occurrence of chewing lice on Spanish raptors. *Ardeola*, **43**(2), 129–138.

Persson, L. (1974) On the occurrence of endoparasites in Eider Ducks in Sweden. *Swedish Wildlife Research Viltrevy*, **9**, 1.

Petrak, M.L. (ed) (1969) *Diseases of Cage and Aviary Birds*, 1st edn. Lea & Febiger, PA, USA.

Petrak, M.L. (ed) (1982) *Diseases of Cage and Aviary Birds*, 2nd edn. Lea & Febiger, PA, USA.

Petrides, G.A. & Bryant, C.R. (1951) An analysis of the 1949–50 fowl cholera epizootic in Texas Panhandle waterfowl. *Transactions of the North American Wildlife Research Conference*, **16**, 193–216.

Petroli, J.C. (1983) *Control of the field vole*. Report of the Neuchâtel Canton Fishing and Hunting Service, Switzerland.

Philips, J.R. (2000) A review and checklist of the parasitic mites (Acarina) of the Falconiformes and Strigiformes. *Journal of Raptor Research*, **34**(3), 210–231.

Pierson, G.P. & Pfow, C.J. (1975) Newcastle disease surveillance in the United States. *Journal of the American Veterinary Medical Association*, **167**, 801–803.

del Pilar Lanzarot, M., Montesinos, A., San Andres, M.I., Rodfiquez, C. & Barahona, M.V. (2001) Hematological, protein electrophoresis and cholinesterase values of free-living nestling peregrine falcons in Spain. *Journal of Wildlife Diseases*, **37**(1), 172–177.

Pinowski, J., Mazurkiewicz, M., Malyszko, E., Pawiak, R., Kozlowski, S., Kruszewicz, A. & Indykiewicz, P. (1988) The effect of micro-organisms on embryo and nestling mortality in House Sparrow (*Passer domesticus*) and Tree Sparrow (*Passer montanus*). Pp. 273–282 in *Proc. Int. 100. Deutsche Ornithologen-Gesellschaft Meeting, Current Topics Avian Biology Bonn 1988* (eds J. Pinowski & D. Summers-Smith).

Poffers, J. & Lumeij, J.T. (2000) Diseases in birds of prey. A partially annotated bibliography. In: *Raptor Biomedicine III* (eds J.T. Lumeij, J.D. Remple, P.T. Redig, M. Lierz & J.E. Cooper). Zoological Education Network, Lake Worth, FL, USA.

Poiani, A. & Wilks, C. (2000) Sexually transmitted diseases: a possible cost of promiscuity in birds? *The Auk*, **117**(4), 1061–1065.

Pokras, M., Karas, A.M., Kirkwood, J.K. & Sedgwick, C.J. (1993) An introduction to allometric scaling and its uses in raptor medicine. In: *Raptor Biomedicine* (eds P.T. Redig, J.E. Cooper, J.D. Remple & D.B. Hunter). University of Minnesota Press, USA.

Pollack, M.P. (2000) Bald eagle deaths – avian vacuolar myelinopathy in South Eastern USA. *Newsletter of the European Association of Zoo and Wildlife Veterinarians*, **2**, 15.

Porter, R.D. & Wiemeyer, S.N. (1970) Propagation of captive American kestrels. *Journal of Wildlife Management*, **34**, 594–604.

Porter, R.D. & Wiemeyer, S.N. (1972) DDE at low dietary levels kills captive American kestrels. *Bulletin of Environmental Contamination and Toxicology*, **8**, 193–199.

Porter, S. (1993) Pesticide poisoning in birds of prey. In: *Raptor Biomedicine* (eds P.T. Redig, J.E. Cooper, J.D. Remple & D.B. Hunter). University of Minnesota Press, USA.

Prakash, V. (1999) Status of vultures in Keoladeo National

Park, Bharatpur, Rajasthan, with special reference to population crash in *Gyps* species. *Journal of the Bombay Natural History Society*, **96**(3), 365–378.

Premovich, M.S. & Chiasson, R.B. (1976) Reproductive tissue activity in hypothyroid or heat stressed hens. *Poultry Science*, **55**, 906–910.

Prestwich, A.A. (1955) *Records of Birds of Prey Bred in Captivity*, 2nd edn. Arthur A Prestwich, London, UK.

Price, P.W. (1980) *Evolutionary Biology of Parasites.* Princeton University Press, NJ, USA.

Proctor, N.S. & Lynch, P.J. (1993) *Manual of Ornithology, Avian Structure and Function*. Yale University Press, New Haven, CT, USA.

Pugh, G.J.F. (1966) Associations between birds' nests, their pH, and keratinophilic fungi. *Sabouraudia*, **5**, 49–53.

Quandt, J.E. & Greenacre, C.B. (1999) Sevoflurane anesthesia in psittacines. *Journal of Zoo and Wildlife Medicine*, **30**(2), 308–309.

Raffe, M.R., Mammel, M., Gordon, M., Duke, G., Redig, P.T. & Boros, S. (1993) Cardiorespiratory effects of ketamine–xylazine in the great horned owl. In: *Raptor Biomedicine* (eds P.T. Redig, J.E. Cooper, J.D. Remple & D.B. Hunter). University of Minnesota Press, USA.

Raidal, S. & Jaensch, S.M. (2000) Central nervous disease and blindness in Nankeen kestrels (*Falco cenchroides*) due to a novel *Leucocytozoon*-like infection. *Avian Pathology*, **29**, 51–56.

Ralph, R. (1993) *William MacGillivray*. HMSO, London, UK.

Ramis, A., Majó, Pumarola, M., Fondevila, D. & Ferrer, L. (1994) Herpesvirus hepatitis in two eagles in Spain. *Avian Diseases*, **38**, 197–200.

Ramos, F., Zurabian, R., Moran, P., *et al.* (1999) The effect of formalin fixation on the polymerase chain reaction characterization of *Entamoeba histolytica*. *Transactions of the Royal Society of Tropical Medicine and Hygiene*, **93**, 335–336.

Ramsay, E.C. & Grindlinger, H.W. (1992) Treatment of feather picking with chlomipramine. *Proceedings of the Association of Avian Veterinarians Annual Conference*, Lake Worth, FL, USA.

Randall, C.J. & Reece, R.L. (1996) *Color Atlas of Avian Histopathology*. Mosby-Wolfe, London and Baltimore.

Ratcliffe, D.A. (1963) The status of the peregrine in Great Britain. *Bird Study*, **10**, 56–90.

Ratcliffe, D.A. (1965) The peregrine situation in Great Britain, 1963–64. *Bird Study*, **12**, 66–82.

Ratcliffe, D.A. (1967) Decrease in eggshell weight in certain birds of prey. *Nature*, **215**, 208–210.

Ratcliffe, D.A. (1970) Changes attributable to pesticides in egg breakage frequency and eggshell thickness in some birds. *Journal of Applied Ecology*, 7, 67–116.

Ratcliffe, D.A. (1993) *The Peregrine Falcon*, 2nd edn. T & A D Poyser, London, UK.

Raynor, P.L., Kollias, G.V. & Krook, L. (1999) Periosseous xanthogranulomatosis in a fledgling great horned owl (*Bubo virginianus*). *Journal of Avian Medicine and Surgery*, **13**(4), 269–274.

RCVS (2000) *Guide to Professional Conduct 2000.* Royal College of Veterinary Surgeons, London, UK.

Real, J., Mañosa, S. & Muñzo, E. (2000) Trichomoniasis in a Bonelli's eagle population in Spain. *Journal of Wildlife Diseases*, **36**, 64–70.

Redig, P.T. (1978) Raptor rehabilitation: diagnosis, prognosis and moral issues. In: *Bird of Prey Management Techniques* (ed. T.A. Geer), pp. 29–41. British Falconers' Club, Oxford, UK.

Redig, P.T. (1981) Aspergillosis in raptors. In: *Recent Advances in the Study of Raptor Diseases* (eds J.E. Cooper & A.G. Greenwood). Chiron Publications, Keighley, Yorkshire, UK.

Redig, P.T. (1986) Mycotic infections of birds of prey. In: *Zoo and Wild Animal Medicine*, (ed. M.E. Fowler). 2nd edn. W.B. Saunders, PA, USA.

Redig, P.T. (1993a) *Medical Management of Birds of Prey. A Collection of Notes on Selected Topics.* The Raptor Center, University of Minnesota, USA.

Redig, P.T. (1993b) A decade of progress in raptor biomedicine. In: *Raptor Biomedicine* (eds P.T. Redig, J.E. Cooper, J.D. Remple & D.B. Hunter). University of Minnesota Press, USA.

Redig, P.T. (1996a) Nursing avian patients. In: *Manual of Raptors, Pigeons and Waterfowl* (eds P.H. Beynon, N.A. Forbes & N.H. Harcourt-Brown). British Small Animal Veterinary Association, Cheltenham, UK.

Redig, P.T. (1996b) Avian emergencies. In: *Manual of Raptors, Pigeons and Waterfowl* (eds P.H. Beynon, N.A. Forbes & N.H. Harcourt-Brown). British Small Animal Veterinary Association, Cheltenham, UK.

Redig, P.T. (1997) Raptors. In: *Avian Medicine and Surgery* (eds R.B. Altman, S.L. Clubb, G.M. Dorrestein & K. Quesenberry). W.B. Saunders, PA, USA.

Redig, P.T. (2000) The use of an external skeletal fixation – intramedullary pin tie – in (ESF-1M fixation) for treatment of longbone fractures in raptors. In: *Raptor Biomedicine III* (eds J.T. Lumeij, J.D. Remple, P.T. Redig, M. Lierz & J.E. Cooper). Zoological Education Network, Lake Worth, FL, USA.

Redig, P. & Ackermann, J. (2000) Raptors. In: *Avian*

Medicine (eds T.N. Tully, M. Lawton & G.M. Dorrestein). Butterworth-Heinemann, Oxford, UK.

Redig, P.T. & Arendt, T.D. (1982) Relay toxicity of strychnine in raptors in relation to a pigeon eradication program. *Veterinary and Human Toxicology*, **24**, 335–336.

Redig, P.T. & Duke, G.E. (1973) Intravenously administered ketamine HCl and diazepam for anesthesia of raptors. *Journal of the American Veterinary Medical Association*, **169**, 886–888.

Redig, P.T., Cooper, J.E., Remple, J.D. & Hunter, D.B. (eds) (1993) *Raptor Biomedicine*. University of Minnesota, MN, USA.

Redig, P.T., Fuller, M.R. & Evans, D.L. (1980a) Prevalence of *Aspergillus fumigatus* in free-living goshawks (*Accipiter gentilis atricapillus*). *Journal of Wildlife Diseases*, **16**, 169–174.

Redig, P.T., Stowe, C.M. & Barnes, D.M. (1980b) Lead toxicosis in raptors. *Journal of the American Veterinary Medical Association*, **177**, 941–943.

Reed, C.I. & Reed, B.P. (1928) The mechanism of pellet formation in the great horned owl (*Bubo virginianus*). *Science, Washington*, **68**, 359–360.

Rees Davies, R. (2000a) A review of nebulisation as a method of both respiratory antibiotic therapy and fluid support to birds. *Proceedings of Autumn Meeting of the British Veterinary Zoological Society*, 41–43.

Rees Davies, R. (2000b) Acute toxicities in birds. *Proceedings of Autumn Meeting of the British Veterinary Zoological Society*, 46–49.

Rehder, N.B. & Bird, D.M. (1983) Annual profiles of blood packed cell volumes of captive American kestrels. *Canadian Journal of Zoology*, **61**, 2550–2555.

Rehder, N.B., Bird, D.M., Laguë, P.C. & Mackay, C. (1982) Variation in selected hematological parameters of captive red-tailed hawks. *Journal of Wildlife Diseases*, **18**, 105–109.

Reiber, M.A., McInroy, J.A. & Conner, D.E. (1995) Enumeration and identification of bacteria in chicken semen. *Poultry Science*, **74**, 795–799.

Reichel, W.L., Schmeling, S.K., Cromartie, E., *et al.* (1984) Pesticide, PCB, and lead residues and necropsy data for Bald Eagles from 32 states – 1978–81. *Environmental Monitoring and Assessment*, **4**, 395–403.

Reid, H.W. (1975) Experimental infection of Red Grouse with louping-ill virus (flavivirus group). I. The viraemia and antibody response. *Journal of Comparative Pathology*, **85**, 223–229.

Reid, H.W., Duncan, J.S., Phillips, J.D.P., Moss, R. & Watson, A. (1978) Studies of louping ill virus (flavivirus group) in wild Red Grouse (*Lagopus lagopus scoticus*). *Journal of Hygiene*, **81**, 321–329.

Reid, H.W., Moss, R., Pow, I. & Buxton, D. (1980) The response of three grouse species (*Tetrao urogallus, Lagopus mutus, Lagopus lagopus*). *Journal of Comparative Pathology*, **90**, 257–263.

Reidarson, T.H., McBain, J. & Burch, L. (1999) A novel approach to the treatment of bumblefoot in penguins. *Journal of Avian Medicine and Surgery*, **13**(2), 124–127.

Reiser, M.H. & Temple, S.A. (1981) Effects of chronic lead ingestion in birds of prey. In: *Recent Advances in the Study of Raptor Diseases* (eds J.E. Cooper & A.G. Greenwood). Chiron Publications, Keighley, Yorkshire, UK.

Remple, J.D. (1981) Avian malaria with comments on other haemosporidia in large falcons. In: *Recent Advances in the Study of Raptor Diseases* (eds J.E. Cooper & A.G. Greenwood). Chiron Publications, Keighley, Yorkshire, UK.

Remple, J.D. (1993) Raptor bumblefoot: a new treatment technique. In: *Raptor Biomedicine* (eds P.T. Redig, J.E. Cooper, J.D. Remple & D.B. Hunter). University of Minnesota Press, USA.

Remple, J.D. (2000) Considerations on the production of a safe and efficacious falcon herpesvirus vaccine. In: *Raptor Biomedicine III* (eds J.T. Lumeij, J.D. Remple, P.T. Redig, M. Lierz & J.E. Cooper). Zoological Education Network, Lake Worth, FL, USA.

Remple, J.D. (2001) Falcon Herpesvirus vaccine. *Falco*, **17**, 19–20.

Remple, J.D. & Al-Ashbal, A.A. (1993) Raptor bumblefoot: another look at histopathology and pathogenesis. In: *Raptor Biomedicine* (eds P.T. Redig, J.E. Cooper, J.D. Remple & D.B. Hunter). University of Minnesota Press, USA.

Remple, J.D. & Forbes, N.A. (2000) Antibiotic-impregnated polymethyl methacrylate beads in the treatment of bumblefoot in raptors. In: *Raptor Biomedicine III* (eds J.T. Lumeij, J.D. Remple, P.T. Redig, M. Lierz & J.E. Cooper). Zoological Education Network, Lake Worth, FL, USA.

Rewell, R.E. (1950) Report of the Society's Pathologist for the year 1949. *Proceedings of the Zoological Society of London*, **120**, 486–595.

Richard, J.L., Thurston, J.R., Cutlip, R.C. & Peir, A.C. (1982) Vaccination studies of aspergillosis in turkeys: subcutaneous inoculation with several vaccine preparations followed by aerosol challenge exposure. *American Journal of Veterinary Research*, **43**, 488–492.

Richardson, P.R.K., Mundy, P.J. & Plug, I. (1986) Bone

crushing carnivores and their significance to osteodystrophy in griffon vulture chicks. *Journal of Zoology,
London*, **210**, 23–43.

Richter, T. & Gerlach, H. (1981) The bacterial flora of
the nasal mucosa of birds of prey. In: *Recent Advances
in the Study of Raptor Diseases* (eds J.E. Cooper &
A.G. Greenwood). Chiron Publications, Keighley,
Yorkshire, UK.

Riemann, H., Behymer, D., Fowler, M., Ley, D., Schultz,
T., Ruppanner, R. & King, J. (1977) Serological investi-
gation of captive and free living raptors. *Raptor
Research*, **11**, 104–110.

van Riper, C., van Riper, S.G., Goff, M.G. & Laird, M.
(1986) The epizootiology and ecological significance of
malaria in Hawaiian land birds. *Ecological Monographs*,
56, 327–344.

Ristow, E. & Xirouchakis, S. (2000) What is killing
Eleonora's falcons? *World Birdwatch*, **22**(1), 14–15.

Ritchie, B.W. (1995) *Avian Viruses. Function and Control*.
Wingers, Lake Worth, FL, USA.

Ritchie, B.W., Harrison, G.J. & Harrison, L.R. (1994)
Avian Medicine: Principles and Application. Wingers,
Lake Worth, FL, USA.

Robbins, P.K., Tell, L.A., Needham, M.L. & Craigmill,
A.L. (2000) Pharmacokinetics of piperacillin after
intramuscular injection in red-tailed hawks (*Buteo
jamaicensis*) and great horned owls (*Bubo virginianus*).
Journal of Zoo and Wildlife Medicine, **31**(1), 47–51.

Roberts, J.C. & Straus, R. (1965) *Comparative
Atherosclerosis*. Harper & Row, New York and London.

Roberts, V. (2000) *Diseases of Free-Range Poultry*. Whittet
Books, Stowmarket, Suffolk, UK.

Robinson, G. (1999) Correspondence. *The Falconer*,
71.

Robinson, I. (2000) Seabirds. In: *Avian Medicine*
(eds T.N. Tully, M.P.C. Lawton & G.M. Dorrestein).
Butterworth-Heinemann, Oxford, UK.

Robinson, P.T. (1975) Unilateral patagiectomy: a technique for deflighting large birds. *Veterinary
Medicine/Small Animal Clinician*, **70**, 143.

Rocke, T.E. & Brand, C.J. (1994) Use of sentinel mallards for epizootiologic studies of avian botulism.
Journal of Wildlife Diseases, **30**(4), 514–522.

Rogers, L.J. (1997) *Minds of their Own – Thinking and
Awareness in Animals*. Allen & Unwin, Australia.

Rosen, M.N. (1971) Avian cholera. In: *Infectious and
Parasitic Diseases of Wild Birds* (eds J.W. Davis, R.C.
Anderson, L. Karstad & D.O. Trainer). Iowa State
University, USA.

Rosen, M.N. & Bischoff, A. (1949) The 1948–49 outbreak of fowl cholera in birds in the San Francisco Bay

area and surrounding counties. *California Fish and
Game*, **35**, 185–192.

Rosen, M.N. & Morse, E.E. (1972) An interspecies chain
in a fowl cholera epizootic. *California Fish and Game*,
45, 51–56.

Rosskopf, W.J., Woerpel, R.W., Reed, S., Snider, K. &
Dispirito, T. (1992) Anesthetic agents: anesthesia
administration for pet birds. *Veterinary Practice Staff*, **4**,
34.

Rothschild, M. & Clay, T. (1952) *Fleas, Flukes and
Cuckoos*. Collins, London, UK.

Royal Society (1999) *Complementary and Alternative
Medicine: Response to the House of Lords Inquiry into
Complementary and Alternative Medicine*, 18/99. The
Royal Society, London, UK.

Rübel, G.A., Isenbügel, E. & Wolvekamp, P. (1991) *Atlas
of Diagnostic Radiology of Exotic Pets*. Wolfe, London,
UK.

Rupley, A.E. (1998) Critical care. *The Veterinary Clinics of
North America. Exotic Animal Practice*, **1**(1), September 1998. W.B. Saunders, PA, USA.

Rushton, R. & Osgood, D.W. (1993) Physiological monitoring of raptors using an automated biotelemetry
system. In: *Raptor Biomedicine* (eds P.T. Redig, J.E.
Cooper, J.D. Remple & D.B. Hunter). University of
Minnesota Press, USA.

Ryder-Davies, P. (1973) The use of metomidate, an intramuscular narcotic for birds. *Veterinary Record*, **92**,
507–509.

Sabisch, G. von (1977) Ornithose bei einem Mäsebussard
(*Buteo buteo*). *Berliner und Münchener Tierärztliche
Wochenschrift*, **90**, 441–442.

Saito, K., Kurosawa, N. & Shimura, R. (2000) Lead poisoning in white-tailed sea-eagle (*Haliaeetus albicilla*)
and Steller's sea-eagle (*Haliaeetus pelagicus*) in Eastern
Hokkaido through ingestion of lead contaminated carcasses from Sika deer (*Cervus nipon*). In: *Raptor Biomedicine III* (eds J.T. Lumeij, J.D. Remple, P.T. Redig,
M. Lierz & J.E. Cooper). Zoological Education
Network, Lake Worth, FL, USA.

Salvin, F.H. & Brodrick, W. (1855) *Falconry in the British
Isles*. John Van Voorst, London, UK.

Samedov, G.A. (1978) Nematody khishchnykh ptits Azer-
baidzhana (Nematodes of birds of prey of Azerbaijan).
Izvestiya Akademii Nauk Azervaidzhnskoi, SSR, **N5**,
70–73.

Samour, J.H. (1999) Serratospiculiasis in falcons in the
Middle East. *Proceedings of the 5th European Association
of Avian Veterinarians Conference*, Pisa, Italy, 178–182.

Samour, J.H. (2000a) *Avian Medicine*. Mosby, London,
UK.

Samour, J.H. (2000b) Supraorbital trichomonas infection in two saker falcons (*Falco cherrug*). *Veterinary Record*, **146**, 139–140.

Samour, J.H. (2000c) *Pseudomonas aeruginosa* stomatitis as a sequel to trichomoniasis in captive, saker falcons (*Falco cherrug*). *Journal of Avian Medicine and Surgery*, **14**, 113–117.

Samour, J.H. & Cooper, J.E. (1993) Avian pox in birds of prey (Order Falconiformes) in Bahrain. *Veterinary Record*, **132**, 343–345.

Samour, J.H. & D'Aloia, M-A. (1996) Normal blood chemistry of the saker falcon (*Falco cherrug*). *Avian Pathology*, **25**, 175–178.

Samour, J.H. & Naldo, J. (2001) Serratospiculiasis in captive falcons in the Middle East: a review. *Journal of Avian Medicine and Surgery*, **15**, 2–9.

Samour, J.H. & Peirce, M.A. (1996) *Babesia shortti* infection in a saker falcon (*Falco cherrug*). *Veterinary Record*, **139**, 167–168.

Samour, J.H., Bailey, T.A. & Cooper, J.E. (1995a) Trichomoniasis in birds of prey (Order Falconiformes) in Bahrain. *Veterinary Record*, **136**, 358–362.

Samour, J.H., Bailey, T.A. & Keymer, I.F. (1995b) Use of ammonium chloride in falconry in the Middle East. *Veterinary Record*, **137**, 269–270.

Samour, J.H., Jones, D.M., Knight, J.A. & Howlett, J.C. (1984) Comparative studies of the use of some injectable anaesthetic agents in birds. *Veterinary Record*, **115**, 6–11.

Sander, O. (1995) *Untersuchungen über die Herpesvirusinfektion der Greifvögel (Falconiformes und Accipitriformes) sowie vergleich ende Studien an 5 Isolaten aus verschiedenen Griefvögeln*. Inaugural dissertation, Justus Liebig Universität, Giessen, Germany.

Santiago, C., Mills, P.A. & Kirkpatrick, C.E. (1985) Oral capillariasis in a red-tailed hawk: Treatment with fenbendazole. *Journal of the American Veterinary Medical Association*, **187**(11), 1205–1206.

Satterfield, W.C. & O'Rourke, K.I. (1981) Immunological considerations in the management of bumblefoot. In: *Recent Advances in the Study of Raptor Diseases* (eds J.E. Cooper & A.G. Greenwood). Chiron Publications, Keighley, Yorkshire, UK.

Savidge, J.A. (1986) *The Role of Disease and Predation in the Decline of Guam's Avifauna*. Dissertation, University of Illinois, USA.

Sawby, S.W. & Gessaman, J.A. (1974) Telemetry of electrocardiograms from free-living birds: a method of electrode placement. *Condor*, **76**, 479–481.

Schell, S.C. (1953) Four new species of *Microtetrameres* (Nematoda: Spiruroidea) from North American birds.

Transactions of the American Microscopical Society, **72**, 227–236.

Schettler, E., Langgemach, T., Sömner, P., Streich, J. & Frölich, K. (2001) Seroepizootiology of selected infectious disease agents in free-living birds of prey in Germany. *Journal of Wildlife Diseases*, **37**(1), 145–150.

Scheuhammer, A.M. & Norris, S.L. (1996) The ecotoxicology of lead shot and lead fishing weights. *Ecotoxicology*, **5**, 279–295.

Schilling, F., Böttcher, M. & Walter, G. (1981) Probleme des Zeckenbefalls bei Nestlingen des Wanderfalken. *Journal für Ornithologie*, **122**, 359–367.

Schneeganß, D. (1990) Demonstration of paramyxovirus 1 in lammergeyers (*Gypaetus barbatus*). *VII. DVG-Tagung über Vogelkrankheiten München*, 262–269.

Schoenbaum, S. (1975) *William Shakespeare, a Documentary Life*. Clarendon Press, Oxford, UK.

Scholander, P.F., Hock, R., Walters, V. & Irving, L. (1950) Adaptation to cold in Arctic and tropical mammals and birds in relation to body temperature, insulation and basal metabolic rate. *Biological Bulletin*, **99**, 259–271.

Schlumberger, H.G. & Henschke, U.K. (1956) Effect of total body x-irradiation of the parakeet. *Proceedings of the Society for Experimental Biology and Medicine*, **92**, 261–266.

Schoon, H.A., Brunckhorst, D. & Pohlenz, J. (1991) Beitrag zur neuropathologic beim rotha lsstrausse (*Struthio camellus*) – spongiforme enzephalopathie. *Verhand lungs bericht des 33 Internationalen Symposiums über die Erkrankungen der Zoo- und Wilttiere*. Akademie-Verlag, Germany.

Schröder, D. (1992) *Untersuchungen über die Hepatosplenitis infectiosa strigum sowie vergleichende Studien an Herpesvirusisolaten aus Uhu (*Bubo bubo*) und Schnee-Eule (*Nyctea scandiaca*)*. Inaugural dissertation, Justus Liebig Universität, Giessen, Germany.

Schulz, T.A., Stewart, J.S. & Fowler, M.E. (1989) Knemidikoptes mutans (Acari: Kniemidocoptidae) in a great-horned owl (*Bubo virginianus*). *Journal of Wildlife Diseases*, **25**(3), 430–432.

Schuster, S. (1996) *Untersuchungen zu Häufigkeit, Lokalisation und Art von Frakturen beim Vogel*. Inaugural dissertation, Justus Liebig Universität, Giessen, Germany.

Schwartz, A., Weaver, J.D., Scott, N.R. & Cade, T.J. (1977) Measuring the temperature of eggs during incubation under captive falcons. *Journal of Wildlife Management*, **41**, 12–17.

Sciple, G.W. (1953) *Avian botulism: information on earlier research*. Special Scientific Report: Wildlife

No. 23, US Department of the Interior, Washington DC, USA.

Scope, A. & Frey, H. (2000) Diseases and mortality causes in captive and free-ranging bearded vultures (*Gypaetus barbatus*). In: *Raptor Biomedicine III* (eds J.T. Lumeij, J.D. Remple, P.T. Redig, M. Lierz & J.E. Cooper). Zoological Education Network, Lake Worth, FL, USA.

Scott, H. & Stewart, J.M. (1972) A new anaesthetic for birds. *British Poultry Science*, **13**, 103–106.

Seal, U.S. & Lacy, R.C. (1989) *Florida panther population viability analysis*. Report to the US Fish and Wildlife Service, Captive Breeding Specialist Group, Species Survival Commission, IUCN, MN, USA.

Sears, J. (1988) Regional and seasonal variations in lead poisoning in the Mute Swan *Cygnus olor* in relation to the distribution of lead and lead weights, in the Thames area, England. *Biological Conservation*, **46**, 115–134.

Seegar, W.S., Schiller, E.L., Sladen, W.J.L. & Trpis, M. (1976) A Mallophaga, *Trinoton anserinum*, as a cyclodevelopmental vector for a heartworm parasite of waterfowl. *Science*, **194**, 739–741.

Seidensticker, J.C. & Reynolds, H.V. (1969) Preliminary studies on the use of a general anesthetic in falconiform birds. *Journal of the American Veterinary Medical Association*, **155**, 1044–1045.

Selye, H. (1950) *The Stress of Life*. McGraw-Hill, New York, USA.

Severino, M.A. (1645) *Zootomia Democritaea*. Noribergae.

Shapiro, C.J. & Weathers, W.W. (1981) Metabolic and behavioral responses of American kestrels to food deprivation. *Comparative Biochemistry and Physiology*, **68A**, 111–114.

Shaw, J. (1988) Arrested development of *Trichostrongylus tenuis* as third stage larvae in Red Grouse. *Research in Veterinary Science*, **45**, 256–258.

Shawyer, C.R. (1987) *The Barn Owl in the British Isles. Its Past, Present and Future*. The Hawk Trust, London, UK.

Shimmel, L. & Snell, K. (1999) Case studies in poisoning – two eagles. *Seminars in Avian and Exotic Pet Medicine*, **8**(1), 12–20.

Shlosberg, A. (1976) Treatment of monocrotophos-poisoned birds of prey with pralidoxime iodide. *Journal of the American Veterinary Medical Association*, **169**, 989–990.

Sibley, C.G. & Monroe, B.L. (1996) *Distribution and Taxonomy of Birds of the World*. Yale University Press, New Haven, CT, USA.

Sibly, R.M., Newton, I. & Walker, C.H. (2000) Effects of dieldrin on population growth rates of sparrowhawks. *Journal of Applied Ecology*, **37**, 540–546.

Sileo, L., Carlson, H.C. & Crumley, S.C. (1975) Inclusion body disease in a great horned owl. *Journal of Wildlife Diseases*, **11**, 92–96.

Sileo, L., Franson, J.C., Graham, D.L., Domermuth, C.H., Rattner, B.A. & Pattee, O.H. (1983) Hemorrhagic enteritis in captive American kestrels (*Falco sparverius*). *Journal of Wildlife Diseases*, **19**, 244–247.

Siller, W.G. (1981) Renal pathology of the fowl – a review. *Avian Pathology*, **10**, 187–260.

Simmons, K.E.C. (1966) Anting and the problem of self-stimulation. *Nature*, **219**, 690–694.

Simpson, G.N. (1996) Wing problems. In: *Manual of Raptors, Pigeons and Waterfowl* (eds P.H. Beynon, N.A. Forbes & N.H. Harcourt-Brown). British Small Animal Veterinary Association, Cheltenham, UK.

Simpson, V.R. & Harris, E.A. (1992) *Cyathostoma lari* (Nematoda) infection in birds of prey. *Journal of Zoology, London*, **227**, 655–659.

Simpson, V.R., Walls, S.S., Cooper, J.E. & Kenward, R.E. (1997) Causes of mortality in radio-tracked Eurasian buzzards (*Buteo buteo*) in Dorset. *Proceedings of the 1997 European Conference on Avian Medicine and Surgery*, 19–24 May 1997, London, UK.

Sitko, J. (1998) Trematodes of birds of prey (Falconiformes) in Czech Republic. *Helminthologica*, **35**(3), 131–146.

Smit, F.G.A.M. (1957) *Handbook for the Identification of British Insects: Series 1, number 16 Siphonaptera*. Royal Entomological Society of London, UK.

Smith, E.E. & Bush, M. (1978) Hematologic parameters on various species of Strigiformes and Falconiformes. *Journal of Wildlife Diseases*, **14**, 447–456.

Smith, G. (1983) Avian sex determination. *Veterinary Record*, **112**, 182.

Smith, G.R. (1975) Recent European outbreaks of botulism in waterfowl. *International Waterfowl Research Bureau Bulletin*, **39/40**, 72–74.

Smith, G.R., Hime, J.M., Keymer, I.F., Graham, J.M., Olney, P.J.S. & Brambell, M.R. (1975) Botulism in captive birds fed commercially bred maggots. *Veterinary Record*, **97**, 204–205.

Smith, G.R., Oliphant, J.C. & Evans, E.D. (1983) Diagnosis of botulism in water birds. *Veterinary Record*, **24**, 457–458.

Smith, R.N., Cain, S.L., Anderson, S.H., Dunk, J.R. & Williams, E.S. (1998) Blackfly-induced mortality of nestling red-tailed hawks. *The Auk*, **115**(2), 368–375.

Smith, S.A. (1993a) Diagnosis and treatment of helminths in birds of prey. In: *Raptor Biomedicine* (eds P.T. Redig, J.E. Cooper, J.D. Remple & D.B. Hunter). University of Minnesota Press, USA.

Smith, S.A. (1993b) Diagnosis of brachial plexus avulsion in three free-living owls. In: *Raptor Biomedicine* (eds P.T. Redig, J.E. Cooper, J.D. Remple & D.B. Hunter). University of Minnesota Press, USA.

Smith, S.A. (1996) Parasites of birds of prey: their diagnosis and treatment. *Seminars in Avian and Exotic Pet Medicine*, **5**(2), 97–105.

Smith, S.A. & Smith B.J. (1988) Lice in birds of prey. *Companion Animal Practice*, **2**(9), 35–37.

Smith, S.A. & Smith, B.J. (1992) *Atlas of Avian Radiographic Anatomy*. W.B. Saunders, PA, USA.

Snow, D.W. (1968) Movements and mortality of British kestrels (*Falco tinnunculus*). *Bird Study*, **15**, 65–83.

Snyder, N. & Snyder, H. (2000) The California Condor: a Saga of Natural History and Conservation. Academic Press, San Diego.

Snyder, B., Thilsted, J., Burgess, B. & Richard, M. (1985) Pigeon herpesvirus mortalities in foster reared Mauritius Pink Pigeons. In: *Proceedings of the American Association of Zoo Veterinarians*. Scottsdale, Arizona (eds M.S. Silbermann & S.D. Silbermann).

Sonin, M.D. (1968) Filariata of animals and man and diseases caused by them. In: *Essentials of Nematodology*, Vol. 21 (ed. K.I. Skrjabin). Akademia Nauk SSSR, Moscow, Union of Socialistic Soviet Republics, pp. 186–190 [English translation].

Soulsby, E.J.L. (1974) *Helminths, Arthropods and Protozoa of Domesticated Animals*. The Williams & Wilkins Co., Baltimore, USA.

Spalding, M.G., Frederick, P.C., McGill, H.C., Bouton, S.N. & McDowell, L.R. (2000a) Methyl mercury accumulation in tissues and its effects on growth and appetite in captive great egrets. *Journal of Wildlife Diseases*, **36**(3), 411–422.

Spalding, M.G., Frederick, P.C., McGill, H.C., *et al.* (2000b) Histologic, neurologic, and immunologic effects of methyl mercury in captive white egrets. *Journal of Wildlife Diseases*, **36**(3), 423–435.

Spearman, R.I.C. & Hardy, J.A. (1985) Integument. In: *Form and Function in Birds*, Vol. 3 (eds A.S. King & J. McLelland). Academic Press, London, UK.

Spray, C.J. & Milne, H. (1988) The incidence of lead poisoning among Whooper and Mute Swans *Cygnus cygnus* and *C. olor* in Scotland. *Biological Conservation*, **44**, 265–281.

Stabler, R.M. (1954) *Trichomonas gallinae* – a review. *Experimental Parasitology*, **III**, 368–402.

Stabler, R.M. & Herman, C.M. (1951) Upper digestive tract trichomoniasis in Mourning Doves and other birds. *Transactions of the North American Wildlife Conference*, **16**, 145–162.

Stabler, R.M. & Holt, P.A. (1965) Hematozoa from Colorado birds. II. Falconiformes and Strigiformes. *Journal of Parasitology*, **51**, 927–928.

Stansley, W. & Roscoe, D.E. (1999) Chlordane poisoning of birds in New Jersey, USA. *Environmental Toxicology and Chemistry*, **18**, 2095–2099.

Stauber, E. (1973) Suspected riboflavin deficiency in a golden eagle. *Journal of the American Veterinary Medical Association*, **163**, 645–646.

Stauber, E.H. (1984) Footprinting of raptors for identification. *Raptor Research*, **18**, 67–71.

Stavy, M., Gilbert, D. & Martin, R.D. (1979) Routine determination of sex in monomorphic bird species using faecal steroid analysis. *International Zoo Yearbook*, **19**, 209–214.

Steadman, D.W., Greiner, E.C. & Wood, C.S. (1990) Absence of blood parasites in indigenous and introduced birds from the Cook Islands, South Pacific. *Conservation Biology*, **4**(4), 398–404.

Steele, K.E., Linn, M.J., Schoepp, R.J., *et al.* (2000) Pathology of fatal west Nile virus infections in native and exotic birds during the 1999 outbreak in New York City, New York. *Veterinary Pathology*, **37**, 208–224.

Stehle, S. (1965) *Krankheiten bei Greifvögeln (Accipitres) und bei Eulen (Striges) mit Ausnahme der parasitären Erkrankungen*. Inaugural dissertation, Tierärztliche Hochschule, Hannover, Germany.

Stehle, S. (1977) Behandlung von Helminthosen bei Greifvögeln (Falconiformes) mit Fenbendazol (Panacur®). *Kleintier Praxis*, **22**, 261–268.

Sterner, M.C. & Espinosa, R.H. (1988) *Serratospiculum amaculata* in a Cooper's hawk (*Accipiter cooperii*). *Journal of Wildlife Diseases*, **24**(2), 378–379.

Stock, A.D. & Worthen, G.L. (1980) Identification of the sex chromosomes of the red-tailed hawk (*Buteo jamaicensis*) by C- and G-banding. *Raptor Research*, **14**, 65–68.

Stone, E.G., Walser, M.M., Redig, P.T., Rings, B. & Howard, D.J. (1999) Synovial chondromatosis in raptors. *Journal of Wildlife Diseases*, **35**, 137–140.

Stone, W.B. & Janes, D.E. (1969) Trichomoniasis in captive sparrowhawks. *Bulletin of the Wildlife Disease Association*, **5**, 147.

Stringfield, C.E. (1998) Medical management of the free-ranging California condor. *Proceedings of the American Association of Zoo Veterinarians and the American Association of Wildlife Veterinarians Joint Conference*. Omaha, Nebraska, USA.

Strouse, S. (1909) Experimental studies on pneumococcus infections. *Journal of Experimental Medicine*, **11**, 743–761.

Suarez, D.L. (1993) Appetite stimulation in raptors. In: *Raptor Biomedicine* (eds P.T. Redig, J.E. Cooper, J.D. Remple & D.B. Hunter). University of Minnesota Press, USA.

Sykes, G., Hardaswick, V. & Heck, W. (1982) Nutritional deficiency and perosis in peregrine falcons. *Hawk Chalk*, **21**, 33–36.

Sykes, G.P., Murphy, C. & Hardaswick, V. (1981) *Salmonella* infection in a captive peregrine falcon. *Journal of the American Veterinary Medical Association*, **179**, 1269–1271.

Tabaka, C.S., Ullrey, D.E., Sikarskie, J.G., DeBar, S.R. & Ku, P.K. (1996) Diet, cast composition, and energy and nutrient intake of red-tailed hawks (*Buteo jamaicensis*), great horned owls (*Bubo virginianus*), and turkey vultures (*Cathartes aura*). *Journal of Zoo and Wildlife Medicine*, **27**(2), 187–196.

Taday, E.M.A. (1998) *Organveränderungen und Enregernachweise nach Infektionen mit* Chlamydia *sp. beim Vogel unter besonderer Berücksichtigung des aviären Wirtsspektrums*. Inaugural dissertation, Justus Liebig Universität, Giessen, Germany.

Taft, S.J. (2000) Host lists of ecto- and endoparasites common to North American raptors, along with useful scientific literature. *Journal of Wildlife Rehabilitation*, **23**(3), 3–7.

Tanabe, M. (1925) The cultivation of trichomonads from man, rat and owl. *Journal of Parasitology*, **12**, 101–104.

Teare, J.A., Agnew, D., Teare, C.S. & Tabaka, C. (1999) *MedARKS Training Manual*. American Association of Zoo Veterinarians' 1999 Workshop. MedARKS Technical Support, Minnesota, USA.

Tella, J.L., Forest, M.G., Gajón, A., Hiraldo, F. & Donázar, J.A. (1996) Absence of blood parasitisation effects on Lesser Kestrel fitness. *The Auk*, **113**, 253–256.

Temple, S.A. (1987) Do predators always capture substandard individuals disproportionately from prey populations? *Ecology*, **68**, 669–674.

Thomsett, S. (1987) Raptor deaths as a result of poisoning quelea in Kenya. *Gabar*, **2**, 33–38.

Thorne, E.T. & Williams, E.S. (1988) Disease and endangered species: the Black-footed Ferret as a recent example. *Conservation Biology*, **2**, 66–74.

Thornton, C.G., Cranfield, M.R., MacLellan, K.M., *et al.* (1999) Processing postmortem specimens with C_{18}-carboxyporpylbetaine and analysis by PCR to develop an antemortem test for *Mycobacterium avium* infections in ducks. *Journal of Zoo and Wildlife Medicine*, **30**(1), 11–24.

Toft, C. (1991) An ecological perspective: the population and community consequences of parasitism. In: *Parasite–Host Association: Coexistence or Conflict* (eds C.A. Toft & A. Aeschlimann), pp. 313–343. University Press, Oxford, UK.

Tompkins, D.M. & Begon, M. (1999) Parasites can regulate wildlife populations. *Parasitology Today*, **15**(8), 311–313.

Toro, H., Pavéz, E.F., Gough, R.E., Montes, G. & Kaleta, E.F. (1997) Serum chemistry and antibody status to some avian pathogens of free-living and captive condors (*Vultur gryphus*) of central Chile. *Avian Pathology*, **26**, 339–345.

Townsend, M.G., Fletcher, M.R., Odam, E.M. & Stanley, P.I. (1981) An assessment of the secondary poisoning hazard of warfarin to tawny owls. *Journal of Wildlife Management*, **45**, 242–248.

Trainer, D.O., Folz, S.D. & Samuel, W.M. (1968) Capillariasis in the gyrfalcon. *Condor*, **70**, 276–277.

Turbervile, G. (1575) *The Booke of Faulconrie or Hawking*. Christopher Barker, London, UK.

Tyler, C. (1966) A study of the egg shells of the Falconiformes. *Journal of Zoology, London*, **150**, 413–425.

Upton, S.J., Campbell, T.W., Weigel, M. & McKown, R.D. (1990) The Eimeriidae (Apicomplexa) of raptors: review of the literature and description of new species of the genera *Caryospora* and *Eimeria*. *Canadian Journal of Zoology*, **68**, 1256–1265.

Urbain, A. & Nouvel, J. (1946) Possibilité de dispersion des bacilles tuberculeux et des spores charbonneuses par les déjections d'oiseaux carnivores. *Bulletin de L'Académie Vétérinaire de France*, **XIX**, 237–239.

Valentin, A., Haberkorn, A. & Jakob, W. (1994) Massive Malaria-infektion mit *Parahaemoproteus* sp. in Schnee-Eulen (*Nyctea scandiaca*) und deren Behandlung mit Primaquin. *Verhandlungsbericht des 36 Internationalen Symposiums über die Erkrankungen der Zoo- und Wildtiere*, **36**, 401–404.

Vallortigara, G., Regolin, L., Rigoni, M. & Zanforlin, M. (1998) Delayed search for a concealed imprinted object in the domestic chick. *Animal Cognition*, **1**, 17–24.

Vallortigara, G., Regolin, L., Tommasi, L. & Zucca, P. (2000) Cervello di Gallina – capacità cognitive degli uccelli. *Le Scienze* (Italian edition of *Scientific American*), **387**, 88–95.

Vallortigara, G., Zanforlin, M. & Compostella, S. (1990) Perceptual organisation in animal learning: cues or objects? *Ethology*, **85**, 89–102.

Van den Abeele, B. (1994) *La Fauconnerie au Moyen Age*. Editions Klincksieck, Paris, France.

Vanden Berge, J.C. & Storer, R.W. (1995) Intratendinous

ossification in birds: a review. *Journal of Morphology*, **226**, 47–77.

Vaughan, G.E. & Coble, P.W. (1975) Sublethal effects of three ectoparasites on fish. *Journal of Fisheries Biology*, **7**, 283–294.

Vaught, R.W., McDougle, H.C. & Burgess, H.H. (1967) Fowl cholera in waterfowl at Squaw Creek National Wildlife Refuge, Missouri. *Journal of Wildlife Management*, **31**, 248–253.

Velasco, M.C. (2000) Candidiasis and cryptococcosis in birds. *Seminars in Avian and Exotic Pet Medicine*, **9**(2), 75–81.

Verwoerd, D. (2000) Observations on the use of azithromycin in falcons. *Falco*, **16**, 19–20.

Verwoerd, D.J. (2001) Aerosol use of a novel disinfectant as part of an integrated approach to aspergillosis in falcons in the UAE. *Falco*, **17**, 15–18.

Vestergaard, K.S. & Sanotra, G.S. (1999) Relationships between leg disorders and changes in the behaviour of broiler chickens. *Veterinary Record*, **144**, 205–209.

Villforth, Y.M. (1995) *Krankheiten und Todesursachen von Greifvögeln und Eulen*. Inaugural dissertation, Justus Liebig Universität, Giessen, Germany.

Virani, M., Watson, R., Risebrough, B. & Oaks, L. (2000) Should Africa brace itself for an imminent vulture epidemic. Lessons from the Asian vulture crisis. *Abstract of paper presented at the Tenth Pan-African Ornithological Congress (PAOC)*. Makerere University, Kampala, Uganda, 3–8 September 2000.

Voitkevich, A.A. (1966) *The Feathers and Plumage of Birds*. Sidgwick & Jackson, London, UK.

Wadsworth, P.F. & Jones, D.M. (1980) A renal carcinoma in an augur buzzard (*Buteo rufofuscus augur*). *Avian Pathology*, **9**, 219–223.

Wadsworth, P.F., Jones, D.M. & Pugsley, S.L. (1984) Fatty liver in birds at the Zoological Society of London. *Avian Pathology*, **13**, 231–239.

Wagner, C., Hochleithner, M. & Rausch, W.D. (1991) Ketoconazole plasma levels in buzzards. *Proceedings of the European Committee of the Association of Avian Veterinarians*, Munich, Germany.

Wagner, U. (1993) *Vergleichende Untersuchunger zur Empfindlichkeit verschiedener aviären Herpesvirusisolate gegenüber chemischen Desinfektionsmitteln*. Inaugural dissertation, Justus Liebig Universität, Giessen, Germany.

Waine, J.C. (1996) *Post-mortem examination technique*. In: *Manual of Raptors, Pigeons and Waterfowl* (eds P.H. Beynon, N.A. Forbes & N.H. Harcourt-Brown). British Small Animal Veterinary Association, Cheltenham, UK.

Walker, A. (1999) *The Encyclopedia of Falconry*. Swan Hill Press, Shrewsbury, UK.

Walker, C.H. & Newton, I. (1999) Effects of cyclodiene insecticides on raptors in Britain – correction and updating an earlier paper by Walker & Newton. *Ecotoxicology*, **7**, 185–189 (1998). *Ecotoxicology*, **8**, 423–427.

Walker, J.B., Mehlitz, D. & Jones, G.E. (1978) *Notes on the Ticks of Botswana*. GTZ Eschborn, Germany.

Wallach, J.D. (1970) Nutritional diseases of exotic animals. *Journal of the American Veterinary Medical Association*, **157**, 583–599.

Wallach, J.D. & Boever, W.J. (1983) *Diseases of Exotic Animals*. W.B. Saunders, PA, USA.

Wallach, J.D. & Flieg, G.M. (1969) Frostbite and its sequelae in captive exotic birds. *Journal of the American Veterinary Medical Association*, **155**, 1035–1038.

Wallach, J.D. & Flieg, G.M. (1970) Cramps and fits in carnivorous birds. *International Zoo Yearbook*, **10**, 3–4.

Wallner-Pendleton, E.A., Rogers, D. & Epple, A. (1993) Diabetes mellitus in a red-tailed hawk (*Buteo jamaicensis*). *Avian Pathology*, **22**, 631–635.

Walter, G. & Hudde, H. (1987) Die Gefiederfliege *Carnus hemapterus* (Milichiidae, Diptera) ein Ektoparasit der Nestlinge. *Journal für Ornithologie*, **128**(2), 251–255.

Walzer, C., Boegel, R., Fluch, G., Karl, E., Schober, F. & Prinzinger, R. (2000) Intra-abdominal implantation of a multi-sensor telemetry system in a free-ranging Eurasian griffon (*Gyps fulvus*). In: *Raptor Biomedicine III* (eds J.T. Lumeij, J.D. Remple, P.T. Redig, M. Lierz & J.E. Cooper). Zoological Education Network, Lake Worth, FL, USA.

Ward, F.P. (1971) Thiamine deficiency in a peregrine falcon. *Journal of the American Veterinary Medical Association*, **159**, 599–601.

Ward, F.P. & Fairchild, D.G. (1972) Air sac parasites of the genus *Serratospiculum* in falcons. *Journal of Wildlife Diseases*, **8**, 165–168.

Ward, F.P. & Slaughter, L.J. (1968) Visceral gout in a captive Cooper's hawk. *Bulletin of the Wildlife Disease Association*, **4**, 91–93.

Ward, F.P., Fairchild, D.G. & Vuicich, J.V. (1970) Pulmonary aspergillosis in prairie falcon nest mates. *Journal of Wildlife Diseases*, **6**, 80–83.

Warner, R.E. (1968) The role of introduced diseases in the extinction of the endemic Hawaiian avifauna. *Condor*, **70**, 101–120.

Wasser, S.K., Bevis, K., King, G. & Hanson, E. (1996) Noninvasive physiological measures of disturbance in the Northern spotted owl. *Conservation Biology*, **11**, 1019–1022.

Weatherhead, P.J. & Bennett, G.T. (1991) Ecology of red-winged blackbird parasitism by haematozoa. *Canadian Journal of Zoology*, **69**, 2352–2359.

Weatherhead, P.J. & Bennett, G.F. (1992) Ecology of parasitism of brown-headed cowbirds by haematozoa. *Canadian Journal of Zoology*, **70**, 1–7.

Weaver, J.D. & Cade, T.J. (1983) *Falcon Propagation: A Manual on Captive Breeding.* The Peregrine Fund Inc., Boise, ID, USA.

Webster, H. (1999) Correspondence. *The Falconer*, 70.

Webster, H.M. (1944) A survey of the Prairie Falcon in Colorado. *The Auk*, **61**, 609–616.

Wehr, E. (1938) New genera and species of the nematode superfamily Filaroididae I. *Serratospiculum amaculata* n. sp. *Proceedings of the Helminthological Society of Washington*, **5**, 59–60.

Weigand-Lommel, S. (1999) *Nachweis und Differenzierung von* Aspergillus *spp. mit der Polymerase – Kettenreaktion zur Etablierung einer neuen Methode für die Diagnostik der Aspergillose bei Vögeln.* Inaugural dissertation, Justus Liebig Universität, Giessen, Germany.

Welle, K.R. (2000) Incorporating behavior services into the avian practice. *Journal of Avian Medicine and Surgery*, **14**(3), 190–193.

Wellstead, G. (1998) Marking time. *Journal of the International Owl Society*, **II**(VI), 116–120.

Wernery, U. & Joseph, S. (1997) Salmonella infections in captive falcons. *Falco*, 9, 10.

Wernery, U., Kinne, J., Sharma, A., Bochnel, H. & Samour, J. (2000) *Clostridium* enterotoxaemia in Falconiformes in the United Arab Emirates. In: *Raptor Biomedicine III* (eds J.T. Lumeij, J.D. Remple, P.T. Redig, M. Lierz & J.E. Cooper). Zoological Education Network, Lake Worth, FL, USA.

Wernery, U., Wernery, R., Kinne, J., *et al.* (1999) Production of a falcon herpesvirus vaccine. *Berliner und Münchener Tierärztliche Wochenschrift*, **112**(9), 339–344.

Wetzel, R. & Enigk, K. (1937) *Caryospora falconis* n. sp. (Eimeridea) aus dem Wanderfalken. *Sitzungsberichte der Gesellschaft naturforschender Freunde Berlin e.V.* January 6–9.

Wheeldon, E.B., Bogan, J.A. & Taylor, D.J. (1975) Dieldrin poisoning in a captive bird of prey. *Veterinary Record*, **97**, 412.

Wheeler, S.J. (ed) (1995) *Manual of Small Animal Neurology.* BSAVA, Cheltenham, UK.

Wheler, C. (1993) Herpesvirus disease in raptors: a review. In: *Raptor Biomedicine* (eds P.T. Redig, J.E. Cooper, J.D. Remple & D.B. Hunter). University of Minnesota Press, USA.

Whiteley, P.L. (1989) *Effects of environmental contaminants, particularly selenium, on waterfowl disease and immunity.* MSc (Veterinary Science) Thesis, University of Wisconsin-Madison, USA.

WHO (1984) *Guidelines for Drinking-Water Quality.* WHO, Geneva, Switzerland.

WHO (2000a) *Danger in the Air.* World Health Organization Press Release WHO/56, Geneva, Switzerland.

WHO (2000b) *Vegetation Fires.* Factsheet WHO/254. World Health Organization, Geneva, Switzerland.

Wiemeyer, S.N., Scott, J.M., Anderson, M.P., Bloom, P.H. & Stafford, C.J. (1988) Environmental contaminants in California Condors. *Journal of Wildlife Management*, **52**, 238–247.

Wijnstekers, W. (1995) *The Evolution of CITES*, 4th edn. CITES Secretariat, Lausanne, Switzerland.

Williams, D.L. (1994) Ophthalmology. In: *Avian Medicine: Principles and Application* (eds B.W. Ritchie, G.J. Harrison & L.R. Harrison). Wingers, Lake Worth, FL, USA.

Williams, D.L. & Cooper, J.E. (1994) Horner's syndrome in an African spotted eagle owl (*Bubo africanus*). *Veterinary Record*, **134**, 64–66.

Williams Smith, H. (1954) Serum levels of penicillin, dihydrostreptomycin, chloramphenicol, aureomycin and terramycin in chickens. *Journal of Comparative Pathology*, **64**, 225–233.

Wilson, J.F. (1989) *Law and Ethics of the Veterinary Profession.* Priority Press, Yardly, PA, USA.

Wilson, M.H., Kepler, C.B., Snyder, N.F.R., *et al.* (1994) Puerto Rican Parrots and potential limitations of the metapopulation approach to species conservation. *Conservation Biology*, **8**, 114–123.

Wilson, R. (1976) Fulmar oils lanneret. *The Falconer*, **VI**, 263–264.

Wimsatt, J., Dresser, P., Dennisson, C. & Turner, A.S. (2000) Ultrasound therapy for the prevention and correction of contractures and bone mineral loss associated with wing bandaging in the domestic pigeon (*Columba livia*). *Journal of Zoo and Wildlife Medicine*, **31**(2), 190–195.

Wingfield, W.E. & DeYoung, D.W. (1972) Anesthetic and surgical management of eagles with orthopedic difficulties. *Veterinary Medicine/Small Animal Clinician*, **67**, 991–993.

Wink, M., Sauer-Guerth, H., Martinez, F., Doval, G., Blanco, G. & Hatzofe, O. (1998) The use of (GACA)$_4$-PCR to sex Old World vultures (Aves: Accipitridae). *Molecular Ecology*, 7, 779–782.

Winteröll, G. (1976) Newcastle-Disease bei Greifen und Eulen. *Der praktische Tierarzt*, **57**, 76–78.

Wisser, J. & Jewgenow, K.N. (1997) PARS – ein Software – programm für die pathologisch–anatomische Diagnostik bei Wildtieren. *Berliner und Münchener Tierärztliche Wochenschrift*, **110**, 461–465.

Wobeser, G. & Saunders, J.R. (1975) Pulmonary oxalosis in association with Aspergillus niger infection in a great horned owl (*Bubo virginianus*). *Avian Diseases*, **19**, 388–392.

Wobeser, G.A. (1981) *Diseases of Wild Waterfowl*. Plenum Press, New York, NY, USA.

Wobeser, G.A. (1994) *Investigation and Management of Disease in Wild Animals*. Plenum Press, New York and London.

Wolff, P.L. & Seal, U.S. (1993) Proceedings issue international conference on implications of infectious disease for captive propagation and reintroduction of threatened species. *Journal of Zoo and Wildlife Medicine*, **24**, 229–408.

Wolfson, F. (1936) *Plasmodium oti* n. sp., a Plasmodium from the eastern screech owl (*Otus asio naevius*), infective to canaries. *American Journal of Hygiene*, **24**, 94–101.

Wong, E., Mikaelian, I., Desnoyers, M. & Fitzgerald, G. (1999) Pansteatitis in a free-ranging red-tailed hawk (*Buteo jamaicensis*). *Journal of Zoo and Wildlife Medicine*, **30**(4), 584–586.

Wood, C.A. (1917) *The Fundus Oculi of Birds*. Lakeside Press, Chicago, IL, USA.

Wood, C.A. & Fyfe, F.M. (1943) *Translation. The Art of Falconry being the 'De Arte Venandi cum Avibus' of Frederick II of Hohenstaufen*. Stanford University Press, USA.

Woodford, M.H. (1960) *A Manual of Falconry*. A & C Black, London, UK.

Woodford, M.H. & Glasier, P.E. (1955) Sub-committee's report on disease in hawks, 1954. *The Falconer*, **III**, 63–65.

Woolfenden, G.E. & Fitzpatrick, J. (1991) Florida Scrub Jay ecology and conservation. In: *Bird Population Studies* (eds C.M. Perrins, J.-D. Lebreton & G.J.M. Hirons), pp. 542–565. University Press, Oxford, UK.

Work, T.M. & Hale, J. (1996) Causes of owl mortality in Hawaii, 1992–1994. *Journal of Wildlife Diseases*, **32**(2), 266–273.

Wyllie, I. (undated) *Guide to Age and Sex in British Birds of Prey*. Institute of Terrestrial Ecology (now Centre for Ecology and Hydrology), Monks Wood Experimental Station, Abbots Ripton, UK.

Wyllie, I. & Newton, I. (1999) Use of carcasses to estimate the proportions of female sparrowhawks and kestrels which bred in their first year of life. *Ibis*, **141**, 504–506.

Wyllie, I., Dale, L. & Newton, I. (1996) Unequal sex-ratio, mortality causes and pollutant residues in Long-eared Owls in Britain. *British Birds*, **89**, 429–436.

Yamamoto, J. & Santolo, G.M. (2000) Body condition effects in American kestrels fed selenomethionine. *Journal of Wildlife Diseases*, **36**(4), 646–652.

Young, K.E., Franklin, A.B. & Ward, J.P. (1993) Infestation of northern spotted owls by hippoboscid (Diptera) flies in northwestern California. *Journal of Wildlife Diseases*, **29**(2), 278–283.

Zaid, Bin Sultan Al Nahayan (1976) *Falconry as a Sport: Our Arab Heritage*. Compiled by Yahya Badr. Published for the International Conference on Falconry and Conservation, Abu Dhabi, 10–18 December, 1976.

Zeigler, H.P. & Karten, H.J. (1973) Brain mechanisms and feeding behavior in the pigeon (*Columba livia*). *The Journal of Comparative Neurology*, **152**, 59–78.

Zenker, W. & Janovsky, M. (1998) Immobilisation of the common buzzard (*Buteo buteo*) with oral tiletamine/zolazepam. *Proceedings European Association of Zoo and Wildlife Veterinarians, Chester*, 449–455.

Zenker, W., Janovsky, M., Kurzwell, J. & Ruf, T. (2000) Immobilisation of the Eurasian buzzard (*Buteo buteo*) with oral tiletamine/zolazepam. In: *Raptor Biomedicine III* (eds J.T. Lumeij, J.D. Remple, P.T. Redig, M. Lierz & J.E. Cooper). Zoological Education Network, Lake Worth, FL, USA.

Zillioux, E.J., Porcella, D.B. & Beoit, J.M. (1993) Mercury cycling and effects in freshwater wetland ecosystems. *Environmental Toxicology and Chemistry*, **12**, 2245–2264.

Zucca, P. (1995) *Prevalence and clinical aspects of wing pathology of European falcons*. Thesis, Parma University, Parma, Italy.

Zucca, P. (2000) Parasitic diseases. Arthropods, Protozoa, Helminths. In: *Avian Medicine* (ed. J.H. Samour). Mosby-Wolfe, London, UK.

Zucca, P. & Cooper, J.E. (2000) Osteological aspects of the falcon wing. In: *Raptor Biomedicine III* (eds J.T. Lumeij, P.T. Redig, J.D. Remple, M. Lierz & J.E. Cooper). Zoological Education Network, Lake Worth, FL, USA.

Index

Road traffic accidents, xi, 72
Roundworms, 116–19, 226–7
Royal College of Veterinary Surgeons, The (RCVS), xvi, 237
Royal Society for the Prevention of Cruelty to Animals (RSPCA), 7, 237
Russia, 7
Rwanda, 267, 270, 279

Scientific names, xv
Samples (specimens)
 clinical, 40–42
 collection of, **Table 4.2**, 50–51, 268–9, **Table AVIII.2**
 posting (mailing) of, 49
 post-mortem, 51, 52
Sardinia, 6
Screening (*see* Health monitoring)
Secretary-bird (*see also* Falconiformes and individual groups and species), 10, 94, 241
Sedation (*see also* Anaesthesia), 172
SEM (*see* Electronmicroscopy)
Semen, **Table 4.2**, 61, 213
Septicaemia, 97, 214
Serum/Serology, **Table 4.2**, 56
Shock, 82, 94, 200, 201–202, 203
SI units, 60
Sicily, 6
Sight (*see also* Eyes *and* Ocular diseases), 23–5
Skeletal disease, 79
Skeleton (*see* Bones)
Skin diseases, 87–8, 121, 131, 192
Skull (*see* Head)
Smell, 26
Snakebite, 158
Solitude, 27
South Africa, 6
Specialisation in avian medicine, 29, 237
 in pathology, 44–6, 62, 281
Species
 of raptor (English and scientific names), 241–2
 protection, 286–7
Specimens (*see* Samples)
Spongiform encephalopathy, 103–104
Stabilisation, 66
Stabler, R. M., 3
Sternum ('keel'), 35, 194
Stomach (*see* Digestive tract)
Stomatitis, 94, 95–7, **Fig. 6.1**
Stress, 34, 202–204
Stressors, 202, 203, 232
Strigidae, 10
Strigiformes, xiv, 207, 241
Sudden death, causes of, 62–3
Surgery, 20, 179–84, **Plate 19**
 asepsis, 180
 history, 179, **Fig. 12.1**
 of the feet, 128–30
 ophthalmological, 196–7, **Plate 25**
 procedures, 181–4
Survival in wild, 80
Swabs, 41

Tags (*see* Identification)
Tail, 21, 36
Talons, 13, 20, **Plate 5**, 34, 36, 74, 78, 131, 209
Tapeworms, 115–16, 228
Tattooing (*see* Identification)
Taxonomy (*see also* Nomenclature), 10
Telemetry, 184
TEM (*see* Electronmicroscopy)
Temperature of body, 34, 37–8, 63–4, 80, 204
Terminology (*see also* Definitions), 9–12
 American terms and spellings, xv, 10–11
 falconry, 10–11
Tethering (*see also* Bating), 207, 237
Thermoregulation, 38, 214
Thorny-headed worms (*see* Acanthocepha)
Thyroid, 186, 204–205, 211
Ticks, 103, 106–107, 143, 196, 200, 218, 233
TOBEC, 40, 47
Toxicology, 51–2, 163–70
Trade in birds, 288–90
Transillumination, 35, 37, 46
Translocation, 5–6, 27, 169–70, 207, 259, 261, 292, 321
Transponder (*see* Microchipping)
Transportation of birds, 73
Trapping, 34–5, 42, 73
Trauma (*see also* Injuries), 14, 68, 71–80, **Figs 5.1**, **5.2**
Treatment
 of diseases, 63–70
 medicines for, 271–6
Trematoda (*see* Flukes)
Trichomoniasis
 characteristics, 112
 elucidation of cause, 3
 threat from food, 161, 233, 228
Tube-feeding (*see* Force-feeding)
Tuberculosis (*see* Mycobacteriosis)
Tytonidae, 10

Uganda, xiii, 215
United Arab Emirates (UAE), 1, 100, 277
United Kingdom (UK), 1–8, 29, 167, 193, 237, 284–93
United States of America (USA), 4, 29, 167, 207, 284–93
Urates, **Figs 4.3**, **4.5**, 41, 79, 198–9
Urban raptors, role as sentinels, 238
Urinary tract conditions, 198–9
Uropygial gland, 36, **Plate 3**, 186

Vaccination (*see* Immunisation)
Van den Abeele, 2
Venereal (sexual) spread of pathogens, 61, 104, 208–209
Veterinarians
 contributions to raptor work, 5–8, 194, 237
Veterinary medicines – not listed separately – *see* 271–7
Veterinary surgeons (*see* Veterinarians)
Virus (viral) disease, **Fig. 6.2**, 84–5, 100–104, 125, 215
Vision (*see also* Eyes), 23–5
Vitamins, 151
Vomiting (vomition) (*see* Regurgitation)
Vortex, 216
Vultures, 10, 20, 26, **Fig. 4.4**, 103, 152–3, 155, 161, 215–16, 232, **Plate 6**